CLINICAL

ASTHMA

CLINICAL

ASTHMA

Mario Castro, MD, MPH
Director, The Asthma & Airway Translational Research Unit
Associate Professor of Medicine and Pediatrics
Division of Pulmonary and Critical Care Medicine
Washington University of St. Louis
Attending Physician
Barnes-Jewish Hospital
St. Louis, Missouri

Monica Kraft, MD
Associate Professor of Medicine
Director, Duke Asthma, Allergy and Airway Center
Duke University Medical Center
Durham, North Carolina

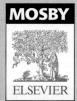

MOSBY

ELSEVIER

ELSEVIER
MOSBY

1600 John F. Kennedy Boulevard
Suite 1800
Philadelphia, PA 19103–2899

CLINICAL ASTHMA   ISBN: 978-0-323-04289-5

Notice

Knowledge and best practice in this field are constantly changing. As new research and experience broaden our knowledge, changes in practice, treatment and drug therapy may become necessary or appropriate. Readers are advised to check the most current information provided (i) on procedures featured or (ii) by the manufacturer of each product to be administered, to verify the recommended dose or formula, the method and duration of administration, and contraindications. It is the responsibility of the practitioner, relying on their own experience and knowledge of the patient, to make diagnoses, to determine dosages and the best treatment for each individual patient, and to take all appropriate safety precautions. To the fullest extent of the law, neither the Publisher nor the Editors assume any liability for any injury and/or damage to persons or property arising out of or related to any use of the material contained in this book.

The Publisher

Library of Congress Cataloging-in-Publication Data

Clinical asthma / editors, Mario Castro, Monica Kraft.—1st ed.
   p. ; cm.
   Includes bibliographical references and index.
   ISBN 978-0-323-04289-5
   1. Asthma. 2. Asthma–Treatment. I. Castro, Mario. II. Kraft, Monica.
   [DNLM: 1. Asthma–diagnosis. 2. Asthma–therapy. WF 553 C641 2008]
RC591.C58 2008
616.2'38–dc22
                                                       2007024850

Acquisitions Editor: Dolores Meloni
Developmental Editor: Mary Beth Murphy
Project Manager: Bryan Hayward

Printed in China

Working together to grow
libraries in developing countries

www.elsevier.com | www.bookaid.org | www.sabre.org

Last digit is the print number: 9 8 7 6 5 4 3 2 1

ELSEVIER   BOOK AID International   Sabre Foundation

Dedications

To my wife, Marianne, and to my sons, Benjamin, Darrian, and Victor; I am so proud of the fine young men you have become. To my parents, Moises and Margot, for all of your love and for all that you have sacrificed as you left Cuba to bring your sons to a better opportunity. Thank you all for the support you have provided through the years of my career. Thanks to my mentors, colleagues, and patients, who have taught me so much.

—MARIO CASTRO, MD, MPH

To my husband, Charles, whose continued love and support I cherish, and to my son, William, who keeps me young and gives me perspective on what matters in this world. To my parents, I thank you for your love and guidance and for instilling in me a strong work ethic, and to my mentors, I thank you for guiding me down the satisfying path of medicine.

—MONICA KRAFT, MD

Contributors

Andrea J. Apter, MD, MA, MSc
Professor of Medicine, University of
Pennsylvania Medical Center, Allergy
and Immunology Section, Pulmonary,
Allergy & Critical Care Division,
Philadelphia, Pennsylvania

Ravi Aysola, MD
Fellow, Washington University School of
Medicine, St. Louis, Missouri

Leonard B. Bacharier, MD
Associate Professor of Pediatrics,
Washington University School of
Medicine; Attending Physician,
Clinical Director, Division of Allergy
and Pulmonary Medicine, Washington
University School of Medicine and
St. Louis Children's Hospital, St. Louis,
Missouri

Ronald C. Balkissoon, MSc, DIH, MD
Associate Professor, Pulmonary Division,
Department of Medicine, University of
Colorado School of Medicine; Associate
Professor, National Jewish Medical and
Research Center, Denver, Colorado

Elisabeth H. Bel, MD, PhD
Professor, Department of Pulmonology,
Academic Medical Centre, Amsterdam,
The Netherlands

Bruce G. Bender, PhD
Head, Pediatric Behavioral Health,
National Jewish Medical and Research
Center, Denver, Colorado

Robyn L. Boedefeld, MD
Assistant Professor, Department
of Medicine, Division of Pulmonary and
Critical Care, University of Virginia
Health System, Charlottesville, Virginia

Larry Borish, MD
Professor of Medicine, University of
Virginia; Staff Physician, Asthma and
Allergic Disease Center, University of
Virginia Health Systems, Charlottesville,
Virginia

Arnaud Bourdin, MD
Associate Professor, Faculté de
Médecine de Montpellier; Consultant,
Hôpital Arnaud de Villeneuve, CHU de
Montpellier, Montpellier, France

Jean Bousquet, MD
Professor, Services des Maladies
Respiratoires, Hôpital Arnaud de
Villeneuve, Montpellier, France

Jessica H. Boyd, MD, MPH
Clinical Fellow, Department of
Pediatrics, Division of Allergy and
Pulmonary Medicine, Washington
University School of Medicine, St. Louis,
Missouri

Jeremy D. Bufford, MD
Associate Physician, Marshfield Clinic,
Marshfield, Wisconsin

William W. Busse, MD
George R. and Elaine Love Professor
of Medicine, Chair, Department of
Medicine, University of Wisconsin
School of Medicine and Public Health,
Madison, Wisconsin

Charles B. Cairns, MD
Associate Professor of Medicine and
Surgery, Duke University School of
Medicine; Associate Chief, Emergency
Medicine, Duke University Medical
Center, Durham, North Carolina

William J. Calhoun, MD
Sealy and Smith Distinguished
Chair of Internal Medicine,
Vice Chair for Research, Department
of Internal Medicine, University of
Texas Medical Branch, Galveston,
Texas

Thomas B. Casale, MD
Professor of Medicine, Creighton
University; Chief, Division of
Allergy/Immunology, Creighton
University Medical Center, Omaha,
Nebraska

Mario Castro, MD, MPH
Director, The Asthma & Airway
Translational Research Unit; Associate
Professor of Medicine and Pediatrics,
Division of Pulmonary and Critical Care
Medicine Washington University School
of Medicine; Attending Physician,
Barnes-Jewish Hospital, St. Louis,
Missouri

Mario Cazzola, MD
Associate Professor of Respiratory
Medicine, University of Rome "Tor
Vergata," Rome, Italy

Pascal Chanez, MD, PhD
Associate Professor, Faculté
de Medecine, Université de la
Mediterannée; Consultant, Department
of Respiratory Diseases, Hôpital Sainte-
Marguerite, Marseille, France

**Reuben Cherniack, MD, Msc. Dsc.
FRCP (Can), MRCP (London), FACP,
FACCP**
Distinguished Professor of Medicine,
University of Colorado, National Jewish
Medical and Research Center, Denver,
Colorado

**Bradley Chipps, MD, FAAP, FAAAI,
FCCP**
Medical Director, Capital Allergy and
Respiratory Disease Center; Medical
Director, Cystic Fibrosis Center and
Respiratory Therapy; Associate Medical
Director, Sleep Lab, Sutter Hospital,
Sacramento, California

Don W. Cockcroft, MD, FRCPC
Professor, University of Saskatchewan;
Active Staff, Royal University Hospital,
Saskatoon, Saskatchewan, Canada

Susan J. Corbridge, RN, MS, CNP
Director, Acute Care Nurse Practitioner
Program, University of Illinois at
Chicago; University of Illinois of
Chicago Medical Center, Chicago,
Illinois

Thomas C. Corbridge, MD, FCCP
Professor of Medicine, Northwestern University, Feinberg School of Medicine; Northwestern Memorial Hospital, Chicago, Illinois

C.J. Corrigan, MA, MSc, PhD, FRCP
Reader and Consultant in Asthma, Allergy & Respiratory Science, King's College London, Division of Asthma, Allergy & Lung Biology; MRC and Asthma UK Centre for Allergic Mechanisms of Asthma, London, United Kingdom

Ronina A. Covar, MD
Assistant Professor of Pediatrics, University of Colorado Health Science Center; Assistant Faculty, National Jewish Medical and Research Center, Denver, Colorado

Danita Czyzewski, PhD
Assistant Professor, Departments of Psychiatry and Behavioral Sciences and Pediatrics, Baylor College of Medicine; Pediatric Psychologist, Texas Children's Hospital, Houston, Texas

Aaron Deykin, MD
The Pulmonary and Critical Care Division, Brigham and Women's Hospital, Harvard Medical School, Boston, Massachusetts

Elizabeth A. Erwin, MD
Assistant Professor of Pediatrics, The Ohio State University; Nationwide Children's Hospital, Columbus, Ohio

David Evans, PhD
Professor of Clinical Sociomedical Sciences (Pediatrics), Columbia University College of Physicians & Surgeons and the Joseph L. Mailman School of Public Health, New York, New York

James B. Fink, MS, PhD
Fellow, Respiratory Science, Nektar Therapeutics, San Carlos, California

James E. Fish, MD
Adjunct Professor of Medicine, Thomas Jefferson University, Philadelphia, Pennsylvania; Senior Medical Director, Genentech, Inc., South San Francisco, California

Anthony J. Frew, MD, FRCP
Professor of Allergy & Respiratory Medicine, Brighton & Sussex Medical School; Consultant Physician, Brighton & Sussex University Hospitals NHS Trust, Brighton, United Kingdom

Anne L. Fuhlbrigge, MD, MS
Assistant Professor, Harvard Medical School; Clinical Director, Pulmonary and Critical Care Division, Respiratory Epidemiology, Channing Laboratory, Brigham and Women's Hospital, Boston, Massachusetts

Maureen George, PhD, RN, AE-C
Assistant Professor, University of Pennsylvania School of Nursing, Philadelphia, Pennsylvania

Lynn B. Gerald, PhD, MSPH
Associate Professor, School of Medicine, University of Alabama at Birmingham, Birmingham, Alabama; Director, Lung Health Center, Associate Scientist, Center for Health Promotion, University of Alabama at Birmingham, Birmingham, Alabama

Peter G. Gibson, MBBS, FRACP
Professor of Medicine, School of Medicine and Public Health; Faculty of Health, University of Newcastle; Senior Staff Specialist, Department of Respiratory and Sleep Medicine, John Hunter Hospital; Director, Asthma and Airways Research Group, Hunter Medical Research Institute, Newcastle, Australia

Stefano Guerra, MD, PhD, MPH
Assistant Professor of Public Health and Medicine, Arizona Respiratory Center and Mel and Enid Zuckerman College of Public Health, University of Arizona, Tucson, Arizona

Nicola A. Hanania, MD, MS
Associate Professor of Medicine, Director, Asthma Clinical Research Center, Baylor College of Medicine, Houston, Texas

Susan M. Harding, MD
Professor of Medicine, School of Medicine; Medical Director, UAB Sleep-Wake Disorder Center, University of Alabama at Birmingham, Birmingham, Alabama

Iftikhar Hussain, MD
Clinical Faculty, Oklahoma University School of Medicine at Tulsa; Active Staff, Saint Francis Hospital, St. John Hospital, SouthCrest Hospital, Tulsa, Oklahoma

Susan L. Janson, DNSc, RN, ANP, FAAN
Professor, University of California, San Francisco, California; Nurse Practitioner and Clinical Nurse Specialist, University of California San Francisco Medical Center, Ambulatory Care Center, San Francisco, California

Nizar N. Jarjour, MD
Professor and Head, Section of Allergy, Pulmonary and Critical Care Medicine, Department of Medicine, University of Wisconsin, Madison, Wisconsin

Sujani Kakumanu, MD
Clinical Instructor, University of Wisconsin Medical School; University of Wisconsin Hospitals and Clinics, Madison, Wisconsin

Kimberly Kelsay, MD
Associate Professor, Department of Psychiatry, University of Colorado Denver School of Medicine; Co-Director, Pediatric Care Unit, National Jewish Medical and Research Center, Denver, Colorado

Sarah B. Knowles, PhD, MPH
Research and Publications Coordinator, Palo Alto Medical Foundation Research Institute, Palo Alto, California

Monica Kraft, MD
Associate Professor of Medicine; Director, Duke Asthma, Allergy, and Airway Center, Duke University Medical Center, Durham, North Carolina

Marzena Krawiec, MD
Assistant Professor of Pediatrics, National Jewish Medical and Research Center, University of Colorado Health Sciences Center, Denver, Colorado

Robert F. Lemanske, Jr., MD
Professor of Pediatrics and Medicine, University of Wisconsin School of Medicine and Public Health; Head, Division of Pediatric Allergy, Immunology and Rheumatology, University of Wisconsin Hospital, Madison, Wisconsin

John J. Lima, PharmD
Director, Clinical Pediatric Pharmacology, Nemours Children's Clinic, Jacksonville, Florida

Njira L. Lugogo, MD
Instructor in Medicine, Division of Pulmonary Allergy and Critical Care Medicine, Duke University Medical Center, Durham, North Carolina

Joan M. Mangan, PhD, MST
Assistant Professor, School of Medicine, School of Public Health, University of Alabama at Birmingham, Birmingham, Alabama; Associate Scientist, Lung Health Center, University of Alabama at Birmingham, Birmingham, Alabama

John G. Mastronarde, MD, MSc
Associate Professor, The Ohio State University Division of Pulmonary, Allergy, Critical Care and Sleep Medicine, Columbus, Ohio

John G. McCartney, MD
Fellow, Department of Medicine, Section of Pulmonary and Critical Care, University of Wisconsin Hospitals and Clinics, Madison, Wisconsin

Elizabeth L. McQuaid, PhD
Associate Professor, Warren Alpert Medical School of Brown University; Staff Psychologist, Rhode Island Hospital, Providence, Rhode Island

Anandhi T. Murugan, MD, MPH
Clinical Postdoctoral Fellow, University of Texas Medical Branch, Galveston, Texas

Jennifer Altamura Namazy, MD
Department of Allergy, Kaiser Permanente Medical Center, San Diego, California

Jonathan P. Parsons, MD
Assistant Professor of Internal Medicine; Associate Director, OSU Asthma Center; Pulmonary, Allergy, Critical Care, and Sleep Medicine, Davis Heart and Lung Research Institute, Ohio State University Medical Center, Columbus, Ohio

Rodolfo M. Pascual, MD, FCCP
Assistant Professor of Medicine, Section on Pulmonary, Critical Care, Allergy and Immunologic Diseases, Department of Internal Medicine, Wake Forest University School of Medicine, Winston-Salem, North Carolina

Anand C. Patel, MD
Instructor in Pediatrics, Division of Pediatric Allergy/Pulmonary Medicine, The Edward Mallinckrodt Department of Pediatrics, Washington University School of Medicine, St. Louis, Missouri

Stephen P. Peters, MD, PhD, FACP, FCCP, FAAAAI, FCPP
Professor of Medicine and Pediatrics, Director of Research, Section on

Pulmonary, Critical Care, Allergy and Immunologic Diseases, Training Program Director, Allergy and Immunology, Department of Internal Medicine and Center for Human Genomics, Wake Forest University, Winston-Salem, North Carolina

Thomas A.E. Platts-Mills, MD, PhD
Head, Division of Allergy and Allergic Disease, University of Virginia, Charlottesville, Virginia

Roy A. Pleasants, PharmD
Associate Professor, Campbell University School of Pharmacy, Buies Creek, North Carolina; Assistant Professor, Duke University School of Medicine; Clinical Pulmonary Specialist, Duke University Medical Center, Durham, North Carolina

Jane Robinson, PhD
Assistant Professor, University of Colorado Health Sciences Center; Clinical Pediatric Psychologist, National Jewish Medical and Research Center, Denver, Colorado

Bruce K. Rubin, MEngr, MD, MBA, FRCPC
Professor and Vice-Chair of Pediatrics; Professor of Physiology and Pharmacology, Wake Forest University School of Medicine, Winston-Salem, North Carolina; Professor of Biomedical Engineering, Virginia Polytechnical Institute and State University/Wake Forest School of Biomedical Engineering Sciences, Blacksburg, Virginia/Winston-Salem, North Carolina

Michael Schatz, MD, MS
Department of Allergy, Kaiser Permanente Medical Center, San Diego, California

Valerie A. Schend, BS
Clinical Instructor, University of Wisconsin School of Pharmacy; Clinical Pharmacist, Department of Asthma/Allergy/Pulmonary Clinical Research, University of Wisconsin School of Medicine and Public Health, Madison, Wisconsin

Phillip E. Silkoff, MD
Medical Director, Clinical Research Symbicort US, Wilmington, Delaware

David Slade, MD
Associate Clinical Instructor/Research Fellow, Duke University Medical Center, Durham, North Carolina

Raymond G. Slavin, MD, MS
Professor of Internal Medicine, Division of Immunobiology, Section of Allergy and Clinical Immunology, St. Louis University School of Medicine, St. Louis, Missouri

Marianna M. Sockrider, MD, DrPH
Associate Professor of Pediatric Pulmonology, Baylor College of Medicine; Adjunct Assistant Professor of Behavioral Sciences, Health Promotion and Behavioral Sciences, University of Texas Health Sciences Center–Houston School of Public Health; Chief of Pediatric Pulmonary Clinic, Texas Children's Hospital, Houston, Texas

Christine A. Sorkness, PharmD
Professor of Pharmacy and Medicine, University of Wisconsin School of Pharmacy; Program Director, Asthma/Allergy/Pulmonary Clinical Research, University of Wisconsin School of Medicine and Public Health, Madison, Wisconsin

Joseph D. Spahn, MD
Associate Professor of Pediatrics, University of Colorado Health Sciences Center; Associate Professor of Pediatrics, National Jewish Medical and Research Center, Denver, Colorado

Jonathan E. Spahr, MD
Assistant Professor of Pediatrics, University of Pittsburgh, Pittsburgh, Pennsylvania

John W. Steinke, PhD
Assistant Professor of Research, Asthma and Allergic Disease Center, University of Virginia Health Systems, Charlottesville, Virginia

Lora Stewart, MD
Division of Allergy–Clinical Immunology, Department of Pediatrics, Ira J. and Jacqueline Neimark Laboratory of Clinical Pharmacology in Pediatrics, National Jewish Medical and Research Center and University of Colorado Health Sciences Center, Denver, Colorado

Jeffrey R. Stokes, MD
Assistant Professor of Medicine, Allergy/Immunology Program Director, Division of Allergy and Immunology, Creighton University, Omaha, Nebraska

Robert C. Strunk, MD
Professor of Pediatrics, Washington
University School of Medicine;
Member, Division of Allergy and
Pulmonary Medicine, St. Louis
Children's Hospital, St. Louis,
Missouri

Stanley J. Szefler, MD
Professor of Pediatrics and
Pharmacology, University of Colorado
Health Science Center; Helen
Wohlberg and Herman Lambert Chair
in Pharmacokinetics, National Jewish
Medical and Research Center, Denver,
Colorado

Laurel R. Talabere, PhD, MA, MS
Professor, Capital University School of
Nursing, Columbus, Ohio

Karen J. Tien, PhD
Senior Instructor, Case Western
Reserve University School of Medicine;
Child Clinical Psychologist, University
Hospitals of Cleveland, Cleveland,
Ohio

Ilonka H. van Veen, MD
Pulmonologist, Medisch Spectrum
Twente, Enschede, The Netherlands

**Christine Waldman Wagner, RN, MSN,
CPNP, FNP-BC, AE-C**
Program Manager, Comprehensive
Asthma Center, Children's Medical
Center, Dallas, Texas

Frederick S. Wamboldt, MD
Professor of Psychiatry, University
of Colorado Health Science Center;
Professor of Medicine and Head,
Division of Psychosocial Medicine,
National Jewish Medical and Research
Center, Denver, Colorado

**John O. Warner, MBChB, MD, FRCP,
FRCPCH, FMedSci**
Professor of Pediatrics, Head of
Department, Faculty of Medicine,
Imperial College London; Honorary
Consultant Paediatrician, St Mary's
Hospital, London, United Kingdom

Michael E. Wechsler, MD, MMSc
Division of Pulmonary and Critical Care,
Brigham and Women's Hospital, Harvard
Medical School, Boston, Massachusetts

Glenn J. Whelan, PharmD
Affiliate Assistant Professor,
AstraZeneca Pharmaceuticals, LLP,
Department of Allergy and Immunology,

University of South Florida; Clinical
Pharmacist, St. Joseph's Hospital,
Tampa, Florida

Larry W. Williams, MD
Associate Professor of Pediatrics, Duke
University Medical Center; Associate
Director, Duke Asthma, Allergy, and
Airway Center, Durham, North Carolina

Sandra R. Wilson, PhD
Adjunct Clinical Professor of Medicine,
Stanford University School of Medicine,
Stanford, California; Senior Staff Scientist,
Chair, Department of Health Services
Research, Palo Alto Medical Foundation
Research Institute, Palo Alto, California

Patrick H. Win, MD
Associate Faculty, Department of
Internal Medicine, Division of Allergy
and Immunology, Washington University
School of Medicine, Barnes-Jewish
Hospital; Active Staff, St. Elizabeth's
Hospital, Memorial Hospital, St. Louis,
Missouri

Anne L. Wright, PhD
Research Professor, Department of
Pediatrics, University of Arizona College
of Medicine, Tucson, Arizona

Preface

Asthma is one of the most common respiratory disorders in the world, yet there is no single comprehensive source to provide assistance to the clinician in the assessment and management of this condition. In *Clinical Asthma*, we have sought to bring together world experts in the field of asthma to provide a practical and useful resource for all who take care of patients affected by this disease. This textbook is written for students, clinicians, educators, and researchers who are seeking an authoritative, up-to-date source about asthma. We believe all individuals working with patients affected by asthma should have ready access to such a resource.

In this first edition of *Clinical Asthma*, we have purposefully incorporated two recently updated international guidelines. The Global Initiative for Asthma (GINA), released in 2006, and the National Asthma Education and Prevention Program (NAEPP) Expert Panel Report 3, released in 2007, have been extensively incorporated throughout each chapter.

Clinical Asthma is divided into seven sections that provide a comprehensive overview. In the first section, the current worldwide epidemic of asthma is described together with intriguing insights into the development of this common disease. In the next two sections, we review current diagnostic and assessment strategies for asthma, including recent concepts from the NAEPP guidelines. The subsequent section deals with practical aspects of asthma management in children and adults and is followed by an overview of current therapies used to treat asthma. We then provide detailed discussions of special situations in asthma such as exercise-induced asthma, rhinosinusitis, vocal cord dysfunction, gastroesophageal reflux, occupational asthma, and the pregnant asthma patient. Last, we dedicate an entire section to the education of the asthma patient, a key area to successful management.

We have asked expert authors to provide a comprehensive yet practical review of the subject matter. In addition, each chapter is preceded by Clinical Pearls of wisdom, which cover key concepts about the subsequent matter to be discussed. Key references and suggested readings are included in each chapter, although they are not meant to be an exhaustive annotation of the subject.

We would like to thank the authors for their outstanding contributions to this first edition of *Clinical Asthma*. We would also like to thank Dolores Meloni and Mary Beth Murphy at Elsevier for their creative guidance and expert input into the development of this book.

Finally, we hope that the readers find this book useful in their daily management of patients to achieve higher quality of life. We believe all of our patients with asthma deserve the best possible education and management of their condition.

MARIO CASTRO, MD, MPH

MONICA KRAFT, MD

Contents

ASTHMA IN THE 21ST CENTURY

Epidemiology of Asthma

Njira L. Lugogo, Monica Kraft, and Mario Castro

Understanding the epidemiology of asthma is essential to decreasing the morbidity and mortality of this common disease. The challenges faced by epidemiologists who study asthma begin with the lack of a pathophysiologically and clinically applicable universal definition for the disease. In 1962, the American Thoracic Society proposed defining asthma as a disease characterized by increased responsiveness of the trachea and bronchi to various stimuli and manifested by widespread narrowing of the airways that changes in severity either spontaneously or as a result of therapy.[1] There is no single physiologic test that is both highly sensitive and specific in diagnosing asthma. The methacholine challenge test is highly sensitive but not specific. In 1975, the World Health Organization described asthma as a chronic condition characterized by recurrent bronchospasm resulting from a tendency to develop reversible narrowing of airway lumina in response to stimuli of a level or intensity not causing such narrowing in most individuals. The emphasis on bronchoconstriction or bronchospasm as the mechanism of asthma is not disputed. Asthma is a far more complicated disease, however, with a complex pathophysiology. Research has proven that asthma involves airway hyperresponsiveness and inflammation. The revised definition of asthma aims to incorporate information obtained from years of extensive research. In 1991, the

National Institutes of Health and the National Heart, Lung, and Blood Institute described asthma as a chronic inflammatory disorder of the airways in which many cells and cellular elements play a role. The chronic inflammation causes an associated increase in airway hyperresponsiveness that leads to recurrent episodes of wheezing, breathlessness, chest tightness, and coughing, particularly in the night and early morning. These episodes are usually associated with widespread but variable airflow obstruction that is often reversible either spontaneously or with treatment.

Most epidemiologic studies in asthma rely on self-reporting by patients regarding whether they have a diagnosis of asthma. There are no standardized questions to be asked or studies that can be done to confirm the diagnosis. The questionnaires used vary from country to country, which makes results more difficult to interpret and generalize to a particular population. This discussion focuses on the prevalence of asthma within the United States and internationally, the morbidity and mortality of asthma, risk factors associated with the development of asthma, and future directions of research in the epidemiology of asthma.

PREVALENCE IN THE UNITED STATES

Asthma prevalence has been increasing despite advances made in treatment over the past 2 decades. The increased prevalence has been accompanied by an increase in morbidity and mortality. In the United States, asthma prevalence has been estimated from surveys using questionnaires, spirometry, and assessment of airway hyperresponsiveness. The National Health Interview Survey (NHIS) collects data on asthma prevalence by conducting annual surveys through the National Center for Health Statistics. From 1980 to 1996 the determination of asthma prevalence relied on a self-reported occurrence of at least one asthma attack within the preceding 12-month period. Asthma prevalence increased 73.9% from 1980 to 1996, with an estimated 6.9 million persons (31.4 per 1000) reporting an episode of asthma in 1980 in comparison with 14.6 million persons (54.6 per 1000 population) in 1996.

The increased prevalence of asthma is multifactorial in etiology. Factors include an epidemic of obesity in the United States, which is an independent risk factor for the development of asthma. The population has become increasingly sedentary, spending more time indoors where the exposure to allergens, such as mold, dust mites, and cockroach dust, is more prevalent. The increased rate of industrialization has increased pollution and consequently increased airway

Note: This chapter is adapted from Lugogo NL, Kraft M: Epidemiology of asthma. Clin Chest Med 2006;27:1–15.

hyperresponsiveness secondary to exposure to environmental triggers. In contrast, the "hygiene hypothesis" suggests that increases in the prevalence of autoimmune and allergic diseases results from a decrease in the prevalence of childhood infections and improved hygiene.[2] Recent studies have provided evidence that innate immunity to bacterial and viral infections induces a T-helper 1 pattern of cytokine release, which potentially would suppress the T-helper 2 immune response of immunoglobulin E–mediated allergic diseases. Therefore, there are many postulated causes for the increased prevalence of asthma, which may vary depending on location, exposures, and how asthma is defined.

In 1997, the asthma questionnaire was changed to include two measures of prevalence. Patients were required to report lifetime asthma prevalence by answering the question, "Have you ever been told by a health care professional that you have asthma?" Second, data were collected on asthma episodes within the preceding 12 months, which was considered to be a surrogate marker of asthma control.[3] In 1997, 11.1 million (40.7 per 1000 population) reported an episode of asthma or asthma attack within the preceding 12-month period. The estimated number reporting asthma was lower than the 12-month estimates obtained in the years before 1997. The data from 1997 were consistent with prior data obtained with higher rates of asthma prevalence in children (5 to 14 years of age), blacks, and females. The lower prevalence of asthma as noted in the 1997 NHIS data may be attributed to the change in the questionnaire used to obtain information about asthma prevalence. The revised questionnaire required reporting a lifetime prevalence of asthma as diagnosed by a medical professional and an episode of asthma or asthma attack within the preceding 12 months. The requirement that the patient have a diagnosis of asthma from a medical professional may have led to more accurate information regarding diagnosis in each individual. Asthma prevalence was noted to be 20% less in 1997 in comparison with 1996. This difference may be a result of the survey redesign.[4] Akinbami and co-workers[5] evaluated data from five sources obtained by the National Center for Health Statistics. The prevalence of

childhood asthma (age 0 to 17 years) increased an average of 4.3% per year from 1980 to 1996, from 3.6% to 6.2%. The peak prevalence was 7.5% in 1995. In 1997 the reported prevalence was 5.4%; however, changes in NHIS survey design precluded one from making any conclusions about changes in prevalence. Data collected since 1997 indicate a plateau in asthma prevalence rates in comparison with the early 1990s, indicating a stabilization of asthma occurrence (Fig. 1-1).

RACIAL AND ETHNICITY ISSUES OF ASTHMA PREVALENCE IN THE UNITED STATES

Data collected by the National Center for Health Statistics indicate that there continue to be racial and ethnic differences in asthma prevalence and health care use and mortality.[6] In 2004, the lifetime prevalence of asthma in persons younger than 14 was highest in the black population with a prevalence of 12.5% versus 7.1% in Hispanics and 7.5% in whites. The lifetime prevalence of asthma in those older than 15 was highest in blacks at 8.1% and lowest in Hispanics at 4.7% (Fig. 1-2). The prevalence of an episode of asthma within the preceding 12-month period was highest in black children younger than 14 at 7.9% versus 4.1% in Hispanic children (Fig. 1-3). The presence of asthma attacks per episodes of asthma in the preceding 12 months is an indicator of asthma control. The increased prevalence of uncontrolled asthma in black children is concerning and is likely caused by lack of access to care, poverty, poor living conditions with exposures to allergens at an early age, and inability to afford medications. The presence of this disparity in care needs urgent evaluation and intervention.

The overall prevalence of asthma in 2004 was highest in black children younger than 14 at 12.5%. Hispanic and white children had similar prevalence rates. The adult prevalence was lowest in Hispanic adults at 4.7%; black and white adults had prevalence rates of 8.1% and 7.4%, respectively (Fig. 1-4). There were no data collected on age of onset of asthma; the higher prevalence in black adults may be secondary to high prevalence of childhood asthma that persists into adulthood. Assessment of racial prevalence of asthma indicates that there are differences in asthma prevalence within the Hispanic population. Data

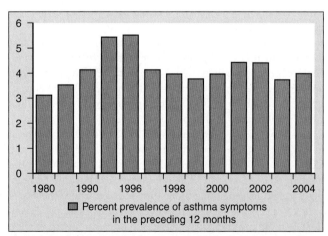

Figure I-I Percent prevalence of self-reported asthma (1980 to 1997) or an episode of asthma or asthma attack within the past 12 months (1997 to 2004): United States. *(Data from Centers for Disease Control and Prevention. Available at www.cdc.gov/nchs/data/nhis/earlyrelease/200412_15.pdf [Fig. 15.1; p 1] and www.cdc.gov/asthma/speakit/slides/slide5.jpg Accessed July 19, 2005.)*

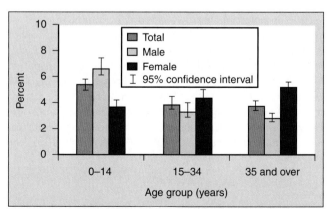

Figure I-2 Percentage of persons of all ages who experienced an asthma episode in the preceding 12 months by age group and sex: United States, 2004. *(From Centers for Disease Control and Prevention. National Health Interview Survey, 2004. Available at www.cdc.gov/nchs/data/nhis/earlyrelease/200503_15.pdf [Fig. 15.2; p 2]. Accessed July 18, 2005.)*

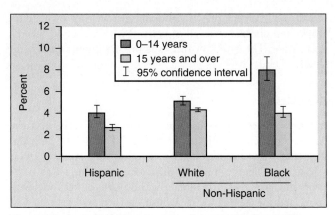

Figure 1-3 Sex-adjusted percentage of persons of all ages who reported an episode of asthma in the preceding 12 months by age group and race or ethnicity: United States, 2004. *(From Centers for Disease Control and Prevention. National Health Interview Survey, 2004. Available at www.cdc.gov/nchs/data/nhis/earlyrelease/200503_15.pdf [Fig. 15.3; p 2]. Accessed July 18, 2005.)*

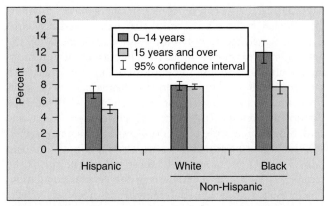

Figure 1-4 Sex-adjusted prevalence of current asthma among groups of all ages, by age group and race or ethnicity: United States, 2004. *(From Centers for Disease Control and Prevention. National Health Interview Survey, 2004. Available at: www.cdc.gov/nchs/data/nhis/earlyrelease/200503_15.pdf [Fig. 15.6; p. 6]. Accessed July 18, 2005.)*

reported by the Centers for Disease Control and Prevention[7] in 2002 revealed a difference that can be masked by grouping all Hispanic ethnicities together. Puerto Ricans have the highest asthma lifetime prevalence rate of 196 per 1000; Mexicans have the lowest asthma prevalence rate of 61 per 1000. Puerto Ricans had the highest asthma attack prevalence, which was 100% higher than non-Hispanic whites and 30% higher than non-Hispanic blacks. The higher prevalence in Puerto Ricans may be related to an underlying genetic predisposition to asthma and environmental factors including access to care. This is an area that requires further evaluation. Risk factors affecting asthma prevalence are areas of ongoing assessment.

RISK FACTORS ASSOCIATED WITH INCREASED ASTHMA PREVALENCE

Income Level and Asthma

Smith and co-workers[8] examined cross-sectional data collected by NHIS in 1997 of 14,244 children younger than 18. Logistic regression was used to analyze the independent and

joint effects of race, ethnicity, and ratio of income to federal poverty level on the prevalence of asthma. The main outcome was a parental report of a lifetime diagnosis of asthma in the group of children. Overall prevalence of asthma was highest in non-Hispanic black children at 13.6% as compared with 11.2% for non-Hispanic white children. The prevalence did not differ significantly between non-Hispanic white children and Hispanic children. The prevalence of asthma was adjusted for sociodemographic variables including the ratio of annual family income to the federal poverty level. There was a statistically significant increase in asthma prevalence in non-Hispanic black children from families with income less than half the federal poverty level. This difference remained significant even in comparison with non-Hispanic white children from very poor families and may be a result of environmental exposures that are unique to children from poor families. This difference in environmental exposures may be related to the percentage of disadvantaged black children who live in urban areas rather than rural areas.

Simon and co-workers[9] analyzed data collected randomly on 6004 children younger than 17 living in Los Angeles County from 1999 to 2000. The prevalence of childhood asthma in the sampled population was highest in blacks at 15.8% compared with 7.3% in whites and 6% in Asians. These differences persisted after correction for income and health care access measures. The asthma rates were highest in children from poor families. These findings illustrate the need for further assessment of high-risk populations to determine the risk factors that can be modified to reduce asthma prevalence.

The population at highest risk for asthma is black children from poor urban neighborhoods. Strategies to curb childhood asthma and decrease long-term morbidity are urgently needed. The Harlem Children's Zone Asthma Initiative is an exemplary intervention program undertaken to address this problem. The current lifetime prevalence of asthma in black children nationally is 8%. The prevalence of asthma in children in New York City was 17% in 2003, with the highest prevalence in central Harlem. The Harlem Initiative began as a comprehensive strategy to improve awareness of asthma treatment and action plans; assist with environmental trigger controls including decreasing exposure to cigarette smoke, dust mites, and cockroaches; to assist with parenting skills; and to assist with technical, public, legal, and housing issues facing the community. This comprehensive intervention has led to improved asthma control, medication compliance, and decreased absenteeism and hospitalizations.[10] This model can be applied to other populations at risk to improve asthma outcomes.

Environmental Allergen Exposure

The effect of environmental tobacco smoke on adult asthma is an area of ongoing investigation. Studies have indicated a relationship between parental smoking and childhood asthma. There seems to be an increased risk of early-onset asthma in children exposed to tobacco smoke with an increased incidence of wheezing until age 6 years.[11,12] The NHIS data collected in 1981 indicate an increased risk of asthma in children younger than 5 whose mothers smoked at least one-half pack per day (odds ratio 2.1, $P = .001$). A prospective cohort study was performed on 451 nonsmoking adults with asthma who were exposed to environmental tobacco. There were three categories of subjects[1]: those with exposure at baseline but none at follow-up,[3] those with no baseline exposure but with new exposure, and those with exposure both at baseline and at follow-up.[4] Subjects with baseline environmental tobacco exposure had greater asthma severity scores and increased emergency room visits and hospitalizations. The subjects who had cessation of environmental tobacco exposure had improved quality-of-life scores and decreased use of emergency room services.[13] Environmental tobacco use continues to be a significant risk factor for asthma and for increased severity of disease.

Arif and co-workers[14] analyzed data from the National Health and Nutrition Examination Survey III to determine the prevalence and risk factors for asthma and wheezing in US adults. The epidemiology of asthma survey was conducted from 1988 to 1994 and collected data on 18,825 adults older than 20. Variables analyzed included demographic factors, socioeconomic status, indoor air quality, allergy or hay fever, and smoking. Overall asthma prevalence was 4.5% and the prevalence of wheezing within the preceding 12 months was 16.4%. Mexican Americans had the lowest overall prevalence of asthma at 2.6% even though they were the largest racial group living below the poverty level. There was no statistically significant difference in the overall prevalence of asthma in non-Hispanic blacks at 5.1% in comparison with non-Hispanic whites at 4.7%. There was no regional variation in overall asthma prevalence and wheezing; however, there was significant regional variation for racial prevalence of asthma (Fig. 1-5). The highest asthma prevalence was in racial and ethnic groups (including Asians and other Hispanics) living in the Northeast and Midwest. Low education status,

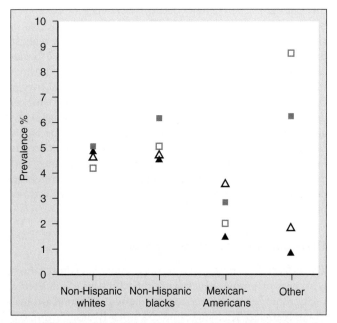

Figure 1-5 Estimated prevalence of asthma across four regions of the United States by race or ethnicity in the National Health and Nutrition Examination Survey III adult study population (1988 to 1994). *Closed square, northeast; open square, midwest; closed triangle, south; open triangle, west. (From Arif AA, Delclos ES, Lee ES, et al: Prevalence and risk factors of asthma and wheezing among US adults: an analysis of the NHANES III data. Eur Respir J 2003;21:829; with permission.)*

female sex, current or past smoking history, pet ownership, atopy, and obesity were all associated with increased asthma prevalence. The effect of race was further illustrated by this study.

Genetics

A family history of asthma in a first-degree relative is the best-recognized risk factor for asthma. The risk of developing asthma was assessed in a population-based study of twins in Norway. The cumulative incidence of asthma was 6.0% for males and 5.4% for females. The relative risk for developing asthma among twins whose co-twin had asthma was 17.9 (95% confidence interval, 10.3–31.0) for identical and 2.3 (95% confidence interval, 1.2–4.4) for fraternal twins. The twins shared similar environments but had varied rates of asthma occurrence. The authors concluded that genetics played a more significant role than environment in the development of asthma.[15]

Recent advances made in genetics and genotype mapping have indicated the presence of various genetic polymorphisms that may be associated with asthma and bronchial hyperresponsiveness. Polymorphisms of the gene for the beta$_2$-adrenergic receptor may be important in determining the clinical response to beta-agonists in individuals with asthma. Single nucleotide polymorphisms have been identified for the beta$_2$-adrenergic receptor with the wild-type pattern of arginine-16-glycine and glutamine-27-glutamic acid. Single nucleotide polymorphisms have been described as homozygous pairs including Arg 16 Arg, Glu 27 Glu, and Gln 27 Gln. The frequency of these polymorphisms is the same in asthmatic individuals as in the general population. The presence of various polymorphisms, however, affects bronchodilator response.[16,17] The discovery of these polymorphisms and their impact on pharmacotherapy in the future has led to increased enthusiasm that genetic mapping will improve asthma management in the future.[18] For a more extensive discussion of pharmacogenetics of asthma, see Chapter 26.

The Salmeterol Multi-Center Asthma Research Trial (SMART) illustrates the likely effects of genetics and race on response to asthma therapy. This trial was a placebo-controlled double-blind study to assess the safety of salmeterol. beta$_2$-agonist–naive patients were enrolled and placed on twice-daily doses of 42 μg of salmeterol for 28 weeks or placebo. Primary end points included respiratory-related deaths or life-threatening events. The interim analysis was performed after 26,353 patients were enrolled. Data analysis revealed a higher number of asthma-related deaths (13 versus 4) or life-threatening experiences (36 versus 23) in patients treated with salmeterol. Post hoc analysis revealed a small but statistically significant difference in primary end points in black persons with asthma. The study did not address whether persons on inhaled corticosteroids and salmeterol are protected by any adverse effect of the salmeterol.[17] The United Kingdom Salmeterol Nationwide Surveillance study showed a numerical but not statistically significant increase in asthma-related deaths in patients treated with salmeterol versus albuterol in addition to standard therapy.[19,20] The current guidelines recommend against the use of salmeterol without concurrent inhaled corticosteroids.

Respiratory Infections

The impact of respiratory infections on asthma incidence is an area of debate. The higher prevalence of asthma in Western countries than in less technologically advanced countries has been explained by the "hygiene hypothesis." The hygiene hypothesis, proposed by Strachan[2] in 1989, is based on the concept that exposure to airway infections and allergens early in life promotes the maturation of T-helper 1 lymphocytes over T-helper 2 lymphocytes, thereby decreasing the risk of developing allergic conditions.[21] Persons living in more rural environments may be exposed to infections early in life with the development of an increased T-helper 1 lymphocyte population and therefore will be less likely to develop atopy and asthma. Several studies support this theory and others contradict the findings.[22,23] The varied conclusions may be a result of the intensity, the timing, and the duration of the exposure. The underlying genetic susceptibility of the individual may also contribute to whether a particular exposure in childhood leads to the development of asthma later in life.[24]

The most frequently cultured infectious pathogens in asthmatic individuals undergoing bronchoscopy with bronchoalveolar lavage are viruses (adenovirus, parainfluenza, influenza, and respiratory synctial virus), *Mycoplasma pneumoniae*, and *Chlamydia pneumoniae*. Studies of patients positive for *M. pneumoniae* by polymerase chain reaction have revealed increased levels of substance P with up-regulation of the NK-1 receptor and increased production of interleukin-8 and epidermal growth factor receptor-β with subsequent increased inflammation and airway remodeling. The effect of *M. pneumoniae* and other chronic infections on asthma and airway inflammation and remodeling is an area of ongoing research.[25–27]

Studies analyzing the National Center for Health Statistics data on asthma prevalence are crucial to enhancing understanding of risk factors that predispose patients to developing asthma and will be instrumental in identifying modifiable risk factors. The ability to adjust risk factors that may influence the development of asthma will lead to decreased prevalence, morbidity, and mortality. The interaction between identified risk factors and race and ethnicity can make it difficult to determine which factors are most important. The heterogeneity of asthma leads to an increased likelihood that the disease is multifactorial in etiology and controlling multiple factors is important in managing patients with the disease.

WORLDWIDE PREVALENCE

The largest study of more than 6000 asthmatic individuals worldwide was performed between 1996 and 1997 in 91 centers in 56 countries in the United Kingdom, Europe, Asia, Africa, and Latin America. There were two age groups: 6- to 7-year-olds and 13- to 14-year-olds. The prevalence of asthma in the 13- to 14-year-olds varied from 2.1% to 4.4% in Albania, China, Greece, and Indonesia to 29.1% to 32.2% in Australia, New Zealand, Republic of Ireland, and the United Kingdom. Countries with a 12-month prevalence of asthma symptoms less than 10% tended to be in Asia, Northern Africa, Eastern Europe, and Eastern Mediterranean areas. North America, Latin America, and Oceania had higher prevalence rates with more than 20% of children reporting asthma symptoms.

The prevalence of asthma in the 6- to 7-year-old group ranged from an average of 4.1% in India, Indonesia, Iran, and Malaysia to 32.1% or lower in Australia, Brazil, New Zealand, and Panama (Fig. 1-6). There was a lower prevalence of all symptoms in the 13- to 14-year-old group except sleep disturbance caused by wheezing, which was more prevalent in the younger age group.[28] There was remarkable consistency of the prevalence rates of asthma, allergic rhinoconjunctivitis, and atopic eczema within countries with low prevalence. There was significant variation between prevalence of asthma within geographic areas, illustrated by high prevalence rates in the United Kingdom and low rates in Albania, Greece, and Italy; however, the prevalence rates varied widely from country to country within the same continent. Studies of asthma prevalence in Europe have revealed similar results, with English-speaking countries having a higher prevalence of asthma than

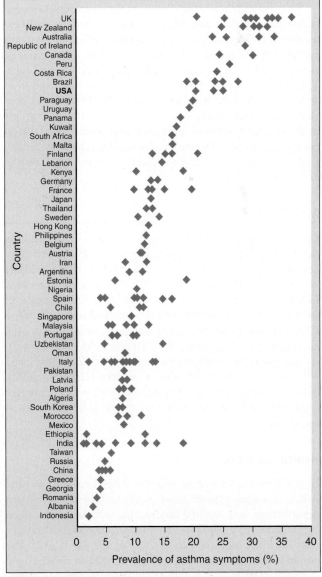

Figure 1-6 Prevalence of 12-month asthma symptoms as reported by written questionnaire. *(From The International Study of Asthma and Allergies in Childhood (ISAAC) Steering Committee: Worldwide variation in prevalence of symptoms of asthma, allergic rhinoconjunctivitis and atopic eczema: ISAAC. Lancet 1998;351:1228; with permission.)*

non–English-speaking countries.[29] Countries ranking highest in prevalence of sleep disturbance and wheeze severe enough to limit speech were different from those with the highest 12-month occurrence of wheezing. There was a higher prevalence of uncontrolled asthma in countries that did not have the highest overall prevalence rates, which may be attributed to the manner in which asthma is managed in different countries. No information was gathered about the management of asthma symptoms, which makes it difficult to come to a definitive conclusion about the etiology of this difference in prevalence. The International Study of Asthma and Allergies in Childhood (ISAAC) trial is assessing the presence of atopy more objectively using skin testing. The varied presence of atopy may indicate a genetic predisposition within the population that increases susceptibility to allergic disease of the upper and lower airways. Genetic factors, although important, cannot completely explain the differences in prevalence rates. There is likely a significant contribution of environment to asthma prevalence.[30]

Basagana and co-workers[31] assessed the association between socioeconomic class and asthma at both individual and center levels in 32 centers in 15 countries in Europe. Asthma prevalence was noted to be higher in lower socioeconomic classes, which was defined by education level or social class. There was an increased prevalence in persons who lived in an area where the education level was lower. The authors concluded that there were exposures to environmental agents in lower socioeconomic areas that may explain the difference in prevalence. The data collected from the next ISAAC trial will explore further the effect of environment on the development of asthma.

MORBIDITY

Data on asthma morbidity have been primarily obtained in the United States, with limited data available from other countries. This information as reported in the *Morbidity and Mortality Weekly Report* in 2002 includes self-reported asthma prevalence, school and work days lost because of asthma, and asthma-associated activity limitations (1980 to 1996); asthma-associated outpatient visits, asthma-associated hospitalizations, and asthma-associated deaths (1980 to 2002); asthma-associated emergency room visits (1992 to 2002); and self-reported asthma episodes or attacks (1997 to 2002). Rates of outpatient and emergency room visits increased from 1980 to 1999 with a decreased rate of hospitalizations and death.[3]

Health Care Use

Health care use for asthma includes outpatient visits to physicians, emergency room visits, visits to hospital outpatient departments, and hospitalizations. There were 13.9 million outpatient visits in 2002, most commonly in children younger than 17, with 5 million visits at a rate of 492 per 10,000. The rate of outpatient visits was 687 per 10,000 in children and 181 per 10,000 in persons older than 18 years. The rate of outpatient visits in patients of different racial and ethnic groups was similar. The number of visits among non-Hispanic blacks was 482 per 10,000, which was similar to that among non-Hispanic whites at 493 per 10,000 (Fig. 1-7). The increase

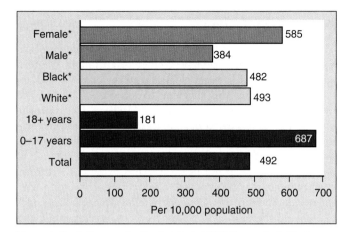

Figure 1-7 Asthma outpatient visits in 2002. *, age adjusted to the 2000 population. *(From Centers for Disease Control and Prevention: National Health Care Use Data. Available at www.cdc.gov/nchs/data/ asthmahealthestat1.pdf [Fig. 5; p 4]. Accessed July 19, 2005.)*

in health care use has occurred concurrently with decreased asthma prevalence rates and may be partly responsible for the decreased prevalence.

Beginning in 1992, information was gathered by the National Hospital Ambulatory Medical Care Survey to determine the reason for hospital emergency room and outpatient visits. There was an increase in emergency room visits from 1980 to 1999 throughout the United States (Fig. 1-8). In 2002, 1.9 million asthma-related emergency room visits were recorded. Children younger than 17 had a rate of 100 per 10,000, with the highest frequency of visits being

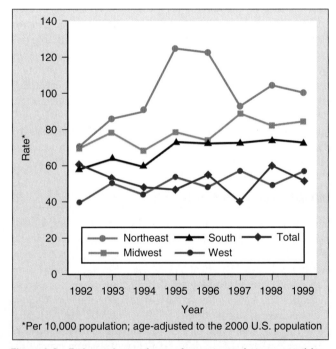

Figure 1-8 Estimated annual rate of emergency department visits for asthma as the first-listed diagnosis by region and year. *(From Centers for Disease Control and Prevention: National Ambulatory Medical Care Survey, 1992–1999. Available at www.cdc.gov/mmwr/preview/mmwrhtml/ss5101a1. htm [Fig. 4]. Accessed July 19, 2005.)*

among children younger than 4. The emergency room visits were four times higher for non-Hispanic blacks with a rate of 217 per 10,000 as compared with whites at a rate of 45 per 10,000.[32] The use of emergency room services can be a marker of uncontrolled or more severe asthma, which is likely caused by poor chronic medical management in this population. The racial differences noted in hospitalization rates and unscheduled emergency room visits are recorded with increased rates in non-Hispanic blacks.

The trend from the 1960s to the 1980s revealed an increase in hospitalizations for persons with asthma of 200% in children and 50% in adults.[33] This trend continued in the 1990s with an increase in the rate of hospitalizations for adults. Rate of hospitalization is higher in persons of non-Hispanic black descent than in non-Hispanic white persons. Information obtained from the National Hospital Discharge Survey in 2002 listed asthma as the cause for admission in 484,000 persons at a rate of 17 per 10,000. There were 187,000 admissions occurring in children younger than 15. The average length of stay was 3.2 days and there were more admissions among females than males. Children younger than 4 years had the highest rate of hospitalization with 59 hospitalizations per 10,000. Non-Hispanic blacks had a 225% higher rate of hospitalization than whites.[32] The hospitalization rate was highest among non-Hispanic blacks at 36 per 10,000 compared with 11 per 10,000 in whites (Fig. 1-9).

The current trend is alarming and emphasizes the importance of addressing health care delivery and risk stratification and modification for all asthmatic individuals. The goal is to optimize outpatient asthma therapy to decrease rates of emergency room use and hospitalization secondary to asthma. The differences in rates of emergency room and hospital use in non-Hispanic blacks with resultant increased risk of severe asthma and death is cause for concern. This may be caused by health care disparities and lack of access to adequate preventive care, leading to more severe uncontrolled asthma. Non-Hispanic black persons living in poverty are more likely to have severe asthma and to die of asthma than non-Hispanic white persons living in poverty. Healthy People 2010 has objectives aimed at addressing asthma prevalence and improving delivery of care and outcome.[34]

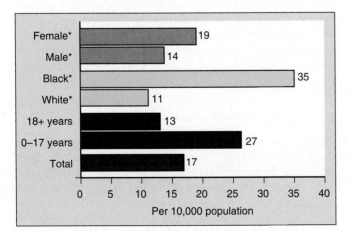

Figure 1-9 Asthma hospitalizations in 2002. *, age adjusted to the 2000 population. *(From Centers for Disease Control and Prevention: National Health Interview Survey. Available at www.cdc.gov/nchs/data/ asthmahealthestat1.pdf [Fig. 6; p. 5]. Accessed July 19, 2005.)*

The National Heart, Lung, and Blood Institute convened a multidisciplinary group of scientists and clinicians to review current research and identify risk factors responsible for health care disparity. The goal is to improve outcomes and to establish priorities for future research aimed at addressing this issue. Clinic- and community-based programs were evaluated to access the efficacy of these programs in reducing the morbidity of asthma. Implementation of various strategies is encouraged to improve the adoption of proven programs by various racial and ethnic groups.[35]

Absenteeism and Decreased Productivity

The morbidity associated with asthma is evident from the increased school absenteeism and loss of work days for adults who are caregivers for children or adults with asthma. The Asthma in America survey documented the severity of symptoms and the requirement for emergency care for more than 2500 adults with asthma or caregivers of children with asthma. During a 12-month period, one half of the children with asthma and one quarter of the adults missed school or work because of their disease. During this period, 9% were hospitalized, 23% required emergency department visits, and 29% had unscheduled emergency visits to a physician's office or clinic related to asthma. Overall, 41% of adults and 54% of children were hospitalized or seen in an emergency room or urgently in an outpatient setting for asthma. These patients had significantly increased morbidity because of sick days and costs associated with seeking care for their asthma.[36] A study of caregivers of children with asthma in France indicated that during a 12-month period 30% of caregivers missed work overall and 13% missed more than 5 days of work because of their child's asthma.[37] Absenteeism due to asthma leads to loss of resources and is a major financial burden to any society.

Financial Burden

Patients with asthma incur a significant financial burden associated with their disease. In 1998, the annual cost of asthma in the United States was estimated to be $11.3 billion with hospitalizations accounting for most of these costs. Current estimates of the cost of medical care in different Western countries ranges from $300 to $1300 per patient per year for asthma. Asthma patients and their families spend on average $1000 per year on medications.[38] Cost of care increased approximately 50% from 1985 to 1994, mostly from indirect costs.[39] The Hunair study evaluated morbidity, cost, and control of asthma in Hungary. The yearly direct and indirect costs (nonmedical output losses that are related to the consequences of illness) averaged $897 for children and $681 for adults. Patients with poorly controlled asthma had increased annual costs associated with their illness.[40] Aggressive management and a focus on stabilization of disease greatly affects the cost of asthma-related medical care and decreases expenditure significantly.

MORTALITY

Asthma-related deaths are a rare occurrence, particularly in children younger than 15. In the United States death rates per 100,000 increased steadily from 0.8 in 1978 to 2 in 1989 and

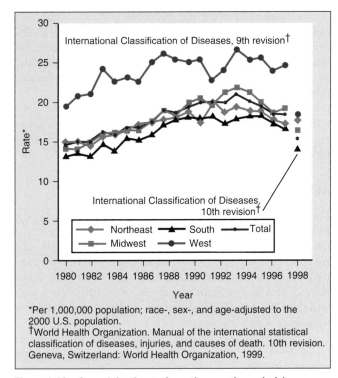

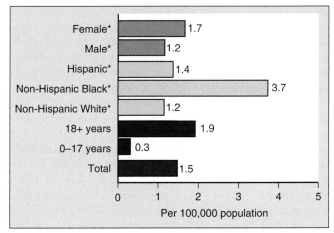

Figure 1-11 **Asthma deaths in 2002.** *, age adjusted to the 2000 population. *(From Centers for Disease Control and Prevention: National Health Interview Survey. Available at: www.cdc.gov/nchs/data/asthmahealthestat1.pdf [Fig. 7; p 6]. Accessed July 19, 2005.)*

Figure 1-10 **Annual death rate for asthma as the underlying cause of death by region and year.** Mortality component of the National Vital Statistics System, United States (1980 to 1999). *(From Mannino DM, Homa DM, Akinbami LJ, et al: Surveillance for asthma—United States, 1980–1999. In MMWR Surveill Summ 2002;51(1):8. Available at www.cdc.gov/mmwr/PDF/ss/ss5101.pdf).*

2.1 in 1994. Death rates plateaued after 1994. Rates in 1998 were 2.5 times higher than in 1979 (Fig. 1-10). The ICD-9 code for asthma-related deaths, which included asthma and chronic obstructive pulmonary disease, was changed in 1999 to the ICD-10 code of other chronic lower respiratory disease. This decreased the number of deaths coded as asthma by 11%. The asthma-related death rate decreased in 2000 to 1.6 per 100,000. This decrease cannot be fully explained by the change in coding.[41]

United States Mortality Statistics

In 2002, 4261 asthma-related deaths were reported, with a death rate of 1.5 per 100,000. Among these, asthma deaths of children were rare, with a death rate of 0.3 per 100,000. The death rate in persons older than 18 is 1.9 deaths per 100,000.[7] Non-Hispanic blacks have the highest death rates at 3.7 deaths per 100,000—a rate over 200% higher than the rate for non-Hispanic whites (Fig. 1-11). The difference between non-Hispanic blacks and non-Hispanic whites is startling: non-Hispanic blacks between the ages of 25 and 34 are six times more likely to die from asthma than non-Hispanic whites in the same age group. The effect of income level and education on the risk of asthma-related death is controversial, but studies have shown that the elevated risk of death is independent of income level and education level.[42] These studies postulate that the increase in asthma mortality rates may be related to the overall increase in prevalence of asthma rather than an increased mortality caused by poor patient care or lack of access to care.

Multiple studies have evaluated the rate of asthma deaths in ethnic minority groups. Death rates have increased dramatically in non-Hispanic blacks from low-income areas.[43,44] These studies conclude that the difference in death rates is likely related to lack of access to health care, more severe disease, and higher prevalence rates of disease. Zoratti and co-workers[45] illustrated the disparity in health care delivery by examining management of asthma in patients enrolled in a Michigan Health Maintenance Organization. The study involved 464 blacks and 1609 whites with asthma between the ages of 15 and 45 who had similar financial resources. Compared with whites, blacks had fewer visits to asthma specialists, fewer inhaled corticosteroids and more oral steroids prescribed, more visits to the emergency room, and more hospitalizations. Black patients were equally likely to have been seen by a primary care physician for asthma. The presence of this health care provision disparity contributes to the staggering difference in outcomes.

A confounding factor that may be contributing to asthma deaths is the misdiagnosis or lack of recognition of a severe asthma attack with lack of early intervention and poor outcome. Near-fatal asthma is the best predictor of future asthma-related deaths. Patients with near-fatal episodes of asthma may not perceive the severity of their disease. Additionally, several studies have shown that physicians underestimate the severity of the symptoms, thereby leading to poor outcomes for patients.[46,47]

Worldwide Mortality Statistics

There is no collective source of data on worldwide asthma death rates; however, international death rates have been decreasing. In the 1980s death rates were high in Australia and New Zealand. The increased death rate in New Zealand was attributed to overuse of the beta-agonist fenoterol. The asthma death rate was 5.8 per 100,000 in 1989 and decreased to 3 per 100,000 by 1996. There has been a significant amount of debate in the literature regarding the validity of this conclusion. A study performed in 1999 by Abramson and co-workers[48] addressed the role of β-agonists in asthma mortality. The study included 322 patients presenting to the hospital with asthma and 89 asthma-related deaths. The subjects who died were less likely to be using corticosteroids and had higher salbutamol blood levels. However, this increased death rate may be confounded by the severity of the patients' asthma. The higher β-agonist levels likely indicate poorer asthma control with increased rescue inhaler usage likely caused by underlying psychosocial stressors. The study further reinforced the importance of asthma action plans, increased use of corticosteroids, and less reliance on β-agonists as a means to improve outcome.

SUMMARY

Asthma is a disease characterized by bronchial hyperresponsiveness and ongoing airway inflammation and remodeling. Asthma prevalence has been steadily increasing over the past 2 decades. Recently, there has been a plateau in asthma prevalence rates in the United States. Asthma is a difficult disease to study epidemiologically secondary to the heterogeneity of the disease and the lack of a uniform means of diagnosis, especially with worldwide comparisons. The lack of a standardized definition and diagnostic tool makes it difficult to accumulate uniform epidemiologic data that can be used to determine the risk factors.

The asthma mortality rate has recently decreased, which may be related to overall decrease in prevalence and advances in diagnosis and pharmacologic management. The ethnic differences in mortality rates are staggering. Non-Hispanic black persons have the highest mortality rates, which are 200% higher than in non-Hispanic whites. Black men between the ages of 25 and 35 are at the greatest risk of dying from asthma. Studies have shown that lack of access to care, tobacco use, environmental exposures particularly in inner-city areas, poor asthma control, and genetic influences likely contribute to this disparity.

Physicians have a large role to play in decreasing the mortality rates associated with asthma. Physicians continue to underprescribe inhaled corticosteroids despite the preponderance of evidence from clinical trials showing significant mortality benefits. Many patients are undereducated about their disease and do not know how to follow an asthma action plan or use a peak flow meter. Physicians can take an active role in educating their patients, prescribing appropriately inhaled corticosteroids, and providing an asthma action plan.

REFERENCES

1. Tang E, Wiesch D, Samet J: Epidemiology of asthma and allergic disease. In Adkinson Jr NF, Yunginger JW, Busse WW, (eds): Middleton's Allergy: Principles and Practice, 6th ed. Philadelphia, Mosby, 2003, pp 1127–1144.
2. Strachan DP: Hay fever, hygiene, and household size. BMJ 1989;299:1259–1260.
3. Centers for Disease Control and Prevention: Measuring childhood asthma prevalence before and after the 1997 redesign of the National Health Interview Survey—United States. MMWR Morb Mortal Wkly Rep 2000;49:908–911.
4. Centers for Disease Control and Prevention: Surveillance for asthma—United States, 1980–1999. MMWR Surveill Summ 2002;51:1–13.
5. Akinbami L, Schoendorf K, Parker J: US childhood asthma prevalence estimates: the impact of the 1997 National Health Interview Survey redesign. Am J Epidemiol 2003;158:99–104.
6. Akinbami L, Schoendorf K: Trends in childhood asthma: prevalence, health care utilization, and mortality. Pediatrics 2002;110(2 pt 1):315–322.
7. Centers for Disease Control and Prevention: Asthma prevalence. Health care use and mortality, 2002. Available at www. cdc.gov/nchs/data/asthmahealthestat1.pdf. Accessed July 19, 2005.
8. Smith LA, Hatcher-Ross, Wertheimer R, et al: Rethinking race/ethnicity, income, and childhood asthma: racial/ethnic disparities concentrated among the very poor. Public Health Rep 2005;120(2):109–116.
9. Simon PA, Zeng Z, Wold CM, et al: Prevalence of childhood asthma and associated morbidity in Los Angeles County: impacts of race/ethnicity and income. J Asthma 2003;40:535–543.
10. Nicholas SW, Ortiz B, Hutchinson V, et al: Addressing the childhood asthma crisis in Harlem: the Harlem Children's Zone Asthma Initiative. Am J Public Health 2005;95:245–249.
11. Weitzman M, Gortmaker S, Walker DK, et al: Maternal smoking and childhood asthma. Pediatrics 1990;85:505–511.
12. Strachan DP, Cook DG: Parental smoking and childhood asthma: longitudinal and case control studies. Thorax 1998;53:204–212.
13. Eisner M, Yelin EH, Henke J, et al: Environmental tobacco smoke and adult asthma: the impact of changing exposure status on health outcomes. Am J Respir Crit Care Med 1998;158:170–175.
14. Arif AA, Delclos ES, Lee ES, et al: Prevalence and risk factors of asthma and wheezing among US adults: an analysis of the NHANES III data. Eur Respir J 2003;21:827–883.
15. Harris JR, Mangus P, Samuelsen SO, et al: No evidence for effects of family environment on asthma. Am J Respir Crit Care Med 1997;156:43–49.
16. Lazarus SC, Boushey HA, Fahy JV, et al: Long acting beta-2 agonist monotherapy vs continued therapy with inhaled corticosteroids in patients with persistent asthma: a randomized controlled trial. JAMA 2001;285:2583–2593.
17. Larj MJ, Bleecker ER: Effects of beta2-agonists on airway tone and bronchial responsiveness. J Allergy Clin Immunol 2002;110 (6 Suppl):S304–S312.
18. Howard TD, Postma DS, Jongepier H, et al: Association of a disintegrin and metalloprotease 33 (ADAM33) gene with asthma in ethnically diverse populations. J Allergy Clin Immunol 2003;112:717–722.
19. GlaxoSmithKline: Salmeterol Multi-Center Asthma Research Trial (SMART Trial). SLGA 5011: a double-blind, randomized, placebo-controlled surveillance study of asthma event outcomes in subjects receiving either usual pharmacotherapy of asthma or usual pharmacotherapy plus salmeterol 42mcg twice daily. Available at ctr.gsk.co.uk/summary/salmeterol/ studylist.asp. Accessed July 22, 2005.
20. Rackemann FM, Edwards MC: Asthma in children. N Engl J Med 1952;246:858–863.
21. Gore C, Custovic A: Can we prevent allergy? Allergy 2004;59:151–161.
22. McDonnell WF, Abbey DE, Nishino N, et al: Long-term ambient ozone concentration and the incidence of asthma in non-smoking adults: the AHSMOG study. Environ Res 1999;80(2 pt 1):110–121.
23. Strachan DP, Butland BK, Anderson HR: Incidence and prognosis of asthma and wheezing illness from early childhood to age 33 in a national British cohort. BMJ 1996;312:1195–1199.

24. King ME, Mannino DM, Holguin F: Risk factors for asthma incidence. Panminerva Med 2004;46:97–111.

25. Kraft M: The role of bacterial infections in asthma. Clin Chest Med 2000;21:301–313.

26. McDonald DM, Schoeb TR, Lindsey JR: *Mycoplasma pulmonis* infections cause long-lasting potentiation of neurogenic inflammation in the respiratory tract of the rat. J Clin Invest 1991;87:787–799.

27. Martin RJ, Kraft M, Chu HW, et al: A link between chronic asthma and chronic infection. J Allergy Clin Immunol 2001;107:595–601.

28. ISAAC Steering Committee: Worldwide variations in the prevalence of asthma symptoms: the International Study of Asthma and Allergies in Childhood (ISAAC). Eur Respir J 1998;12:315–335.

29. European Community Respiratory Health Survey (ECRHS): Variations in the prevalence of respiratory symptoms, self reported asthma attacks, and use of asthma medication in the European Community Respiratory Health Survey. Eur Respir J 1996;9:687–695.

30. Worldwide variation in prevalence of symptoms of asthma, allergic rhinoconjunctivitis and atopic eczema: ISAAC. The International Study of Asthma and Allergies in Childhood (ISAAC) Steering Committee. Lancet 1998;351:1225–1232.

31. Basagana X, Sunyer J, Kogevinas M, et al: Socioeconomic status and asthma prevalence in young adults. Am J Epidemiol 2004;160:178–188.

32. Centers for Disease Control and Prevention: National Center for Health Statistics, 2002. Available at www.cdc.gov/mmwr/preview/mmwrhtml/ss5101a1.htm. Accessed July 19, 2005.

33. Evans R III, Mullally DI, Wilson RW, et al: National trends in the morbidity and mortality of asthma in the US. Chest 1987;91:65S–73S.

34. US Department of Health and Human Services: Respiratory diseases (goal 24). In Healthy People 2010 (conference edition, volume 2). Washington, DC, US Department of Health and Human Services, 2000, pp 1–27.

35. Strunk RC, Ford JG, Taggart V: Reducing disparities in asthma care: priorities for research—National Heart, Lung, and Blood Institute workshop report. J Allergy Clin Immunol 2002;109:229–237.

36. Beasley R: The burden of asthma with specific reference to the United States. J Allergy Clin Immunol 2002;109:S482–S489.

37. Laforest L, Yin D, Kocevar VS, et al: Association between asthma control in children and loss of workdays by caregivers. Ann Allergy Asthma Immunol 2004;93:265–271.

38. Sullivan S, Elixhauser A, Buist AS, et al: National Asthma Education and Prevention Program working group report on the cost effectiveness of asthma care. Am J Respir Crit Care Med 1996;154:S84–S95.

39. Weiss KB, Sullivan SD, Lyttle CS: Trends in the cost of illness for asthma in the United States, 1985–1994. J Allergy Clin Immunol 2000;106:493–499.

40. Herjavecz I, Nagy GB, Gyurkovits K, et al: Cost, morbidity, and cost of asthma in Hungary: The Hunair Study. J Asthma 2003;40:673–681.

41. Sly RM: Continuing decreases in asthma mortality in the United States. Ann Allergy Asthma Immunol 2004;92:313–318.

42. Grant EN, Lyttle CS, Weiss KB: The relation of socioeconomic factors and racial/ethnic differences in US asthma mortality. Am J Public Health 2000;90(12):1923–1925.

43. Weiss KB, Wagener DK: Changing patterns of asthma mortality: identifying target populations at high risk. JAMA 1990;264(13):1683–1687.

44. Lang DM, Polansky M: Patterns of asthma mortality in Philadelphia from 1969 to 1991. N Engl J Med 1994;331(23):1542–1546.

45. Zoratti EM, Havstad S, Rodriguez J, et al: Health service use by African Americans and Caucasians with asthma in a managed care setting. Am J Respir Crit Care Med 1998;158(2):371–377.

46. McFadden ER, Warren EL: Observations on asthma mortality. Ann Intern Med 1997;127:142–147.

47. American College of Physicians: Inner city health care. Ann Intern Med 1997;126:48–90.

48. Abramson MJ, Bailey MJ, Couper FJ, et al: Are asthma medications and management related to deaths from asthma? Am J Respir Crit Care Med 2001;163:12–18.

Development of Asthma in Early Life

John O. Warner

- Airway inflammation and airway remodeling are under separate genetic and environmental influences
- Environmental factors influence the risk of allergic sensitization and the phenotypic manifestations of genetic polymorphisms
- Protection of the fetus against maternal TH1 immune responses is in part orchestrated by TH2 cytokines generated at the feto-maternal interface
- The newborn infant has a TH2-polarized immune response that is down-regulated by exposure to microbial factors postnatally
- Wheezing infants who also have developed allergic sensitization will have the most persistent form of asthma

Asthma may be defined as a chronic disorder of conducting airways associated with both inflammation and structural changes in the airway wall. As a consequence there is variable airflow limitation that is manifest by recurrent cough and wheeze. Interaction between genotype and environment contributes both to the changes in airway wall structure and independently to the induction of inflammation. However, all asthma guidelines emphasize the importance of treating the underlying inflammation as well as just relieving the symptoms of asthma. It has been assumed that by suppressing the inflammation, structural changes to the airway wall will be improved as well and perhaps if the treatment is introduced early enough, also prevented. However, there is no evidence that any form of pharmacotherapy modifies the natural history of the disease or ever effects a cure. With the possible exception of immunotherapy, no treatment has been shown to modify the natural course of the disease and certainly no cure has been identified. Indeed, beyond the use of inhaled corticosteroids (ICS) and beta$_2$-adrenoceptor agonists, which were introduced 30 to 40 years ago, there has been very little change to the therapeutic algorithm other than so called "add-on therapy" with leukotriene-receptor antagonists and long-acting beta-agonists.

Most asthma has its origins in early life and the best predictors of continuation into adulthood are an early age of onset, sensitization to house-dust mite and/or *Alternaria* mold in environments where these are the major allergens, reduced lung function, and increased bronchial hyperresponsiveness (BHR) in early life.[1] Even employment of ICS at a very early stage in the disease evolution does not appear to influence outcome. While it is clear that ICSs given to preschool children

reduce symptoms and exacerbations, they also slow growth and have no carryover effect after the treatment is stopped. Compared with placebo, there are no significant differences in symptoms, lung function, or BHR once ICSs are stopped after 2 years of treatment.[2] Thus it becomes imperative to understand the early life origins of the disease to identify targets for prevention and/or early intervention.

EPIDEMIOLOGY OF ALLERGY AND ASTHMA

There has been a progressively increasing prevalence rate for asthma and all related allergic diseases over the past 30 to 40 years[3] (Fig. 2-1). These changes cannot be attributable to any genetic differences. It is far more likely to have been a result of a shift in environmental influences acting on a pre-existing genetic susceptibility. Most studies have focused on the genetic and environmental influences that affect allergic sensitization. Much less attention has been focused on airway wall structure. It has now become clear that concentrating on the cellular and mediator pathways producing an allergic inflammatory response falls short of explaining the origins of the disease. There are independent genetic and environmental factors affecting airway wall structure. Thus it has, for instance, been shown that increased BHR at 4 weeks of age is predictive of asthma at 6 years of age independent of allergic sensitization.[4] This chapter will, therefore, present the development of asthma in relation to the early life origins of allergy and its influence of airway inflammation and separately in relation to the evolution of changes to airway wall structure.

ALLERGY AND ASTHMA

Allergy has long been viewed as one of the major risk factors for the development of asthma. Once the disease has manifested, allergy predicts its persistence from childhood through adolescence and into adulthood. Successive studies have demonstrated that both the prevalence and severity of asthma and the related allergic disorders rhinitis and eczema have increased in many countries. However, it is important to note that very recent studies are suggesting that the increase may be coming to an end at least in some developed countries.[5] So far this is exclusively in relation to asthma and not to the other allergic conditions such as eczema and rhinitis, which continue to increase in all environments. The International Study of Asthma and Allergies in Children (ISAAC) highlighted enormous differences in prevalence rates of the allergic conditions with the highest being in Australia, New Zealand, United Kingdom, United States, and Canada. There are progressively diminishing prevalence rates through southern Europe and eastward through India and China. While ethnic

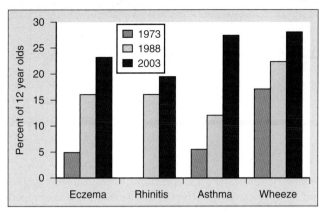

Figure 2-1   Prevalence of atopic diseases in 12-year-olds in South Wales. Three consecutive prevalence of allergic diseases studies in 12-year-olds in the same stable population in South Wales using identical ascertainment. The considerable and parallel increases in all allergic conditions over the past 3 decades are shown. The only redeeming feature, from a medical perspective, is that as of 2003, virtually all individuals who wheeze are now labeled as asthmatic. *(Data from Burr ML, et al: Thorax 2006;61:296–299.)*

and therefore genetic differences might account for some of the variation, even within countries among the same ethnic groups there are considerable differences dependent on environment and particularly the degree of affluence of the community. Asthma and allergies may be viewed worldwide as a disease of the affluent despite that when the disease occurs, it is often more severe and potentially life threatening among those in more deprived circumstances.

The presence of sensitization to common environmental allergens is commonly associated with the presence of asthma. Epidemiological evidence would suggest that about 50% of asthma may be attributable to allergy. There is a strong association between the presence of allergy as demonstrated either by raised total immunoglobulin E (IgE) or specific IgE antibodies or positive skin prick tests and asthma. Up to 85% of children with asthma have allergies as compared with only 25% to 30% of the whole population. Furthermore, most children who become sensitized to aeroallergens during the first years of life will develop asthma, whereas those children who become sensitized beyond 8 to 10 years of age have no greater risk of developing asthma than children who have no allergy whatsoever.

Exposure to allergens is a risk factor for the development of allergic sensitization to those allergens and exposure to allergens in sensitized individuals is a risk factor for exacerbations of asthma, particularly if combined with additional exposure to viruses. There is a significant association between increasing degrees of allergy as represented either by total IgE levels or skin prick test weal sizes and severity of asthma.

The one consistent factor that predicts ongoing disease in infants who wheeze is the presence of allergy. Allergen avoidance studies in established asthma have shown that it is possible to achieve improvements in control of symptoms with associated reductions in BHR and the need for concomitant asthma therapy. Furthermore, the use of anti-IgE therapy has been shown to have appreciable beneficial effects in the management, particularly of more severe disease. However, against this background, it is clear that many allergic individuals do not have asthma. Therefore, there are additional components

to the disease process, other than those that result in allergy, contributing considerably to the development, persistence, and severity of disease.[6]

THE IMMUNOLOGY OF ALLERGY

The underlying immunological paradigm associated with allergy is the expression of a subtype of T-helper lymphocytes labeled TH2, which respond to common allergens by generating a cytokine profile including interleukin 4 (IL4), IL5, IL9, and IL13 as opposed to a TH1 profile generating IL2 and interferon γ, which is more associated with the normal response to infection and with autoimmune disease. The cytokines IL4 and IL13 promote the production of IgE, and IL5, among other cytokines, activates eosinophils. There is a mutual exclusivity between TH1 and TH2 activity with IL4 suppressing TH1 responses and interferon γ suppressing TH2 responses. However, the paradigm has now extended because it is clear that autoimmune disease can coexist more frequently than by chance with allergic disease. Both TH1 and TH2 activity are regulated by the nature of the antigen, the site of exposure (airway, skin, gut, and so forth) and a range of costimulatory signals and cytokines transmitted from antigen-presenting cells (APCs) to T lymphocytes. An additional group of T lymphocytes with regulatory function downregulates TH1 and TH2 responses both through the generation of the cytokines IL10 and transforming growth factor β (TGFβ) and by cell/cell contact. Thus, dysregulation may well explain the demographic trends with increasing prevalence rates for both allergy and autoimmune disease (Fig. 2-2).

THE ONTOGENY OF ALLERGIC IMMUNE RESPONSES

Fetal development occurs in an environment biased toward the TH2 and T-regulatory cell immune responses. Both in murine and human pregnancies, a maternal TH1 response to fetopaternal antigens is associated with recurrent early miscarriage or intrauterine growth retardation. That this does not occur is a consequence of regulation of the maternal immune response to fetopaternal antigens by the generation of IL4, IL13, IL10, and TGFβ at the maternofetal interface. It is rare to find any TH1 cytokines at this location. Inevitably the cytokines that regulate the maternal immune response during pregnancy will have some impact on the developing fetal immune system.

It has been commonly considered that the newborn infant is immunologically naïve. However, it is obvious that the fetus is capable of mounting a significant immune response and pediatricians will be familiar with the demonstration of immunoglobulin M (IgM) antibodies in relation to maternal infection during pregnancy with rubella, cytomegalovirus (CMV), and toxoplasma, as well as similar responses after maternal immunizations. Studies in fetal baboons immunized with recombinant hepatitis B surface antigen have shown that they are capable of mounting an IgG antibody response where none has occurred in the mother and that this leads to enhanced postnatal responsiveness to repeat immunization.

There are APCs and T and B lymphocytes detectable from 14 weeks' gestation in rudimentary lymphoid follicles in the small bowel. Surface markers on these cells suggest that

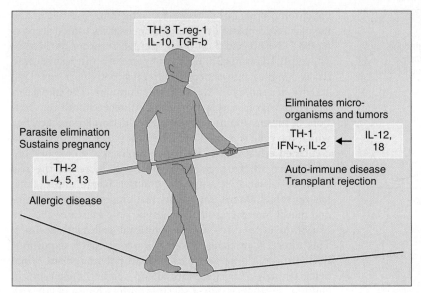

Figure 2-2 The extended TH1-TH2 paradigm.
Representation of the balance of T-helper (TH) lymphocyte responses with their cytokine profiles in various situations. TH-1 responses with the generation of interferon (IFN)-γ and interleukin (IL)-2 initiated by IL-12 and 18 among many other cytokines from antigen presenting cells are associated with a normal response to infection but also autoimmune disease. TH2 cytokines, IL-4, 5, and 13, are normally released during parasite infestation but also orchestrate an allergic response. These latter factors also protect the pregnancy against a maternal TH1-mediated rejection of feto paternal antigens (equivalent to that of transplant rejection). Exerting a regulatory effect on both TH1 and TH2 activity are another group of lymphocytes designated as TH3 and T-regulatory cells, which generate IL-10 and transforming growth factor (TGF)-β.

antigen presentation has occurred with appropriate costimulatory signaling to promote a sensitizing immune response in T lymphocytes. Furthermore, allergen is detectable in amniotic fluid at about 10% of maternal circulating levels. Similarly, IgE can also be detected in amniotic fluid again at 10% of maternal levels and will thus be higher in mothers who either have parasitic infestation or allergy. Dendritic cells in the fetal gut express both the high- and low-affinity IgE receptors. It can be hypothesized that a phenomenon known as IgE antigen focusing will facilitate sensitization to extremely low concentrations of allergen. Thus, swallowed maternal IgE will fix to high- and low-affinity IgE receptors on fetal dendritic cells in the small bowel and facilitate the pickup of allergens by dendritic cells allowing them to respond to a 100- to 1000-fold lower concentration than would be the case in the absence of IgE. That this phenomenon occurs has perhaps most compellingly been shown in a recent study using proteomic techniques to detect low levels of IgE antibody to specific cow's milk proteins and demonstrating a strong association between the presence of such IgE antibodies in the mother during pregnancy and the cord blood of the resulting infant. As IgE does not cross the placenta into the fetal circulation, it must have been generated by the fetus.[7]

By 16 weeks' gestation, circulating B lymphocytes can be detected with surface IgM. It is, therefore, not surprising that circulating blood mononuclear cells are capable of mounting a specific proliferative response to allergens such as ovalbumin from hen's egg and even the major house-dust mite allergen from as early as 22 weeks' gestation. By full term, the overwhelming majority of newborns are able to mount specific responses to common environmental factors. It has even been shown that a high proliferative response to an allergen at birth is associated with a higher probability of allergic disease later in childhood. Clearly in the presence of TH2-promoting cytokines, it is likely that this neonatal response will be TH2 biased. Indeed this has been well demonstrated, in that stimulated cord blood mononuclear cells have a dominant production of TH2 rather than TH1 cytokines.

This sophisticated system for sensitizing the fetus with a TH2-biased response may not just be a bystander effect of protecting the pregnancy against maternal TH1 responses. It might also have an evolutionary relevant role in protecting the newborn infant against parasitosis. Clearly this mechanism will facilitate the fetal response to maternal helminth infection. Infants born to helminth-infected mothers have a specific TH2-biased immune response to maternal helminth antigens and detectable IgE antibodies to these antigens at birth. Furthermore, although the newborn baby has an obligate exposure to its mother's parasites, it is exceedingly rare for the infant to become infected by these parasites, implying a mature immune response preventing such infection. It is possible that certain properties of allergens have counterparts to parasite antigens leading to stimulation of the same immune response in the parasite-free environment.[8]

While the likely route of primary sensitization to allergen in pregnancy is via the fetal gut, predominantly during the second trimester of pregnancy, there is also exposure to allergen directly from maternal to fetal circulation. This is a consequence of active transport of IgG antibody across the placenta complexed with antigens and allergens, predominantly during the third trimester. Studies suggest that the higher the IgG antibody to an allergen, the less likelihood of subsequent allergic sensitization to those allergens. Variation in timing and concentration of exposure during pregnancy will have subtly different influences on outcomes. Thus, there is one study of birch and timothy grass pollen exposure in pregnancy suggesting that the fetus only mounts a sensitizing cellular response if the pollen season occurs during the first 6 months of pregnancy while exposure in the last 3 months results in tolerance. Concentration of exposure will affect the maternal IgG antibody levels and therefore it follows that high-dose exposure might have a tolerizing effect by generation of high levels of IgG allergen-specific antibody and allergen complexes. One study of the children of mothers who had undergone rye grass allergen immunotherapy during pregnancy and consequently had high IgG antibody levels compared with children born to rye grass–allergic mothers who did not receive immunotherapy showed fewer positive skin tests to rye grass 3 to 12 years later. Newborn babies with high levels of IgG antibody to cat and/or pollens

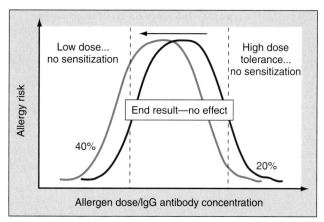

Figure 2-3 The effect of allergen avoidance. A hypothetical representation of the effect of an increasing dose of allergen exposure on the risks of allergic sensitization. Very low doses are not sufficient to trigger a response, whereas very large doses induce tolerance, similar to that achieved by immunotherapy, perhaps through the generation of IgG antibodies. Introducing attempts at allergen avoidance usually result in reduced exposure and thus in a whole population there will be no overall reduction in allergy risk, although some individuals may benefit while others suffer, dependent on the level of exposure before introduction of attempts at avoidance.

have been shown to have a lower probability of generating IgE antibodies to those allergens up to 8 years later. Similarly a study of egg exposure during pregnancy has shown that both very high and very low dose exposure is associated with less allergy in the offspring than in those where the mother had a moderate to low exposure. These observations might explain the remarkable effect of cat and dog ownership during pregnancy and postnatally being associated with less sensitization to these allergens subsequently.

The above studies imply that attempts to reduce allergen exposure in pregnancy might have an adverse rather than favorable effect. Two recent publications suggested that this may be the case. While at 1 year of age house-dust mite avoidance has been shown to be associated with somewhat less wheezing by 3 years of age, there was an increased rate of sensitization to house-dust mite. Most studies have failed to demonstrate any consistent effect of house-dust mite avoidance in preventing sensitization or asthma and low-level exposure to house-dust mite has been associated with a greater risk of IgE sensitization and asthma than higher levels. Thus there is currently no justification for making any recommendations about environmental modification during pregnancy to prevent the onset of allergic disease[9] (Fig. 2-3).

GENETIC POLYMORPHISMS AND ALLERGY

Asthma and associated allergic diseases are highly hereditable. Genetic polymorphisms have been demonstrated, on virtually every chromosome, to be associated with an increased risk of asthma and allergy. Many have highly credible mechanistic explanations. Thus there is a significant focus on the cytokine gene cluster on the long arm of chromosome 5 (5q31–33). This chromosome region contains the genes for many TH2 cytokines and also the gene for the endotoxin receptor CD14. Polymorphisms in this chromosome region are more strongly associated with allergy than asthma. Other associations have been with the common subunit of the IL4 and IL13 receptor

on chromosome 6p12, those for interferon γ on 12q, the major histocompatibility complex molecules, tumor necrosis factor (TNF) α and β on 6p21, the IgE receptor on 11q12–13, and IL18 on 11q22. IL18 is of particular interest because it has complex interactions in affecting both TH1 and TH2 activity depending on the antigenic stimulus. The impact of any genetic polymorphism will be influenced both by variations in the environment and the stage in development during which the gene is expressed. Thus it has been shown that the combined effect of a TNFα polymorphism and environmental tobacco smoke exposure significantly increases the risk of school absence in asthmatic children where either alone has no effect. More important, the presence of a glutathione methyl transferase null genotype only increases the risk of asthma in the presence of significant pollutant exposure. This effect is particularly relevant to antenatal exposures. Furthermore, the presence of an IL13 polymorphism, while being strongly associated with allergy-related phenotypes in children, in adults is only associated with asthma and not with raised IgE. Toll-like receptor 4 polymorphisms are associated with increasing allergy severity, based on a cumulative skin prick test positivity score but are not associated with asthma severity or lung function abnormality in asthmatic individuals. Toll-like receptor 2 polymorphisms have a negative impact on the beneficial effect of being conceived, born, and bred on a farm compared with any other environment.[10]

FETAL GROWTH AND NUTRITION

It is clear that fetal nutrient delivery and its effect on fetal growth will have a significant impact on the ontogeny of immune responses. There have been some odd associations between large head circumference at birth and levels of total IgE at birth, in childhood, and even adulthood. Furthermore, there is an association between large head circumference at birth and asthma requiring medical attention. It is possible that good nutrient delivery to the fetus in early pregnancy programs for a rapid growth trajectory. This means that the fetus has a continuing high nutrient demand. If this is not met in the latter stages of pregnancy, there will be continued head growth at the expense of relatively poorer nutrition to the body with consequent effects on rapidly dividing tissues such as those in the immune system. This raises the question whether there are any pivotal nutrients that might be important in this process.

Reduced intake of fresh fruit and vegetables is associated with a higher rate of allergic sensitization comparing different populations in Europe. Low cord blood selenium and iron are associated with higher subsequent risk of persistent wheeze for the former and both wheeze and eczema for the latter. High fish intake during pregnancy is associated with less food allergy in offspring. Two recent studies that focused on fish oil supplementation during pregnancy produced rather variable results but showed some effects both on cord blood mononuclear cell responses to allergen and on some atopic manifestations; however, the overall effect was small. Other studies have shown that there are even variations in the polyunsaturated fatty acid constituents of colostrum and mature human milk in allergic rather than nonallergic mothers and these variations in turn have an impact on allergy risk in the infant.[11]

One other component of the diet that has been suggested as possibly having an impact on allergy risk is vitamin D. This has immunoregulatory properties with actions via a vitamin D receptor that is present on monocytes and activated T and B lymphocytes. Vitamin D inhibits in vitro T-cell proliferation and TH1 cytokine production and therefore has the potential to allow up-regulation of TH2 activity. It has been hypothesized that the increase in prevalence of allergic diseases runs in parallel with the increase in vitamin D supplementation particularly during pregnancy.[12] Whether or not there is a relationship, however, remains to be established.

Infant feeding practices clearly have been investigated in great detail in relation to allergy outcomes. The proposed beneficial effect of breastfeeding in preventing allergic disease has generated some controversy. A number of studies have suggested significant protective effects, whereas others have either shown no effect or actually increased risks of allergy particularly with duration of breastfeeding beyond 4 months of age. However, these studies are subject to methodological problems not the least of which is the potential for inverse causality in that families with the highest allergy risk are likely to attempt to breastfeed for the longest amount of time, thereby showing a direct relationship between prolonged breastfeeding and allergy. What is more consistent in systematically reviewing the literature is that breastfeeding does reduce the risks of early food allergy and childhood eczema but it is doubtful whether there are any effects that extend beyond the first 2 to 3 years of life.[13] Variations in constituents of human breast milk among lactating mothers may account for lesser protective effects in some circumstances rather than others. This, for instance, may relate to the polyunsaturated fatty acid constituents that, in turn, may be affected by maternal health and nutrition.

In situations where breastfeeding is not possible, it is usually recommended that infants at high risk of developing allergy should be fed with a hydrolyzed milk formula. A recent systematic review suggested that extensively hydrolyzed casein formulae and partially hydrolyzed whey formulae may have some degree of protective effect if breastfeeding is not possible. This appears to be most relevant in relation to the use of extensively hydrolyzed casein formulae in high-risk babies. Whether expensive alternative formulae should be recommended as a whole population intervention to reduce the impact of allergic disease is highly questionable.[14]

The other contentious area in relation to infant feeding practices has been the timing of solid food introduction (Table 2-1). Most guidelines suggest that weaning onto the more allergenic foods, such as milk, egg, wheat, peanut, tree nut, and so forth, should be significantly delayed and that the weaning process should be very slow in high-risk infants. However, the evidence base for this recommendation is highly tenuous and one or two recent studies have suggested that there is no evidence to support delayed introductions of solids beyond 6 months of life in the prevention of eczema or allergic sensitization. Although more studies are required in this area, the concept of high dose tolerance is one that needs to be considered. Mothers of cystic fibrosis children who required treatment with pancreatic extract in the form of a powder often became allergically sensitized to the pancreatic extract with symptoms of rhinitis and asthma while they were mixing the powder into a paste. Despite the fact that children with cystic fibrosis have a high prevalence of allergy, however, no children were ever shown to have allergic problems with the pancreatic extract. They, of course, were being fed this product in large doses, which one might suggest was inducing tolerance. In keeping with this concept is some evidence that high full-cream milk intake at 2 years of age is associated with less asthma at 3 years of age compared with having a low intake. Furthermore, there is a suggestion that the switch from using butter to margarine has increased asthma and allergy rates.

HYGIENE HYPOTHESIS

The hygiene hypothesis was originally proposed following the observation of an inverse relationship between birth order and the subsequent prevalence of rhinoconjunctivitis. It was suggested that older siblings were transmitting infections to young babies whose immune response was therefore switched from its neonatal TH2-biased pattern to one in which a TH1 response predominated. This, therefore, has a very credible mechanistic explanation. Subsequent studies have shown inverse relationships between the prevalence of a wide range of infections and allergy, including typhoid, tuberculosis, measles, and hepatitis. Whether or not this is a pre- or a postnatal effect could be disputed as the sibling effect may also affect cord blood IgE levels. There is, however, also a problem of defining whether the observations relate to inverse causality. It is possible that, for instance, the inverse relationship between tuberculin responsiveness and allergy is because allergic individuals are unable to mount an efficient tuberculin response as a consequence of their immune dysregulation. BCG has not been shown to have a significant effect on subsequent development of allergy in Europe, although there may be some effects observed in developing countries.

There is an inverse relationship between antibiotic use both during pregnancy and in infancy and the prevalence of allergy. Such antibiotic use has a potent influence on gut microflora. Thus, if this is changed in the mother, it will alter the organisms that will colonize the newborn infant's gut. Certainly the composition of gastrointestinal flora has been shown to be different in allergic compared with nonallergic infants.

The above observations led to studies of the use of probiotics in pregnancy and infancy in an attempt to reduce allergic disease. One study showed that in a parallel group, double-blind, placebo-controlled trial of lactobacillus GG administered to mothers during pregnancy and the infant postnatally there was less atopic eczema up to 3 years of age compared with the group receiving placebo. However, there was no difference in the degree of allergic sensitization between the two

Table 2-1
PUTATIVE EFFECTS, BOTH BENEFICIAL AND DELETERIOUS, OF DIET ON THE DEVELOPMENT OF ALLERGIC SENSITIZATION AND DISEASE

Beneficial	Deleterious
Fresh fruit and vegetables	High salt intake
Selenium	Obesity
Vitamins A, C, E	Vitamin D?
Breastfeeding	Unmodified cow's milk formulae
Milk and butter	n-6 polyunsaturated fatty acids
Magnesium	
n-3 polyunsaturated fatty acids	

groups. Clearly much larger studies are required to elaborate on this. It is perhaps naïve to think that administration of a single probiotic organism will change outcomes, as the gut flora is a complex combination of up to 200 different bacteria. The diverse range of colonizing organisms exists in ecological balance and it is impossible to say which is more important in relation to modulation of immune responses. Furthermore, probiotic bacteria do not achieve long-lasting colonization and it may be important to use pre- and probiotics to encourage rather more permanent colonization. As such, children brought up in families that adopt an anthroposophic lifestyle having a diet consisting mainly of fermented vegetables high in probiotics, have a very different gut flora and much lower prevalence of allergic disease.

The lay media is full of concerns about immunization schedules and their impact in adversely affecting the health of infants, including suggestions that immunizations might increase allergy. There is no evidence to support this contention. Indeed, in children with high vaccine coverage, there is transiently a better protection against development of allergy in the first years of life. This is an extremely important public health message.

The hygiene hypothesis has been used to explain the differences in the development of allergy and allergic diseases in children born and raised on farms. It has been suggested that the farming effect is a consequence of exposure to a number of organisms including *Toxoplasma gondii*. Clearly there are higher levels of exposure to aeroallergens as well as to endotoxin. Furthermore, if infants are fed on milk from the farm, which one assumes based on studies from central Europe is nonpasteurized, then there are gut exposures to a wider range of organisms. To what extent these effects are moderated by genotype, such as polymorphisms in the *TLR2* gene, is currently being investigated.

It will be important to establish whether there are any interventions that will negate the effect of excessive hygiene. Factors considered have been the use of TH1 immune stimulators such as *Mycobacterium vaccae* or bacterial DNA CpG-motifs. Murine studies have shown dramatic effects but it remains to be established whether it will be safe to proceed to human studies.

It is important to note that exposure to early infection may be a two-edged sword. Certain viral respiratory tract infections have a positive association with subsequent asthma. Whether this is a consequence of an underlying immunological aberration increasing the risks of infection as well as allergy and asthma remains to be established. Thus, infants infected with respiratory syncytial virus (RSV) are more likely to develop bronchiolitis if they come from atopic families and are themselves atopic. The immune response to RSV in those developing bronchiolitis is TH2 biased compared with infants who have RSV upper respiratory tract infection alone who are more likely to generate interferon γ in response to the infection. Thus, the same immune response that leads to bronchiolitis may also lead to allergy, linking the two conditions. Furthermore, recurrent rhinovirus-associated wheeze in infancy is a strong predictor of subsequent asthma. It has now been established that asthmatic airway epithelial cells have an innate inability to generate interferon β in response to rhinovirus infection. This in turn results in an impairment of cell apoptosis and, therefore, failed clearance of the virus.

Whether or not this defect antedates the onset of asthma remains to be established. It might explain the association between susceptibility to early recurrent rhinovirus infection, wheezing, and subsequent asthma.

While the concept of the hygiene hypothesis has had a considerable beneficial influence on epidemiological and immunological investigation into the origins of allergy over the past 15 years, the term has perhaps outlived its usefulness. Sadly by focusing public attention on the potential allergy-promoting effects of cleanliness and avoidance of infection it has had the potential to adversely affect rates of acute infection. It has therefore been suggested that we now remove the focus on hygiene and consider how to capitalize on the components of microbes that reduce allergy risk.[15]

The mechanisms by which microbial factors provide a TH1 stimulation is through pattern recognition molecules. CD14 is one such molecule, which specifically recognizes endotoxin (lipopolysaccharide). Studies have identified a polymorphism in the promoter region of the *CD14* gene, which manifests as diminished levels of the soluble component of this molecule and is associated with increased intensity of allergy expression in many but not all populations. CD14 is poorly expressed by fetuses and neonates but is present in a soluble form in amniotic fluid and at high levels in human breast milk. A reduced supply of this molecule from the mother, either in amniotic fluid or breast milk, is associated with a higher probability of early-onset atopic eczema. Another pattern recognition molecule, TLR4, is also important in binding endotoxin when complexed with CD14 to initiate a cytoplasmic signal leading to IL12 production, which in turn promotes IFNγ generation. A study in Swedish schoolchildren has shown a polymorphism of *TLR4* gene to be associated with a higher prevalence of asthma. To what extent these polymorphisms can be overcome by relevant microbial exposure remains to be established. There has been an association between levels of soluble CD14 in breast milk and n-3 polyunsaturated fatty acid levels. Thus, supplementation of the maternal diet could conceivably raise levels, which might explain the effect of a high fish oil intake in reducing some allergic manifestations.[11]

AIRWAY REMODELING AND THE DEVELOPMENT OF ASTHMA

BHR is the one noninvasive measure that has been associated with the pathological changes of remodeling. Increased BHR at 4 weeks of age is associated with asthma at 6 years of age independent of atopy. Furthermore, reduced airway function at 4 weeks is also associated with persistent wheeze at 11 years and this is independent of both atopy and increased BHR. Increased specific airway resistance and allergic sensitization at 3 years of age in children who had wheeze before 3 years were independent predictors of persistent wheeze at 5 years. One potential interpretation of these observations is that the remodeling process occurs long before the onset of disease or any evidence of allergic inflammation. It is even possible that the changes had occurred antenatally. TGFβ is a key factor involved in the regulation of lung airway branching morphogenesis in the first trimester of pregnancy. There is a variable spatial expression of isoforms of TGFβ during lung development. TGFβ1 colocalizes to the branch clefts with collagen 1 and 3 and fibronectin. TGFβ2 and 3 are expressed in epithelial cells at the tips of the growing lung buds, which has led to the proposal that the remodeled asthmatic airway is the result of reactivation of fetal airway modeling processes. The other possibility is that the modeling process in utero has already been adversely affected by the intrauterine environment interacting with genetic factors. Indeed, the whole concept of the immunopathology of asthma could be turned on its head in that rather than eosinophilic inflammation inducing remodeling, it is possible that the remodeled or improperly modeled fetal airway increases the risks of persistent inflammation. Thus it has been shown that inflammatory cells will behave very differently depending on the nature of the collagen matrix.[11]

While anti-IL4 and -IL5 clearly reduce allergic airway inflammation, there are rather disappointing effects on asthma and BHR. It is likely that these modalities of treatment will not have any significant effect on the remodeled airway. This may also explain why the very early use of inhaled steroids in preschool children with wheezing does not have any carryover effects once the treatment is stopped.

GENETIC POLYMORPHISMS AND AIRWAY REMODELING

Polymorphisms in the beta$_2$ adrenoceptor gene were the first to be associated with variations in structure and function of the airway rather than with inflammation. Thus polymorphisms have been associated with susceptibility to subsensitization when short-acting beta-agonists are used continuously with consequent increases in BHR and disease severity. Interestingly, this gene is also located in the same region as the cytokine gene cluster on the long arm of chromosome 5. Since then a number of other novel genes associated with airway epithelium and fibroblasts rather than inflammatory cells have been identified.

A disintegrin and metalloprotease 33 (ADAM33) has been identified as a major candidate gene for asthma and BHR on chromosome 20p13. The strength of associations of the polymorphisms in this gene is highest when BHR is included in the definition of asthma and weakest if allergy is incorporated into the phenotype. Expression of the gene product is restricted to mesenchymal cells such as fibroblasts and smooth muscle. It is not expressed in any inflammatory cells. Thus it is likely that disturbance of function will influence smooth muscle hypertrophy and other components of the airway remodeling process, thereby affecting BHR. Indeed the mouse equivalent of the polymorphisms in this gene has been linked with BHR. This gene is also preferentially expressed during branching morphogenesis in lung development and thereby provides the linking concept of airway remodeling as perhaps a reactivation of the process of airway modeling during embryonic life. It is also possible to hypothesize that polymorphisms in the gene will result in abnormal airway modeling and thereby initiate changes in airway structure and perhaps function at an early stage antenatally. It remains to be seen whether this is indeed the case. However, polymorphisms in the gene have been associated with reduced lung function in children aged both 3 and 5. It has also been associated with a more accelerated decline in lung function in asthmatic adults. As the name of the gene product suggests, it

has a number of functions. It has proteolytic activity and can release a range of pro-inflammatory mediators from anchor sites. It also has functions in relation to binding of cell surface proteins and, therefore, will affect cell adhesion and signaling events. It may well also have a role in myogenesis thereby contributing to smooth muscle hypertrophy. However, much has yet to be achieved in identifying the impact of polymorphisms on the function of the gene product and the way in which environmental factors might interact with it.

Other genes selectively expressed in epithelial cells include those coding for proteins designated ESE-2 and ESE-3 on the short arm of chromosome 11, polymorphisms of which have been linked to BHR and asthma. ESE-3 may be involved in epithelial cell differentiation toward a mucus-secreting phenotype and is also up-regulated in fibroblasts and smooth muscle when they are exposed to pro-inflammatory cytokines.

SPINK-5, a gene encoding a serine protease inhibitor Kazal type 5, has been associated with a condition known as Netherton syndrome, which in part is characterized by eczema. Polymorphisms in the gene have been associated with asthma and eczema. The gene product is expressed in epithelial cells and protects against the effect of proteases such as those generated by mast cells and some that are present directly in allergen such as those in house-dust mite. Thus, polymorphisms might be expected to render the airway epithelium more susceptible to proteolysis and therefore shedding of the cells, which is a feature of a pathology of asthma. In eczema rather than affecting allergic susceptibility it may affect skin barrier functions.

Glutathione is an important antioxidant particularly in intracellular oxidant defenses. A number of genes coding for glutathione S-transferases (GSTs) are components of defense pathways. There have been some intriguing associations between variations in the genes and susceptibility to airway disease. There is a common null allele of GST-M1 and polymorphisms of GST-P1 associated with decreased lung function and increased susceptibility to environmental pollutants. The combination of GST-M1 null allele and exposure to environmental pollution significantly increases the risks of asthma. One study has suggested that it might be possible to increase antioxidant activity by supplementing the diet with vitamin C and vitamin E, bypassing the defect of an absent GST-M1 protein. Even more intriguingly this null genotype increases the likelihood that pregnancy smoking increases the prevalence of asthma in the offspring. There is even a suggestion that a polymorphism of the GST-P1 gene present in mothers results in reduced lung function in the infant irrespective of whether the infant has the same genotype. How this interacts with the environment of the mother requires further investigation.[16]

ENVIRONMENT AND AIRWAY STRUCTURE

Maternal pregnancy smoking has diverse effects on fetal health including lung growth and development. There are significant differences in lung function in newborn and 4-week-old infants born to smoking mothers compared with nonsmoking mothers. This in turn is associated with a significantly higher risk of wheezing illnesses in the first year of life. As interactions have been shown with GST-M1 null genotype, it is likely there will be other interactions identified in the future. While maternal pregnancy smoking has primarily been associated with early rather than later wheeze and one systematic review suggested that it does not increase the risks of allergy, more recent studies would suggest otherwise. There certainly are interactions between atopy in the family, pregnancy smoking, and increased risks of later atopic asthma. Indeed, maternal pregnancy smoking has been associated with modification of fetal immune response. It remains to be established whether exposure to other pollutants such as ozone might also have an interactive effect promoting susceptibility to asthma.

The interaction between diet and genotype in affecting airway structure and function has yet to be investigated. Selenium deficiency, which is relatively common, has been associated with an increased risk of persistent asthma and could well interact with GST polymorphisms, as selenium is an important substrate for the antioxidant system. Mild vitamin A deficiency in murine models has been associated with reduced expression of lung surfactant and delayed maturation of lung function. To what extent this might contribute to abnormalities of airway structure in humans remains to be established and may again interact with genetic factors.[17]

Recent studies on the association between obesity and asthma have reported a strong relationship between body mass index and asthma risk in children as well as adults. One study suggested that weight loss improves asthma control in obese subjects. However, there is also a possibility that the relationship has its origins in early life. Two studies have shown a significant correlation between reduced lung function in infancy and rapid early postnatal weight gain. This latter phenomenon may represent catch-up growth as a consequence of late intrauterine growth faltering. This impaired fetal growth may affect lung development. Rapid postnatal weight gain following lower birth weight often translates into later obesity and may explain the relationship between obesity and asthma, these effects being independent of the presence of atopy.[18]

SUMMARY

The two main components of the pathology of asthma, namely airway eosinophilic inflammation and remodeling, are both under separate genetic and environmental influences. Both are affected by events occurring from conception onwards and the seeds of both atopy and asthma are sown in early fetal life (Fig. 2-4).

Some genetic polymorphisms increase the risks of allergic sensitization when associated with environmental factors such as timing and concentration of allergen exposure and variations in the nutrition and health of the mother during pregnancy

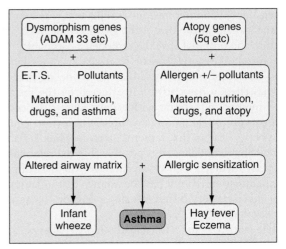

Figure 2-4 The pathology of asthma begins in early fetal life. An algorithm demonstrating the two independent influences, which, if they coincide, lead to the development of asthma. While genetic factors are distinct there are *common environmental determinants*. E.T.S., environmental tobacco smoke exposure.

and lactation. Postnatally, further exposure to allergen in the absence of infection polarizes the immune responses toward an allergic phenotype. Some components of a range of organisms would appear to have a down-regulatory effect on allergic susceptibility.

Additional gene environment interactions affect the development of asthma and airway wall structure and function. These interactions antenatally affect the modeling of the airway in the first place and if reactivated postnatally lead to an abnormal remodeling process. Here the major interactions would appear to be with environmental pollutants such as tobacco smoke, diesel particulates, and ozone. However, there may also be interactions with nutritional aberrations.

Postnatally, infections, pollutants, and allergens can promote an inflammatory immune response not only associated with eosinophilic infiltration but also with activation of neutrophils. The latter have the apparatus to induce proteolysis of matrix proteins and activation of fibrogenesis. This in turn accentuates the abnormalities in airway wall structure and function. Variations in tissue matrix proteins also then adversely affect inflammatory cells thereby creating a vicious cycle of inflammation and remodeling.[19]

Understanding the interactions between genes and environment in relation to the generation of the two major abnormalities associated with asthma will, in time, lead to the identification of targets for therapeutic intervention. It is hoped that in the future it will be possible to interrupt the inexorable progression to chronic airway disease before it has actually started.

REFERENCES

1. Sears MR, Greene JM, Willan AR, et al: Longitudinal, population based, cohort study of childhood asthma followed to adulthood. New Engl J Med 2003;349:1414–1422.
2. Guilbert TW, Morgan WJ, Zeiger RS, et al: Long-term inhaled corticosteroids in pre-school children at high risk for asthma. New Engl J Med 2006;354:1985–1997.
3. Burr ML, Wat D, Evans C, Dunstan FDJ, Doull IJM on behalf of the British Thoracic Society Research Committee: Asthma prevalence in 1973, 1988 and 2003. Thorax 2006;62:296–299.
4. Palmer LJ, Rye PJ, Gibson NA, et al: Airway responsiveness in early infancy predicts asthma, lung function and respiratory symptoms by school age. Am J Respir Crit Care Med 2001;163:37–42.

5. Hess J, deJongste JC: Epidemiological aspects of paediatric asthma. Clin Exp Allergy 2004;34:680–685.
6. Holgate ST, Puddicombe SM, Mullings RE, et al: New insight into asthma pathogenesis. Allergy Clin Immunol Int 2004;16:196–201.
7. Bertino E, Bisson C, Martano C, et al: Relationship between maternal and fetal specific IgE. Pediatr Allergy Immunol 2006;17:484–488.
8. Holt P, Warner JO: Early immunological influences. Chem Immunol Allergy 2004;84:102–127.
9. Warner JO: Can we prevent allergies and asthma? Allergy Clin Immunol Int 2004;16:186–191.
10. Holloway JW, Holgate ST: Genetics. Chem Immunol Allergy 2004;84:1–35.
11. Warner JO: Developmental origins of asthma and related allergic disorders. In Gluckmann P, Hanson M (eds). Developmental Origins of Health and Disease. Cambridge University Press, 2006, pp 349–369.
12. Wjst M: The vitamin D slant on allergy. Pediatr Allergy Immunol 2006;17:477–483.
13. Kull I, Bohme M, Wahlgren C-F, et al: Breast feeding reduces the risk for childhood eczema. J Allergy Clin Immunol 2005;116:657–661.
14. Hays T, Wood RA: A systematic review of the role of hydrolyzed infant formulas in allergy prevention. Arch Pediatr Adolesc Med 2005;159:810–816.
15. Bloomfield SF, Stanwell-Smith R, Crevel RWR, Pickup J: To clean or not to clean: The hygiene hypothesis and home hygiene. Clin Exp Allergy 2006;36:402–425.
16. Kleeberger SR, Peden D: Gene-environment interactions in asthma and other respiratory diseases. Annu Rev Med 2005;56:383–400.
17. Warner JO, Jones CA: Foetal origins of lung disease. In Barkere DJP (ed). Foetal Origins of Cardiovascular and Lung Disease. Lung Biology in Health and Disease. New York, Marcell Dekker Inc, 2001, pp 297–322.
18. Lucas JS, Inskip HM, Godfrey KM, et al: Small size at birth and greater postnatal weight gain: Relationships to diminished infant lung function. Am J Respir Crit Care Med 2004;170:534–540.
19. Beeh KM, Beier J: Handle with care: Targeting neutrophils in chronic obstructive pulmonary disease and severe asthma? Clin Exp Allergy 2006;36:142–157.

Pathophysiology of Asthma

Pascal Chanez and Arnaud Bourdin

Asthma is a heterogeneous and variable inflammatory disease of the airways that causes recurrent symptoms of brief duration and exacerbations. It is a systemic disease involving the activation of many inflammatory cells in the lungs. Within the airways, eosinophils in untreated patients are conspicuous in association with mast cells, lymphocytes, and other mononuclear cells. This inflammatory infiltrate is associated with marked changes in the structure of the bronchi. These structural changes include denuded epithelium and altered subepithelium characterized by collagen deposition, smooth muscle hypertrophia, and hyperplasia (Fig. 3-1).

The mechanisms underlying asthma are complex and intricate. Primary abnormalities of smooth muscle cell activity have received much attention. A neural persistent abnormality involving the cholinergic and noncholinergic nonadrenergic bronchospastic tone has been linked to inflammation. A complex activation of T lymphocytes, which drives the paradigm that asthma is a "T-helper 2 (Th2)-associated disease," is suggested by T-lymphocyte production of Th2-type cytokines (e.g., interleukin [IL]-4, -13), immunoglobulin E (IgE)-mediated mast cell activation, and mediator release. Recently, the chronic decline of lung function noted in asthma brought attention to early and permanent changes of the structure of the airways called airway remodeling. The bronchial epithelium is at the interface between the external environment and the internal milieu and may play a central role in orchestrating many of the pathophysiologic manifestations of asthma. The submucosa of the bronchi, which includes the extracellular matrix (ECM), vessels, glands, and smooth muscle, appears to be modified in asthmatic as compared with healthy individuals. These changes have been observed

even in milder forms or at an early stage of the disease. These pathophysiologic mechanisms and their relationship to the clinical manifestations of asthma will be discussed.

The effects of therapeutic interventions on inflammation and structural changes have been investigated using endobronchial biopsy analysis in asthma (Fig. 3-2). These studies have been important in confirming the potential involvement of different pathways in the pathophysiology of the disease (Fig. 3-3). Noninvasive measures of airway inflammation, including sputum, exhaled nitric oxide, and breath condensates, may provide further insight into the pathophysiology of this disease. In this review, we will discuss immunopathologic and molecular approaches to better understand the mechanisms leading to the clinical picture of asthma.

AIRWAY EPITHELIUM

The bronchial epithelium is a complex structure involving goblet, ciliated, and basal cells (Fig. 3-4). In endobronchial biopsies, airway epithelium appears fragile as demonstrated by partially or completely denuded areas. There are increased epithelial cells in the bronchoalveolar lavage of asthmatic individuals, which reflects the potential for epithelial desquamation in the airway lumen. Some authors have suggested that this epithelial disruption could be attributed to a sampling artifact, but current data suggest that there is increased epithelial fragility. This loss of mechanical and biochemical dynamic barrier can lead to subsequent submucosal cellular activation, referred to as an abnormal epithelial mesenchymal unit.

The mechanisms underlying the fragility of epithelium in asthma are still a matter of debate. Plasma exudation may facilitate the detachment of epithelium from the submucosa. A direct effect of proinflammatory mediators such as metalloproteinases (MMP) or tumor necrosis factor (TNF)-α can induce cell death by necrosis. Epithelial damage may lead to heightened airway responsiveness by the depletion of relaxant factors and loss of enzymes degrading proinflammatory neuropeptides (e.g., substance P). The integrity of airway epithelium may influence the sensitivity of the airways to provocative stimuli by liberating a variety of broncho-active mediators such as lipoxygenase- and cyclooxygenase-derived products.

Epithelial cells are recognized as key players of the inflammatory process by producing proinflammatory products, including cytokines and proteases, and expressing various adhesion molecules. Different triggers, including allergens, pollutants, and microorganisms, can activate epithelial cells. Epithelial cells can generate inflammatory signals that are able to activate various structural and inflammatory cells. These

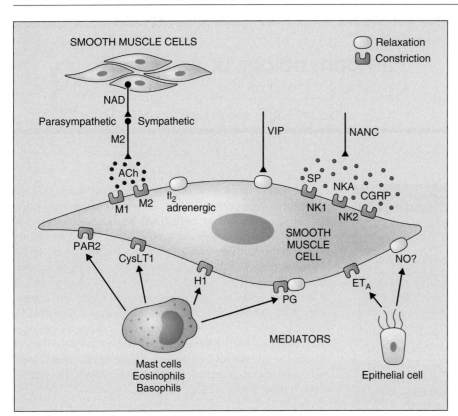

Figure 3-1 Role of smooth muscle in asthma.

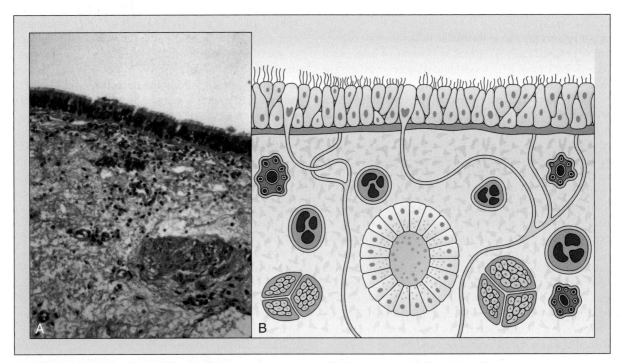

Figure 3-2 Normal bronchus from endobronchial biopsy. (**A,** H&E stain, ×400.) *(Photomicrograph © Pascal Chanez.)*

signals can then increase leukocyte recruitment from the blood and allow longer survival of inflammatory cells within the bronchi by altering cell apoptosis. The bronchial epithelial cells can perpetuate activation, as shown by the overexpression of transcription factors such as nuclear factor kappa B (NFκB), which leads to a constant state of inflammation within the bronchial structures.

Both repair and inflammatory processes are present in the asthmatic bronchial epithelium. The number of goblet cells in the airway epithelium is increased in asthma. Hypersecretion is a common endoscopic finding in asthmatic airways related to the overproduction of mucus. On the other hand, mucus clearance is altered, contributing to an excessive mucus accumulation, implicated in airway obstruction. This can be due

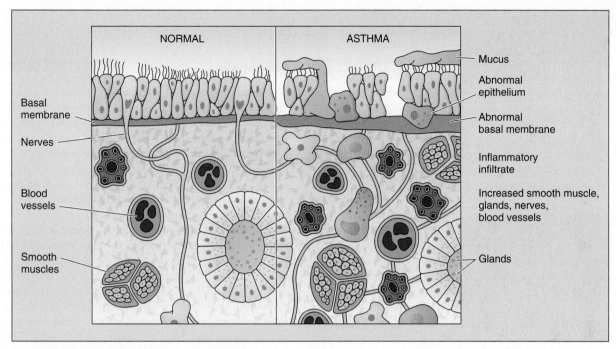

Figure 3-3   **Endobronchial biopsies depicting asthma pathology.**

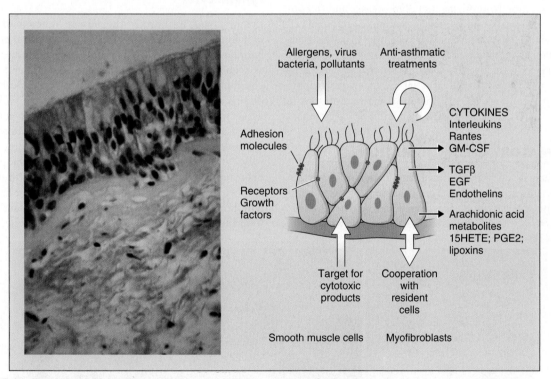

Figure 3-4   **Epithelium in bronchial asthma.** (**A,** H&E stain, x400.) *(Photomicrograph © Pascal Chanez.)*

in part to a diminution in ciliated cells, or a different secretory phenotype with increased goblet cells, and/or decreased cilia viability. Mucins and many other products are dysregulated and contribute to the phenotypic modifications of the asthmatic bronchi. In fact, goblet cell hyperplasia would be the consequence of epithelial cell activation via the up-regulation of mucin genes (MUC5AC). Various cytokines, derived from the epithelium, such as IL-4 and IL-13, can contribute to goblet cell hyperplasia as shown in animal (in vivo) and cellular (ex vivo) models.

The epithelial cells release different mediators involved in regeneration, proliferation, and differentiation. Activated epithelial cells are involved in every stage of the inflammatory reaction by the release of mediators including lipid-derived proinflammatory molecules, such as leukotrienes, prostaglandins, and cytokines. Epithelial cells are also involved in the recruitment and activation of leukocytes, release of extracellular matrix components and growth factors, and expression of adhesion molecules contributing to cell-cell interactions.

The epithelial cells are at the interface between airspace and the internal milieu. They act as a physical and biochemical barrier to ensure the best transition between compartments. Many stimuli activate epithelial cells including noxious agents, infections (viruses, bacteria, or fungi), allergens in atopic patients, air pollutants such as diesel particulates or ozone, and cigarette smoke. Once activated, these epithelial cells produce many mediators, such as cytokines, growth factors, inflammatory and anti-inflammatory products, chemokines, and others. Through these mediators, epithelial cells provide an adaptive response that is important in antigen neutralization, elimination, and wound healing in case of injury. In some cases, the stimuli can provide a sufficiently intense signal to generate a systemic response.

When chronic stimulation of epithelial cells is maintained and the local response insufficient, these cells can induce a proinflammatory response, by recruiting leukocytes and promoting interactions with structural cells, and a profibrotic response leading to airway remodeling. Submucosal fibroblasts and myofibroblasts are able to synthesize large amounts of ECM components. The shedding of the epithelium can be supposed as a manifestation of a failed accelerated repair process. Activated epithelial cells may be responsible for their own desquamation by inducing metalloproteases and disruption of the cell-matrix bridges. The induction of epithelial cell activation via specific or nonspecific receptors usually signals downstream events such as through the NFκB, AP1, and signal transducer and activator of transcription (STAT) pathways. The activation of this epithelial-mesenchymal trophic unit has thus been suggested as a potential mechanism for the exaggerated physiological response characteristic of asthma.

INFLAMMATORY CELL INFILTRATION

In the bronchial submucosa of asthmatic individuals, one can observe an inflammatory infiltrate consisting of eosinophils (Fig. 3-5), mast cells, lymphocytes, monocytes, and neutrophils. This infiltration of inflammatory cells can vary with time,

symptoms, treatments, and severity. We will review the respective roles of each of these cell types.

Eosinophils

Eosinophils are recruited in the airway epithelium under chemotactic signals including cytokines, chemokines, and cell surface adhesion molecules. CD11b, very late antigen 4 (VLA4), intercellular adhesion molecule-1 (ICAM1), and vascular cell adhesion molecule-1 (VCAM1) are involved in this process and are upregulated in asthma. IL-5, granulocyte-macrophage colony-stimulating factor (GM-CSF), eotaxin, and Regulated on Activation, Normal T-cells Expressed and Secreted (RANTES) (now known as CCL5) are known mediators implicated in the recruitment of eosinophils and lymphocytes into the airway wall of asthmatic individuals. These eosinophils appear to be stimulated within the bronchial tissue as suggested by their degranulation. The activated eosinophil products release proinflammatory mediators such as eosinophil cationic protein (ECP) and major basic protein (MBP) in secretory granules, oxygen free radicals, cytokines, eicosanoids, and others known to induce epithelial injury, smooth muscle contraction, bronchial hyperresponsiveness (BHR), and increased vascular permeability with mucosal edema (Fig. 3-6).

Lymphocytes

Lymphocytes infiltrating the airway mucosa of asthmatic individuals express CD4+ (Fig. 3-7). Functional properties of lymphocytes are assessed by their cytokine production profile as a Th1 or Th2. Th2 cytokines and IL-4, -5, and -13 induce eosinophil recruitment and activation and differentiation of plasma cells into an IgE secretory phenotype. However, this Th1-Th2 dichotomy does not fully explain the pathophysiology of asthma. Other T cells with regulatory function (Th0, T regulatory cells [Treg]) are involved, releasing inflammatory cytokines such IL-10. In endobronchial biopsies, it has been reported that CD4+ T cells in the epithelium could amplify the inflammatory process. On the other hand, CD8+ lymphocytes may play a role in severe asthma and have been found to be associated with lung function decline.

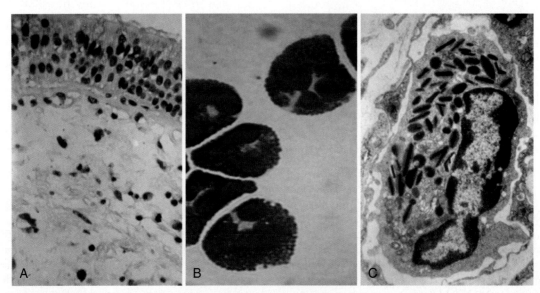

Figure 3-5   Eosinophils. A, Eosinophils in endobronchial biopsy (Anti-FG₂ mab stain, x400). **B,** Blood eosinophils (May-Grunwald-Giemsa stain, x800).
C, Transmission electronic microscopy of blood eosinophils. *(Photomicrograph © Pascal Chanez.)*

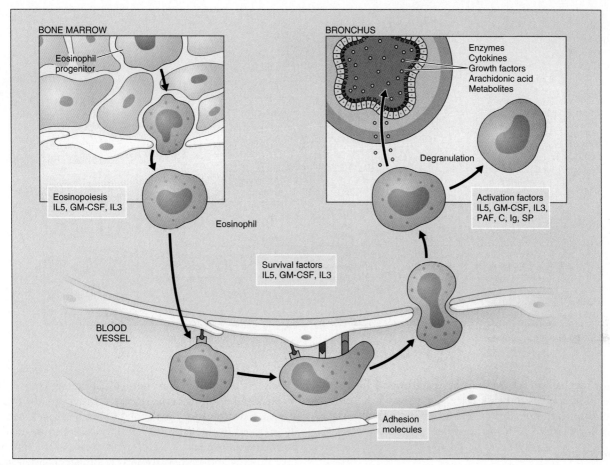

Figure 3-6   Fate of eosinophils in asthma.

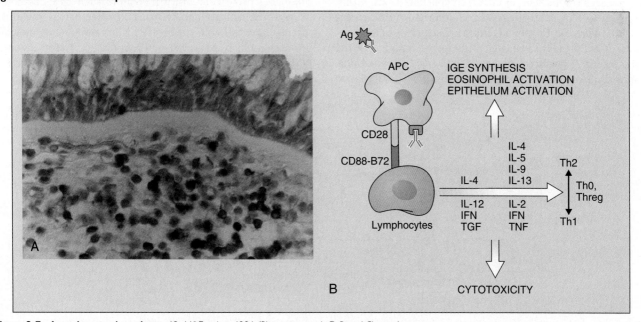

Figure 3-7   Lymphocytes in asthma. (**A**, H&E stain, ×400.) *(Photomicrograph © Pascal Chanez.)*

Mast Cells

Mast cells are leukocytes that are effectors of the inflammatory process (Fig. 3-8). Rarely observed directly in the epithelium, they have been shown to have direct relationships with smooth muscle cells. They are often degranulated, having liberated amounts of proinflammatory mediators such as histamine, proteases like tryptase, lipid bronchoconstric-

tor mediators known as cysteinyl-leukotrienes (LTD_4, LTE_4), and prostaglandin (PG)-D_2. Mast cells can also contribute to epithelial CD40-dependent IgE secretion. Profibrogenic intermediates, transforming growth factor (TGF)-β and ECM products such as laminins, are released by mast cells. Tryptase, a serine protease, is a potent stimulant of fibroblast and smooth muscle cell proliferation and is capable of stimulating synthesis of type I collagen by human fibroblasts.

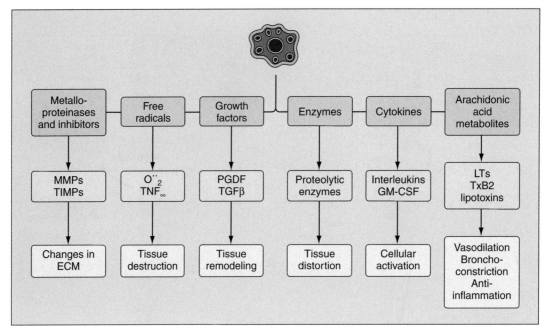

Figure 3-8   Mast cells in asthma.

A major mechanism involved in the regulation of fibroblast proliferation appears to be cleavage and activation of protease-activated-receptor (PAR)-2 expressed on the cell surface of lung fibroblasts.

Macrophages

Macrophages can be seen in increased concentrations within the airway wall of asthmatic subjects, even though this level is far under what can be seen in chronic obstructive pulmonary disease (COPD) (Fig. 3-9). Macrophages are mainly derived from recently migrated blood monocytes. They exhibit abnormal functions even though their gross morphology is not clearly different from the "normal" situation. They seem to be activated resulting in the release of many proinflammatory signals. Co-stimulatory molecules on macrophages, necessarily involved in the activation of T cells, are up-regulated in asthmatic individuals. They can participate in the inflammatory process and perpetuate airway bronchoconstriction by producing proinflammatory mediators such as eicosanoids, oxygen-free radicals, and cytokines. In asthmatic individuals, macrophages are able to secrete higher amounts of metalloproteases, which are growth and chemotactic factors involved in the extracellular matrix and in the recruitment and activation of other leukocytes.

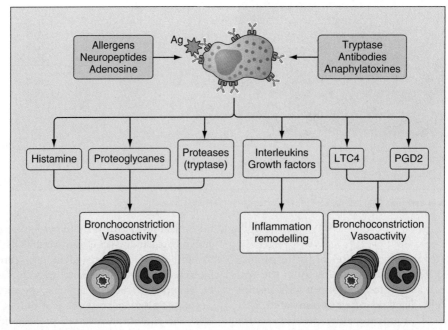

Figure 3-9   Airway macrophages in asthma.

Dendritic Cells

Dendritic cells are largely involved in presenting antigens and the perpetuation of an intense inflammatory response. In the airway epithelium, they constitutively express HLA DR class molecules and are specialized in the initiation of the immune response. Corticosteroids are thought to actively modify this function. Increased immunolocalization of dendritic cells is described in asthma biopsies, although their exact role in the pathophysiology of the disease remains a subject of debate (Fig. 3-10).

Neutrophils

Airway diseases, such as COPD, bronchiectasis with or without cystic fibrosis, and bronchiolitis, share with severe asthma a prominent neutrophilic response. Induced sputum and bronchial biopsies obtained from severely asthmatic patients, including those dying from acute fatal episodes, demonstrate high degrees of chemotactic activity and proactivating molecules for neutrophils. IL-8 and other agonists for CXCR chemokines are largely increased and unregulated by conventional treatments. When activated, they can be responsible for oxygen burst reactions and the release of neutrophil elastase and oxidants. Mostly, neutrophilic inflammation in the airway is corticosteroid resistant. The relationships between neutrophilic bronchitis and the persistence of microorganisms, especially bacteria and viruses, are under investigation in severe asthma.

EXTRACELLULAR MATRIX

The extracellular matrix (ECM) is a prominent structural feature in the asthmatic airway. Thickening of the lamina reticularis has been described in asthma, even early in the disease process. The denuded epithelium found in asthmatic patients exposes the basement membrane directly to the airspace. The real basement membrane in asthma is not abnormal. The sub-basement membrane is abnormally enlarged and densified. The acellular zone is thickened even in the milder forms of the disease when compared with controls. Collagen, fibronectin, laminin, tenascin, entactin-nidogen, but also growth factors, syndecan, and heparan sulfate proteoglycan, are the main components of this zone. Few fibrils are overexpressed. Epithelial cells and myofibroblasts contribute to this thickening, potentially in a synergistic way. Growth factors, including TGF-β, platelet-derived growth factor (PDGF), endothelin, and fibroblast growth factor (FGF), are involved in this process, counterbalanced by prostaglandin 2 (PGE2) and others.

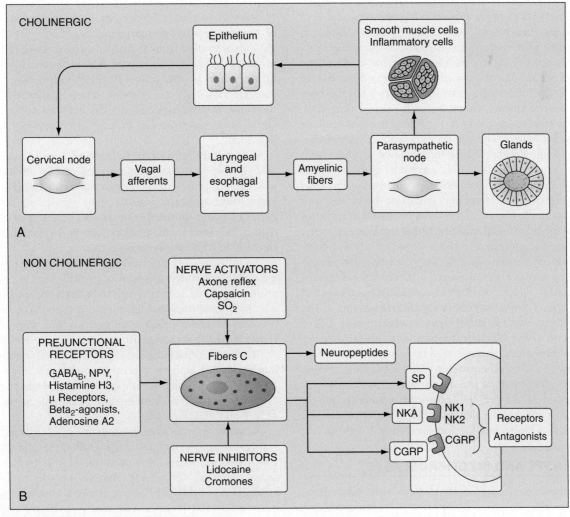

Figure 3-10 Potential neural pathways involved in asthma.

Thickening of the lamina reticularis is specifically associated with asthma, although thickening to a lesser extent is seen in COPD patients. The consequences of thickening of the lamina reticularis are being investigated. Mathematical models suggest that this enlarged fibrillar zone surrounding the airway lumen can protect against excessive airway narrowing due to bronchoconstriction. The presence of large amounts of growth factors and syndecan suggest a putative role in leukocyte trafficking and communication with airway epithelial cells.

ECM components can lead to epithelial cell activation by overstimulating differentiation, migration, and attachment. The interrelations established between ECM components and the basal side of the epithelial cells are complex and dynamically regulated. Integrins and the dystroglycan-dystrophin complex are thought to play a role. Metalloproteases and matrix-metalloproteases (MT-MMP) can promote leukocyte trafficking and epithelial cell shedding. The excessive deposition of ECM components leads to airway remodeling and unclear physiologic manifestations.

Several studies have reported marginal and likely clinically insignificant decreases in lamina reticularis thickness in subjects treated with inhaled corticosteroids (ICSs). Signaling pathways involved in the formation of ECM (e.g., TGF-β) are mainly unaffected by steroids. Whether ICSs can interfere with excessive growth and profibrogenic factor release at the mucosal level is not clearly supported.

Asthmatic individuals have an abnormal elastic fiber network with superficial fibers appearing fragmented and deeper layers that are often patchy, tangled, and thickened, similar in appearance to solar elastolysis in the skin. Transmission electron microscopy (TEM) studies have shown that an elastolytic process occurs in asthmatic patients resulting in disruption of fibers. In fatal asthma, elastic fiber fragmentation has also been found in central airways associated with marked elastolysis. These fiber bundles appear to be hypertrophied as a result of an increased amount of collagen and myofibroblast deposition.

Loss of lung elastic recoil has been shown in adults with chronic persistent asthma and fixed expiratory airflow obstruction. Interestingly, these subjects show markedly abnormal maximal expiratory flow-volume curves at both high and low lung volumes. Hyperinflation can be found at residual volume, at forced residual capacity, and at total lung capacity. The increased elastolysis in asthma is part of a more complex process. The submucosal network in asthmatic airways is formed by elastic fibers dispersed in a collagen and myofibroblast matrix, which constitutes longitudinal bundles in the bronchial tree. Chronic inflammation and remodeling of the airway wall may result in stiffer dynamic elastic properties of the asthmatic airway. These features cause a change in airway mechanical properties demonstrated by reduced airway compliance, particularly in the patients with long-lasting asthma. In addition, disruption of the elastic fibers may contribute to a reduction of the pre- and post-load of smooth muscle contraction, a mechanism that may play a major role in the development of exaggerated airway narrowing in asthma.

FIBROBLASTS AND MYOFIBROBLASTS

The aforementioned cellular interactions may be responsible for an abnormal mesenchymal cell proliferation and for the increased number of fibroblasts and myofibroblasts found in the airways of asthmatic patients. Although they are regarded as fixed cells of ECM, fibroblasts retain the capacity for growth and regeneration and may evolve into various cell types, including smooth muscle cells becoming myofibroblasts. Myofibroblasts can contribute to tissue remodeling by releasing ECM components such as elastin, fibronectin, and laminin. Increased numbers of myofibroblasts are found in the airways of asthmatic subjects, and their number appears to correlate with the size of the basement reticular membrane. Following bronchial allergen challenge, myofibroblast numbers are increased and the cells undergo a differentiation process and present with structural and ultrastructural features similar to those of smooth muscle cells. Myofibroblasts, in addition to contractile responses and mitogenesis, have synthetic and secretory potential, as they can release CCL5 (RANTES). Myofibroblasts participate in chronic airway inflammation by interacting with both Th1- and Th2-derived cytokines to modulate chemoattractant activity for eosinophils, activated T lymphocytes, and monocytes/macrophages. Therefore, smooth muscle cells have the potential to alter the composition of the ECM environment and orchestrate key events in the process of chronic airway remodeling.

SMOOTH MUSCLE CELLS

Excess accumulation of bronchial smooth muscle cells is another prominent feature of airway wall remodeling that is believed to play a fundamental role in the pathogenesis of exaggerated airway narrowing in asthma (Fig. 3-11). In patients who died from an asthma exacerbation, the increase in smooth muscle is far greater than in those who died from other causes. In vivo animal studies confirm that prolonged allergen exposure can increase smooth muscle thickness. Recently, muscle hypertrophia has been found in the muscle layer in endobronchial biopsies from severely asthmatic individuals.

Cell culture studies have disclosed a wide range of soluble factors that can promote proliferation of human airway smooth muscle cells, suggesting that, through autocrine loops, these cells can regulate their own proliferative rate. Airway smooth muscle cells may also be a source of inflammatory mediators and cytokines, in particular chemokines, thus implicating airway smooth muscle cells as contributors to the inflammatory mechanisms of asthma. The pro-activating signals for converting airway smooth muscle cells into a proliferative and secretory cell in asthma are unknown, but may include viruses and IgE. Some authors have shown the presence of smooth muscle mitogens in the bronchoalveolar lavage (BAL) from asthmatic subjects who underwent allergen challenge. Molecular sieving of BAL fluids demonstrates that mitogenic activity is present exclusively in a less than 10-kD fraction, which is compatible with a series of potential candidate factors, such as epidermal growth factor (EGF), TGF-β and PDGF.

An additional mechanism regulating smooth muscle proliferation is through production of metalloproteinase (MMP)-2, which has been demonstrated to be an important autocrine factor required for airway smooth muscle proliferation. Production of MMP-2 by airway smooth muscle suggests that it contributes to extracellular matrix turnover and airway remodeling. Furthermore, in vivo MMP-2 may be produced

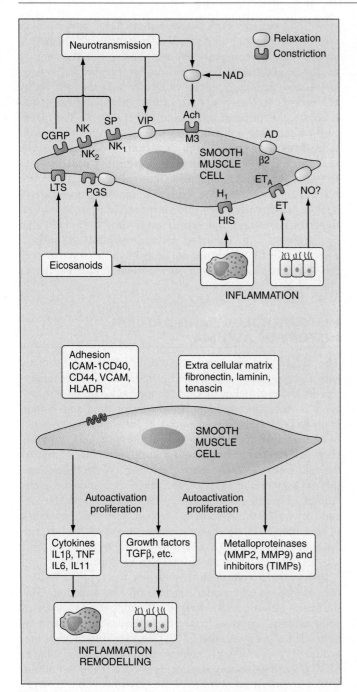

Figure 3-11 Role of smooth muscle cells in inflammation.

by other airway cells including fibroblasts and macrophages, indicating that other airway cells may interact to support airway smooth muscle proliferation in asthma.

It is also conceivable that abnormal smooth muscle cell proliferation may represent a failure of the antiproliferative mechanisms that limit the quantity of smooth muscle in the airways. In this regard, an important homeostatic mechanism seems to be apoptosis, a form of programmed cell death that represents a pathway by which tissues can eliminate unhealthy, harmful, or excess cells. Interestingly, it has recently been shown that Fas cross-linking induces apoptosis in cultured human smooth muscle cells, suggesting a mechanism by which Fas-mediated apoptosis could act to oppose excess smooth muscle accumulation during airway remodeling in asthma.

Although nonspecific BHR is a basic mechanism underlying the excessive smooth muscle contraction and airway narrowing that is characteristic of asthma, its mechanism remains unknown. It is still unclear if the phenomenon is due to fundamental changes in the phenotype of the smooth muscle or is caused by structural and/or mechanical changes in the noncontractile elements of the airway wall or by alterations in the relationship of the airway wall to the surrounding lung parenchyma. Previous studies found that the volume fraction of smooth muscle in the submucosa correlated with BHR but not in the asthmatic group. Although airway wall remodeling may contribute to BHR, there is increasing evidence that the bronchodilating response to cyclic and periodic stretch is impaired in asthma. There are at least two different mechanisms by which periodic length and force oscillations could influence airway smooth muscle shortening and airway narrowing. These processes, called "perturbed equilibrium of myosin binding" and "plasticity," have different biochemical and mechanical mechanisms and consequences. They have the potential to interact and to have a fundamental effect on the shortening capacity of airway smooth muscle and its ultimate ability to cause excessive airway narrowing.

NERVES

Dysfunction of the airway innervation in asthma contributes to its pathophysiology. β-Adrenergic blockers and cholinergic agonists are known to induce bronchoconstriction and produce symptoms of asthma. Blockade of these two pathways is insufficient to prevent the in vitro ability of bronchial ring to contract. This led to the discovery of nonadrenergic noncholinergic (NANC) neural pathways involving new neuromediators, such as bradykinin, neurokinin, vasoactive intestinal peptide (VIP), and substance P. These neuromediators produce in vitro and in vivo features of clinical asthma involving bronchoconstriction, vasodilation, and inflammation. The NANC system has been proposed as an explanation for bronchial hyperreactivity but has never been fully demonstrated in the human disease because of the failure to develop potent and safe antagonists.

BLOOD VESSELS

Airway wall remodeling in asthma involves a number of changes including increased vascularity, vasodilation, and microvascular leakage. Evidence suggests that the number and size of bronchial vessels is moderately increased in patients with asthma compared with healthy controls. In particular, there may be increased numbers of vessels in patients with uncontrolled disease or fatal asthma, but the extent of neovascularization or angiogenesis is still unclear. Vascular endothelial growth factor (VEGF) levels are variable in asthmatic airways suggesting a low degree of angiogenesis in patients with controlled asthma.

GLANDS

Bronchial hypersecretion is observed at bronchoscopy in patients with asthma (Fig. 3-12). Although increased luminal mucus is seen in postmortem cases of mild asthma, cough with sputum production is not a common symptom of mild asthma. In fact, the collection of spontaneously produced

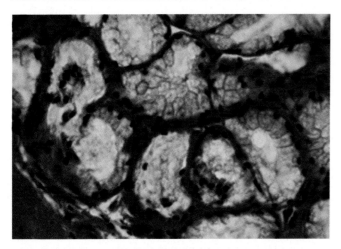

Figure 3-12   Glands hypertrophia in asthma: endobronchial biopsies. (H&E stain, x400.) *(Photomicrograph © Pascal Chanez.)*

sputum samples from asthma is difficult and induction with agents such as hypertonic saline is necessary. Bronchial hypersecretion is the consequence of hypertrophy and hyperplasia of submucosal glands and epithelial goblet cells. Increased mucus will certainly result in sputum production and contribute to excessive airway narrowing. The replacement of ciliated cells by goblet cells contributes to airway remodeling in asthma. Impaired clearance of mucus is present during exacerbations and is a potential important contributor to fatal asthma.

LOCALIZATION OF ABNORMALITIES

The small airway, known as the silent part of the airway tree, has been postulated to be involved in asthma. Transbronchial biopsies have demonstrated that the distal airways are involved in the inflammatory and remodeling changes associated with asthma. The immunohistochemistry analysis performed on small airways demonstrates increased infiltration by eosinophils, CD4+ T cells, and mast cells. Computed tomography (CT) of the chest shows that these abnormalities are associated with airway trapping during expiration. Thus, small airways play a significant role in the perpetuation and chronicity of asthma symptoms.

In fatal asthma cases, inflammation has been observed in bronchioli and alveoli with neutrophils found at the deepest level. Mucus, apoptotic eosinophils, leukocyte debris, and shed epithelium are found to occlude the small airway lumen. The airway wall is thickened by edema, smooth muscle and gland enlargement, and increased extracellular matrix thickness and density. Some emphysematous lesions have been described related to severe asthma. Modifications of the epithelium at the bronchiolar level have also been described: decreased Clara cells and modification of surfactant protein functions. The specificity of such findings should be better characterized and the consequences analyzed to propose new therapeutic avenues.

SIZE OF THE AIRWAY WALL IN ASTHMA

Asthmatic individuals have greater airway wall thickening than healthy subjects as assessed by high-resolution CT of the

chest, and patients with severe asthma have greater airway wall thickening than those with mild asthma. The degree of airway wall thickening may relate to the duration and severity of disease and the degree of airflow obstruction. It has been postulated that the increase in airway wall area shown by CT reflects increased smooth muscle, mucosal glands, submucosal and epithelial thickening, and the ECM. The observation that total wall thickness was not greater in younger individuals with fatal asthma than control subjects suggests that factors other than airway wall geometry contribute to the pathogenesis of fatal attacks in this age group. These features of airway remodeling result in an increased resistance to airflow, particularly when there is bronchial constriction and hyperresponsiveness. The effect on airflow is compounded by the presence of increased mucous secretion and inflammatory exudate, which not only blocks the airway passages but also causes an increase in surface tension favoring airway closure.

HISTOPATHOLOGY AND NATURAL HISTORY OF ASTHMA

The structural changes that occur in the airways of asthmatic subjects result from interdependent and highly variable inflammatory and remodeling processes leading to common features, such as vascular congestion, exudation of fluid and protein from blood vessels, and migration of inflammatory cells out of the microvessels into the interstitial tissue. In addition, there is increased secretion of mucus and sloughing of epithelial cells from the surface into the lumen. When this inflammatory response becomes chronic, there is an increase in the amount of collagen close to the epithelium leading to the concept of epithelial-mesenchymal trophic unit and remodeling of the airways. These changes in structure likely lead to various functional consequences involved in the severity of asthma attacks and may affect the natural history of asthma.

Many epidemiologic studies suggest that asthma is associated with an accelerated decline of lung function. This decline is heterogeneous among patients; whereas it seems to be minimal in some, it is quite extensive in others, similar to that of patients with COPD. Indeed, during adult life, asthma is associated with an increase in the rate of decline in FEV_1 (forced expiratory volume in 1 second) and in middle-aged and elderly smokers it is virtually impossible to separate chronic bronchitis and asthma by means of FEV_1. Many asthmatic subjects are smokers and the combination of both risk factors appears to have a major impact on the decline of FEV_1. Another risk factor for an accelerated decline in lung function is bronchial hyperreactivity. Nonspecific bronchial hyperreactivity appears to be associated with airway remodeling and accelerated decline in lung function.

These observations support the concept that airway remodeling in asthma starts early in life, even before the onset of asthma in children. The Childhood Asthma Management Program (CAMP) of 1041 children demonstrated that inhaled corticosteroids did not modify decline in FEV_1 after bronchodilators in comparison to placebo, suggesting that structural changes of the airways occur at an early stage of the natural history of the disease.

On the other hand, the airways of elderly subjects who have had persistent asthma for decades are likely candidates for airway remodeling. Because the duration of asthma in the elderly can range from several months to many decades, this has been considered an ideal population in which to study the consequence of long-standing asthma. By comparing airflow and lung volumes in a cohort of elderly asthmatic subjects, it has been shown that those with asthma of long duration had a significantly lower FEV_1 than those with asthma of short duration. Interestingly, the duration of asthma was found to be inversely associated with FEV_1 and lung hyperinflation. Most subjects with asthma of long duration fail to achieve normal airflow after bronchodilator administration, indicating that severe decrements in pulmonary function associated with long-term asthma can become irreversible.

There is a common agreement that changes in lung function may be the consequence of the underlying remodeling of the entire airway wall, and not of a single airway structure. The increased thickness of the lamina reticularis has long been considered *the* marker of airway remodeling; however, the clinical impact of this specific structural change of the airway remains poorly understood. Indeed, the thickness of the lamina reticularis is not influenced by the duration of asthma.

It is likely that repetitive injury to the airway wall, and the ensuing tissue-repair process, may establish, through autocrine and paracrine immune-regulatory mechanisms, the extent of airway remodeling in asthma. There are many proinflammatory agents to which the airways are continuously exposed. Repeated inhalation of large amounts of cold air, as occurs in ski athletes during strenuous training, has been shown to induce airway inflammation and remodeling. Similarly, repeated exposures to allergens likely lead to the maintenance of a persistent inflammatory process leading to structural airway changes. This possibility was tested using an animal model, such as sensitized brown Norway rats. Following repeated allergen exposure for periods of 2, 4, or 12 weeks to aerosolized ovalbumin (OA), serum IgE and a number of peribronchial eosinophils significantly increased because of the development of an inflammatory response. Of note, after 2 weeks of OA exposure, structural airway changes occurred, such as goblet cell hyperplasia, an increase in airway epithelium proliferation, increased fibronectin deposition, thickening of the airway wall, and airway hyperresponsiveness. These histologic alterations were not influenced by an additional 10 weeks of exposure to allergen. This finding shows that some tissue alterations occur at a very early stage of the remodeling process, whereas "chronic" exposure to inflammatory agents may lead to its expansion to the submucosal structures and subsequent increase in the amount of collagen within the impaired tissue. These pieces of evidence support the concept that remodeling of the airways is a multistep process, in which changes in the inner airway wall, and particularly of the bronchial epithelium, may play a fundamental role.

CLINICAL CORRELATES

In asthma, cough, dyspnea, and sputum production are frequent symptoms. Cough is usually described as a symptom of brief duration along with shortness of breath. Chest tightness and wheeze may be related to airway narrowing. Stimulation of cough receptors in the central airways may be important. However, the stimulation may be related to air-trapping/hyperinflation with activation of stretch fibers, as a consequence of occlusion of distal airways. The increased number of inflammatory cells (neutrophils, eosinophils), goblet cells, and submucosal mucous glands is a well-established pathological feature and explains the potential productive cough of patients with asthma. Asthma perception of symptoms is variable and may be related to lung hyperinflation and abnormalities of C-reactive fibers. On the other hand, bronchial eosinophilic inflammation is associated with poor perception of asthma symptoms with anti-inflammatory treatment improving this perception.

NONSPECIFIC BRONCHIAL HYPERRESPONSIVENESS

Nonspecific BHR is a major functional abnormality in asthma. BHR appears related to severity of symptoms over long periods (months) rather than days or weeks. This suggests that BHR is at least related to the natural history of the disease rather than an episode of acute inflammation. BHR can be a response to a wide range of stimuli such as methacholine, histamine, cold/dry air, exercise, nonisotonic stimuli, or specific allergens to which the patient is sensitized. BHR may vary during allergy seasons and after viral infections. The degree of BHR is loosely related to severity of asthma although not to baseline lung function.

BHR does not appear to be completely related to bronchial eosinophilic inflammation. Some studies suggest that easier access of the stimulus to epithelial and submucosal sites may enhance BHR, as demonstrated by a positive correlation between the loss of epithelial tight junctions and BHR. A number of studies have shown that the thickness of the reticular basement membrane (lamina reticularis) measured on biopsy is related to BHR; however, a number of studies have not shown such a relationship. With more prolonged exposure, scarring occurs with increased fibronectin and collagen deposition mainly in the outer airway wall. At the same time, BHR wanes and even turns into a slight hyporesponsiveness. These findings support the mathematically derived concepts relating airway responsiveness to wall thickness.

CORRELATES WITH CHRONICITY AND SEVERITY

Although many factors contribute to asthma severity, airway inflammation and structural changes are almost certainly important factors. CT scan and morphometric studies of the proximal airways in asthma have shown a relation between increased severity of disease and increased thickness of the airway wall. The pathologic changes include thickness of the total airway wall, inner airway wall, the smooth muscle, and mucous glands. Deposition of extracellular matrix proteins such as collagen results in increased thickness of the reticular basement membrane in asthma, which has been shown to be related to severity. More severe cases have been characterized by increased airway smooth muscle. The degree of air trapping or hyperinflation (measured physiologically or radiologically) contributes to asthma severity.

FATAL ASTHMA

The pathology of asthma was initially described in case series of fatal asthma. These largely qualitative descriptions highlighted common features including the infiltration of the airway wall with eosinophils, neutrophils, and lympho-mononuclear cells both in the epithelium and in the submucosa; occlusion of airway lumens with mucus; cellular debris and eosinophil products; and thickening of the airway wall with prominence of the smooth muscle and mucous glands. The pathology of fatal asthma appears similar to that of asthma in general. These observations suggest that overall, clinically severe asthma is not always fatal asthma. However, one of the strongest risk factors for a near-fatal or fatal asthma attack is a previous near-fatal event, which supports an underlying inflammatory or structural change in the lungs that contributes to the risk. It has been shown that increased numbers of eosinophils and CD3+ cells in large, but not small, airways in fatal asthma were comparable to mild-moderate asthma cases in patients who died from nonrespiratory causes. Exposure to a number of triggers, often as a massive exposure (allergens, occupational) can lead to asthma deaths. Neutrophilic and eosinophilic inflammation has been associated with fatal asthma. Mucus plugs are almost always present in most of the bronchial tree. Bronchial epithelium, smooth muscle, and glands are clearly damaged and abnormal in most of the autopsy studies. Some abnormalities from the outer airway wall have been reported where no airway inflammation can be found. In addition, loss of alveolar attachments indicates a potential mechanism for asthma to induce parenchymal destruction.

THERAPEUTIC CORRELATES TO ASTHMA PATHOPHYSIOLOGY

Although the exact clinical relevance of airway inflammation and remodeling to disease expression is not completely clear, it is proposed that treatment or prevention of inflammation and remodeling is a crucial element in asthma management (Fig. 3-13). Current data indicate that treatment

with ICS does decrease eosinophilic inflammation but weakly affects bronchial remodeling in established asthma. In a single study, it was shown that if the dose of ICS is modified based on the degree of BHR, a reduction in lamina reticularis thickening can be achieved. However, the doses of ICS used in this study were far higher than usually recommended in mild asthma. In addition, high doses of ICS significantly reduce airway vascularity. These morphological data correspond to the clinical observation that prolonged treatment with ICS improves both hypersensitivity and hyperreactivity of the airways, thus suggesting an effect on components of structure of the bronchi. However, in most studies BHR improves, but does not return to within normal limits, indicating that corticosteroids cannot fully reverse the abnormal tissue.

This raises the question of whether it would not be more beneficial to start ICS at an early stage of asthma to prevent the inflammatory cascade leading to structural remodeling, instead of reversing established lesions. This hypothesis has been tested in a rat model in which pretreatment with fluticasone proprionate reduces airway inflammation and partly prevents goblet cell hyperplasia, fibronectin deposition, thickening of the airway wall, and the accompanying increase in BHR. However, treatment with fluticasone after allergen exposure, although preventing further progression of structural airway changes, does not reverse already established alterations. The CAMP study showed that continuous, long-term treatment with budesonide in a large cohort of mild-to-moderate asthmatic children is not associated with long-term improvement in lung growth. This evidence further supports the hypothesis that airway wall remodeling in asthma occurs very early in the natural history of the disease and that early treatment with corticosteroids may not significantly reverse the development of airway wall remodeling. Large clinical studies, including not only evaluation of efficacy but also side effects and a pharmaco-economical evaluation, together with a better insight in the phenomena of remodeling, are needed to further address this important issue. In addition, the effect of other forms of controller medication remains to be examined. Pharmacological interventions that interfere with the natural history of the disease should be developed.

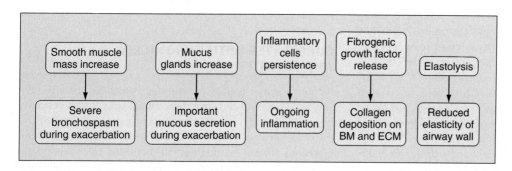

Figure 3-13 Clinical correlates for remodeling in asthma.

SUGGESTED READING

Bousquet J, Jeffery PK, Busse WW, Johnson M, Vignola AM: Asthma. From bronchoconstriction to airways inflammation and remodeling. Am J Respir Crit Care Med 2000;161:1720–1745.
Busse WW, Rosenwasser LJ: Mechanisms of asthma. J Allergy Clin Immunol 2003;111(3 Suppl):S799–804.

James A: Airway remodeling in asthma. Curr Opin Pulm Med 2005;11(1):1–6.
Wenzel SE: Asthma: Defining of the persistent adult phenotypes. Lancet 2006;368(9537):804–813.

The Natural History of Asthma into Adulthood

Stefano Guerra and Anne L. Wright

CHAPTER

4

CLINICAL PEARLS

- Although most children with early wheezing are symptom-free by school age, the presence of early wheezing increases the risk of having active wheezing at school age by approximately 80% and is associated with lung function deficits up to age 16.

- Complete remission of asthma after the onset of puberty is not as common as previously believed.

- Low lung function, bronchial hyperresponsiveness, female gender, atopy, upper airway disease, obesity, and positive family history of asthma are significant risk factors for the persistence of the disease.

- Children with severe and/or persistent asthma show deficits of lung function by the end of childhood that may track, or even worsen, over time during adult life.

- Patients with severe and/or persistent asthma are at increased risk of developing non–fully reversible airflow limitation, the defining functional feature of chronic obstructive pulmonary disease.

Several lines of evidence suggest that, in most cases, asthma has its origin and onset in childhood. First, up to one third of children experience wheezing episodes by 3 years of age and population-based longitudinal studies have shown that the presence of wheezing by school age significantly increases the risk of having persistent asthma and airflow limitation both in adolescence and adult life. Second, allergy-related immune responses that are strongly linked to asthma appear to begin in many cases in early life, when the maturation of the immune system is influenced by the complex interplay between inherited predisposition and specific environmental stimuli. Consistent with this scenario, exposures that exert their effects in infancy and childhood—such as attending day care or having older siblings—have been associated with protection against asthma later in life. Similarly, the risk for wheezing in adulthood is significantly increased for subjects who develop early allergic sensitization but not for subjects who develop allergic sensitization after age 8.

Although most asthma begins in childhood, the disease can begin at any stage in life including adulthood, and, regardless of when the clinical onset of disease occurs, its natural history can be quite difficult to predict. Asthma is a variable disease that can present with any possible combination of remissions and relapses over time. Because the long-term sequelae of asthma on lung health are likely to be quite different depending on the pattern of remission and relapse, understanding the factors that affect the natural history of the disease is of great interest from both a public health

and clinical standpoint. Yet, many vital questions remain unsolved. The following are just a few of them, which will be addressed in this chapter:

- A positive history for wheezing is reported by the parents of up to one third of children by age 3 and 50% of children by age 6. This observation raises questions regarding the specificity of these reports for identifying the children destined to develop asthma later in life. *Can we identify profiles of risk factors that predict which children with early wheezing will go on to develop asthma and which ones will not?*
- A question that parents quite commonly ask the physician is: *When a child is diagnosed with asthma, is it possible to predict the long-term course of the disease in his or her adult life?*
- *Does epidemiological evidence substantiate that childhood asthma is likely to remit during adolescence? What are the factors affecting asthma remission/persistence from childhood to adult life?*
- *Can long-term persistent asthma progress into chronic obstructive pulmonary disease (COPD)? And how does the prognosis of these asthma-related COPD cases compare to the prognosis of smoking-related COPD cases?*
- *Finally, how can we translate what we learn from epidemiological studies into interventions to prevent the onset of asthma and/or affect its clinical course?*

ASTHMA PHENOTYPES IN INFANCY AND CHILDHOOD

Wheezing is a common symptom in infancy, when it is usually associated with viral lower respiratory illnesses (LRI). In most cases, early wheezing is a transitory condition that will remit conclusively once the child reaches school age. However, for some children early wheezing may represent the first sign of a predisposition to develop asthma later in life. In addition, the occurrence of wheezing in the first years of life has been linked to early deficits of lung function that may track over time and affect susceptibility to lung damage by noxious agents in adult life.

The prevalence of early wheezing and its relationship to asthma risk and lung function later in life have been studied in a population-based birth cohort, the Tucson Children's Respiratory Study (CRS)[1] (Fig. 4-1). In the CRS cohort, 277 (34%) of 826 children had at least one lower respiratory tract illness with wheezing in the first 3 years of life. Among these 277 children, 164 (59%) reported no wheezing at 6 years of age and were defined as "transient early wheezers," while 113 (41%) reported wheezing at age 6 and were defined as "persistent wheezers." As expected, most children (549 out of 826: 66%) had no wheezing before the age of 3 years. Among

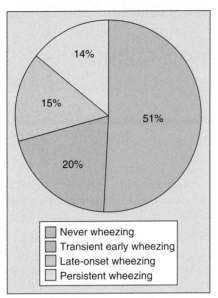

Figure 4-1 Proportion of children with no wheezing from birth to age 6 years (never wheezing), wheezing lower respiratory illness (LRI) before age 3 years only (transient early wheezing), wheezing at age 6 years only (late-onset wheezing), and wheezing both with LRI before age 3 years and at age 6 years (persistent wheezing) in the CRS birth cohort. (*Data derived from Martinez FD, Wright AL, Taussig LM, Holberg CJ, Halonen M, Morgan WJ: Asthma and wheezing in the first six years of life. The Group Health Medical Associates. N Engl J Med 1995;332:133–138.*)

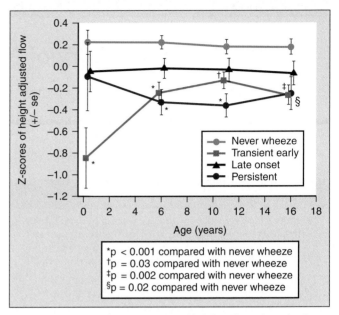

Figure 4-2 Cross-sectional *z* scores of height-adjusted maximal expiratory flows at ages 2.4 months and 6, 11, and 16 years for the preschool wheeze phenotypes. The preschool wheeze phenotypes were defined as follows: no wheeze from birth to age 6 years (Never Wheeze), wheezing LRI before age 3 years only (Transient Early), wheeze at age 6 years only (Late Onset), and wheezing LRI before age 3 years and wheeze at age 6 years (Persistent). (*Data from Morgan WJ, Stern DA, Sherrill DL, et al: Outcome of asthma and wheezing in the first 6 years of life: follow-up through adolescence. Am J Respir Crit Care Med 2005;172:1253–1258.*)

them, 425 (77%) reported no wheezing at 6 years of age and were defined as "never wheezers" while 124 (23%) reported wheezing at age 6 and were defined as "late-onset wheezers." These findings point toward two important and apparently conflicting conclusions. First, most children with early wheezing are symptom-free by school age. Second, early wheezing increases the risk of having active wheezing at 6 years of age by approximately 80%.

In addition, early wheezing, whether it is transient or persistent, appears to be associated with deleterious effects on later lung health. Children who wheeze in the first 3 years of life have lower forced expiratory flows (FEF_{25-75}), forced expiratory volume in 1 second (FEV_1), and FEV_1/forced vital capacity (FVC) ratio values up to age 16, as compared with their peers who did not wheeze in the first 3 years of life[2] (Fig. 4-2). This association is *independent* of the presence of wheezing at age 6, as children with either transient early wheezing or persistent wheezing show comparable levels of lung function deficit. In contrast, these two groups can be differentiated based on maximal expiratory flow at 3 months of age (before any LRI), when transient wheezers, but not persistent wheezers, show significantly lower values, as compared with never wheezers.

Thus, it appears that there are at least two mechanisms by which early wheezing may affect lower levels of lung function in school age and adolescence. One mechanism, observed in early transient wheezers, pertains to reduced lung function as early as the third month of life, which is associated with maternal smoking during pregnancy, but is unrelated to the likelihood of wheezing and atopy during school years. A different mechanism may be present in persistent wheezers, whose lung function is normal in the first months

of life. For this group, lower lung function in childhood is linked to the traditional risk factors of atopic asthma, such as increased immunoglobulin (Ig)E levels, positive skin prick tests, history of eczema and allergic rhinitis, and family history of asthma.

By the time of school age, the vast majority of children with asthma have increased plasma total IgE levels and specific IgE directed against aeroallergens, as compared with healthy children. Yet not all atopic children have asthma. In children with asthma, atopic sensitization has at least three differentiating characteristics, as compared with atopic sensitization in children with no asthma: it is more intense, it has an earlier onset, and it is preferentially directed against specific perennial aeroallergens. However, the specific aeroallergens associated with asthma differ by geographic area. For example, sensitization to indoor allergens such as the house-dust mites, *Dermatophagoides pteronyssinus* and *Dermatophagoides farinae*, cockroaches, and cat allergens has been most commonly associated with asthma worldwide. However, we have consistently found these allergens to play a secondary role in children with asthma in the desert environment of Tucson, Arizona, where sensitization to the mold *Alternaria* shows by far the strongest association with the disease. Whether these different sensitization patterns are related to different levels of exposure to specific allergens in different environments remains unknown. However, this observation suggests that whatever the nature of the association between elevated IgE and asthma, this link is not allergen-specific.

Traditionally, atopy has been causally linked to asthma. The postulated mechanism by which atopy and asthma are linked is that allergen exposure results in sensitization and that continued exposure to specific allergens in sensitized individuals leads to airway allergic inflammation and asthma symptoms. However, recent epidemiological studies have challenged this view of a unidirectional link between atopy and asthma. It has been shown that the presence of asthma in the mother or father is not only associated with asthma in the child (as one would expect), but it is also a strong predictor of the child's total IgE levels and skin test reactivity.[3] Of note, these associations hold true after adjusting for the intensity and other characteristics of parental atopy, suggesting that parental asthma may independently predispose the child to the development of atopy. In addition, although the level of allergen exposure early in life appears related to the development of allergic sensitization, and allergic sensitization is a risk factor for development of asthma, epidemiological studies have failed to find a direct link between allergen exposure early in life and subsequent development of asthma.

A possible explanation for these puzzling epidemiological findings is that the link between atopy and asthma, rather than being a straightforward cause-effect relationship, is at least partly explained by some yet unknown shared factors. It is tempting to postulate that an immunological deviation is among these shared factors. Using the Tucson cohorts of the CRS and the Infant Immune Study (IIS), we found that reduced interferon (IFN)-γ production from polyclonally stimulated peripheral blood mononuclear cells in the first year of life predicts the subsequent development of both allergic sensitization and asthma-related symptoms, such as recurrent wheezing.[4,5] Reduced IFN-γ responses might be related to genetic mechanisms or to a delayed maturation of the immune system. In turn, they may predispose to viral infections, airway growth alterations, and/or T-helper 2 (Th2)-skewed polarization of the immune system. It should be acknowledged that the deficit of early IFN-γ responses is only one of many possible pathways that could be shared by atopy and asthma, or it might simply act as a surrogate for some other factor. Whatever the nature of these shared pathways, they are likely to hold the key to understanding the link between atopy and asthma, and thus represent a promising area for future research in asthma epidemiology.

PERSISTENCE AND REMISSION OF ASTHMA IN ADOLESCENCE

Adolescence is a period of transition during which rapid hormonal, developmental, and behavioral changes can affect the natural history of asthma. It has been long accepted that most children with asthma outgrow the disease after the onset of puberty. However, this belief has been challenged by several lines of evidence from recent studies, which suggest that complete remission of asthma in adolescence may be the exception rather than the rule. For example, in the CRS cohort we found remission of wheezing after puberty to be quite common among children who experienced only infrequent wheezing during childhood.[6] However, up to 58% of children with frequent wheezing and/or a physician-confirmed diagnosis of asthma acquired between age 6 and the onset of puberty experienced wheezing at some point after the onset of puberty by age 16. Further, relapse of asthma in adulthood even after prolonged periods of disease

remission appears to be a relatively common event. Investigators from the Dunedin Multidisciplinary Health and Development Study found that up to one third of subjects with asthma in remission at 18 years of age had disease relapses by 26 years of age.[7] This proportion is likely to be even higher when longer periods of follow-up are considered.

Finally, many asthmatic individuals in clinical remission (as defined by the absence of symptoms and medication use) may still have subclinical but active forms of the disease. In a cohort of 119 subjects who were diagnosed with asthma during school age and reexamined 30 years later (at age 32 to 42), 57% of those who were in clinical remission as adults had bronchial hyperresponsiveness and/or reduced lung function.[8] This finding is consistent with those from other studies supporting a clear distinction between clinical and complete remission of asthma, with the possibility that an underlying inflammatory process remains active in the airways of subjects during periods of apparent remission of asthma. Several indicators of airway inflammation, including eosinophils and interleukin (IL)-5 in bronchial biopsies, eosinophil percentage in bronchoalveolar lavage, and exhaled nitric oxide levels, as well as bronchial responsiveness to adenosine-5′-monophosphate, have been shown to be higher in children and adolescents with remitting asthma than in peer controls. It remains unclear whether an anti-inflammatory treatment would be beneficial in cases of subclinical asthma. Further, whether bronchial hyperresponsiveness and reduced lung function among these apparently remitting asthma cases represent manifestations of an underlying ongoing airway inflammation, irreversible structural sequelae of the disease, or both, is unknown. In any case, the evidence on inflammation and airway remodeling in asthma suggests the importance of monitoring patients with asthma in clinical remission over time.

Potential factors that might influence the patterns of remission and persistence of asthma in adolescence hold great interest (see "Predictors of Asthma Persistence from Childhood to Adult Age"). Among these factors, gender is likely to play a key role. Indeed, the male:female ratio shows inverse trends in asthma prevalence before and after puberty, reflecting an increased risk among males during childhood and among females after adolescence. The specific reasons for these trends remain unknown because, in addition to hormonal factors, many other physical and behavioral changes associated with puberty might affect the natural history of asthma differentially in the two genders. For example, the height and weight spurts show gender-specific patterns and may have a more beneficial impact on the course of asthma among boys than girls, because boys are known to have narrower airways than girls before puberty. Of note, the increase in asthma risk among females after puberty might be related to higher rates of incidence of asthma, higher rates of persistence of asthma, or both. Findings from previous studies have been somewhat conflicting on a female predominance in asthma persistence, but they appear consistent in pointing toward a strong gender effect on asthma incidence. In the British 1958 Birth Cohort, the male:female incidence ratio for asthma was found to rise from 1.23 in the 0- to 7-year period to 1.48 at 12 to 16 years, but to reverse to 0.59 at 17 to 23 years.[9]

Although gender differences in asthma rates reflect mainly true differences in rates of respiratory symptoms between males and females, evidence is emerging that they may also be related to some diagnostic bias. Among children with asthma symptoms, boys appear more likely to receive a diagnosis of asthma than girls, a finding quite consistent across epidemiological studies, including the CRS cohort. There are many possible reasons for this gender difference. First, the asthma-related phenotypes might be different between boys and girls. For example, as compared with girls, in childhood boys have higher levels of atopic sensitization and, thus, they may be more likely to experience hay fever and other atopy-related phenotypes that support the label of asthma diagnosis in a wheezing child. In a cohort of 662 13-year-old children, gender differences in allergen sensitivities were found to explain only partly gender differences in diagnosed asthma.[10] Wheezing boys differ from wheezing girls also in the severity and onset of their disease. Boys are more likely to have frequent wheezing and the first onset of wheezing at an earlier age than girls and, thus, they may have more time and more opportunities to consult a physician. Alternatively, these differences might reflect different health-seeking behaviors by the parents and/or gender-specific diagnostic bias by the physicians. Interestingly, it has been hypothesized that physicians may be influenced by their adult patient's gender in labeling the case as asthma, emphysema, or chronic bronchitis. Regardless of their reasons, it is becoming increasingly evident that these gender-specific differences need to be taken into account when assessing the role of sex in asthma prevalence before and after the onset of puberty.

INCIDENCE AND PERSISTENCE OF ASTHMA IN ADULT AGE

Asthma in adult age can be either (1) truly adult-onset asthma or (2) a persistent or relapsing form of asthma that began in childhood.

Compared to asthma that begins in childhood, adult-onset asthma has been relatively little studied, partly because it is difficult to say what percentage of adult asthma truly began in adult life since most studies are retrospective and thus subject to errors in recall. Indeed, prospective studies have shown that, when previous early wheezing in preschool age is not taken into account, incident wheezing in adolescence is not uncommon. In the CRS cohort, approximately one in five subjects who had never wheezed between age 5 and the onset of puberty reported at least one wheezing episode after the onset of puberty and before age 16. In the British 1958 cohort study, the percentage of incident cases of asthma or wheezy bronchitis between the ages of 17 and 33 years was 24%.[11] In the Dunedin cohort[12] 28% of subjects who had no wheezing by age 10 reported incident wheezing between age 10 and 26 and 95% of them developed symptoms between 10 and 18 years, suggesting that most postpuberty incident cases may occur in early adult life. However, when adult-onset asthma is defined by a physician-confirmed report of asthma in mid- to late adult life, estimates are definitely lower and range from 1 to 12 cases/1000 subject years. These cases appear to be often quite severe, raising the possibility that mild cases of adult-onset asthma may be underdiagnosed.

Virtually all studies find that asthma incidence is greater for adult females than for adult males, with the difference being almost twofold in most populations. Adult-onset asthma may actually encompass several distinct subphenotypes, some of which may be particularly severe and refractory to treatment and show a weaker association with atopy as compared with cases of childhood asthma. In different individuals, adult-onset asthma may be triggered by aspirin sensitivity, chronic respiratory infections, smoking, allergic or nonallergic exposures in the workplace, or inhalation of irritants. These subphenotypes may differ in typical age of onset, associated comorbidities, and pathophysiologic mechanisms and, in turn, in their long-term sequelae (see "Long-term Sequelae of Asthma in Adult Life").

However, many cases of asthma in adult age are persistent or relapsing forms of asthma that began in childhood. Findings from the major long-term longitudinal cohorts on the natural history of asthma have consistently indicated that, in the general population, approximately one third of subjects who had episodes of wheezing in childhood report active asthma symptoms when surveyed in their young to mid-adult life. This proportion is markedly higher among subjects whose childhood asthma was severe, persisted over time, started early in life, and/or was characterized by reduced lung function. In this respect, data from the Melbourne Asthma Study, in which several groups of school-age children were enrolled based on their wheezing/asthma history and followed over time into their adulthood, are illustrative[13] (Fig. 4-3). At age 42, 15% of controls reported wheezing episodes in the preceding 3 years compared with 40% of subjects who, during childhood, had wheezing associated with bronchitis or respiratory tract

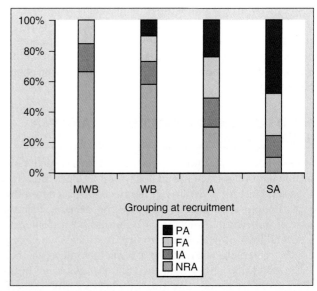

Figure 4-3   Clinical expression of childhood asthma at age 42 years. Histogram showing pattern of asthma at age 42 years in subjects from original recruitment groups in the Melbourne Epidemiological Study of Childhood Asthma. MWB, mild wheezy bronchitis; WB, wheezy bronchitis; A, asthma; SA, severe asthma; PA, persistent asthma; FA, frequent episodic asthma; IA, infrequent episodic asthma; NRA, no recent asthma. *(Data from Phelan PD, Robertson CF, Olinsky A: The Melbourne Asthma Study: 1964–1999. J Allergy Clin Immunol 2002;109:189–194.)*

infection. However, among subjects who had asthma or severe asthma during childhood, wheezing episodes were reported by 70% and 90%, respectively. In that study, childhood asthma was defined as wheezing in the absence of respiratory tract infection and severe childhood asthma was defined by a combination of criteria related to persistence of symptoms (persistent symptoms at 10 years of age), early onset of symptoms (before 3 years of age), and reduced lung function at 10 years of age (FEV_1/FVC ratio $\leq$ 50%). Of note, children in the group with severe asthma continued to show lower levels of lung function (including FEV_1 percentage predicted and the ratio FEV_1/FVC) throughout their adult life up to age 42 and the magnitude of these deficits in lung function was already established by the time they entered adult life (Fig. 4-4).

In the Melbourne Asthma Study, children with wheezing associated only with "bronchitis or respiratory tract infection" did not show significant lung function deficits in their adult life as compared with healthy peers. These findings appear to conflict to some extent with results from the CRS cohort, in which children with transient early wheezing had lower FEV_1, FEF_{25-75}, and FEV_1/FVC ratio at age 16, as compared with those who never wheezed. However, in the Melbourne Study wheezing history was assessed when the children were already 7 years old and, thus, the "wheezy bronchitis" groups in that study could be a mixture of transient early wheezers and children with mild asthma. These and other questions on the long-term consequences of early wheezing on adult lung function will have definite answers when children from ongoing birth cohort studies that assessed wheezing history in the first 3 years of life prospectively enter their mid-adult life.

PREDICTORS OF ASTHMA PERSISTENCE FROM CHILDHOOD TO ADULT AGE

Various longitudinal studies have investigated factors affecting persistence of asthma. When addressing specifically the outcome of childhood asthma in adolescence, we found that having frequent prepuberty wheezing, prepuberty bronchial hyperresponsiveness, early age at onset of puberty, prepuberty sinusitis, and being overweight and skin test positive at age 11 predicted the persistence of wheezing after the onset of puberty in a group of 166 children with asthma.[6] With the exception of the age at onset of puberty, all these factors had been previously reported as significant predictors of incidence and/or persistence of asthma in childhood and/or adult age, suggesting that adolescence may be mainly characterized by a change in the baseline risk for asthma in the two genders. Furthermore, findings from this and other studies indicate that risk factors for persistence and incidence of asthma overlap to some extent. In this section, we will review some of these factors (Table 4-1 shows a complete list of asthma risk factors discussed in this chapter).

Atopy

Atopy, as assessed by positive skin prick tests to aeroallergens or elevated serum IgE levels, has been consistently associated not only with incidence (see "Asthma Phenotypes in Infancy and Childhood"), but also with persistence and relapse of asthma. In the CRS cohort, children with asthma with positive skin prick tests to *Alternaria* had fourfold increased odds for persistent wheezing after the onset of puberty as compared with their peers with asthma and no sensitization to *Alternaria*.[6] In the Dunedin cohort, the corresponding odds ratios (OR) associated with positive skin prick tests for house-dust mites and cat allergen were 3.4 and 2.8, respectively, for persistence of asthma by age 26.[12] In that study, sensitization to house-dust mites and cat allergens was also associated

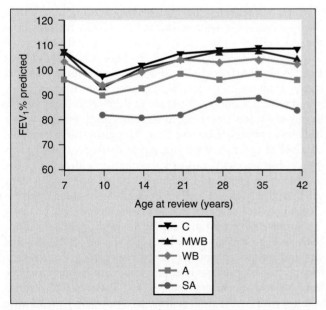

Figure 4-4   Lung function over time by classification at recruitment. FEV_1 percent predicted at ages 7, 10, 14, 21, 28, 35, and 42 years in subjects in their recruitment groups in the Melbourne Epidemiological Study of Childhood Asthma. C, control; MWB, mild wheezy bronchitis; WB, wheezy bronchitis; A, asthma; SA, severe asthma. *(Data from Phelan PD, Robertson CF, Olinsky A. The Melbourne Asthma Study: 1964–1999. J Allergy Clin Immunol 2002;109:189–194.)*

Table 4-1 RISK FACTORS FOR PERSISTENCE OF ASTHMA	
Risk Factor	**Chapter Section**
Female gender	Persistence and Remission of Asthma in Adolescence; Incidence and Persistence of Asthma in Adult Age
Severity and age at onset of wheezing	Incidence and Persistence of Asthma in Adult Age
Low lung function	Incidence and Persistence of Asthma in Adult Age
Bronchial hyperresponsiveness	Predictors of Asthma Persistence from Childhood to Adult Age
Atopy and atopic diseases	Asthma Phenotypes in Infancy and Childhood; Predictors of Asthma Persistence from Childhood to Adult Age
Upper airway disease	Predictors of Asthma Persistence from Childhood to Adult Age
Obesity	Predictors of Asthma Persistence from Childhood to Adult Age
Family history of asthma and atopy	Predictors of Asthma Persistence from Childhood to Adult Age
Smoking	Long-term Sequelae of Asthma in Adult Life

with threefold to fourfold increases in the odds for relapses of asthma. The mechanisms by which atopy increases the risk for asthma remain largely unknown.

Upper Airway Disease

Atopy may be also involved in the association between upper airway disease and asthma (see Chapter 44). In a group of 3371 consecutive patients from two asthma and allergy clinics in Sainte-Foy, Québec, approximately 59% of patients with asthma had a coexisting diagnosis of rhinitis.[14] The proportion of asthma patients reporting rhinitis symptoms varies to some extent across different studies, but the existence of a strong link between rhinitis (and sinusitis) and asthma has been consistently described in literature. Because of its postulated direct effects on asthma risk, atopy has been long believed to be the factor truly responsible for this association, but several recent lines of evidence suggest that the link between upper airway disease and asthma cannot be completely explained by confounding by atopy. Several studies have shown that rhinitis and asthma remain significantly associated after adjusting for skin prick tests results or IgE levels. Even more importantly, rhinitis has been linked to asthma both among atopic and non-atopic subjects. In the European Community Respiratory Health Survey, subjects with perennial rhinitis were found to have 16-fold increased odds of having asthma as compared with subjects with no rhinitis.[15] Surprisingly, the association between rhinitis and asthma was stronger among non-atopic subjects (adjusted OR: 11.6) as compared with atopic subjects (OR 8.1). Although any temporal relationship between the two diseases is possible, longitudinal studies have shown that the onset of rhinitis tends to precede the onset of asthma and that the presence of rhinitis increases the risk for both incidence and persistence of asthma. In the large British 1958 birth cohort, a prior report of hay fever increased the risk for asthma or wheeze up to age 23 by a factor between 1.9 and 2.3.[9] The predictive value of rhinitis for asthma has been confirmed in adult cohorts. Odds ratios for the association between rhinitis and subsequent development of asthma among adults were found to be very similar (between 4 and 5) in a random population sample in Sweden and in the Tucson Epidemiologic Study of Airway Obstructive Disease (TESAOD).[16,17] In the latter study, we found the risk of being diagnosed with asthma to increase as the duration and severity of nasal symptoms increased, according to a linear dose-response relationship (Fig. 4-5).

The possible causal nature of the association between rhinitis and asthma remains debated. Several mechanisms, including a neural nasal-bronchial reflex, postnasal drip of inflammatory cells and mediators, and mouth breathing caused by nasal obstruction, have been suggested to support direct effects of nasal dysfunction on the lower airway. There is also convincing experimental evidence that rhinitis treatment can play a direct role in modulating asthma among patients with both diseases. Intranasal use of corticosteroids, independent of the deposition of the drug into the lower airway, can reduce asthma symptoms and bronchial reactivity in patients with respiratory allergy. Consistently, large studies using claims databases have shown that, in patients with asthma, treatment of concomitant rhinitis results in lower risk for emergency department visits and hospitalizations for asthma.

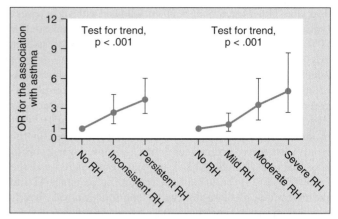

Figure 4-5 Odds ratios (ORs) for the association with asthma and 95% confidence intervals across different levels of duration and severity of rhinitis (RH) among adult participants in the Tucson Epidemiological Study of Airway Obstructive Disease. ORs were adjusted for years of follow-up, age, sex, atopic status, smoking status, and presence of COPD. Rhinitis was coded as mild (severity of nasal symptoms ranked 1 or 2 by the patient on a 5-level ranking scale), moderate (rank 3), or severe (rank 4 or 5). *(Data from Guerra S, Sherrill DL, Martinez FD, Barbee RA: Rhinitis as an independent risk factor for adult-onset asthma. J Allergy Clin Immunol 2002;109:419–425.)*

Based on the existing evidence, the workshop group Allergic Rhinitis and its Impact on Asthma (ARIA) recommended a combined strategy to treat the upper and lower airway diseases in patients with coexisting diseases.[18] Questions that still remain open are whether early treatment of nasal symptoms can modify the progression from rhinitis to asthma and to what extent it can affect the clinical course of asthma once the disease has occurred.

Obesity and Age at Onset of Puberty

Obesity has recently received much attention as a potential risk factor for asthma. In the late 1990s, findings from the longitudinal cohort of the Nurses' Health Study pointed toward a strong, independent, and positive association of body mass index (BMI) with risk of adult-onset asthma.[19] In that study, adult women with BMI greater than 30kg/m^2 were found to be 2.7 times more likely to develop incident asthma during the study follow-up, as compared with women whose BMI was between 20.0 and 22.4. This association was independent of age, race, smoking, physical activity, total energy intake, birth weight, and other potential confounders. The link between obesity and asthma has been confirmed in many other studies. Taken together, evidence from these epidemiological studies suggests that (1) being overweight or obese is a strong risk factor for acquiring a new diagnosis of asthma both among children and adults; (2) the link between obesity and asthma appears to be stronger among women than men; (3) obesity is associated not only with incident asthma, but also with persistent asthma (i.e., patients with asthma who are overweight are less likely to remit than patients with asthma who are not overweight).

As in the case of rhinitis, the possible causal nature of the relationship of obesity with asthma remains debated. It has been argued that patients with asthma might be less likely to exercise and, in turn, more likely to gain weight and be exposed to environmental tobacco and indoor allergens, as compared with healthy peers; i.e., obesity might be the effect rather than the cause of asthma (reverse causation). Data from longitudinal studies, however, do not support this hypothesis since elevated BMI levels among disease-free subjects have been found to be predictive of subsequent development of new asthma, supporting a specific obesity→asthma temporal sequence. In the TESAOD cohort, for example, we assessed the presence of an elevated BMI among asthmatic patients both before the asthma diagnosis and before the onset of respiratory symptoms (first report of shortness of breath with wheezing).[20] In both cases, the proportion of overweight or obese subjects (BMI > 28) was significantly higher among patients than among control subjects, with the corresponding ORs for asthma being 2.25 and 2.29, respectively.

Obesity may be linked to asthma also through its effects on disease perception and/or lung function. Being overweight may lead to an increased work of breathing, predispose to sleep disorders and gastroesophageal reflux disease, and directly affect lung function and airway caliber through chest wall restriction. Alternatively, specific molecular mechanisms involving leptin and/or sex hormones may be part of the possible causal pathway from obesity to asthma. The latter hypothesis is supported by two observations. First, the link between obesity and asthma appears stronger among women than men, suggesting an important role of sex hormones. In this respect, it is known that the course of asthma can be affected by pregnancy and the menstrual cycle because of hormonal fluctuations, and that sex hormones can alter cytokine production from peripheral blood mononuclear cells. Second, age at onset of puberty has been correlated inversely with risk and severity of asthma in several studies. In the CRS cohort, we found that the odds of having persistent asthma were reduced by 35% for every 1-year increase in the age at onset of puberty.[6] In the same cohort, a strong interaction exists between obesity and age at onset of puberty in affecting the risk of incident wheezing in girls. Consistent with these findings, investigators from the Epidemiological Study on the Genetics and Environment of Asthma found that, in a group of 177 asthmatic women, BMI was directly correlated with severity of asthma but only among women with early menarche (menarche at 11 years or earlier).[21]

Dissecting the independent contributions of obesity and early menarche to asthma risk is difficult because obesity strongly increases the likelihood of early menarche itself. Nevertheless, these associations suggest the possibility that molecular factors (e.g., sex hormones, hormonal disruptors, leptin) may mediate complex interactions between the developmental processes of body growth and sexual maturation and their impact on the natural history of asthma. Among these factors, leptin represents an interesting candidate molecule. It is secreted by adipocytes, is increased in obese subjects, and appears to be one of the signals controlling sexual maturation. Receptors for leptin have been shown to be present in the airways, and, thus, this molecule might be involved in the regulation of lung physiology and airway inflammation. Whether the effects of overweight on asthma are mediated by structural or molecular mechanisms, optimal weight control of patients with (or at risk of) asthma should always be a specific goal of the physician. Weight reduction in obese asthma patients can lead to better lung function, but educating patients about weight control has multiple health benefits.

Bronchial Hyperresponsiveness

Bronchial hyperresponsiveness (BHR) has been linked to both incidence and persistence of asthma. Positive responses to methacholine challenge tests are more common among children having wheezing (especially if persistent or relapsing wheezing) than healthy peers. In a longitudinal cohort of third- and fourth-grade schoolchildren in Australia, children with a positive histamine challenge test at age 8 to 12 were at significantly increased risk for persistence of wheeze up to age 27.[22] In the same cohort, severity of BHR at school age was correlated with persistence of both BHR and respiratory symptoms at age 12 to 14. Further research is required to determine whether and to what extent the predictive value of BHR for persistence of asthma is independent of the well-known effects of severity of the disease and low lung function (see "Incidence and Persistence of Asthma in Adult Age").

Positive Family History

Almost invariably, studies have shown that a positive family history of asthma or asthma-related phenotypes (such as atopic diseases) strongly increases the risk of a child developing asthma and experiencing persistent symptoms. In the Tasmanian Asthma Survey, among subjects who did not have childhood asthma, maternal hay fever was associated with an 80% increase in the odds of having active asthma at age 30.[23] In addition, among subjects who had childhood asthma, both maternal and paternal asthma were associated with significantly increased odds for active asthma at age 30. Of note, all these factors remained significant in multivariate models adjusting for other predictors of asthma. The familiar aggregation of asthma (and related atopic phenotypes) can reflect either genetic or environmental factors (or both) that are shared within families. In asthma, there is evidence to believe that the predictive value of a positive family history for asthma mainly reflects the strong genetic component of the disease. The search for the genes whose variation is involved in asthma has not provided definitive answers yet and continues to be at the forefront of asthma research. In this framework, it is noteworthy that, all evidence considered, it is likely that genetic variation may affect not only the risk for incident asthma, but also the natural history of the disease. Both genes directly affecting the airways and their responses to asthma treatment (e.g., the beta$_2$-adrenoceptor) and genes affecting some of the aforementioned risk factors for asthma (e.g., genes associated with atopy or obesity) could play an important role in determining which patients outgrow their asthma and which ones do not.

LONG-TERM SEQUELAE OF ASTHMA IN ADULT LIFE

In asthma epidemiology, some of the most compelling questions relate to the possible sequelae of the disease: to what extent is asthma associated with long-term sequelae in adult life? Is it possible to identify at an early stage patients destined to progress to non–fully reversible airflow limitation? Can asthma treatment affect the natural history of the disease at all?

The two long-term outcomes that have received the most attention are reduced lung function and comorbidity with COPD, both of which represent important risk factors for mortality in adult populations. Reduced lung function in adult patients with asthma can be due to deficits that are established by the end of childhood or an accelerated decline of lung function once the patient has entered adult life, or both. Prospective studies that have followed samples of the general population in the transition from childhood into adult life have provided solid evidence that, in cases of severe and/or persistent asthma, lung function deficits are already present before adult life begins and track strongly over time. In this regard, some of the most illustrative data come from the Dunedin Study[13] (Fig. 4-6). In that study,

children with persistent wheezing had consistently lower values of the FEV_1/FVC ratio as compared with controls, with a mean deficit of almost 7%. These deficits were present from age 9 up to age 26, with no significant difference in the slopes of change in the FEV_1/FVC ratio between persistent wheezers and controls. In contrast, in the Busselton Health Study and in the Copenhagen City Heart Study, two prospective cohort studies on adults, asthma was associated with both initial FEV_1 deficits at age 20 years and an increased slope of FEV_1 decline in adulthood.[24,25] However, the magnitude of the FEV_1 decline associated with asthma was quite different in the two studies, being only 4 mL per year in the Busselton Study. In the TESAOD Study, after taking into account comorbidity with COPD, we found that FEV_1 levels were lower but the slopes of FEV_1 decline were not steeper in asthmatic individuals, as compared with controls.[26] Taken together, these findings suggest that (1) significant deficits in lung function are already present in early adult life in those with severe and persistent asthma in childhood, suggesting the existence of early damage to lung growth and/or early airway remodeling; (2) during adulthood accelerated decline of FEV_1 might be present for subgroups of asthmatic individuals, but, once the effects of smoking are removed, this accelerated decline is likely to account for a limited proportion of the asthma-related deficits in lung function.

The deficits in lung function associated with asthma are strictly related to another issue of considerable importance in terms of prognosis of asthma: the overlap between asthma and COPD in adult life.[27] At the population level, adult subjects who report asthma are more likely to also report chronic bronchitis and/or emphysema than are subjects with no asthma. That individual patients can have different combinations of asthma, chronic bronchitis, and emphysema can be effectively illustrated using a Venn diagram[28] (Fig. 4-7). In the US National Health and Nutrition

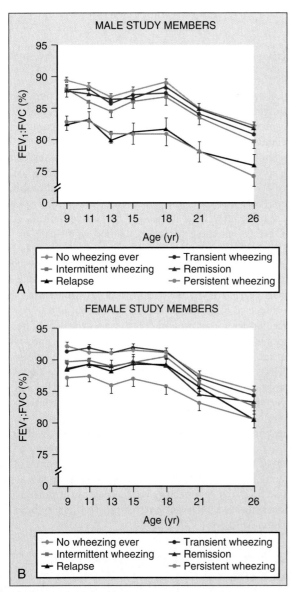

Figure 4-6 Mean (± SE) FEV_1/FVC ratios measured at 9, 11, 13, 15, 18, 21, and 26 years in male (Panel A) and female (Panel B) participants in the Dunedin Multidisciplinary Health and Development Study, according to the pattern of wheezing. (Data from Sears MR, Greene JM, Willan AR, et al: A longitudinal, population-based, cohort study of childhood asthma followed to adulthood. N Engl J Med 2003;349:1414–1422.)

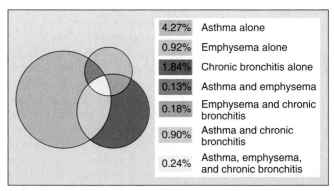

Figure 4-7 Proportional Venn diagram of obstructive lung disease (asthma, chronic bronchitis, and emphysema) in the United States (National Health and Nutrition Examination Survey [NHANES] III, 1988–1994) for all ages. The circle areas are a proportional representation of the prevalence of asthma, chronic bronchitis, and emphysema in the US NHANES III population. The areas of intersection represent subjects with more than one condition. Prevalence rates are listed for each of the seven possible combinations. (Adapted with permission from Guerra S: Overlap of asthma and chronic obstructive pulmonary disease. Curr Opin Pulm Med 2005;11:7–13. Data from Soriano JB, Davis KJ, Coleman B, et al: The proportional Venn diagram of obstructive lung disease: two approximations from the United States and the United Kingdom. Chest 2003;124:474–481.)

Examination Survey (NHANES) III, 8.5% of the participants reported asthma, chronic bronchitis, or emphysema. Of these subjects, approximately 17% reported more than one of these conditions. As compared with subjects reporting only one condition, those who reported having two or three obstructive lung diseases are older, have higher prevalence of airflow limitation, and are at increased risk for mortality.

The overlap of asthma, chronic bronchitis, and emphysema can have several explanations. First, part of this overlap may be explained by confusion in terminology. For example, it has been shown that only a minority of subjects reporting chronic bronchitis in epidemiological surveys meet the criteria for the presence of chronic cough and phlegm that define the disease. Similarly, assessment of emphysema is challenging in the epidemiological setting.

Alternatively, the overlap between these obstructive lung diseases may be explained by the fact that they share common risk factors. Genetic variation in key genes, for instance, might be involved in the pathogenesis and clinical progression of more than one of these diseases. Occupation exposures are important risk factors in adult age for asthma, chronic bronchitis, and emphysema. Asthma-related intermediate phenotypes, such as BHR and elevated IgE, may be significant predictors of the clinical progression of COPD. Conversely, smoking, the long-recognized major risk factor for COPD, may be also associated with elevated IgE, eosinophilia, and BHR. Of note, active smoking was strongly associated with adult-onset wheezing in the British 1958 Birth Cohort, showing a clear dose-response relationship. In that same cohort as well as in the Dunedin Study, active smoking was also associated with an almost twofold increase of the odds for persistent wheezing. Indeed, dissecting the relation of smoking to asthma is complicated by the overlap between obstructive lung diseases, which makes it difficult to distinguish what effects of smoking are specific to asthma as opposed to the related diseases of chronic bronchitis and emphysema. In addition, the existence of a "healthy smoker" effect should be always taken into account as patients with severe asthma may be less likely to engage in cigarette smoking and the association between smoking and asthma might, in turn, be underestimated because of this.

Finally, the overlap of asthma, chronic bronchitis, and emphysema might be explained by the possible progression of asthma into COPD. This hypothesis appears supported by recent studies. In the TESAOD cohort, adult subjects with active asthma were found to have a 10-times higher risk of acquiring chronic bronchitis and a 17-times higher risk of acquiring emphysema over time than subjects with no asthma, even after adjusting for smoking.[29] In that study, chronic bronchitis and emphysema were defined by the presence of chronic symptoms, a physician-confirmed diagnosis, and objective lung function measurements, such as FEV_1 or diffusing capacity of the lung for carbon monoxide of less than 80% predicted. However, no information on response to bronchodilator was available.

The fact that the definitions of asthma, chronic bronchitis, and emphysema are not mutually exclusive and are differentially based on clinical, anatomic, or functional conditions has been a major source of confusion in estimating and understanding the overlap of these diseases. In addition, chronic bronchitis and emphysema have been traditionally considered two phenotypes of COPD, but these terms are often used incorrectly and capture only some of the complex structural abnormalities and clinical symptoms associated with the disease. Recently, the Scientific Committee of the National Heart, Lung, and Blood Institute/World Health Organization (NHLBI/WHO) Global Initiative for Chronic Obstructive Lung Disease (GOLD) defined COPD as a disease state characterized by airflow limitation that is not fully reversible, and recommended the use of post-bronchodilator values of the FEV_1/FVC ratio to confirm the existence of such non–fully reversible airflow limitation.[30]

When using the GOLD definition of COPD, the evidence in support of the possible progression of asthma into COPD appears even stronger. Once again, findings from the Dunedin Study are illustrative (Fig. 4-6). In that study, children with persistent and relapsing wheezing had consistently lower FEV_1/FVC ratio from age 9 up to age 26, suggesting that they are at increased risk for falling below the level of 70% (the GOLD defining cut-off level of FEV_1/FVC for COPD) at an earlier age, as compared with other children. These data also suggest that, if any preventive interventions are to effectively reduce this risk, they need to be started early, as lung function deficits are already established by the end of childhood.

Whether these asthma-related deficits are still completely responsive to bronchodilators as the children enter adult life remains to be determined. In the Melbourne Study, subjects who were originally classified as children with severe asthma at the beginning of the study had a mean FEV_1/FVC ratio below 70% and accounted for most of those with moderate-to-severe airflow limitation at age 35. However, only 14% of subjects with FEV_1% predicted <70% had an improvement of less than 10% after inhaled salbutamol. Interestingly, at 42 years of age, 50% of subjects who had FEV_1% predicted <70% had an improvement of less than 10% and/or FEV_1 values that remained below 70% after inhaled salbutamol. These data suggest that, although most cases of moderate-to-severe airflow limitation in mid-adult life associated with childhood asthma are limited to subjects with severe forms of the disease, in this subgroup progressive loss of responsiveness to bronchodilators and the onset of non–fully reversible airflow limitation are not uncommon events.

In summary, although the epidemiological evidence available to date on the long-term sequelae of asthma is limited, most studies appear to support one of the two hypothetical scenarios depicted in Figure 4-8. In children with severe and/or persistent asthma, significant deficits of lung function are established by the time the lung growth is completed. As compared with lung function of healthy peers, these asthma-related deficits can either track over time throughout adult life (Fig. 4-8A) or they can worsen during adulthood because of an accelerated decline of lung function (Fig. 4-8B). The latter scenario likely applies to specific subphenotypes of asthma or to synergistic effects of asthma with exposure to noxious agents, such as smoking. It is likely that, for each patient with asthma, the magnitude of the asthma-related deficits in lung function can take any value between the levels of healthy peers (blue

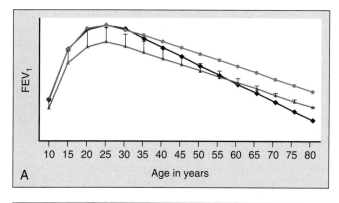

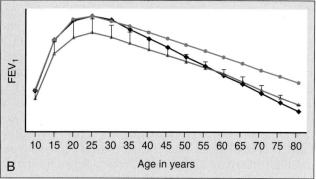

Figure 4-8   Possible scenarios of growth and decline of FEV₁ values over time in healthy subjects (blue line; • symbol), subjects with severe and/or persistent asthma that began in childhood (orange line; ▲ symbol), and subjects with COPD associated with exposure to noxious agents such as smoking (red line; ♦ symbol). Black error bars associated with orange lines represent the level of FEV₁ that can be attained after bronchodilator among patients with persistent asthma (responsiveness to bronchodilator). **A,** Persistent asthma is associated with lower levels of FEV₁ but not with steeper slopes of FEV₁ decline in adult age. **B,** Persistent asthma is associated with both lower levels and steeper slopes of decline of FEV₁ in adult age.

line; • symbol) and those of severely asthmatic individuals (orange line; ▲ symbol), depending on the severity and persistence of the disease. In addition, the clinical course of persistent asthma can be characterized by a progressive loss of responsiveness to bronchodilator and, in turn, development of non–fully reversible airflow limitation. Thus, as severely asthmatic patients grow older, they can show profiles of non–fully reversible airflow limitation that are indistinguishable from those of patients with COPD, most of whom, however, experience a different natural history of the disease (red line; ♦symbol), starting adult life with normal lung function and showing subsequently an accelerated decline of lung function because of their exposure to noxious agents such as smoking.

Finally, it is noteworthy that the possible progression of persistent asthma into irreversible airflow limitation depicted in Figure 4-8 appears to support the central idea of the so-called Dutch Hypothesis: "The asthmatic child becomes the father of the COPD man." However, it should also be acknowledged that the development of COPD-like signs occurs only in subgroups of patients with asthma and that these patients can still be differentiated from patients with smoking-related COPD based on many other functional, morphological, and immunological factors. Research is very much needed to determine whether early treatment and optimal management of asthma might reduce the proportion of asthma cases that ultimately develop persistent airflow limitation and whether patients with coexisting signs of asthma and COPD may benefit from management strategies that are based on multiple functional, morphologic, and immunologic assessments rather than on a categorization into rigid diagnostic labels of either asthma or COPD.

REFERENCES

1. Martinez FD, Wright AL, Taussig LM, et al: Asthma and wheezing in the first six years of life. The Group Health Medical Associates. N Engl J Med 1995;332:133–138.
2. Morgan WJ, Stern DA, Sherrill DL, et al: Outcome of asthma and wheezing in the first 6 years of life: Follow-up through adolescence. Am J Respir Crit Care Med 2005;172:1253–1258.
3. Crestani E, Guerra S, Wright AL, et al: Parental asthma as a risk factor for the development of early skin test sensitization in children. J Allergy Clin Immunol 2004;113:284–290.
4. Martinez FD, Stern DA, Wright AL, et al: Association of interleukin-2 and interferon-gamma production by blood mononuclear cells in infancy with parental allergy skin tests and with subsequent development of atopy. J Allergy Clin Immunol 1995;96(5 Pt 1):652–660.
5. Guerra S, Lohman IC, Halonen M, et al: Reduced interferon gamma production and soluble CD14 levels in early life predict recurrent wheezing by 1 year of age. Am J Respir Crit Care Med 2004;169:70–76.
6. Guerra S, Wright AL, Morgan WJ, et al: Persistence of asthma symptoms during adolescence: role of obesity and age at the onset of puberty. Am J Respir Crit Care Med 2004;170:78–85.
7. Taylor DR, Cowan JO, Greene JM, et al: Asthma in remission: can relapse in early adulthood be predicted at 18 years of age? Chest 2005;127:845–850.
8. Vonk JM, Postma DS, Boezen HM, et al: Childhood factors associated with asthma remission after 30 year follow up. Thorax 2004;59:925–929.
9. Anderson HR, Pottier AC, Strachan DP: Asthma from birth to age 23: Incidence and relation to prior and concurrent atopic disease. Thorax 1992;47:537–542.
10. Sears MR, Burrows B, Flannery EM, et al: Atopy in childhood. I. Gender and allergen related risks for development of hay fever and asthma. Clin Exp Allergy 1993;23:941–948.
11. Strachan DP, Butland BK, Anderson HR: Incidence and prognosis of asthma and wheezing illness from early childhood to age 33 in a national British cohort. BMJ 1996;312:1195–1199.
12. Sears MR, Greene JM, Willan AR, et al: A longitudinal, population-based, cohort study of childhood asthma followed to adulthood. N Engl J Med 2003;349:1414–1422.
13. Phelan PD, Robertson CF, Olinsky A: The Melbourne Asthma Study: 1964–1999. J Allergy Clin Immunol 2002;109:189–194.
14. Boulet LP, Turcotte H, Laprise C, et al: Comparative degree and type of sensitization to common indoor and outdoor allergens in subjects with allergic rhinitis and/or asthma. Clin Exp Allergy 1997;27:52–59.
15. Leynaert B, Bousquet J, Neukirch C, et al: Perennial rhinitis: An independent risk factor for asthma in nonatopic subjects: results from the European Community Respiratory Health Survey. J Allergy Clin Immunol 1999;104(2 Pt. 1):301–304.

16. Plaschke PP, Janson C, Norrman E, et al: Onset and remission of allergic rhinitis and asthma and the relationship with atopic sensitization and smoking. Am J Respir Crit Care Med 2000;162(3 Pt 1):920–924.

17. Guerra S, Sherrill DL, Martinez FD, Barbee RA: Rhinitis as an independent risk factor for adult-onset asthma. J Allergy Clin Immunol 2002;109:419–425.

18. Bousquet J, Van Cauwenberge P, Khaltaev N: Allergic rhinitis and its impact on asthma. J Allergy Clin Immunol 2001;108 (5 Suppl):S147–S334.

19. Camargo CA, Jr., Weiss ST, Zhang S, et al: Prospective study of body mass index, weight change, and risk of adult-onset asthma in women [see comments]. Arch Intern Med 1999;159:2582–2588.

20. Guerra S, Sherrill DL, Bobadilla A, et al: The relation of body mass index to asthma, chronic bronchitis, and emphysema. Chest 2002;122:1256–1263.

21. Varraso R, Siroux V, Maccario J, et al: Asthma severity is associated with body mass index and early menarche in women. Am J Respir Crit Care Med 2005;171:334–339.

22. Xuan W, Marks GB, Toelle BG, et al: Risk factors for onset and remission of atopy, wheeze, and airway hyperresponsiveness. Thorax 2002;57:104–109.

23. Jenkins MA, Hopper JL, Bowes G, et al: Factors in childhood as predictors of asthma in adult life. BMJ 1994;309:90–93.

24. James AL, Palmer LJ, Kicic E, et al: Decline in lung function in the Busselton Health Study: The effects of asthma and cigarette smoking. Am J Respir Crit Care Med 2005;171:109–114.

25. Lange P, Parner J, Vestbo J, et al: A 15-year follow-up study of ventilatory function in adults with asthma. N Engl J Med 1998;339:1194–1200.

26. Sherrill D, Guerra S, Bobadilla A, Barbee R: The role of concomitant respiratory diseases on the rate of decline in FEV1 among adult asthmatics. Eur Respir J 2003;21:95–100.

27. Guerra S: Overlap of asthma and chronic obstructive pulmonary disease. Curr Opin Pulm Med 2005;11:7–13.

28. Soriano JB, Davis KJ, Coleman B, et al: The proportional Venn diagram of obstructive lung disease: Two approximations from the United States and the United Kingdom. Chest 2003;124:474–481.

29. Silva GE, Sherrill DL, Guerra S, Barbee RA: Asthma as a risk factor for COPD in a longitudinal study. Chest 2004;126: 59–65.

30. Pauwels RA, Buist AS, Calverley PM, et al: Global strategy for the diagnosis, management, and prevention of chronic obstructive pulmonary disease. NHLBI/WHO Global Initiative for Chronic Obstructive Lung Disease (GOLD) Workshop summary. Am J Respir Crit Care Med 2001;163: 1256–1276.

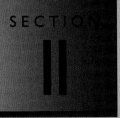

SECTION

II

DIAGNOSIS OF ASTHMA

What Is Asthma?

Jessica H. Boyd and Robert C. Strunk

CLINICAL PEARLS

- There is no pathognomic set of clinical characteristics or diagnostic test for asthma that is not shared by other disease entities.

- In the natural history of asthma, there is improvement in morbidity in late adolescence with relapse in later decades when airway size decreases as part of normal aging. During remission of symptoms in adolescence, evidence of asthma is present during testing of pulmonary function.

- Persistence of symptoms and associated airway responsiveness are promoted by ongoing exposure to perennial allergens to which the patient is sensitized. Keeping furry pets is a major factor in persistence.

- Clinicians generally agree that asthma is a wheezing disease (recognizing that not all that wheezes is asthma), but patients with asthma can also have other symptoms, cough being most prominent.

- All that wheezes is not asthma. Making a diagnosis of asthma often requires consideration of differential diagnoses.

"What is asthma?" may be the most difficult question to be answered in this book. Clinicians in both primary care and subspecialty medicine know what asthma is when they sit in front of a patient presenting with frequent wheeze at times other than with colds. However, there is no universally agreed-upon definition of asthma and there is no pathognomic set of clinical features and no diagnostic test that is not positive in diseases other than asthma. This chapter will undertake a careful consideration of the different aspects of the disease that we all know to be asthma.

WHAT EXACTLY IS ASTHMA?

Asthma is a chronic disease of the airways with tremendous public health implications that affects an estimated 20 million people in the United States and 100 to 150 million people worldwide. In 2002, asthma contributed to 14.7 million missed school days, 11.8 million lost work days, 13.9 million outpatient visits, 1.9 million emergency room visits, 484,000 hospitalizations, and 4261 deaths.[1] The economic impact of asthma was estimated at more than $12.5 billion per year in 1998.[2]

The impact of asthma is unquestionable, but what exactly is asthma? In general, asthma is characterized by recurrent episodes of wheezing, cough, breathlessness, and chest tightness. The episodes most often begin in childhood, frequently with a period of apparent remission of symptoms during adolescence and then resurgence in adulthood as lung function declines as a part of the normal aging process. Airway inflammation

and associated bronchial hyperresponsiveness can be initiated acutely by exposure to allergens to which the person is sensitized or viral infection, and result in at least partly reversible airway obstruction. Asthma can also be a persistent disease with chronic airway inflammation and airway remodeling contributing to the clinical course. The symptoms and clinical presentation of asthma are highly variable and defining asthma is complex with the expression of multiple phenotypes.

Clinical, pathophysiologic, and epidemiologic definitions have emerged describing asthma at the individual, cellular, and population levels. The National Heart, Lung, and Blood Institute (NHLBI) and the National Asthma Education and Prevention Program (NAEPP) Expert Panel put forth this comprehensive working definition, which serves as an important starting point in the discussion of what is asthma:

Asthma is a chronic inflammatory disorder of the airways in which many cells and cellular elements play a role, in particular, mast cells, eosinophils, T lymphocytes, neutrophils, and epithelial cells. In susceptible individuals, this inflammation causes recurrent episodes of wheezing, breathlessness, chest tightness, and cough, particularly at night and in the early morning. These episodes are usually associated with widespread but variable airflow obstruction that is often reversible either spontaneously or with treatment. The inflammation also causes an associated increase in the existing bronchial hyperresponsiveness to a variety of stimuli.[3]

In this chapter, various definitions of asthma will be explored, with particular emphasis on the elements outlined in the NHLBI working definition. At the cellular level, changes occur in the airway as a result of acute and chronic airway inflammation resulting in the symptoms of asthma. At the individual level, recurrent episodes of wheezing and other symptoms reflect the cellular level changes associated with asthma as it presents to the physician or health care provider. Additionally, the various phenotypes of asthma present differently on a population level, affecting how we think about the impact of asthma.

PATHOPHYSIOLOGIC DEFINITION OF ASTHMA

What causes the symptoms of asthma and what are the changes that occur in the lungs of patients with asthma? Asthma is characterized by several changes in the airways including smooth muscle hyperplasia, thickening of the basement membrane, denudation of epithelial cells, airway tissue edema, and mucosal gland hypertrophy, all of which contribute to the composite of clinical symptoms that characterize asthma. Numerous cell types contribute to asthma. Of particular importance are T-helper 2 (TH2) cells, eosinophils, antigen-presenting macrophages, mast cells, and respiratory epithelial cells.

Airway Inflammation

Airway inflammation plays a central role in asthma (Fig. 5-1). Acutely, airway inflammation contributes to airflow limitation through bronchoconstriction, mucus production, and airway edema. Allergic inflammation, characterized by elevated levels of immunoglobulin E, stimulates an immune response driven by TH2 lymphocytes, which activate airway mast cells, macrophages, and other proinflammatory mediators. This cascade leads to the contraction of the smooth muscle in the airways, increased secretion of mucus into the airway, and vasodilation of airway vessels. Exposure to exacerbating factors such as allergens, irritants, and viruses results in a bronchoconstrictive response and consequently acute asthma exacerbations with wheezing and respiratory distress. In conjunction with airway hyperresponsiveness, the changes result in narrowing of the airways and airflow obstruction, which in the acute setting of asthma is at least partly reversible.

Chronic inflammation also plays a role in asthma by producing abnormalities of airway obstruction and chronic symptomatology and predisposition to exacerbations with exposure to relevant allergens and irritants, and recurrence of viral infection. Chronic inflammation also modifies nonspecific bronchial hyperresponsiveness, which facilitates airway narrowing in response to these exacerbating factors. Eosinophils are key cells in chronic inflammation, promoting the release of proinflammatory mediators and cytokines that results in changes in the airways. Chronic inflammation is associated pathologically with hyperplasia of the smooth muscle of the airway, increased number of goblet cells, basement membrane thickening, and shedding of epithelial cells with loss of cilia. Chronic inflammation represents persistent damage to the airway, and as the airway is healed, remodeling occurs.

Airway Obstruction

In patients with asthma, airway inflammation leads to variable levels of lower airway obstruction that affects both the small and large airways. Recurrent airflow limitation is caused by bronchoconstriction, airway edema, chronic mucus plug

formation, and airway remodeling. Usually, the obstruction can be improved with bronchodilators and corticosteroids; however, in the setting of chronic inflammation and airway remodeling, airway obstruction may be persistent and irreversible. Spirometry is an important tool to identify lower airway obstruction, helping to support a diagnosis of asthma.

Airway Hyperresponsiveness

Airway hyperresponsiveness is associated with airway inflammation and underlies the presentation of symptoms in asthma. It also contributes to acute exacerbations and bronchoconstriction when the airways are exposed to a stimulant, such as relevant allergens, environmental irritants, cold air, and exercise among others. Hyperresponsiveness not only contributes to the acute symptoms of bronchoconstriction and airflow limitation, but has also been shown to be associated with a decline in lung function in adulthood.[4] For diagnostic purposes, bronchoconstrictive agents such as methacholine may be used to determine the presence of hyperresponsiveness and to define its level, which is associated with the severity of asthma.

Airway Remodeling

Airway remodeling, as previously described, represents the healing and alteration in the airway that occur as a consequence of chronic inflammation. The airway wall becomes thickened with the increase in smooth muscle in the airway. Mucous glands are increased in number, affecting the thickness of the airway wall and increasing mucus secretion and inflammatory exudate that increase surface tension and promote closure of the airway. The reticular basement membrane also becomes thickened with the deposition of collagens. Changes that result in increasing thickness of the airway wall exaggerate the degree of airway obstruction with any given stimulus. With ongoing exposure to factors producing inflammation, disorder in the healing process as a result of ongoing inflammation produces changes in the airway that become irreversible. This airway remodeling results in persistent disease and is associated with ongoing presence of asthma symptoms and increased frequency of exacerbations.[5]

CLINICAL COURSE OF ASTHMA

Symptoms

The cardinal symptom of asthma is recurrent wheezing, but all that wheezes is not asthma and not all asthma wheezes. According to the NHLBI expert panel report, a history of recurrent wheezing, cough, breathlessness, or chest tightness suggests a possible diagnosis of asthma.[3] Taking a good history of symptoms, precipitating factors, and development of the disease and its prior response to treatment are extremely important in the process of understanding asthma in an individual patient (Box 5-1). Symptoms may be precipitated by factors such as exercise, allergic stimuli, viral infections, cold air, and tobacco smoke. Weather change is also a commonly reported precipitating factor. It may be difficult for children and their caregivers to recognize or describe the classic symptoms, and the context of symptoms is important in diagnosis. For example, eliciting a history of coughing particularly

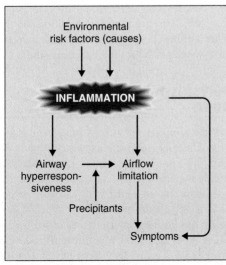

Figure 5-1 Schematic diagram of asthma.

BOX 5-1 Suggested Items for Medical History

A detailed medical history of the new patient who is known or thought to have asthma should address the following items*:

1. Symptoms

   Cough
   Wheezing
   Shortness of breath
   Chest tightness
   Sputum production

2. Pattern of symptoms

   Perennial, seasonal, or both
   Continual, episodic, or both
   Onset, duration, frequency (number of days or nights, per week or month)
   Diurnal variations, especially nocturnal and on awakening in early morning

3. Precipitating and/or aggravating factors

   Viral respiratory infections
   Environmental allergens, indoor (e.g., mold, house-dust mite, cockroach, animal dander or secretory products) and outdoor (e.g., pollen)
   Exercise
   Occupational chemicals or allergens
   Environmental change (e.g., moving to new home; going on vacation; and/or alterations in workplace, work processes, or materials used)
   Irritants (e.g., tobacco smoke, strong odors, air pollutants, occupational chemicals, dusts and particulates, vapors, gases, and aerosols)
   Emotional expressions (e.g., fear, anger, frustration, hard crying or laughing)
   Drugs (e.g., aspirin; beta-blockers, including eye drops; nonsteroidal anti-inflammatory drugs; others)
   Food, food additives, and preservatives (e.g., sulfites)
   Changes in weather, exposure to cold air
   Endocrine factors (e.g., menses, pregnancy, thyroid disease)

4. Development of disease and treatment

   Age of onset and diagnosis
   History of early-life injury to airways (e.g., bronchopulmonary dysplasia, pneumonia, parental smoking)
   Progress of disease (better or worse)
   Present management and response, including plans for managing exacerbations
   Need for oral corticosteroids and frequency of use
   Comorbid conditions

5. Family history

   History of asthma, allergy, sinusitis, rhinitis, or nasal polyps in close relatives

6. Social history

   Characteristics of home including age, location, cooling and heating system, wood-burning stove, humidifier, carpeting over concrete, presence of molds or mildew, characteristics of rooms where patient spends time (e.g., bedroom and living room with attention to bedding, floor covering, stuffed furniture)
   Smoking (patient and others in home or day care)
   Day care, workplace, and school characteristics that may interfere with adherence
   Social factors that interfere with adherence, such as substance abuse
   Social support/social networks
   Level of education completed
   Employment (if employed, characteristics of work environment)

7. Profile of typical exacerbation

   Usual prodromal signs and symptoms
   Usual patterns and management (what works?)

8. Impact of asthma on patient and family

   Episodes of unscheduled care (emergency department, urgent care, hospitalization)
   Life-threatening exacerbations (e.g., intubation, intensive care unit admission)
   Number of days missed from school/work
   Limitation of activity, especially sports and strenuous work
   History of nocturnal awakening
   Effect on growth, development, behavior, school or work performance, and lifestyle
   Impact on family routines, activities, or dynamics
   Economic impact

9. Assessment of patient's and family's perceptions of disease

   Patient, parental, and spouse's or partner's knowledge of asthma and belief in the chronicity of asthma and in the efficacy of treatment
   Patient perception and beliefs regarding use and long-term effects of medications
   Ability of patient and parents, spouse, or partner to cope with disease
   Level of family support and patient's and parents', spouse's, or partner's capacity to recognize severity of an exacerbation
   Economic resources
   Sociocultural beliefs

*This list does not represent a standardized assessment or diagnostic instrument. The validity and reliability of this list have not been assessed.

at night or following exercise may increase specificity of the diagnosis. Also, the symptoms may be difficult to describe, but the consequences may provide a clue to symptoms. The child or caregiver may describe difficulty sleeping or that the child "has a cold all of the time" or "colds last a lot longer than anyone else in the family." The clinical course and expression of symptoms is highly variable, with some patients experiencing daily symptoms and others with episodes only with upper respiratory tract infections. The initial history gives the opportunity to teach patients and family members to recognize symptoms that might be signs of asthma, and begins the process of partnership between physician and patient to understand the disease and its impact.

NATURAL HISTORY

Most patients with asthma begin to have symptoms in childhood. The symptoms may persist through adolescence and young adulthood or go into remission with some patients relapsing following a period of remission. In the Tucson Childhood Respiratory Study, approximately one third of children enrolled in the study wheezed before 3 years of age, and about 40% of these children went on to persistently wheeze.[6] An additional 15% of children developed wheezing after 3 years of age.[6] Follow-up studies demonstrated that children who wheezed at 6 years of age were more likely to continue wheezing than children who never wheezed or wheezed transiently.[7] Figure 5-2 represents the relative prevalences of transient, nonatopic, and atopic (asthma) wheezing in the first years of life as defined in the Tucson study. In a population-based, longitudinal study conducted in New Zealand, approximately half of the patients with more than one episode of wheezing before age 13 years were asymptomatic in young adulthood.[8] Approximately half of the patients who were currently experiencing wheezing episodes had persistent asthma, and the other half had been in remission from symptoms and relapsed before age 26 years.[8]

Wheezing and asthma are often categorized by the duration, age at onset, and the association with atopy. Wheezing may be transient or persistent, early-onset or late-onset, and atopic or nonatopic.

TRANSIENT WHEEZING

Transient wheezing describes children who wheeze early in life (before 3 years of age) but not into childhood. In the Tucson Children's Respiratory Study, approximately 20% of children were classified as having transient wheezing. Risk factors for transient wheezing include maternal smoking during pregnancy and a younger mother. Even though symptoms may not persist into childhood, children with transient wheezing had persistently low lung function shortly after birth, before lower respiratory infection, and at 6 years of age.[6] Unlike children with persistent wheezing and asthma, children with transient wheezing were not more likely to have a family history of asthma, atopic dermatitis, eosinophilia, or high levels of serum immunoglobulin (Ig) E.

ATOPIC ASTHMA

Atopy is the major predisposing factor for developing asthma. Of children who were wheezing persistently at both 3 and at 6 years of age, 60% of the children had evidence of atopy.[9] Most often, sensitization to allergens such as dust mite, cockroach, trees, and animal dander occurs after 2 years of age in genetically predisposed individuals. For that reason, asthma symptoms in children with atopic asthma usually present after 2 to 3 years of age with most patients exhibiting symptoms within the first 6 years of life. Serum IgE levels have been shown to be closely related to the prevalence of asthma and airway inflammation.[10] A parental history of asthma and patient history of eczema or allergic sensitization have been identified as risk factors for asthma in children.

NONATOPIC ASTHMA

Respiratory tract infections, in particular viral infections such as respiratory syncytial virus (RSV) and *Mycoplasma pneumoniae* and *Chlamydia pneumoniae*, contribute to wheezing in children and are associated with the development of asthma. Taussig et al[9] suggest that children with nonatopic asthma may have an alteration in airway tone, which in the setting of a viral infection results in acute airway obstruction.

Risk Factors

The Tucson Childhood Respiratory Study found that wheezing that continues into the school-age years was associated with a history of allergy in the child and a parental history of asthma.[6] An Asthma Predictive Index was determined as a part of this study. Children with recurrent wheezing in the previous year and who had one of two major criteria (physician-diagnosed atopic dermatitis or parental asthma) or two minor criteria (peripheral blood eosinophilia, wheezing apart from colds, or physician-diagnosed allergic rhinitis) were more likely to have wheeze continue and acquire a diagnosis of asthma.[9]

Several other demographic and environmental risk factors for asthma have been identified. Low socioeconomic status and non-white race have been linked to increased asthma prevalence. Male gender is a risk factor for asthma in early childhood; however, asthma is more common in female adolescents and adults. Viral infections of the lower respiratory tract resulting in wheezing during infancy, in particular respiratory syncytial virus, significantly increase the risk of developing asthma. Exposure to environmental factors such

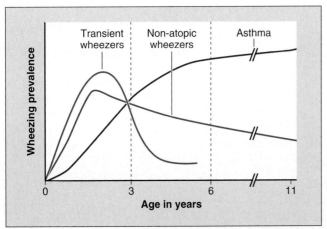

Figure 5-2 Hypothetical peak prevalence by age for the different wheezing phenotypes. The prevalence of each age interval should be the area under the curve. This does not imply that the groups are exclusive.

as tobacco smoke, dust, or cockroaches plays a key role in the development of asthma. Prenatal exposure to environmental tobacco smoke has also been associated with recurrent wheezing and a physician diagnosis of asthma in young children; however, this may represent transient wheezing, as the association does not persist.[9,11] In adults, cigarette smoke, rhinitis, obesity, and occupational exposures to relevant allergens or respiratory irritants have also been identified as risk factors for the development of asthma. In general, sensitization to aeroallergens is associated with presence of asthma, and exposure to allergens to which a person is sensitized increases severity of symptoms. The link to worsened symptoms is especially true for sensitized individuals who live with furry pets. There is a link between sensitization to *Alternaria* mold and severity of asthma; sleeping with open windows during periods of high mold counts can be particularly troublesome.

EPIDEMIOLOGIC DEFINITIONS OF ASTHMA

As discussed in the previous sections of this chapter, asthma is a complex and variable disease. In what ways do epidemiologists capture asthma prevalence on a population level? Commonly, two questions are used to determine if a child has asthma[1]: "Has a doctor or other health professional ever told you that your child has asthma?" and[2] "During the past 12 months, has your child had an episode of asthma or an asthma attack?" This self-report of a physician diagnosis of asthma has been used to differentiate lifetime asthma from current asthma and is used in multiple asthma prevalence studies.

The National Health and Nutrition Examination Survey (NHANES) survey conducted by the National Center for Health Statistics (NCHS) and the Centers for Disease Control and Prevention (CDC) allows asthma to be categorized into five phenotypes: current physician-diagnosed atopic asthma, current physician-diagnosed nonatopic asthma, resolved physician-diagnosed asthma, frequent respiratory symptoms with no asthma diagnosis, and normal. To make these delineations the following questions were asked: "Has a doctor ever told you that your child has asthma?" and "Does the child still have asthma?" Allergy skin testing was used to differentiate between atopic and nonatopic children. Report of 12 or more episodes of coughing, wheezing, or upper respiratory tract infection in the past 12 months without a physician diagnosis of asthma has been used to describe moderate to severe undiagnosed asthma.[12]

The International Study of Asthma and Allergies in Childhood (ISAAC) written questionnaire was developed and validated to determine international asthma prevalence in a systematic manner (Box 5-2). This tool has been applied to more than 750,000 children to determine asthma prevalence globally.[13] The questionnaire consists of eight questions used to describe asthma (see Box 5-1). Self-report of lifetime and current asthma is included, as well as questions to assess severity, nocturnal symptoms, and exercise-associated symptoms. A video questionnaire was also developed as a part of this study to allow for a standard approach to the understanding of what constitutes wheezing.

The Epidemiologic Section of the American Public Health Association puts forth that a diagnosis of asthma based on self-report alone represents probable asthma.[14] Clinical

---

BOX 5-2 Core Questionnaire Wheezing Module for 13 to 14 Year Olds from ISAAC

1. Have you ever had wheezing or whistling in the chest at any time in the past?
2. Have you ever had wheezing or whistling in the chest in the last two months?
3. How many attacks of wheezing have you had in the last 12 months?
4. In the last 12 months, how often, on average, has your sleep been disturbed due to wheezing?
5. In the last 12 months, has wheezing ever been severe enough to limit your speech to only one or two words at a time between breaths?
6. Have you ever had asthma?
7. In the last 12 months, has your chest sounded wheezy during or after exercise?
8. In the last 12 months, have you had a dry cough at night, apart from a cough associated with a cold or a chest infection?

---

information in conjunction with objective assessments of lung function and airway lability are essential in making the diagnosis of asthma.

MAKING A DIAGNOSIS OF ASTHMA

In making a diagnosis of asthma, the clinician should determine if symptoms of airflow obstruction are present, demonstrate the obstruction and at least partial improvement with bronchodilator, and exclude alternative diagnoses. The evaluation starts with a careful history (see Box 5-1), starting with a standard set of questions (Boxes 5-3 and 5-4) that will focus the discussion and begin to define the severity and degree of interference of the disease in the patient's life. The history elicits the nature of symptoms, age of onset and general course over time, clinical status when the patient is at his or her best, how symptoms start from complete wellness or worsen and progress from the best status to sick, therapies used, and response of chronic and acute symptoms to these therapies. Possible precipitating factors need to be carefully reviewed both to determine the roles of specific factors in the course of the disease and to begin a process of education of the patient and parent about possible relationships between exposures and symptoms. Presence of airway obstruction can be determined if the patient has wheeze at the time of the examination or its presence on spirometry. Reversibility can be established by elimination of wheeze clinically after admission of bronchodilator or a 12% or greater improvement in FEV_1 (forced expiratory volume in 1 second) with administration of bronchodilator during pulmonary function testing. Use of a peak flow meter to define reversible airflow limitation in diurnal variation is presented in Box 5-3.

Differential Diagnosis of Asthma

All that wheezes is not asthma (Box 5-5). Since wheezing with characteristics identical to asthma can occur in multiple disease settings, a necessary first step in making a diagnosis

BOX 5-3 Key Indicators for Considering a Diagnosis of Asthma

Consider asthma and performing spirometry if any of these indicators are present.* These indicators are not diagnostic by themselves, but the presence of multiple key indicators increases the probability of a diagnosis of asthma. Spirometry is needed to establish a diagnosis of asthma.

■ Wheezing—high-pitched whistling sounds when breathing out—especially in children. (Lack of wheezing and a normal chest examination do not exclude asthma.)
■ History of any of the following:

   Cough, worse particularly at night
   Recurrent wheeze
   Recurrent difficulty in breathing
   Recurrent chest tightness

■ Reversible airflow limitation and diurnal variation as measured by using a peak flow meter, for example:

   Peak expiratory flow (PEF) varies 20 percent or more from PEF measurement on arising in the morning (before taking an inhaled short-acting beta$_2$-agonist) to PEF measurement in the early afternoon (after taking an inhaled short-acting beta$_2$-agonist).

■ Symptoms occur or worsen in the presence of:

   Exercise
   Viral infection
   Animals with fur or feathers
   House-dust mites (in mattresses, pillows, upholstered furniture, carpets)
   Mold
   Smoke (tobacco, wood)
   Pollen
   Changes in weather
   Strong emotional expression (laughing or crying hard)
   Airborne chemicals or dusts
   Menses

■ Symptoms occur or worsen at night, awakening the patient.

*Eczema, hay fever, or a family history of asthma or atopic diseases are often associated with asthma, but they are not key indicators.

BOX 5-4 Sample Questions for the Diagnosis and Initial Assessment of Asthma*

A "yes" answer to any question suggests that an asthma diagnosis is likely.

In the past 12 months,...

■ Have you had a sudden severe episode or recurrent episodes of coughing, wheezing (high-pitched whistling sounds when breathing out), or shortness of breath?
■ Have you had colds that "go to the chest" or take more than 10 days to get over?
■ Have you had coughing, wheezing, or shortness of breath during a particular season or time of the year?
■ Have you had coughing, wheezing, or shortness of breath in certain places or when exposed to certain things (e.g., animals, tobacco smoke, perfumes)?
■ Have you used any medications that help you breathe better? How often?
■ Are your symptoms relieved when the medications are used?

In the past 4 weeks, have you had coughing, wheezing, or shortness of breath...

■ At night that has awakened you?
■ In the early morning?
■ After running, moderate exercise, or other physical activity?

*These questions are examples and do not represent a standardized assessment or diagnostic Instrument. The validity and reliability of these questions have not been assessed.

out a mediastinal mass impinging on the airway may be indicated in a child with more persistent wheeze. A history of choking followed by a period of wellness in the past is important in a younger child with a persistent infiltrate that may be caused by a foreign body.

In adolescents and adults, the differential diagnosis of asthma includes the aforementioned possibilities, but also includes vocal cord dysfunction and other chronic obstructive diseases such as chronic bronchitis and emphysema, although overlap may occur. Allergic bronchopulmonary aspergillosis, chronic eosinophilic pneumonia, and Churg-Strauss may also present similarly to asthma. To distinguish these diseases, chest radiography and pulmonary function tests, as well as careful history and physical examination are essential.

Initial Assessment of a Patient Presenting With Cough Without Wheeze: Controversies in Diagnosis and Different Modalities to Diagnose

Clinicians generally agree that asthma is a wheezing disease (recognizing that not all that wheezes is asthma). But patients with asthma also have other symptoms, most prominently being cough. A problem in diagnosis arises when a patient presents with just cough. Cough-variant asthma is known to

of asthma is ruling out other diseases (Box 5-5). This is most important in young children and older adults, for whom differential diagnoses are more common and asthma more difficult to diagnose even with a history very consistent with the disease. In children with frequent wheezing and coughing, cystic fibrosis, anatomical abnormalities that impinge on the bronchial tree, and the possibility of a foreign body must be excluded. A sweat test to diagnose cystic fibrosis is indicated in a young child with difficult to control wheezing episodes even if not accompanied by infiltrates on a chest radiograph or failure to thrive. A chest radiograph is required in any child with severe or frequent wheeze to rule out the myriad of other causes of wheezing. A barium swallow to rule

BOX 5-5 Differential Diagnostic Possibilities for Asthma

Infants and Children

Upper airway diseases
- Allergic rhinitis and sinusitis

Obstructions involving large airways

- Foreign body in trachea or bronchus
- Vocal cord dysfunction
- Vascular rings or laryngeal webs
- Laryngotracheomalacia, tracheal stenosis, or bronchostenosis
- Enlarged lymph nodes or tumor

Obstructions involving small airways

- Viral bronchiolitis or obliterative bronchiolitis
- Cystic fibrosis
- Bronchopulmonary dysplasia
- Heart disease

Other causes

- Recurrent cough not due to asthma
- Aspiration from swallowing mechanism dysfunction or gastroesophageal reflux

Adults

- Chronic obstructive pulmonary disease (chronic bronchitis or emphysema)
- Congestive heart failure
- Pulmonary embolism
- Laryngeal dysfunction
- Mechanical obstruction of the airways (benign and malignant tumors)
- Pulmonary infiltration with eosinophilia
- Cough secondary to drugs (angiotensin-converting enzyme [ACE] inhibitors)
- Vocal cord dysfunction

of airway obstruction can be helpful in making a diagnosis of asthma, and a negative challenge is very useful in pointing thinking in another direction. Unfortunately, making a diagnosis of asthma in an individual with only cough is most problematic in young children in whom it is also difficult to perform pulmonary function testing. In such a young person, the presence of a family history of asthma and other atopic disease (such as eczema), or positive allergy skin tests, peripheral blood eosinophilia, or an elevated total serum IgE support a diagnosis of asthma but do not eliminate the possibility of other diseases that can be coexisting. The Tucson Childhood Respiratory Study noted that children with cough but not wheeze were most often from homes with smoking parents and had minimal evidence of atopic disease. When other diseases were not present, these young children tended to improve by age 6 years.

CONCLUSION

Asthma is a common chronic disease with multiple presentations and a variable course. In spite of increasing attention to asthma prevalence, a remarkable number of children have frequent wheeze without colds that likely represents undiagnosed asthma. Asthma surveillance studies suggest that undiagnosed asthma affects at least 10% of urban children, irrespective of gender and race.[14–16] Studies suggest that children with undiagnosed asthma are more likely to be nonatopic and have milder disease with less intense symptoms.[16] However, among those with symptoms of cough and wheeze but no diagnosis, there are individuals with moderate or severe asthma who would benefit from intervention.

There is no gold standard or single diagnostic test to determine if a person has asthma. Primary care physicians, emergency medicine physicians, and specialists in any area of medicine may encounter a patient with symptoms of wheeze and cough. Understanding the natural history of asthma including risk factors and clinical course is critical in first identifying and then obtaining management for these individuals. A comprehensive history to assess symptoms, presence of atopy, and pulmonary function testing to assess bronchodilator response and airway responsiveness to methacholine are important tools to decide if what they are seeing is asthma.

exist, but must be confirmed by other studies. The best of such studies would be pulmonary function testing to examine for the presence of airway obstruction accompanied by an evaluation of improvement after bronchodilator administration. A methacholine challenge showing development

REFERENCES

1. Asthma Prevalence, Health Care Use and Mortality, 2002. Available at http://www.cdc.gov/nchs/products/pubs/pubd/hestats/asthma/asthma.htm: National Center for Health Statistics.
2. Weiss KB, Sullivan SD: The health economics of asthma and rhinitis. I. Assessing the economic impact. J Allergy Clin Immunol 2001;107:3–8.
3. U.S. Department of Health and Human Services, National Institutes of Health: Guidelines for the Diagnosis and Management of Asthma (NIH Publication No. 97–4051). NHLBI, National Asthma Education and Prevention Program. Rockville, MD, U.S. Department of Health and Human Services, 1997.
4. Grol MH, Gerritsen J, Vonk JM, et al: Risk factors for growth and decline of lung function in asthmatic individuals up to age 42 years. A 30-year follow-up study. Am J Respir Crit Care Med 1999;160:1830–1837.
5. Bousquet J, Jeffery PK, Busse WW, et al: Asthma: From bronchoconstriction to airways inflammation and remodeling. Am J Respir Crit Care Med 2000;161: 1720–1745.
6. Martinez FD, Wright AL, Taussig LM, et al: Asthma and wheezing in the first six years of life. N Engl J Med 1995;332:133–138.
7. Morgan WJ, Stern DA, Sherrill DL, et al: Outcome of asthma and wheezing in the first 6 years of life: Follow-up through adolescence. Am J Respir Crit Care Med 2005;172:1253–1258.
8. Sears MR, Greene JM, Willan AR, et al: A longitudinal, population-based, cohort study of childhood asthma followed to adulthood. N Engl J Med 2003;349:1414–1422.
9. Taussig LM, Wright AL, Holberg CJ, et al: Tucson Children's Respiratory Study: 1980 to present. J Allergy Clin Immunol 2003;111:661–675.

10. Burrows B, Martinez FD, Halonen M, et al: Association of asthma with serum IgE levels and skin-test reactivity to allergens. N Engl J Med 1989;320:271–277.

11. Lannero E, Wickman M, Pershagen G, Nordvall L: Maternal smoking during pregnancy increases the risk of recurrent wheezing during the first years of life. Respir Res 2006;7:3.

12. Kelley CF, Mannino DM, Homa DM, et al: Asthma phenotypes, risk factors, and measures of severity in a national sample of US children. Pediatrics 2005;115:726–731.

13. Beasley R, Ellwood P, Asher I: International patterns of the prevalence of pediatric asthma the ISAAC program. Pediatr Clin North Am 2003;50:539–553.

14. Clark NM, Brown R, Joseph CL, et al: Issues in identifying asthma and estimating prevalence in an urban school population. J Clin Epidemiol 2002;55:870–881.

15. Mvula M, Larzelere M, Kraus M, et al: Prevalence of asthma and asthma-like symptoms in inner-city schoolchildren. J Asthma 2005;1:9–16.

16. Joseph CL, Havstad S, Anderson EW, et al: Effect of asthma intervention on children with undiagnosed asthma. J Pediatr 2005;146:96–104.

How Do You Diagnose Asthma in the Child?

Joseph D. Spahn, Lora Stewart, and Bradley Chipps

DIAGNOSIS OF ASTHMA IN PRESCHOOL CHILDREN

The diagnosis of asthma in preschool children is a challenge for many reasons. First and foremost, many preschool children with wheezing will not persist to be diagnosed with asthma. Large birth cohorts have shown that approximately 50% of preschool children with recurrent wheezing episodes will have only transient wheezing of childhood.[1] There is no single diagnostic test for asthma at any age group. Evaluations used in older patients to support an asthma diagnosis such as spirometry, exhaled nitric oxide, and sputum samples are not feasible in the preschool population. When considering a diagnosis of asthma in a younger child, many aspects of the current history, past history, and physical exam aid in distinguishing between transient wheezing and persistent asthma.

Important Aspects of the History of Present Illness

Recurrent or persistent respiratory symptoms often prompt consideration of a diagnosis of asthma. The most frequent presenting symptom is recurrent wheeze. Although many parents confuse wheeze with upper airway congestion or noise, previous physician-documented wheezing is helpful in confirming the presence of true wheeze. Often wheezing has been associated only with previous viral respiratory tract infections; however, it is important to clarify if any wheezing has been appreciated independent of obvious infection. Additional triggers of wheeze or respiratory symptoms may include exercise or activity, exposure to a furred or feathered animal, and environmental tobacco smoke. Cough is another important

symptom that is often reported by caregivers. Persistent cough can be a sign of active disease. Unfortunately, cough is rather nonspecific, as most children will cough during childhood, especially with viral respiratory tract illnesses. A characteristic asthma cough is often described as dry and will often respond to bronchodilator therapy. Additionally, persistent cough apart from viral illness, especially nocturnal cough, is consistent with a diagnosis of asthma and a frequent nocturnal cough may be associated with more severe disease. Cough associated with activity such as exercise, laughing, or tickling is often related to asthma. Furthermore, a history of tachypnea, respiratory distress, or hypoxia is very helpful in assessing the severity of an episode and may help distinguish a simple upper respiratory infection from an episode of bronchospasm.

Important Aspects of Past Medical History

Birth history, specifically prematurity and a history of oxygen requirement and/or mechanical ventilation, is important to clarify in patients undergoing evaluation for recurrent respiratory symptoms. Patients born prematurely often develop chronic lung disease or bronchopulmonary dysplasia (BPD) and many also have airway hyperresponsiveness characteristic of asthma. Some studies have shown a lack of persistent inflammation in former premature infants with current asthma, and the condition may be different in this population compared with former term infants with current asthma. Nonetheless, former premature infant status is associated with increased risk of asthma, although prematurity is not associated with an increased risk of allergy. Additional risk factors in this population include very low birth weight, prolonged mechanical ventilation, and prolonged oxygen requirement.

Table 6-1
ASTHMA PREDICTED INDEX VERSUS THE MODIFIED ASTHMA PREDICTIVE INDEX

Asthma Predictive Index (2)	Modified Asthma Predictive Index (3)
Major Criteria	*Major Criteria*
• Parental history of asthma	• Parental history of asthma
• Physician-diagnosed atopic dermatitis	• Physician-diagnosed atopic dermatitis
	• Allergic sensitization to ≥1 aeroallergen
Minor Criteria	*Minor Criteria*
• Physician-diagnosed allergic rhinitis	• Allergic sensitization to egg, milk, or peanut
• Wheezing apart from colds	• Wheezing apart from colds
• Blood eosinophilia (>4%)	• Blood eosinophilia (>4%)

Table 6-2
DIFFERENTIAL DIAGNOSIS OF RECURRENT WHEEZING

I. Upper Airway Conditions
  A. Allergic rhinitis
  B. Sinusitis
  C. Adenoidal hypertrophy
II. Large Airway Conditions
  A. Laryngotracheomalacia
  B. Vascular rings, laryngeal webs
  C. Tracheoesophageal fistula
  D. Foreign body aspiration
  E. Vocal cord dysfunction
  F. Vocal cord paresis/paralysis
  G. External mass compressing airway (e.g., tumor, or enlarged lymph nodes, congenital heart disease)
III. Small Airway Conditions
  A. Viral bronchiolitis (e.g., respiratory syncytial virus)
  B. Bronchopulmonary dysplasia
  C. Gastroesophageal reflux
  D. Bronchiolitis obliterans
  E. Diseases associated with bronchiectasis

  1. Cystic fibrosis
  2. B-cell immune deficiency
  3. Alpha$_1$-antitrypsin deficiency
  4. Primary ciliary dyskinesia

  F. Medications associated with chronic cough (e.g., angiotensin converting enzyme [ACE] inhibitors and beta-adrenergic antagonists)

It is important to clarify the details regarding the child's respiratory status during viral upper respiratory infections (URI) and when well. Children who have a history of cough or wheeze between episodes of URI are more likely to have persistent wheezing in the future compared to children with symptoms associated only with viral URIs. Additionally, children with frequent episodes of recurrent wheeze or cough (more than three per year) are more likely to have persistent disease.

The number of unscheduled visits to the primary physician, emergency or urgent care center visits, and hospitalizations can help determine the severity of the symptoms. Finally, a good response to previous therapies including bronchodilators and inhaled and systemic steroids is helpful in assessing the etiology of respiratory symptoms because a simple URI without associated bronchospasm will not be improved with the use of bronchodilator therapy or systemic steroids.

Infants and young children with the combination of atopic dermatitis and recurrent respiratory symptoms are at an increased risk for developing asthma. In the Tucson birth cohort, the presence of eczema was a major risk factor in predicting the likelihood of persistent disease.[2] Based on this cohort, an Asthma Predictive Index (API) was developed, as listed in Table 6-1. Major risk factors (only one is required) include parental asthma and physician-diagnosed atopic dermatitis. Minor risk factors (two are required) include physician-diagnosed allergic rhinitis, wheezing unrelated to colds, and blood eosinophilia (greater than or equal to 4%). The API has recently been modified based on a large early intervention study called the Prevention of Early Asthma in Kids (PEAK) study.[3] In this study, 2- to 3-year-old children with recurrent wheeze at risk for the development of persistent asthma were enrolled to receive 2 years of therapy with placebo or an inhaled glucocorticoid. Entry criteria included presence of one of three major criteria (parental history of asthma, physician-diagnosed atopic dermatitis, or allergic sensitization

to 1 aeroallergen) or two minor criteria (allergic sensitization to milk, egg, or peanut; wheezing unrelated to colds; or blood eosinophils equal to 4%). As both eczema and asthma are atopic diseases, many children initially present with eczema with or without food allergies and then progress to develop asthma and finally allergic rhinitis or the so-called "atopic march."

Studies have shown that previous severe infection with respiratory syncytial virus (RSV), including hospitalization and/or oxygen requirement, is an independent risk factor for the development of asthma. It is still unclear whether the infection itself results in damage of the airway, which then results in the development of asthma, or if children predisposed to developing asthma are more vulnerable to experience a severe course when faced with infection by RSV. In either case, a history of a significant RSV infection may support a prediction of persistent disease.[4]

Important Aspects of the Family History

The evaluation of a child with recurrent respiratory symptoms should include a thorough review of the family medical history. Parental physician-diagnosed asthma is a major risk factor for persistent wheezing in a preschool-aged child with both infrequent and frequent episodes of wheezing. Reviewing the family history for the presence of other atopic disease such as allergic rhinitis, food allergy, and eczema will help establish a potential atopic genetic background for the patient.

Important Aspects of the Environmental History

An environmental history should be obtained to determine the presence of potential perennial allergens in the home; specifically, types of family pets both furred and feathered, whether the pets are indoor or outdoor, and if they sleep in the child's bedroom. In dust mite–endemic regions, the use of mattress and pillow covers; the frequency and manner of cleaning bedding; and the presence of carpeting, curtains, upholstered furniture, and stuffed animals should be included in an environmental history. Additional questions should address the presence of other potential irritants such as fireplaces or wood-burning stoves and the type of heat and air-cooling systems. Finally, the history should include environmental tobacco smoke exposure. Previous studies have shown that children who are sensitized to the allergens of house-dust mite and to the mold *Alternaria* are more likely to have asthma as documented by bronchial hyperresponsiveness.

Important Aspects of the Physical Exam

There are several portions of the physical exam that may support atopic disease in a young child with recurrent wheeze. Examination of the nose will often reveal edema and rhinorrhea, but unfortunately it is nearly impossible to differentiate allergic rhinitis from viral upper respiratory illnesses. When performing a lung exam on a well-appearing child, the respiratory rate, inspiratory-to-expiratory phase ratio, oxygen saturation, and auscultation will likely be normal. As such, a normal lung exam during a well time does not rule in or rule out the diagnosis of asthma. During an acute episode, the lung exam will be most helpful. Documentation of wheezing, tachypnea, retractions, and/or hypoxia is important in characterizing the symptoms and severity of an episode. Skin examination is important in determining whether the child has any concomitant atopic dermatitis, specifically looking for erythema, excoriations, thickening, or lichenification. In the preschool age group, the distribution of eczema may include the face and extensor regions seen in infancy or be transitioning to the flexor regions as seen with the older age groups.

Testing Options in the Younger Child

LUNG FUNCTION TESTING

In the older child, lung function tests such as spirometry and lung volume measurements (body plethysmography) are often helpful in confirming or excluding a diagnosis of asthma. In this situation, improvement in airflow obstruction by 12% is supportive of the diagnosis. Unfortunately, these tests require both cooperation and coordination to complete. In the preschool-aged child, lung function testing is possible, but its regular application is limited by the requirement for sedation, costly equipment, and specialized personnel.

Infant Pulmonary Function Tests

In infants, several techniques are available to quantitate lower airway function. At present, these techniques are used in research and normative values are not available from large cohorts. The available techniques include measurement of lung volumes (body plethysmography or gas dilution), partial expiratory flow volume curves (thoraco-abdominal compression), or rapid interruption of expiratory flow to measure airway resistance (Rint). These methods are labor intensive and usually require sedation of the infant. These tests may be used in clinical situations such as (1) unexplained tachypnea, cough, hypoxemia, or respiratory distress where a definitive diagnosis is not clear; (2) in children with lower airway symptoms who are not responding to standard therapy; (3) to determine the severity of lower airway obstruction and provide basis for follow-up after intervention; and (4) in research studies to better define the course of diseases and response to therapy. It is hoped that further advances will allow for wider application of this technology as equipment becomes more affordable and easier to use, and better normative standards become available.

Impulse Oscillometry

Impulse oscillometry (IOS) is a newer technology that uses small-amplitude pressure oscillations to determine the resistance of the airway. It is largely independent of effort and does not require coordination, but does require cooperation of the child, which is a limiting factor for routine use. To perform IOS, the child holds a mouthpiece in place over a 30-second period of time while breathing normally (tidal breathing). Sound impulses of various frequencies from 5 to 35 Hz are applied to the airway through the mouthpiece with total respiratory system resistance (Rrs) and reactance (Xrs) determined at the various frequencies. IOS has been studied in young children with suspected asthma with conflicting results obtained. While some investigators have not found IOS to be useful in differentiating recurrent wheezers from healthy preschool children, others have found significant differences in both baseline Rrs and change in Rrs following inhalation of a beta-agonist in asthmatic compared with nonasthmatic children. Last, young children at risk for asthma have a significant change in Rrs following bronchodilator compared with age-matched control children. Thus, IOS may become a useful measure in young children with suspected asthma, but at present it remains largely a research tool.

In older children and adults who are able to complete spirometry, a bronchial challenge (methacholine, histamine, or exercise) demonstrating airway hyperresponsiveness is strongly supportive of a diagnosis of asthma. Younger children are unable to voluntarily complete spirometry; therefore, the bronchial challenge has been modified by incorporating auscultation and pulse oximetry monitoring. Currently, the presence of wheeze, significant tachypnea, and/or a 5% or more decrease in oxygen saturation from baseline constitutes a positive challenge. Unfortunately the test is not standardized and there has been dispute as to the best parameter to confirm positivity. These issues aside, there is evidence that more severe degrees of airway hyperresponsiveness are correlated with increased likelihood of disease persistence or development.

OTHER TESTS

Radiographic studies such as chest x-rays and chest computed tomography (CT) scans of young children with a history of recurrent wheezing or cough are not routinely obtained during well periods. The usefulness of radiographic studies during acute wheezing episodes has been debated and is usually reserved for patients with significant tachypnea, localized findings on auscultation, associated fever, or significant hypoxemia. Additionally, chest radiographs can be useful when concern exists about a foreign body or the presence of an anatomical abnormality.

Demonstration of specific immunoglobulin (Ig) E either by percutaneous skin prick testing or radioallergosorbent test (RAST) of serum can confirm atopy in a child. Because it takes several seasons to develop sensitization to seasonal aeroallergens, skin testing in the preschool-aged child is confined to perennial allergens (dust mite, mold, and pet dander) or food allergens if this is a concern for an individual patient. Unfortunately, negative testing does not rule out atopy but merely confirms that there is currently no sensitization to the allergens tested. A negative test at a young age does not predict whether the child might develop sensitization in the future.

Additional laboratory results such as an elevated eosinophil count or elevated serum IgE level may suggest atopy, but are much less specific. An elevated eosinophil count is considered a minor criterion for predicting persistence as defined by the API and modified API.[2,3]

In patients in whom there is concern for recurrent infection as the etiology of recurrent wheeze or cough, an immune system evaluation may be warranted including quantitative immunoglobulin levels (IgG, IgM, and IgA) and assays for functional antibody. Typically, patients with underlying immunodeficiency have additional signs and symptoms apart from recurrent wheeze or cough such as recurrent fever, failure to thrive, and documented bacterial infections. Cystic fibrosis (CF) must also be considered in any young child presenting with a history of recurrent or persistent respiratory symptoms. Classically, CF presents with additional symptoms of failure to thrive or evidence of pancreatic insufficiency, but milder variants of CF exist and can be ruled out by a normal sweat test (<30 mEq/L Cl⁻ in children <2 years old) or demonstration of the absence of a CF DNA mutation.

Some patients will present with recurrent episodes of choking or aspiration or a history of gastroesophageal reflux symptoms in addition to recurrent wheeze or cough. These patients warrant evaluation for swallowing dysfunction, aspiration, or gastroesophageal reflux disease (GERD) by barium swallow and/or pH probe study. These problems are not infrequently found in combination with underlying bronchial hyperresponsiveness and treatment often results in improvement of both problems.

Finally, in patients with a history of inspiratory stridor or wheeze, or patients who have failed to respond to bronchodilator therapy or a short course of systemic steroids, tracheomalacia must be considered. Although diagnosis can often be made clinically, the diagnosis and severity assessment can also be made by bronchoscopy.[5]

Summary

Although predicting the likelihood of persistent asthma in a preschool-aged child with recurrent or persistent respiratory symptoms is difficult, the presence of several risk factors including personal history of eczema or allergic rhinitis, parental history of asthma, positive allergy skin tests, and persistence of symptoms without viral illnesses will aid in the diagnosis. Additionally, one must consider other potential causes of recurrent respiratory symptoms, including GERD, tracheomalacia, or cystic fibrosis. Finally, a number of tests are available to support a diagnosis of asthma or the risk of future asthma such as skin prick testing, blood work documenting atopy (eosinophilia or elevated IgE level), or even documentation of bronchial hyperresponsiveness.

DIFFERENTIAL DIAGNOSIS OF RECURRENT WHEEZE IN PRESCHOOL CHILDREN

When evaluating a preschool-aged child with recurrent wheezing or other respiratory symptoms, the differential diagnosis is quite extensive, but it can be narrowed based on a thorough history and physical examination (see Table 6-2). Additionally, the practitioner should focus on common conditions such as asthma, GERD, and upper airway diseases such as rhinitis and sinusitis unless the evaluation supports pursuing rare etiologies.

GERD is a common diagnosis in young children. Often this age group does not complain of the classic symptoms of heartburn or abdominal pain, but rather presents with excess burping or emesis, coughing after meals, or nocturnal cough or wheeze. Diagnosis can be suspected clinically and confirmed with positive response to empiric therapy with an acid suppression regimen. Alternatively, a pH probe to document increased or prolonged events of acid in the esophagus or radiographic studies may be used before treatment is started. Because GERD and asthma symptoms may coexist, a diagnosis of one or the other is not mutually exclusive, but previous studies have shown that treatment of GERD may result in improved asthma symptoms and decreased need for asthma medication.

Chronic sinusitis or rhinitis with associated postnasal drip may contribute to persistent cough in the preschool-aged patient. Typically, patients have evidence of persistent nasal congestion or drainage in association with the cough. The cough is more likely to be wet and/or productive and worse at night or early morning. This type of cough will not improve with bronchodilator therapy or inhaled corticosteroid therapy, but does often improve with treatment of the underlying condition. Treatment can be started empirically, but a sinus CT may also be useful if considering a prolonged antibiotic course.

Tracheomalacia, or abnormal tracheal cartilage, is a common anatomic defect seen in young children. Patients often present with recurrent episodes of stridor, wheeze, or barky cough, which is worsened by crying and concurrent respiratory infection. Respiratory symptoms often subside while sleeping, in contrast to asthma where symptoms often worsen at night. In many patients the symptoms are present between episodes of infection, but mild cases may only be symptomatic with infection or vigorous crying. Additionally, treatment with a bronchodilator results in no change or even worsens symptoms because it results in diminished tone in the presence of malacia. Glucocorticoids, both systemic and inhaled, are also ineffective. For most patients the symptoms will resolve by age 2, but more persistent disease can occur. Evaluation for potential etiologies, including tracheoesophageal fistula, vascular ring, or underlying connective tissue disorder, should be pursued for severe or persistent presentations. Bronchoscopy is the study of choice in the diagnosis and assessment of tracheomalacia.

Mechanical airway compression due to congenital cardiac anomalies should be considered in a patient with recurrent respiratory symptoms that have failed to improve with bronchodilator or corticosteroid therapy. Anatomic compression is obviously a less common etiology for recurrent wheeze compared to asthma, but is often unrecognized in this age group. Compression can occur due to vascular rings or slings (right-sided or double aortic arch, anomalous innominate artery, or pulmonary artery sling) or enlargement of cardiac and/or pulmonary vasculature (dilated pulmonary arteries, left atrial enlargement, or massive cardiomegaly). A classic presentation includes recurrent respiratory difficulties with wheezing and stridor. Many patients have associated dysphagia or apnea. The symptoms are usually aggravated by crying and concurrent respiratory viral infections. The severity of symptoms is dependent on the location and the degree of the anomaly. When this diagnosis is suspected, a chest x-ray should be obtained with close attention to the side of the aortic arch, size and shape of the cardiac silhouette, and for the presence of tracheal deviation or constriction. Esophagrams are often used to evaluate for vascular rings and slings, but are nonspecific and may be normal despite the presence of an anomaly if that anomaly does not compress the esophagus. Of note, bronchoscopy is not diagnostic; magnetic resonance imaging (MRI) of the chest or angiography is required to confirm the diagnosis. Finally, congestive heart failure in young children rarely presents with wheezing, but may present with a history of increased work of breathing.

The rare H-type tracheoesophageal fistula (TEF) may need to be considered in a patient with recurrent respiratory symptoms, usually recurrent pneumonia or persistent infiltrate on chest radiograph. These patients will not respond to conventional therapies including bronchodilators and corticosteroids. The vast majority of patients with TEF have additional birth anomalies. This type of TEF is often difficult to demonstrate by conventional radiographic studies and may require bronchoscopy, possibly in combination with esophageal motility studies, as GERD is a common comorbidity.

In a preschool-aged patient with acute onset of wheeze and/or cough, foreign body (FB) aspiration must be considered. On physical exam, the wheezing will often be unilateral or localized. A forced expiratory chest radiograph may demonstrate air trapping behind the foreign body. The diagnosis is confirmed by bronchoscopy and removal of the FB. Typically, patients present with acute respiratory symptoms, but chronic symptoms or a history of infiltrate or pneumonia that fails to clear can occur as well.

Patients with CF classically present with a history of recurrent respiratory symptoms in association with systemic symptoms of failure to thrive, diarrhea, and recurrent sinus and ear infections. Additionally, there are many more mild variants to classic CF that may not have associated systemic symptoms. Therefore, in a patient with recurrent pneumonia or who has failed to respond to conventional therapies, one should consider CF in the differential diagnosis.

Immunodeficiency presenting with only recurrent wheeze and/or cough without superimposed infections, diarrhea, rash, or failure to thrive is quite rare. Immunodeficiency should not be considered in the initial differential diagnosis of a young child with only recurrent wheeze and/or cough.

Summary

In summary, when evaluating a preschool-aged child with recurrent wheezing or other respiratory symptoms, first consider the most common etiologies unless there are additional findings in the history or physical that point to a more rare explanation for the symptoms.

DIAGNOSIS OF ASTHMA IN SCHOOL-AGED CHILDREN

Important Aspects of the History of Present Illness

Similar to those in younger children, recurrent or persistent respiratory symptoms often prompt the consideration of asthma in school-aged children. The most frequent presenting symptoms are recurrent cough and wheeze. As many parents confuse wheeze with upper airway congestion, previous physician-documented wheezing is most helpful in confirming the presence of true wheeze. Wheezing may occur only with viral respiratory tract infections, but the parents may have noted wheezing or other respiratory symptoms with exercise, animal exposure, cold air, or environmental tobacco smoke exposure. Cough is another important symptom as persistent cough can be a sign of active disease. Although very sensitive, cough is nonspecific, as most children will cough during childhood. Important clues to cough being associated with asthma include a nocturnal predominance, exaggerated cough with exercise or cold air, and cough that improves in frequency and/or severity following controller therapy. Chest tightness is another symptom reported by children. The location of chest tightness is also important to delineate, as it can be helpful in differentiating tightness associated with vocal cord dysfunction, which is localized to the neck and throat, from

chest tightness associated with lower airway flow limitation. Last, the presence of eczema or nasal symptoms consistent with allergic rhinitis strengthens the likelihood of asthma in a child with recurrent cough or wheeze, as 80% to 90% of all school-aged children with asthma have an allergic diathesis.

Important Aspects of Past Medical History

As mentioned previously, history of preterm birth and a history of oxygen requirement and/or mechanical ventilation are important to clarify in patients undergoing evaluation for possible asthma. Inquiry into the frequency and severity of past wheezing episodes provides information with respect to level of severity and control. Has the child ever required an urgent care or emergency room visit or hospitalization for respiratory difficulties? Equally important is determining whether the child's respiratory symptoms worsen with viral respiratory tract infections and whether wheezing occurs apart from colds. Other important questions include the following: Does the child have a seasonal component to his or her symptoms? Has the child ever been treated with bronchodilators or controller therapy for previous episodes? If so, has the treatment resulted in improvement? Last, has the child's lung function ever been tested? If so, was the lung function diminished and did it improve with bronchodilator?

Important Aspects of the Family History

The evaluation of a child with recurrent respiratory symptoms should include a thorough review of the family medical history. The presence of nasal allergies, food allergy, eczema, or asthma in siblings, grandparents, or parents is often noted in children with asthma.

Important Aspects of the Physical Exam

There are several components of the physical exam that can aid in the diagnosis of asthma. When examining the eyes and nose, look for the presence of conjunctival injection, allergic shiners, a nasal crease, and the presence of boggy, pale inferior turbinate edema with clear nasal discharge, which are the classic features of allergic rhinoconjunctivitis. As roughly 70% of children with asthma have allergic rhinitis, the presence of rhinitis in a child with lower respiratory symptoms supports asthma as the diagnosis. The presence of nasal polyps should always prompt evaluation for CF, as polyps are far more frequently encountered in children with CF compared with allergic rhinitis and asthma. Nasal polyps in childhood asthma are relatively rare. They are much more commonly encountered in adults with aspirin-sensitive asthma.

When performing a lung exam on a well-appearing child, respiratory rate, inspiratory-to-expiratory phase ratio, chest auscultation, and oxygen saturation will often be normal. As such, a normal lung exam does not exclude the diagnosis of asthma. In fact, many children with chronic severe, yet stable asthma will have clear lungs on auscultation despite having significant airflow limitation. In contrast to the lung exam in stable asthma, it is helpful during acute attacks where diminished air exchange, wheezing, tachypnea, retractions, and/or hypoxia are often present and can be used to characterize the severity of the episode. In some children, wheezing may be absent despite significant respiratory distress. Only after several bronchodilator treatments does air exchange improve enough for wheezing to be appreciated.

Examination of the skin should always be performed, as the presence of atopic dermatitis in a child with recurrent wheezing strongly supports the diagnosis of asthma. One should specifically look for erythema, excoriations, and thickening or lichenification of the skin. The distribution of skin involvement is largely age dependent. In the preschool age group, the distribution of eczema often includes the face and extensor regions, while the flexor regions and neck are often involved in school-aged children and adolescents.

Testing Options in the Older Child

LUNG FUNCTION TESTING

Peak Expiratory Flow
The peak expiratory flow (PEF) is the maximum flow obtained within the first 200 milliseconds of a forced expiratory maneuver after inhalation to total lung capacity (TLC). PEF meters are portable, inexpensive, and easily used. Peak flow monitoring in patients with known asthma is useful in monitoring disease activity and response to pharmacologic intervention.

Whether it is useful as a diagnostic tool is less clear. A recent study comparing PEF variability to methacholine responsiveness in subjects with suspected asthma found PEF variability a poor substitute for methacholine challenge.[6]

Spirometry
Spirometry is among the most important tests of lung function in asthma. With adequate coaching, children as young as 5 years can perform the maneuver. When performing spirometry, inspection of the volume-time curve allows an assessment of the adequacy of the child's expiratory effort (Fig. 6-1). An acceptable test requires an older child to exhale for at least 6 seconds. Patients with airflow limitation will have a characteristic concave or "scooped out" expiratory flow-volume loop as seen in Figure 6-1. The inspiratory flow volume loop should have the appearance of a semicircle. A blunted or scalloped appearance, as illustrated in Figure 6-2, is suggestive of inappropriate closure of the vocal cords as is seen in vocal cord dysfunction (VCD), a frequent masquerader of asthma.

The FEV_1 (forced expiratory volume in 1 second) is the gold standard measure for diseases characterized by airflow limitation such as asthma, CF, and chronic lung disease of prematurity. According to NHLBI asthma guidelines,[7] patients

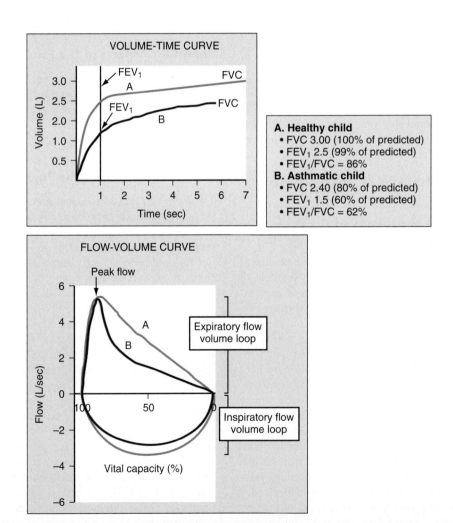

Figure 6-1 **Volume-time and flow-volumes curves from a healthy control and an asthmatic child demonstrating significant decrease in FEV_1 in the asthmatic child compared with the nonasthmatic child.** Both children have adequate expiratory times. The flow-volume curve in the asthmatic child demonstrates airflow obstruction with the characteristic concave appearing expiratory flow volume loop. Both children have normal inspiratory flow volume loops. Of note, despite the diminished FEV_1 and FEV_1/FVC ratio, the asthmatic child had a normal PEF.

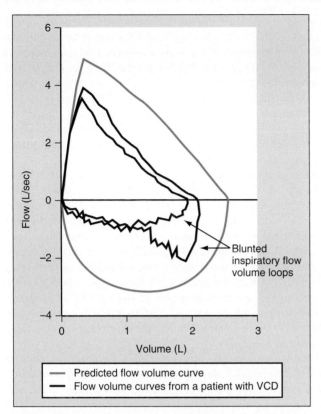

Figure 6-2   Flow volume curves from a patient with vocal cord dysfunction. The FEV₁ and FVC are proportionally impaired at 75% of predicted while the FEV₁/FVC ratio is normal, indicating the absence of flow limitation. Evaluation of the inspiratory flow-volume loop reveals significant blunting caused by inappropriate closure of the vocal cords.

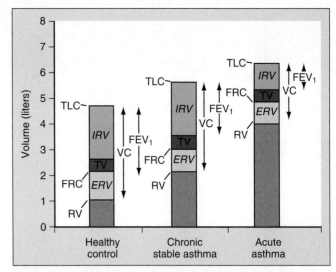

Figure 6-3   Lung volume measurements in a nonasthmatic individual, a chronic yet stable asthmatic individual, and in an asthmatic patient during an acute asthma attack. Note that the RV is most profoundly affected during an acute asthma attack. Also note that the RV increases more disproportionately than the TLC. As a result, the patient's inspiratory and expiratory reserve volumes (IRV, ERV) shrink substantially.

lyzed over 24,000 lung function measures in 2728 asthmatic children evaluated at a tertiary referral center. The mean FEV₁ of the cohort studied was 92.7% of predicted, with 77% of the values within the normal range (>80% of predicted). In contrast, the mean FEF₂₅₋₇₅ was 78% with only 27.7% of the values greater than 80% of predicted, while 30.4% were between 60% and 80%, and 40.9% were less than 60% of predicted.

Assessment of Lung Volumes
There are two ways to assess lung volume: helium dilution and body box plethysmography. Of the two techniques, body plethysmography is the preferred method as helium dilution can underestimate air trapping in patients with severe airflow obstruction. The first and most consistently elevated lung volume measure in asthma is the residual volume (RV) (Fig. 6-3). With increasing asthma severity, the RV increases followed by an increase in the functional residual capacity (FRC) and the total lung capacity (TLC). The RV is also the last measure to normalize following an asthma exacerbation.

MEASURES OF AIRWAY HYPERRESPONSIVENESS
Airway Hyperresponsiveness
Airway hyperresponsiveness (AHR) can be measured by naturally occurring stimuli (cold air challenge or exercise) or pharmacologic stimuli (methacholine, histamine, mannitol, and adenosine monophosphate [AMP]). These measurements may be used to establish the diagnosis of asthma and monitor disease progression and response to therapy. The two most commonly employed tests in children are exercise and methacholine challenge. The methacholine challenge has both high sensitivity and specificity making it the gold standard measure to diagnose asthma. A positive challenge is noted when the FEV₁ falls 20% or more at no more than 8 mg/mL of methacholine (Fig. 6-4). When a methacholine challenge is negative (<20% drop in FEV₁ at 8 mg/mL), the diagnosis of asthma is in doubt.

with mild asthma have FEV₁ values of more than 80%, those with moderate persistent asthma have values 60% to 80%, and those with severe persistent asthma have FEV₁ values of less than 60% of predicted. The FEV₁ primarily measures flow through the mid- to large-sized airways. Of importance, children with asthma often have normal FEV₁ values when well. As a result, a normal value does not rule out asthma.

The FEV₁/FVC ratio is the amount of air exhaled in the first second divided by all of the air exhaled during a maximal exhalation. The FEV₁/FVC ratio is highest in young children (>90%) and decreases with increasing age. A normal FEV₁/FVC ratio in children is 86%, with values below 80% indicative of airflow limitation. Studies evaluating the association between lung function and asthma severity based on the NHLBI asthma guidelines have found the FEV₁/FVC ratio to be a more sensitive measure of severity versus the FEV₁.

The forced expiratory flow between 25% and 75% of vital capacity (FEF₂₅₋₇₅) measures airflow in the mid-portion of the vital capacity. It is largely effort independent and it is thought to be a measure of peripheral airway obstruction. The FEF₂₅₋₇₅ is among the first parameters to be abnormal in pediatric asthma, and it is often the most significantly impaired of all of the spirometric measures. It is the impairment in the FEF₂₅₋₇₅ that gives the expiratory flow volume curve the characteristic scooped out or concave appearance (see Fig. 6-1). The FEF₂₅₋₇₅ is another sensitive measure of airflow limitation in children as demonstrated by Paull and co-workers,[8] who ana-

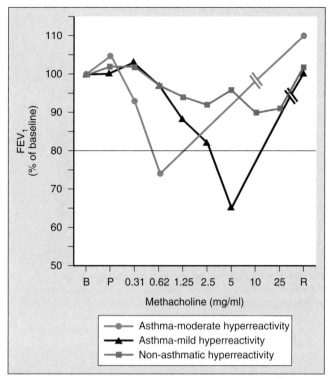

Figure 6-4 Methacholine dose response curves from three children. Two of the children had methacholine PC$_{20}$ FEV$_1$ values of less than 8 mg/mL and were known asthmatic patients. The third child had recurrent cough, normal spirometry, and no beta-agonist reversibility. A methacholine challenge revealed the child to have normal airway reactivity with a PC$_{20}$ value of greater than 25 mg/mL making the diagnosis of asthma unlikely.

Methacholine challenges are not widely performed in clinical practice because of their high cost, need for trained personnel, and limited availability.

Exercise-induced asthma is a common trigger for asthma with a prevalence of exercise-induced bronchospasm (EIB) of up to 80% in young asthmatic patients. Standard exercise protocols require patients to exercise at 85% of maximum predicted heart rate for 6 to 10 minutes while continuously monitoring heart rate and Sa$_{O_2}$. Spirometry is done at baseline and 1, 5, and 10 minutes after exercise. A positive test is defined as a 15% drop in FEV$_1$ or 20% drop in peak flow from baseline.

Beta-Agonist Reversibility

Beta-agonist reversibility allows for assessment of reversibility of airflow limitation and should be done even if the baseline FEV$_1$ is within the normal limits. Not only is beta-agonist responsiveness (12% improvement in FEV$_1$ or an increase of 200 mL) helpful in making the diagnosis of asthma, but the degree of beta-agonist reversibility also correlates with airway inflammation. Covar and colleagues[9] evaluated the clinical utility of two noninvasive measures of airway inflammation, exhaled nitric oxide (eNO) and sputum eosinophils, in children with mild to moderate asthma and found neither sputum eosinophilia nor eNO levels to correlate with baseline FEV$_1$ values, while both correlated with the change in FEV$_1$ following a bronchodilator.

OTHER TESTS

Radiographic studies such as chest x-rays are often performed in children with suspected asthma mainly to rule out other causes of cough or wheeze and have little diagnostic utility. The usefulness of radiographic studies during acute episodes has been debated and is usually reserved for patients with significant tachypnea or hypoxemia, localized findings on auscultation, or associated fever.

Demonstration of specific IgE either by percutaneous skin prick testing or RAST testing of serum is important in ascertaining atopy. Skin testing in the school-aged child should include a panel of seasonal aeroallergens including representative trees, grasses, and weeds in addition to outdoor molds. Perennial allergens such as dust mite, cockroach, molds, and pet dander should also be evaluated. Food allergens should be tested only if food allergy is suspected. Not only do the presence of positive skin tests indicate the presence of atopy, but they also identify triggers for both upper and lower airway symptoms.

Elevated circulating eosinophil counts or elevated serum IgE levels may suggest atopy, but are neither sensitive nor specific markers for asthma. In patients in whom there is concern for recurrent infection as the etiology of recurrent wheeze or cough, an immune system evaluation may be warranted including quantitative immunoglobulin levels (IgG, IgM, and IgA).

Gastroesophageal reflux (GER) is common in children with asthma. GER should be considered in children with difficult to control asthma and in children with significant nocturnal symptoms. These patients warrant evaluation for GER by barium swallow and/or pH probe study.

Finally, in patients with a history of inspiratory stridor or audible wheeze, or patients who have failed to respond to bronchodilator therapy, vocal cord dysfunction (VCD) must be considered. VCD is among the most common masqueraders of asthma in older children and adolescents.[10] Although diagnosis can often be made from the characteristic blunting of the inspiratory flow volume loop, the diagnosis and severity of paradoxical vocal cord closure is made by flexible laryngoscopy.

Summary

Making the diagnosis of asthma in a school-aged child is accomplished by obtaining pertinent information regarding type, frequency, and severity of symptoms in addition to determining the presence of risk factors, such as a parent with asthma or the coexistence of atopic dermatitis. Additionally, airflow limitation that improves following bronchodilator in a child with lower respiratory symptoms strongly supports the diagnosis of asthma. The presence of atopy and associated allergic conditions such as allergic rhinitis also lends support to the diagnosis of asthma. Last, in cases that remain difficult to determine, a methacholine challenge can be performed. A positive methacholine challenge in a child with lower respiratory symptoms is diagnostic of asthma, whereas a negative test does not support the diagnosis.

DIFFERENTIAL DIAGNOSIS OF RECURRENT WHEEZE OR COUGH IN SCHOOL-AGED CHILDREN

When evaluating a school-aged child with recurrent cough or wheezing, the differential diagnosis is not as extensive as it is for young children and it can be narrowed based on a thorough history and physical examination. The most common conditions include asthma, gastroesophageal reflux, sinus disease, vocal cord dysfunction, and chronic cough, unless the evaluation supports pursuing rare etiologies.

Gastroesophageal Reflux Disease

Recent studies show a general prevalence of gastroesophageal reflux in school-aged children with asthma of between 47% and 75%, which is similar to adults with asthma, and about two to four times the prevalence in the general population. Although respiratory symptoms in asthmatic adults are often associated with reflux, asthmatic children often deny heartburn, regurgitation, and dysphagia. As such, GER must always be considered, even in the absence of symptoms, in children with asthma or suspected asthma, particularly in children who have difficult-to-control asthma. As the case for young children with asthma, 24-hour pH monitoring is considered the gold standard for documenting the presence of GER. Other tests, such as barium swallow and endoscopy, while providing important data, are neither sensitive nor specific for the diagnosis of GER.

Sinusitis

Radiographic evidence for sinus disease is often noted in children with asthma. Mounting data link the physiology of the upper and lower airways and support the hypothesis that the same pathology underlies both sinusitis and asthma. Studies demonstrate that inflammation of the nose and sinuses is associated with lower airway hyperresponsiveness, and that nasal allergen challenge results in airway hyperresponsiveness and eosinophilia of both the upper and lower airways.

Treatment of the upper airway, generally with nasal glucocorticoids, has been shown to ameliorate lower airway hyperreactivity in children with asthma. In addition, significant improvement in asthma control can occur when sinus disease is recognized and appropriately treated. A screening CT scan of the sinuses provides greater resolution and thus greater sensitivity than conventional sinus radiographs and should be used when evaluating for sinusitis.

Vocal Cord Dysfunction

VCD, defined as inappropriate or paradoxical adduction of the vocal cords during inspiration, is among the most common masqueraders of asthma in older children and adults. In addition, children can have both VCD and asthma. VCD must be suspected in all patients who have frequent or unremitting symptoms, as this condition can be misdiagnosed as refractory asthma leading to overtreatment.[10]

VCD is frequently triggered by many of the same triggers as asthma (e.g., irritants, exercise, postnasal drip, GERD, emotions) and as such is easily mistaken by patients and physicians as asthma. Questioning the patient for symptoms prominent in the throat and on inspiration may reveal this diagnosis, although many patients are unable to localize symptoms to the throat. Importantly, a history of nocturnal abatement of symptoms and lack of response to bronchodilators may guide the physician to this diagnosis. The finding of stridor or inspiratory wheeze that is loudest at the neck, but often radiating throughout the chest during an acute episode is also suggestive of the diagnosis.

Because all routine monitoring of expiratory function in asthma requires maximal inspiration before a maximal expiratory effort, both PEF and FEV_1 measures can be falsely decreased and misleading. The FVC may also be falsely diminished, and hence, the FEV_1/FVC ratio will often remain in the normal range and not show evidence of obstruction typical of asthma (Fig. 6-2). Inspiratory flow volume loops are indispensable for the interpretation of the forced expiratory maneuvers. Truncation or irregularity of the flow volume loop on inspiration, and a forced inspiratory fraction and forced expiratory fraction at 50% of vital capacity (FIF_{50}/FEF_{50}) of greater than 1 is highly suggestive of obstruction of the extrathoracic airway, but like the findings above, may only be present during a symptomatic episode. Although evaluation of the inspiratory flow volume loop is suggestive of VCD, the gold standard remains direct visualization of vocal cord motion by flexible rhinolaryngoscopy during a symptomatic episode.

Summary

The diagnosis of asthma in childhood is primarily based on frequency, quality, and severity of symptoms in addition to family history and other allergic comorbidities (see Table 6-1). Response to therapy can be especially helpful as a diagnostic tool in younger children where pulmonary function testing can be a challenge. The differential diagnosis of recurrent wheezing is especially large in infants and toddlers and testing to rule out other conditions should be performed in a thoughtful manner (see Table 6-2). Alternative diagnoses or comorbid conditions must be appropriately evaluated and treated. The key to the diagnosis of asthma in children includes a high index of suspicion, as 80% of asthma starts before the age of 5 years. The clinical course will reflect the variability of childhood asthma, with some patients having long periods of quiescent symptoms, but this should not prevent appropriate diagnoses and treatment when supported by the appropriate clinical presentation.

REFERENCES

1. Martinez FD, Wright AL, Taussig LM, Holberg CJ, Halonen M, Morgan WJ: Asthma and wheezing in the first six years of life. N Eng J Med 1995;332:133–138.
2. Castro-Rodriquez JA, Holberg CJ, Wright AL, Martinez FD: A clinical index to define risk of asthma in young children with recurrent wheezing. Am J Respir Crit Care Med 2000;162:1403–1406.
3. Guilbert TW, Morgan WJ, Zeiger RS, et al: Atopic characteristics of children with recurrent wheezing at high risk for the development of childhood asthma. J Clin Immunol 2004;114:1282–1287.
4. Sigurs N, Bjarnason R, Sigurbergsson F, Kjellman B: Respiratory syncytial virus bronchiolitis in infancy is an important risk factor for asthma and allergy at age 7. Am J Respir Crit Care Med 2000;161:1501–1507.

5. Saglani S, Nicholson AG, Scallon M, et al: Investigation of young children with severe recurrent wheeze: any clinical benefit? Eur Respir J 2006;27:29–35.

6. Goldstein MF, Veza BA, Dunsky EH, Dvorin DJ, Belecanech GA, Haralabatos IC: Comparisons of peak flow diurnal expiratory flow variation, postbronchodilator FEV1 responses and methacholine inhalation challenges in the evaluation of suspected asthma. Chest 2001;119:1001–1010.

7. National Institutes of Health, National Heart, Lung, and Blood Institute: National Asthma Education and Prevention Program. Executive summary of the NAEPP expert panel report. Guidelines for the diagnosis and management of asthma—update on selected topics 2002 (NIH Publication No. 02-5075). Rockville, Md, U.S. Department of Health and Human Services, June 2002.

8. Paull K, Covar R, Jain N, Gelfand EW, Spahn JD. Do the NHLBI lung function criteria apply to children? A cross-sectional evaluation of childhood asthma at National Jewish Medical Center 1999–2002. Pediatr Pulmonol 2005;39:311–317.

9. Covar RA, Szefler SJ, Martin R, et al: Relationships between exhaled nitric oxide and measures of disease activity among children with mild to moderate asthma. J Pediatr 2003;142:469–475.

10. Christopher KL, Wood RP, Eckert RC, et al: Vocal-cord dysfunction presenting as asthma. N Engl J Med 1983;308:1566–1570.

Diagnosis of Asthma in Adults

Njira L. Lugogo and Monica Kraft

CLINICAL PEARLS

- Asthma occurs at high frequency in young and older adults.
- The recognition and accurate diagnosis of asthma is critical in decreasing the morbidity and mortality associated with the disease.
- Various modalities exist to aid in the diagnosis of asthma in adults.
- Contributing factors affecting the severity of asthma must be recognized and managed to enhance asthma control.
- The differential diagnosis can be extensive, as all wheezing is not asthma.
- The use of lung function testing early can aid in the diagnosis of asthma.

The diagnosis of asthma in adults can be a challenging endeavor, as most patients present with nonspecific symptoms and have multiple other medical problems that may be contributing to their clinical presentation. This is particularly true in older patients who typically have comorbid diseases. The morbidity and mortality associated with asthma can be significantly reduced by making the diagnosis early and by aggressively treating patients. Delays in diagnosis may lead to serious consequences including decreased lung function with possible airway remodeling, reduced quality of life, significant time away from work, and, in severe cases, death.

DEFINITION

Asthma is a disease of variable airway obstruction and inflammation with resultant bronchial hyperreactivity and wheezing. The National Institutes of Health/National Heart, Lung, and Blood Institute described asthma as a chronic inflammatory disorder of the airways in which many cells and cellular elements play a role. The chronic inflammation causes an associated increase in airway hyperresponsiveness that leads to recurrent episodes of wheezing, breathlessness, chest tightness, and coughing, particularly in the night and early morning. These episodes are usually associated with widespread but variable airflow obstruction that is often reversible either spontaneously or with treatment. The onset of asthma occurs most commonly in childhood and adolescence; however, it can occur anytime during one's lifetime.

The challenges faced by epidemiologists who study asthma begin with the lack of a universal definition for the disease that is pathophysiologically and clinically applicable. Epidemiologic studies define asthma based on the presence

of wheezing and on a diagnosis of asthma by a health professional, relying on self-reporting by study participants. The prevalence of asthma is reported yearly by the Centers for Disease Control and Prevention and is based on data collected by the National Health Interview Survey. The prevalence rates of asthma increased from 1980 to 1996, with a peak prevalence rate of 5.4% reported in 1996. The prevalence rates of asthma have decreased since 1996 with a reported prevalence of 4.0% in 2004 (Fig. 7-1).

NATURAL HISTORY

Several factors that influence the prevalence of asthma include obesity, atopy and allergic rhinitis, genetics/family history, exposure to allergens at an early age, and smoking history. Thomsen and colleagues[1] assessed the incidence of asthma in young adults by performing a longitudinal study on birth cohorts in the Danish Twin Registry over a period of 29 years, from 1953 to 1982. The subjects were surveyed using standard instruments including a questionnaire focused on the presence of asthma symptoms over a 12-month period. The initial survey was performed in 1994 with a follow-up survey in 2002. The subjects who answered "no" in 1994 to the question, "Do you have, or have you ever had asthma?" but "yes" in 2002 were considered incident cases of asthma. These subjects were categorized as having adult-onset asthma.[2] The overall prevalence in this cohort was 4.5 per 1000 person-years in males and 6.4 per 1000 person-years in females. The risk factors for the development of asthma as identified in the study included increased body mass index (BMI) (particularly important in female subjects) with an odds ratio of 1.05. Asthma prevalence was higher in females and subjects with a history of hay fever, eczema, or both. There was no association between the increased asthma prevalence rates and a sedentary lifestyle. Sedentary lifestyle had been postulated as the etiology for increased incidence of asthma in obese adults, due to increased exposure to allergens while spending time indoors.

CLINICAL PRESENTATION

Classic Presentation

The hallmark of classic presentation of adult-onset asthma includes the presence of episodic symptoms that are at least partially reversible.[3] Young adults are more likely to present with classic asthma symptoms. Initial assessment should include determining the presence of wheeze, dyspnea, chest tightness, or cough. These symptoms are often triggered by allergens or sinusitis/rhinitis. Patients typically have subacute onset of symptoms and present months into their disease process.

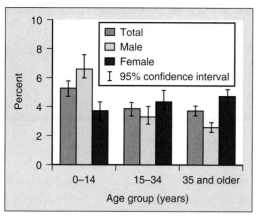

Figure 7-1 Percentage of persons of all ages who experienced an asthma episode in the preceding 12 months, by age group and sex: United States, 2004. *(Data from Centers for Disease Control and Prevention: National Health Interview Survey, 2004. Available at http://www.cdc.gov/nchs/data/ nhis/earlyrelease/200503_15.pdf [Fig 15.2; p. 2]. Accessed July 18, 2005.)*

Physical examination demonstrates nasal turbinate erythema and induration with evidence of retropharyngeal cobblestoning due to postnasal drip. The lung examination is critical in the diagnosis of asthma, as patients often have wheezing, prolonged end-expiration, and decreased air movement. However, the examination can be normal. There is no tympany or egophany. The presence of crackles should prompt an evaluation to rule out cardiac etiologies, infection, and interstitial lung disease. Clubbing, cyanosis, and edema are usually absent.

Patients respond well to bronchodilators and have reversibility of their airway obstruction (as demonstrated by spirometry). The addition of corticosteroids results in decreased frequency of symptoms and improved control of symptoms in the vast majority of asthmatics. Uncontrolled symptoms in spite of aggressive therapy warrant evaluation to rule out other etiologies of the patient's symptoms and assess whether there are any triggers that can be controlled.

Atypical Presentation

Atypical presentations include dyspnea without wheezing, chronic cough, increased shortness of breath that is particularly severe at nighttime, dyspnea on exertion (especially present with exercise), and the presence of allergic rhinitis with subsequent wheezing. The presentation is usually subacute with an indolent course and most patients have seen several physicians before being diagnosed with asthma. Asthma should be considered for any patients with dyspnea and chronic cough that has not responded to conventional therapy for reflux and allergic rhinitis. Older adults typically present with atypical symptoms of asthma. Mortality data in the United States from 1977 and 1982, respectively, demonstrated a higher mortality rate for older adults aged 65 to 74 years old at 4.9 per 100,000 in comparison with 3.0 per 100,000 in adults younger than 35.[4] A study of older adult participants in the Cardiovascular Health Study Research Group revealed a definite diagnosis of asthma in 4% with an additional 4% of participants having a probable diagnosis of asthma. Participants with a definite diagnosis of asthma were

defined by positive responses to questions about lifetime prevalence of asthma, current asthma symptoms, and a physician diagnosis of asthma. There were significantly decreased quality of life scores, fewer patients on inhaled corticosteroids, and increased risk of uncontrolled asthma symptoms. More importantly, the patients with probable asthma, based on positive responses to questions addressing the presence of wheezing and dyspnea, appeared to have obstruction on spirometry, persistent symptoms, and lower quality of life scores.[2,5] This study indicated the underdiagnosis of asthma in older adults and demonstrated the significant morbidity faced by these patients.

Physical examination differs from typical presentation of asthma, most importantly by the lack of wheezing that is noted in most patients. The nasopharyngeal examination may or may not include increased nasal turbinate induration and erythema and the lung examination may be rather unremarkable. There may be a prolonged expiratory phase that can be overlooked if it is not specifically focused on during the examination. Patients usually have lower extremity edema and obesity, which makes clinicians suspicious of cardiac etiologies for the patient's symptoms. Response to medications is variable with a lower incidence of airway reversibility noted on spirometry with bronchodilator responsiveness.

DIAGNOSTIC STUDIES

Diagnostic studies are crucial in aiding with the diagnosis of asthma in adults. Asthma is generally a clinical diagnosis and the presence of classic symptoms in a young adult with response to bronchodilators can be relied upon solely to make the diagnosis of asthma. Any patients who do not present with typical symptoms and have variable response to medications should undergo further evaluation. The following studies should be used in this population of patients. Each modality will be discussed in greater detail in subsequent chapters of this text.

Chest Radiography

All patients who present with dyspnea must have chest radiography performed on initial evaluation. Chest radiography is essential in evaluating the patient and provides a wealth of information regarding the extensive list of etiologies that can result in dyspnea. The appearance of the lung fields is usually normal in asthma. The presence of infiltrates, nodules, and consolidation of effusions should raise the possibility of an alternate diagnosis. The presence of infiltrates increases the likelihood of infection and interstitial lung diseases including pulmonary fibrosis, sarcoidosis, and bronchiolitis obliterans. The presence of a smoking history should lead to further evaluation to rule out chronic obstructive pulmonary disease (COPD). The ability to differentiate asthma from COPD is difficult because of the presence of hyperresponsiveness and bronchodilator responsiveness in both diseases. Patients with COPD are more likely to have fixed airway obstruction. There is also an increased incidence of hyperinflation and emphysematous changes noted on chest radiography, but these findings are neither sensitive nor specific. The presence of cardiomegaly and pleural effusions should lead to the evaluation for cardiac etiologies.

Chest CT Scan

The utility of chest computed tomography (CT) scanning in the diagnosis of asthma is limited. This modality should be used primarily when emphysema, pulmonary embolism, and interstitial lung disease are considered on the differential diagnosis. Routine chest CT scanning is not recommended in the diagnosis of asthma in adults.

Pulmonary Function Testing: Simple Spirometry

Spirometry is useful in establishing the presence of airflow obstruction. Obstruction is described by forced expiratory volume in 1 second/forced vital capacity (FEV_1/FVC) ratio less than 70%; the severity of obstruction is determined by the decrease in FEV_1. The curvature of the expiratory loop demonstrates the presence of airflow obstruction (Fig. 7-2B). Reversibility of airflow obstruction is thought to be an important aspect of the pathophysiology of asthma. Reversibility is defined as a 12% improvement and an increase of 200 mL in FEV_1 for FVC in comparison to baseline spirometry.

Methacholine Challenge Testing

Methacholine challenge testing (MCT) is one method of assessing airway responsiveness. MCT is often useful in establishing the diagnosis of asthma in patients with normal spirometry without reversibility and symptoms suggestive of asthma. The patients receive methacholine doses in varying concentrations followed by the obtaining of flow volume loops. A positive test result is a 20% decrease in the FEV_1 noted at less than or equal to an 8-mg/mL concentration of methacholine, but there is a spectrum of responsiveness according to American Thoracic Society/European Respiratory Society guidelines. The optimal diagnostic value of MCT occurs when the pretest probability of asthma is 30% to 70%.[6] MCT is more useful in excluding a diagnosis of asthma because of a greater negative predictive value (Fig. 7-3). A negative MCT excludes the diagnosis of asthma but should be repeated if there is a high pretest probability of

asthma. A false-negative MCT can occur in patients with variable episodes of airway hyperresponsiveness, or if deep inspiration results in bronchodilation. This event is rare and occurs in less than 5% of patients.

Allergy Skin Testing

Allergy skin testing is important particularly in patients with allergic rhinitis and atopy. Management of seasonal allergic rhinitis is critical in preventing frequent or persistent asthma exacerbations. Positive results are a mean wheal of 3 mm or greater in diameter. Allergy skin testing can be used to guide

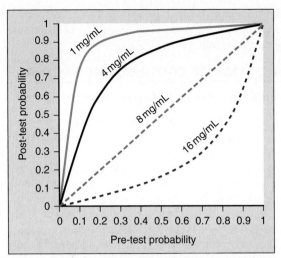

Figure 7-3 Curves illustrating pretest and posttest probability of asthma after a methacholine challenge test with four PC$_{20}$ values. The curves represent a compilation of information from several sources.[10] They are approximations presented to illustrate the relationships and principles of decision analysis. They are not intended to calculate precise posttest probabilities in patients. (Data from Crapo RO, Casaburi R, Coates AL, et al: Guidelines for methacholine and exercise challenge testing, 1999. This official statement of the American Thoracic Society was adopted by the ATS Board of Directors, July 1999. Am J Respir Crit Care Med 2000;161[1]:309–329.)

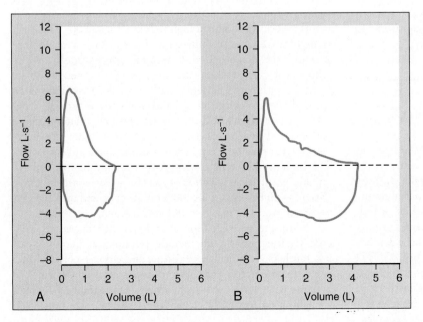

Figure 7-2 Spirometry is useful in establishing airflow obstruction. A, Normal spirometry. **B**, Moderate obstruction in an asthmatic patient.

allergy immunotherapy in patients with uncontrolled symptoms in spite of aggressive nasal lavage and antihistamine and nasal corticosteroid use.

EVALUATION OF CONTRIBUTING FACTORS

Chronic Sinusitis and Allergic Rhinitis

Allergic rhinitis frequently occurs in patients with asthma. Adults with asthma are more likely to have developed allergic rhinitis initially with the appearance of airway hyper-responsiveness and asthma symptoms thereafter. Asthma control is enhanced by aggressive management of allergic rhinitis. Patients without adequate control with antihistamines and nasal steroids warrant further investigation. Obtaining a sinus CT scan in these patients will help to establish the presence of chronic sinusitis, which would result in improved symptom control with treatment. Patients with evidence of chronic sinusitis necessitate endoscopic evaluation and sampling of the sinuses to rule out infection and nasal polyps or other abnormalities.

Gastroesophageal Reflux Disease

Gastroesophageal reflux disease (GERD) can lead to bronchial hyperresponsiveness due to acid contact times in the trachea and bronchial tree. These patients present with dyspnea, cough, and wheezing, with a higher prevalence of symptoms at night. Asthmatic individuals with GERD may not have classic symptoms including heartburn and indigestion. Patients may report hoarseness, increased asthma symptoms with increased frequency of exacerbations requiring steroid therapy, and increased rescue inhaler use. Empiric therapy with proton pump inhibitors for patients with symptoms consistent with GERD has been shown to significantly reduce frequency of asthma exacerbations and improve quality of life scores. There was no significant improvement in pulmonary function or rescue inhaler usage.[7] Further evaluation to rule out silent GERD is warranted in patients with moderate to severe asthma with uncontrolled symptoms in spite of therapy with inhaled corticosteroids and long-acting beta agonists. The evaluation should include a pH probe study and a barium swallow test, the former to determine if reflux is present and the latter to rule out any esophageal pathology or dysmotility that may contribute to the presence of GERD.

DIFFERENTIAL DIAGNOSIS

Chronic Obstructive Pulmonary Disease

COPD is a disease characterized by fixed airflow obstruction without bronchodilator responsiveness. COPD encompasses two distinct disorders, chronic bronchitis defined as a chronic cough productive of sputum for 3 consecutive months at least 2 years in a row and emphysema defined pathologically by destruction of the airway parenchyma distal to the terminal bronchiole with the presence of bullae. A diagnosis of COPD should be considered in patients with cough, sputum production, or dyspnea and a history of exposure to risk factors including tobacco use. COPD typically occurs in persons aged 45 and older, and is associated with a prior history of cigarette smoking in the vast majority of patients, usually more than 10 pack-years.

Patients typically report having dyspnea on exertion that limits exercise tolerance. Risk factors for the development of COPD include tobacco smoke, occupational dusts, and smoke from cooking. A small proportion of patients have COPD secondary to α_1 antitrypsin deficiency. The Dutch hypothesis postulates that COPD and asthma are two diseases on the same spectrum with a great degree of overlap. Typically, patients with COPD are thought to have irreversible airflow obstruction without a response to bronchodilators. However, a small proportion of patients with COPD can have reversibility with bronchodilators as demonstrated by spirometry. The ability to differentiate COPD from asthma is particularly challenging in older adults who present with dyspnea and wheezing. The management of COPD includes strategies to enhance tobacco cessation, use of inhaled bronchodilators and anticholinergic medications, and vaccination against influenza and pneumococcus, as well as pulmonary rehabilitation and management of psychological stressors that are associated with the presence of the disease.

GERD Without Bronchial Hyperreactivity

GERD can present with minimal or no gastrointestinal symptoms but rather as a persistent cough. This phenomenon is referred to as silent reflux. The cough can be productive or nonproductive and can be associated with chest discomfort and a feeling of breathlessness.[8] Differentiating this phenomenon from asthma can be challenging and necessitates a methacholine challenge test. Patients with GERD-related cough will not have bronchial hyperreactivity on methacholine challenge testing. There is a considerable degree of overlap in the causes of chronic cough and a positive methacholine challenge in a patient with GERD may signify the presence of asthma.

Vocal Cord Dysfunction

The clinical presentation of vocal cord dysfunction (VCD) mimics asthma with the presence of cough, shortness of breath, dyspnea on exertion, throat clearing, throat and chest tightness, and occasionally wheezing. Making the diagnosis is difficult and requires a high index of suspicion. The diagnosis of VCD is often missed and it can take years before patients are diagnosed and treated appropriately. Those with vocal cord dysfunction are frequently thought to be severely asthmatic patients with persistent symptoms in spite of therapy with inhaled and oral corticosteroids, long-acting beta-agonists, and short-acting bronchodilators. These patients may even present with near fatal episodes of exacerbation with resultant intubation and mechanical ventilation. The patients immediately improve after intubation and are quickly extubated, which is atypical for status asthmaticus. Patients will have exercise-induced dyspnea and may present with symptoms of exercise-induced asthma.

The diagnostic evaluation of patients with suspected vocal cord dysfunction should include pulmonary function testing, methacholine challenge testing and laryngoscopy. Morris et al demonstrated that spirometry is typically normal in patients with vocal cord dysfunction.[9] Forty military recruits were studied for VCD; 15 of the recruits were diagnosed

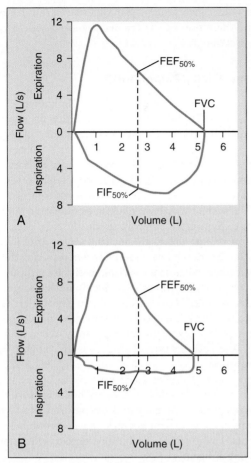

Figure 7-4 **A,** Normal spirometry. **B,** Fixed extra-thoracic obstruction with flattening of the inspiratory loop.

with VCD. All of these patients had normal baseline spirometry. These patients underwent methacholine challenge testing and 60% had abnormal flow volume loops suggestive of VCD (Fig. 7-4B). The methacholine challenge test results in reduced inspiratory flow rather than airway obstruction that occurs in asthmatic patients. The reduced inspiratory flow is secondary to the adduction of the vocal cords with inspiration as demonstrated in Figure 7-5B.

The gold standard test for diagnosing VCD is direct laryngoscopy. The use of exercise or methacholine challenge to induce VCD before laryngoscopy increases the yield of the evaluation and should be pursued whenever possible. Evaluation of vocal cord movement in an asymptomatic patient leads to a low diagnostic yield. Patients with suspected VCD should be referred to a practitioner who specializes in the diagnosis of VCD. These practitioners are often pulmonologists or speech pathologists.

The treatment of VCD includes speech therapy with laryngeal breathing techniques, behavior modification therapy, and occasionally botulinum toxin A injections of the vocal cords. Patients may warrant psychiatric evaluation and management of anxiety and depression, which usually results from the distress caused by the presence of symptoms related to VCD.

INTERSTITIAL LUNG DISEASES WITH AIRFLOW OBSTRUCTION

Sarcoidosis

Sarcoidosis is characterized by the presence of noncaseating granulomatous inflammation and typically presents with pulmonary involvement (Fig. 7-6). Sarcoidosis is frequently found incidentally on chest radiography with the mediastinal adenopathy being the most common finding.

Sarcoidosis is staged using a chest radiograph.

Stage 1: Mediastinal adenopathy and bilateral hilar adenopathy only (Fig. 7-7).
Stage 2: Parenchymal infiltrates bilaterally without mediastinal adenopathy.
Stage 3: Both mediastinal and parenchymal abnormalities.
Stage 4: Includes the presence of upper lobe predominant fibrosis and extrapulmonary manifestations such as the presence of ocular, cranial, hepatic, renal, cardiac, and skin involvement.

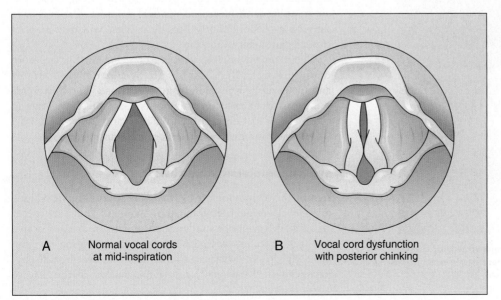

A Normal vocal cords at mid-inspiration

B Vocal cord dysfunction with posterior chinking

Figure 7-5 **A,** Normal vocal cords at mid-inspiration. **B,** Adducted vocal cords on inspiration in a patient with vocal cord dysfunction.

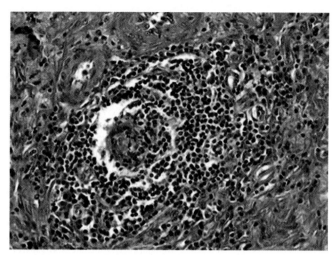

Figure 7-6 Noncaseating granulomas in the airway of a patient with sarcoidosis. *(From Nikon Microscopy U: Human pathology digital image gallery. Sarcoidosis. Available at http://www.microscopyu.com/galleries/pathology/ sarcoidosis.html. Accessed April 17, 2006.)*

The diagnosis of sarcoidosis requires a biopsy of the affected organ. The yield of transbronchial biopsy in the diagnosis of sarcoidosis is high, approaching 85%, and a referral should be made for bronchoscopy if the patient has findings suspicious for sarcoidosis. Patients with sarcoidosis require full pulmonary function testing to determine the degree of respiratory function impairment. The degree of severity of respiratory impairment and the presence or absence of symptoms dictates whether patients require therapy. Patients are often treated with oral corticosteroids and inhaled steroids for patients with obstruction noted on pulmonary function testing. Patients should be followed closely with pulmonary function tests at least yearly and routine eye examinations to

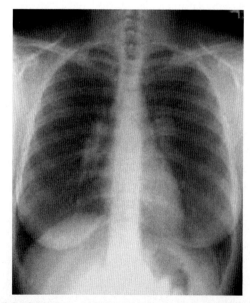

Figure 7-7 Stage I sarcoidosis as demonstrated by chest radiography with bilateral hilar adenopathy. *(From http://www.emedicine. com/med/images/2586pasarc1.jpg. Accessed April 28, 2006.)*

rule out ocular involvement. Sarcoidosis can remit spontaneously and therefore not all patients diagnosed with sarcoidosis require treatment.

Hypersensitivity Pneumonitis

Hypersensitivity pneumonitis (HP) is also known as allergic intrinsic alveolitis and represents a reaction to a particular environmental irritant. Clinical manifestations of hypersensitivity pneumonitis are divided into acute, subacute, and chronic. Acute hypersensitivity pneumonitis is characterized by acute onset of fever, chills, malaise, cough, severe dyspnea, and tachypnea 4 to 6 hours after exposure to an inciting agent. The patient may have rales on examination but wheezing is rare. Symptoms improve gradually over days but can recur after reexposure to the inciting agent. Antibiotic therapy is often instituted but is ineffective in resolving the symptoms. Subacute HP is characterized by similar symptoms that occur over weeks to months of continued exposure. Most patients have fever, dyspnea, and cough. Chronic HP is a consequence of either low-level exposure over a long period of time or high-level exposure intermittently over a long period of time. The patients typically have cough, fatigue, malaise, and weight loss.

Diagnosis of HP relies on history taking, focusing particularly on occupational and environmental exposures. Acute HP is suspected when there is an exposure history, flu-like syndrome, increased lymphocytes and neutrophils on bronchoalveolar lavage (BAL), and improvement with removal of the inciting antigen.

Conventional radiographs demonstrate low sensitivity in subacute disease (Fig. 7-8). Acute HP presents with bilateral infiltrates and ground-glass opacities.[10] Subacute HP is associated with exposure history, BAL with increased lymphocytes (>50%), and a diffuse micronodular pattern on CT scanning with air trapping and ground-glass attenuation. Pathologically, acute HP is characterized by interstitial infiltration by neutrophils, lymphocytes, and plasma cells. Subacute and chronic HP is a bronchiolocentric interstitial granulomatous pneumonitis. Chronic HP can lead to fibrosis, which would be evident pathologically. Pulmonary function testing typically reveals airway obstruction and air trapping with increased residual volumes. Patients who develop a predominantly fibrotic process will have restriction on pulmonary function tests.

The mainstay of treatment is to prevent further exposure to the inciting antigen. This is critically important in achieving and maintaining remission from the disease. Corticosteroids can be used to induce remission and are most effective in acute HP. In patients with chronic HP and fibrosis, the only treatment option is evaluation for lung transplantation.

Lymphangioleiomyomatosis

Lymphangioleiomyomatosis (LAM) is a rare interstitial lung disease affecting premenopausal women. The pathogenesis of LAM is poorly understood and is an area of active research. Patients with LAM are of childbearing age and typically present with exertional dyspnea, cough, and chylous pleural effusions. The pathophysiology of the disease

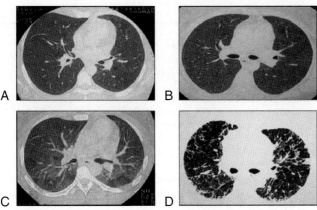

Figure 7-8 **A,** High-resolution CT (HRCT) scan of a patient with subacute HP shows ground-glass attenuation and bronchiolocentric micronodules. **B,** HRCT demonstrates diffuse, small, poorly defined nodules. C, HRCT at expiration of the same patient in A reveals patchy air trapping images (mosaic pattern). D, HRCT scan in a patient with chronic HP exhibits reticular fibrotic opacities with few areas of ground-glass attenuation. *(From Glassberg MK: Lymphangioleiomyomatosis. Clin Chest Med 2004;25:536.)*

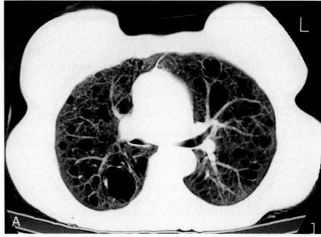

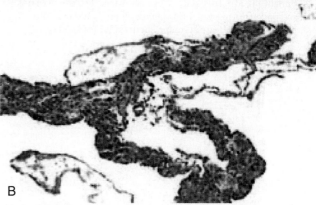

Figure 7-9 HRCT of the chest demonstrates multiple cysts of varying sizes (**A**). Pathology reveals LAM cellular infiltrate with large cystic airspaces (**B**). *(From Glassberg MK: Lymphangioleiomyomatosis. Clin Chest Med 2004;25:577.)*

includes peribronchial, perivascular, and smooth muscle–like cell proliferation in the lymphatics that results in vascular and airway obstruction and cyst formation. Patients can develop spontaneous pneumothorax secondary to the underlying cysts.[11]

Radiographically, patients present with pleural effusions and interstitial infiltrates with reticulonodular infiltrates and associated cysts (Fig. 7-9). CT scans reveal numerous thin-walled cysts throughout the lungs without any particular distribution. Pulmonary function tests reveal obstruction and air trapping, with a decreased DLCO (diffusing capacity of the lung for carbon monoxide). LAM is a clinical diagnosis and no pathology specimen is required if the radiographic and clinical picture are consistent with the disease. Diagnosis is often delayed due to insidious onset and misdiagnosis of the condition.

LAM is treated with hormone therapy, specifically progesterone and oophorectomy. The response to therapy is variable. Patients diagnosed at an earlier age tend to have progressive disease with subsequent loss of lung function. Progressive LAM can lead to the development of end-stage lung disease that necessitates lung transplantation.

Pulmonary Langerhans Cell Histiocytosis

Pulmonary Langerhans cell histiocytosis is a disease that is prevalent in young adults with a current or prior history of smoking. Pathologic evaluation reveals clusters of Langerhans cells in the distal bronchioles with associated eosinophils, neutrophils and lymphocytes. Most patients are between the ages of 20 and 40 years old and there is an equal gender distribution. The presentations vary from incidental findings to respiratory symptoms and spontaneous pneumothorax. The most common symptoms are fatigue, dyspnea, and cough. Diabetes insipidus can occur because of hypothalamic involvement and bone pain due to cystic bone disease should increase suspicion for this diagnosis. High-resolution

CT (HRCT) scan reveals multiple cysts and nodules with a predilection for the upper lobe in a smoker, which is classic for pulmonary Langerhans histiocytosis and is adequate for making the diagnosis. Pulmonary function testing demonstrates preserved lung volumes and no obstruction with a decreased diffusion capacity. Therapy is focused on encouraging and achieving smoking cessation. The disease may regress with smoking cessation but some patients continue to have progressive loss of lung function. Corticosteroids and cytotoxic agents are of limited value and do not result in remission of the disease. Progressive disease necessitates evaluation for lung transplantation.

SUMMARY

Diagnosis of asthma in adults can be challenging, as comorbid conditions can mask signs and symptoms and make lung function measurements difficult to interpret. In addition, contributing factors such as vocal cord dysfunction, GERD, and sinusitis/rhinitis can exacerbate and/or mimic symptoms of asthma. Careful history and physical examination combined with lung function measurements and radiography can suggest the diagnosis such that appropriate therapy can be instituted.

REFERENCES

1. Thomsen SF, Ulrik CS, Kyvik KO, et al: Risk factors for asthma in young adults: A co-twin control study. Allergy 2006;61(2):229–233.

2. Morris MJ: Difficulties with diagnosing asthma in the elderly. Chest 1999;116(3):591–593.

3. National Institutes of Health, National Heart, Lung, and Blood Institute: National Asthma Education and Prevention Program. Executive summary of the NAEPP expert panel report. Guidelines for the diagnosis and management of asthma— update on selected topics 2002 (NIH Publication No. 02-5075). Rockville, MD, U.S. Department of Health and Human Services, June 2002, pp 1–23.

4. Evans R 3rd, Mullally DI, Wilson RW, et al: National trends in the morbidity and mortality of asthma in the US. Prevalence, hospitalization and death from asthma over two decades: 1965-1984. Chest 1987;91(6 Suppl):65S–74S.

5. Enright PL, McClelland RL, Newman AB, et al: Underdiagnosis and undertreatment of asthma in the elderly. Cardiovascular Health Study Research Group. Chest 1999;116(3):603–613.

6. Crapo RO, Casaburi R, Coates AL, et al: Guidelines for methacholine and exercise challenge testing—1999. This official statement of the American Thoracic Society was adopted by the ATS Board of Directors, July 1999. Am J Respir Crit Care Med 2000;161(1):309–329.

7. Littner MR, Leung FW, Ballard ED 2nd, et al: Effects of 24 weeks of lansoprazole therapy on asthma symptoms, exacerbations, quality of life, and pulmonary function in adult asthmatic patients with acid reflux symptoms. Chest 2005;128(3):1128–1135.

8. Pratter MR: Overview of common causes of chronic cough: ACCP evidence-based clinical practice guidelines. Chest 2006;129 (1 Suppl):59S–62S.

9. Morris MJ, Deal LE, Bean DR, et al: Vocal cord dysfunction in patients with exertional dyspnea. Chest 1999;116(6):1676–1682.

10. Selman M: Hypersensitivity pneumonitis: a multifaceted deceiving disorder. Clin Chest Med 2004;25(3):531–547.

11. Glassberg MK: Lymphangioleiomyomatosis. Clin Chest Med 2004;25(3):573–582.

Pulmonary Function Tests: How Do I Interpret Them?

Reuben Cherniack

From a conceptual standpoint, pulmonary function tests can be divided into those that assess the ventilatory function of the lungs and those that are concerned with gas exchange. In the majority of patients the assessment of ventilatory function provides sufficient delineation of the impairment present, while assessment of gas exchange is essential in acute situations. Before discussing my approach to the interpretation of ventilatory function tests it is important to review the underlying basis of these tests.

VENTILATORY FUNCTION TESTS

Ventilatory function tests reflect alterations of the elastic resistance of the respiratory apparatus (the lungs, the chest cage, and the abdominal contents) as well as the resistance to airflow in the airways, both of which are related intimately to the volume of air in the lungs. Thus, knowledge of the absolute lung volume is essential for a proper assessment of the mechanical properties of the respiratory system.

LUNG VOLUME

The subdivisions of lung volume are indicated in Figure 8-1. The functional residual capacity (FRC), which is the amount of air in the lungs at the end of a normal expiration, is

particularly critical as it is necessary in order to calculate two other important volumes: the total lung capacity (TLC) and the residual volume (RV). Fortunately the FRC is remarkably constant in any one individual because, at FRC, the lung elastic force, which acts to deflate the lungs, is exactly balanced by the elastic force of the chest cage, which acts to inflate the lungs.

The TLC is the maximum amount of air that can be present in the lungs. It is determined by the ability of the respiratory muscles to maximally expand the chest, and is limited by the intrinsic elastic recoil of the lungs and chest wall, both of which are acting in an expiratory direction at TLC. In healthy individuals, the magnitude of the TLC, and its subdivisions or compartments, is related to the height, age, gender, and ethnic origin. To determine the TLC, one must add the FRC and the inspiratory capacity (IC), which is the maximum amount of air that can be inspired from the FRC (i.e., to TLC).

The residual volume (RV) is the amount of air remaining in the lungs at the end of a maximal expiration. To determine the RV, one must subtract the maximum amount that can be expired from the FRC, which is called the expiratory reserve volume (ERV), from the FRC. It is largely determined by the extent of airway narrowing and closure, which, in turn, is related to the extent of airway obstruction and the lung elastic recoil.

The vital capacity (VC) is the maximum volume of air that can be expired from TLC, and clearly is composed of the IC and ERV. The VC and its subdivisions can be determined with a spirometer. The TLC and RV cannot be measured directly, but as indicated above, must be calculated with reference to the FRC. In practice, the FRC is determined either by body plethysmography, through application of Boyle's Law, or by a gas dilution technique by breathing helium or some other tracer gas.

LUNG ELASTIC PROPERTIES

One can assess the elastic properties or dispensability of an object by determining its stress/strain relationship, or its change in length or size when a given force is applied. However, assessment of the change in both length and the force applied is not feasible in the respiratory system. Instead, the pressure difference between that in the esophagus, which reflects that in the pleura, and that at the mouth serves as a surrogate for force, and the volume change serves as a surrogate for length. Thus, in practice, the elastic properties of the lungs are assessed by determining the pressure/volume (PV) relationship of the lungs. The esophageal-mouth differential pressure is measured under static conditions (i.e., no airflow) at decrements of lung volume between the TLC and RV. As is seen in Figure 8-2, knowledge of the absolute lung volume

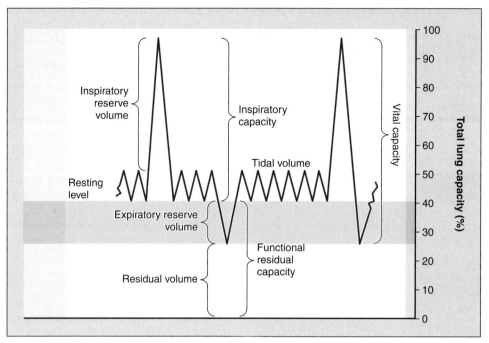

Figure 8-1 **Total lung capacity and its subdivisions.** *(Adapted with permission from Cherniack RM, ed: Pulmonary Function Testing, 2nd ed. Philadelphia, WB Saunders, 1997.)*

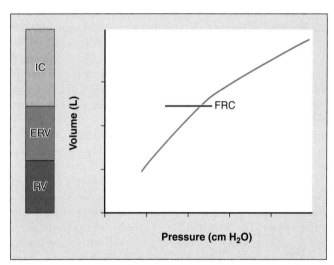

Figure 8-2 **The relationship between the pressure across the lungs and lung volume when there is no airflow (static pressure/volume curve) in a healthy individual.** *(Adapted with permission from Cherniack RM, ed: Pulmonary Function Testing, 2nd ed. Philadelphia, WB Saunders, 1997.)*

is important because the lung elastic recoil pressure (Pel) is greater with increasing lung volume and the PV relationship is not linear, even in healthy individuals.

AIRFLOW RESISTANCE

The resistance to flow in the airways (Raw) is assessed by determining the relationship between the driving pressure for airflow (the pressure difference between the alveoli and the mouth) and airflow rate. Since the airway size is related to lung volume (and lung elastic recoil), the Raw depends on the volume at which it is determined, being lowest at high lung volumes and increasing disproportionately at low lung volume. On the other hand, the reciprocal of the Raw, which is

called airway conductance (Gaw), is linearly related to lung volume. Accordingly, what is generally determined in practice is the specific airway conductance (sGaw), which is the conductance expressed per unit of lung volume. This can be calculated relatively simply by the body plethysmographic technique, where both airway resistance and lung volume can be determined virtually simultaneously.

In clinical practice, the degree of airflow resistance is frequently estimated indirectly by evaluation of the airflow rates during a forced expiratory vital capacity (FVC) maneuver. The volume expired during the first second (FEV_1), the FEV_1/FVC ratio, and the mean rate of airflow during the middle half of the FVC (FEF_{25-75} or MMEF), along with the maximum expiratory flow/volume relationship, are frequently examined. It is important to recognize that a lower than expected maximal expiratory flow rate may be due to increased airway resistance, reduced driving pressure (including reduced lung elastic recoil pressure), or both. Most importantly, like Raw, the flow rates achieved during the forced expiration depend on the lung volume at which they are achieved. Finally, it must be emphasized that the parameters calculated from the forced expiratory maneuver assess something quite different from the Raw determination, which is estimated during panting.

HOW DO I INTERPRET VENTILATORY FUNCTION TESTS?

My approach to interpretation of ventilatory function tests proceeds, whenever possible, in the following sequential manner:

1. Since ventilatory function tests reflect alterations of the elastic properties of the lungs and/or chest cage, as well as airway resistance, and since these, in turn, depend on lung volume, I examine lung volume first. Based on the TLC, I visualize in my mind's eye what the underlying

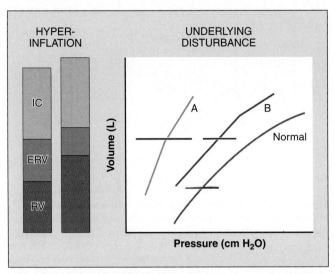

Figure 8-3   Potential underlying static pressure/volume relationship of the lungs associated with hyperinflation. The yellow line labeled A indicates emphysema and the green line labeled B indicates asthma or bronchitis. Note that the PV curves are shifted upward and to the left with the resultant increase of the FRC and TLC. The slope of the curve is greater in emphysema, and is normal in asthma and bronchitis

pressure/volume (PV) relationship of the lungs could be, and compare that with the position and shape of the PV curve seen in healthy people. As is seen in Figures 8-3 and 8-4, a greater than predicted TLC indicates that the PV curve of the lungs has shifted upward and that the lung elastic recoil pressure is reduced, while a reduced TLC indicates that the PV curve has shifted downward and the lung elastic recoil pressure is increased. Also, I examine the FRC, which will be altered by a change in the elastic properties of either the lungs or chest wall.

2. I then examine the maximal expiratory flow rates to determine if there is airflow limitation. In evaluating the flow rates, it is particularly important that they are compared at equivalent lung volume (isovolume). Lower than expected

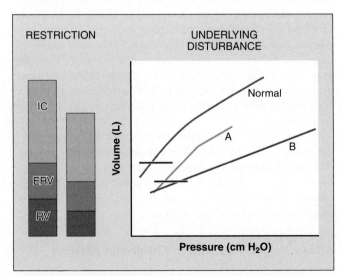

Figure 8-4   Potential underlying pressure/volume relationship associated with reduced TLC. The yellow line labeled A indicates obesity and the green line labeled B indicates interstitial lung disease (ILD). Note that the PV curves are shifted downward and to the left with the resultant decrease of the FRC and TLC. The slope of the curve is reduced in ILD, and is normal in obesity.

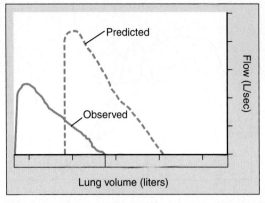

Figure 8-5   Lung volume and flow/volume characteristics in airflow limitation. Note that volume (TLC) is increased and isovolume flow rates are lower than expected. (*Adapted with permission from Cherniack RM, ed: Pulmonary Function Testing, 2nd ed. Philadelphia, WB Saunders, 1997.*)

isovolume expiratory flow rates (Fig. 8-5) are indicative of flow limitation, while greater than expected isovolume flow rates (Fig. 8-6) are consistent with a restrictive process.

The FVC and FEV_1 of the three best attempts must be within 200 mL of each other. It is particularly important that the FVC maneuver is truly maximal. As is shown in Figure 8-7, a less than maximal inspiration (efforts 4, 5, and 6) or less than maximal expiratory effort (efforts 2, 3, and 7) will result in lower volume and flow parameters calculated from the spirometric trace.

When lung volume has not been determined, as is frequently the case in practice, the percent predicted FEV_1 and the FEV_1/FVC ratio are used as surrogates. A lower than expected FEV_1 and FEV_1/FVC ratio suggests airflow limitation, while a low FEV_1 and normal FEV_1/FVC ratio suggests a restrictive process.

3. I then look to see if there is improvement following inhalation of a bronchodilator. It is generally accepted that a 12% improvement in FEV_1 is indicative of reversible airway obstruction; however, I call a beneficial effect of inhaled bronchodilator if the post-bronchodilator is consistently greater than baseline. Most important, changes in lung

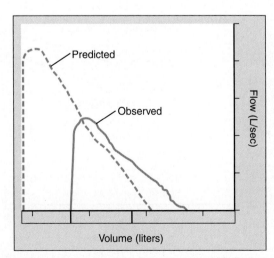

Figure 8-6   Lung volume and flow/volume characteristics in restriction. Note that volume (TLC) is decreased and isovolume flow rates are higher than expected. (*Adapted with permission from Cherniack RM, ed: Pulmonary Function Testing, 2nd ed. Philadelphia, WB Saunders, 1997.*)

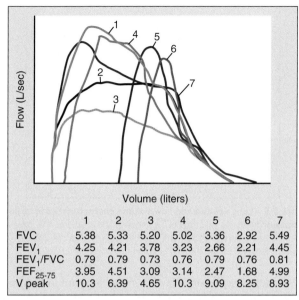

	1	2	3	4	5	6	7
FVC	5.38	5.33	5.20	5.02	3.36	2.92	5.49
FEV$_1$	4.25	4.21	3.78	3.23	2.66	2.21	4.45
FEV$_1$/FVC	0.79	0.79	0.73	0.76	0.79	0.76	0.81
FEF$_{25-75}$	3.95	4.51	3.09	3.14	2.47	1.68	4.99
V peak	10.3	6.39	4.65	10.3	9.09	8.25	8.93

Figure 8-7   The effect of less than maximal expiratory and inspiratory effort on flow/volume relationship and spirometric parameters. Note that a poor inspiration (4, 5, and 6) and a less than maximal expiratory effort (2, 3, and 7) result in reduced spirometric values.

volume (and thus in lung elastic recoil pressure) must be taken into account when assessing the impact of therapy. In many patients, lessening of bronchospasm results in a shift of the PV curve downward toward the normal position (Fig. 8-8), that is, the TLC falls and the driving pressure at any lung volume is increased. As a consequence, isovolume flow increases. The effect of this volume shift on isovolume flow following inhalation of a nebulized beta-agonist in a patient whose FEV$_1$ or flow/volume relationship did not improve is shown in Figure 8-9.

4. While examining expiratory flow rates, I also examine the inspiratory flow rates, as they may reflect an upper airway disturbance. Reduction of both inspiratory and expiratory maximal flow rates almost equally suggests a fixed airway obstruction, while a markedly reduced inspiratory flow

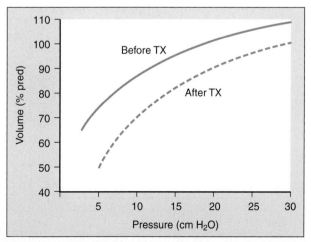

Figure 8-8   The effect of therapy on the pressure/volume relationship of the lungs in a patient with asthma. Note the shift of the curve downward and the resultant decrease in volume (TLC). The increase in lung elastic recoil will also result in a fall in FRC. TX, bronchodilator.

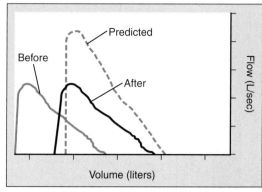

Figure 8-9   Volume shift and flow/volume relationship following inhaled beta-agonist in a patient whose FEV$_1$ and spirometric values did not change following inhaled bronchodilator. Note the volume shift and improvement in isovolume flow. *(Adapted with permission from Cherniack RM, ed: Pulmonary Function Testing, 2nd ed. Philadelphia, WB Saunders, 1997.)*

and relatively uninhibited expiratory flow indicate a variable extrathoracic obstruction. Finally, a slightly reduced inspiratory flow and an early plateau of expiratory flow suggest a carinal lesion.

5. When lung function is normal or responsiveness to bronchodilator is equivocal in a patient who has a history suggestive of asthma, I inspect the results of a bronchial challenge. Airway hyperreactivity is indicated if there is a 20% fall of FEV$_1$ or a 35% fall of sGaw following the inhalation of a nonspecific agonist (histamine and methacholine) or exposure to "real life" stimuli such as exercise, cold air, hyperventilation, a specific antigen, or occupational irritant.

Alterations in Function in Adult Asthma

In adult asthma, lung volume is generally increased and the pressure/volume curve is shifted upward and to the left (see Fig. 8-8). The resistance to airflow is increased and the FEV$_1$ and FEV$_1$/FVC ratio are reduced. The increased FRC indicates that the equilibrium between the elastic forces of the lung and chest wall have been reset at a new volume, usually because of the shift of the pressure/volume curve of the lungs and the reduced lung elastic recoil pressure. The FRC may also be increased because the elevated flow resistance prolongs the overall time constant of the respiratory system (i.e., resistance × compliance) so that there is a shorter time for deflation.

The increased lung volume is accompanied by expiratory airflow rates that are lower than expected at any lung volume. As is seen in Figure 8-9, bronchodilator therapy is frequently followed by a shift of the pressure/volume curve (and lung volume) downward toward that of a healthy individual and improvement in isovolume airflow.

Alterations in Function in Childhood Asthma

It is important to note that in children with persistent asthma, even in those with severe persistent asthma, a significantly reduced FEV$_1$ when clinically stable is the exception, rather than the rule. In a significant number of children with asthma, the FVC, FEV$_1$, and lung volume are greater than expected.

The increased lung volume is frequently associated with a loss of lung elastic recoil as well as enlarged airways. Thus, lung function tests may be misinterpreted if one relies solely on the FEV_1, especially if it has not been assessed pre- and post-bronchodilator.

Alterations in Function in Acute Exacerbations

Most importantly, an acute exacerbation may not be recognized in the early stages because the physiologic disturbances that are present may be particularly subtle. Because the cross-sectional area of the peripheral airways is significantly greater than that in the large central airways, the resistance to airflow is only about 10% of the total airway resistance. As is seen in Figure 8-10, even complete obstruction in one half of the peripheral airways may result in a virtually unrecognizable increase in total airway resistance (or fall in specific conductance). Thus, mucous plugging and constriction in the very small peripheral airways may not be recognizable. On the other hand, even minimal alterations in the peripheral airways may have a significant effect on the homogeneity of regional time constants (airway resistance × alveolar compliance) and consequently on the intrapulmonary distribution of gas. If there is continued perfusion of

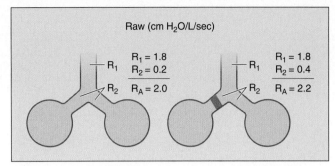

Figure 8-10   The effect of peripheral airway obstruction on total airway resistance. Note that the flow resistance in the small peripheral airways is only about 10% of the total airway resistance, and that a doubling of the flow resistance in these peripheral airways has a minimal effect on the total airway resistance.

the poorly ventilated alveoli, PaO_2 will fall and the $PAO_2 - PaO_2$ gradient will increase.

As the exacerbation progresses, airflow resistance and TLC, FRC, and RV increase and maximal expiratory flow rates fall. In those patients, both children and adults, in whom lung elastic recoil pressure is reduced, an increase in airway obstruction during acute exacerbations may be particularly serious.

BIBLIOGRAPHY

American Thoracic Society: Standardization of spirometry—1987 update. Am Rev Respir Dis 1987;136:1285–1298.

Cherniack RM, ed: Pulmonary Function Testing, 2nd ed. Philadelphia, WB Saunders, 1997.

Cherniack RM, Raber MB: Normal standards for ventilatory function using an automated wedge spirometer. Am Rev Respir Dis 1972;106:38–46.

Coates AL, Peslin R, Rodenstein DO, et al: ERS/ATS Workshop Series: Measurement of lung volumes by plethysmography. Eur Respir J 1997;10:1415–1427.

Hankinson JL, Odencrantz JR, Fedan KB: Spirometric reference values from a sample of the general U.S. population. Am J Respir Crit Care Med 1999;159:179–187.

Jenkins HA, Cherniack RM, Szefler SJ, et al: A comparison of the clinical characteristics of children and adults with severe asthma. Chest 2003;124:1318–1324.

Macklem PT: New tests to assess lung function. N Engl J Med 1975;293:339–342.

Mead J: Mechanical properties of lungs. Physiol Rev 1961;41:281–330.

Bronchoprovocation Tests: When and How Should I Use Them?

Don W. Cockcroft

BACKGROUND

Bronchoprovocation tests are tests in which subjects are challenged with a stimulus with a goal of inducing broncho-constriction. Bronchoprovocation tests have a wide use in asthma both in clinical evaluation of patients with (possible) asthma and in asthma research. Challenges can range from simple challenges with natural stimuli (e.g., free-range running) to complex challenges with expensive equipment (e.g., carefully monitored occupational exposure chambers with diisocyanates).

Various stimuli can be used for bronchoprovocation. These are initially characterized as sensitizing or nonsensitizing (Table 9-1). The *sensitizing* stimuli provoke symptoms in a (generally small) subset of asthma patients who have some form of sensitivity. The mechanism of sensitivity can vary from immunologic (e.g., immunoglobulin E (IgE)-mediated sensitivity to inhalant allergens) and presumed immunologic (sensitization to low molecular weight occupational chemicals such as toluene diisocyanate) to uncertain but nonimmunologic (acetylsalicylic acid [ASA]/nonsteroidal anti-inflammatory drug [NSAID] sensitivity, food additives, and so forth). Since allergen challenges have limited if any clinical role and occupational challenges are limited to a small number of highly specialized centers, the selective challenges will not be further discussed here.

Nonselective stimuli have the potential to provoke bronchoconstriction in many if not all subjects with asthma. The nonselective stimuli are subcategorized into *direct* and *indirect* (see Table 9-1). The direct stimuli provoke airway smooth muscle contraction by directly stimulating receptors on airway smooth muscle. This includes muscarinic agonists (e.g., methacholine) stimulating muscarinic receptors, histamine-

stimulating H$_1$ receptors, and leukotrienes. The indirect stimuli involve one or more intermediate steps leading up to the bronchoconstriction. Frequently, this involves the release of mediators from inflammatory cells such as mast cells. Examples include physical stimuli (exercise, cold air, hyperventilation, nonisotonic aerosols) and number of chemical stimuli such as AMP, propranolol, and mannitol.

For clinical purposes, bronchoprovocation is usually done using direct stimuli. Only methacholine (Provocholine, Methapharm Inc.) has been approved for use in North America. Chemical agents used for indirect challenges have not yet received approval and consequently these challenges are currently limited to research settings. Exercise and EVH (eucapnic voluntary hyperpnea) are available in some areas. Because direct and indirect stimuli have different clinical significance and different clinical availability, they will be considered separately.

METHACHOLINE CHALLENGE

Introduction

Airway hyperresponsiveness (AHR) is a characteristic feature of asthma and is now part of the definition of asthma. The direct stimulus, methacholine, is the most widely used

Table 9-1
BRONCHOPROVOCATION TESTS

Nonselective
Direct
Methacholine
Histamine
Leukotriene
Prostaglandin
Indirect
Exercise
Cold air
EVH
Nonisotonic aerosols
AMP
Mannitol
Propranolol
Etc.
Selective
Immunologic
Allergen
Occupational
Nonimmunologic
ASA
Food additives (?)

for assessing and quantitating AHR. With attention to certain methodologic considerations, methacholine tests are highly *sensitive* but not that *specific* for a diagnosis of asthma. It seems likely that data obtained from methacholine challenges are occasionally misinterpreted and perhaps often overinterpreted. This review of methacholine challenges will highlight some important caveats regarding interpretation (termed *pearls and pitfalls*) as background in understanding when and how they should be used.

History

It is only in the past 60 years that spirometric technology has allowed measurement of expiratory flow rates, e.g., forced expired volume in 1 second (FEV_1). Shortly after this technology became available, it was suggested that measurement of FEV_1 before and after both bronchodilators and bronchoconstrictors might have some role in the clinical assessment of patients with airways disease, particularly asthma. Initial studies measured FEV_1 before and after the bronchodilator (isoproterenol) and the bronchoconstrictor (acetylcholine). In the early years, challenge tests targeted a *significant* change in FEV_1; it became customary to look for a 20% change. While bronchodilator responsiveness could be done with a single dose, bronchoconstrictor challenges were done with a dose step-up, primarily for safety purposes. Consequently, a 20% FEV_1 fall was considered a positive test, independent of the dose at which it was achieved.

It is now appreciated that airway responsiveness (e.g., the provocation concentration causing a 20% fall in FEV_1 or PC_{20}) is distributed in a log-normal fashion in the population. There is no sharp cutpoint between normal and asthmatic. Furthermore, the measurement is not particularly precise. In the best of laboratories with the best of trained subjects, methacholine PC_{20} repeatability is within ± one doubling concentration or dose with the mean difference between two measurements being slightly less than one-half a doubling concentration or dose. For all these reasons, it is important to identify and regulate the methacholine dose as closely and reproducibly as possible in order to best identify the cutoff between normal and asthma and to allow comparison between laboratories and between different methods. Since the requirement for careful standardization was recognized after the fact, there still are many varied and different methods for performing methacholine challenge, many of which are difficult to compare.

Standardization

For reasons noted previously, standardization of methods for methacholine challenge is very important and is aimed at achieving a known repeatable dose of methacholine at each step. Detailed outline of the two most commonly used methods (the five-breath dosimeter method and the 2-minute tidal breathing method) have recently been published by the American Thoracic Society (ATS). The specific details are available (see "Suggested Reading") and will not be repeated here. However, the principles will be reviewed. Both methods recommend either doubling or quadrupling methacholine concentrations administered at a fixed (5-minute) time interval followed by appropriately timed carefully measured determinations of FEV_1. The results are expressed as the methacholine

Table 9-2 METHACHOLINE PC_{20} DEFINITIONS	
Methacholine PC_{20}	**Definition**
> 16 mg/mL	Normal
> 4 to 16 mg/mL	Borderline
> 1 to 4 mg/mL	Mild AHR
> 0.25 to 1 mg/mL	Moderate AHR
≤ 0.25 mg/mL	Marked AHR

PC_{20} or dose (PD_{20}). The two methods were considered to give equivalent results based on one small study.

Recent studies in a larger number of individuals have compared the two methods. These studies have demonstrated that the two methods give reasonably comparable results in subjects with moderate to marked AHR. However, in some subjects with asthma and mild AHR, the five total lung capacity (TLC) inhalations and breathholds required for the dosimeter method result in inhibition of methacholine-induced bronchoconstriction and false-negative tests. Unfortunately, this loss of diagnostic sensitivity occurs in the range of AHR, which would be seen in most positive challenges done in a clinical laboratory. When the dosimeter method is modified so that methacholine is inhaled by half-TLC breaths, the PC_{20} approximates that of the tidal breathing method.

Therefore, when deep breaths are avoided for the inhalation of methacholine, the two ATS methods produce similar results. The arbitrary definitions are outlined in Table 9-2 with *normal* being defined as a methacholine PC_{20} above 16 mg/mL and increasing levels of AHR severity based on values below 16 mg/mL.

Sensitivity and Specificity

The clinical value of a diagnostic or screening test is based on critical evaluation of its sensitivity and specificity and their more practical derivatives, the negative predictive value (NPV) and positive predictive value (PPV). Sensitivity-specificity evaluation of methacholine challenge has been hindered first by the lack of an independent gold standard for defining asthma in subjects whose baseline lung function is normal and, second, by the many different methods used to perform the methacholine challenge. Contradictory results in the literature can likely be explained in part by methodological differences (note TLC inhalation false-negative challenges in the previous section) and also by performance of challenges at times when symptoms are not clinically current (discussed in the following section). There is, however, a consensus that the methacholine challenge, particularly done by the tidal breathing non-TLC breath method, is highly sensitive. There are data showing that a methacholine PC_{20} has sensitivity and negative predictive values both approaching 100% for current symptomatic asthma. These are the features of a test that will function best to *rule out* (current) disease when the test is negative. The test has a mediocre specificity and a variable but frequently low positive predictive value for identifying disease when it is positive. The specificity and positive predictive value will vary depending on the *pretest probability*, that is, depending on the population studied and the (likely) prevalence of asthma in that population. Thus, the positive predictive value for a methacholine PC_{20} of less than 16 to signify current symptomatic asthma in a random population of individuals is likely around 35% or less. However, in a population of subjects with symptoms suggestive of asthma, the positive predictive value will increase. Although not validated, to our knowledge, the positive predictive value may further increase if the methacholine-induced symptoms mimic the symptoms for which the test was ordered.

As with all medical tests, altering the cutpoint used for definition will alter the sensitivity and specificity. For example, a methacholine PC_{20} of 1 mg/mL is a level with an extremely high specificity (and positive predictive value) and an extremely low sensitivity (and negative predictive value). Almost all subjects with normal resting spirometry and a methacholine PC_{20} below 1 mg/mL will have asthma.

Pearls and Pitfalls

There are a number of important caveats (see "Clinical Pearls") that must be borne in mind before performing and interpreting methacholine challenges. These are frequently overlooked. This has led to some confusion and probably misinterpretation (often overinterpretation) of methacholine challenges. Some important pearls and pitfalls are outlined below in approximate order of importance.

1. *Symptoms and exposures should be clinically current:* The mechanisms of airway hyperresponsiveness are not completely understood and will not be discussed in any detail here. However, there are two important pathophysiologic features that probably have independent effects on airway responsiveness. The first is airway inflammation, which is associated with both airway hyperresponsiveness and also with *current* asthma activity and severity. The second is structural (and perhaps physiologic) airway changes, the *airway remodeling* that is likely to be associated with *chronicity* rather than current activity of asthma. Structural airway changes are also seen in subjects with nonasthmatic airways disease (see point 2). Inflammation-associated AHR consequently will wax and wane with inflammatory exposures and anti-inflammatory treatments and may be absent when the asthmatic subject is unexposed and asymptomatic. This is particularly a feature of subjects with seasonal allergic asthma and occupational asthma. Because of AHR due to chronicity, AHR that is absent when away from exposures is more likely to be a feature in subjects whose allergic or occupational asthma is of relatively brief duration. Interestingly, in recent-onset occupational asthma (months or less duration), removal from exposure can result in normalization of methacholine challenge in as short a period as 2 days. Subjects with asthma and AHR exclusively related to recurrent (viral) infections, although less common, may also have normalization of their AHR when they are asymptomatic. The important clinical message is that a negative methacholine challenge done at a time when symptoms and exposures are remote, even as remote as a few days or a few weeks, does not exclude asthma, be it episodic allergic asthma or occupational asthma. Physicians should consider this when timing the ordering of their methacholine challenges and should

appreciate that a normal methacholine PC_{20} excludes only *current* asthma.

2. *Expiratory flow rates (FEV_1) must be (near) normal:* Much has been discussed about baseline lung function and methacholine challenge, particularly with regard to safety. There are no data to suggest that methacholine challenges are particularly dangerous in subjects with even very low FEV_1 and indeed our experience is that subjects with FEV_1 as low as 1 L (research studies only) tolerate methacholine-induced bronchoconstriction surprisingly well. The major concern with low baseline FEV_1 relates to difficulty in interpretation of the methacholine challenge. Subjects with nonasthmatic airways obstruction (e.g., chronic obstructive pulmonary disease [COPD]) exhibit positive responses to the direct bronchoconstricting agents histamine and methacholine, which appears to be a *geometric* phenomenon in that it is closely related to the degree of airflow obstruction, that is, to the reduced cross-sectional area of the airway(s). For this reason, there are interpretation difficulties when subjects with reduced baseline FEV_1 have a positive methacholine challenge. It is, therefore, not possible to use the methacholine challenge to differentiate asthma from COPD.

3. *Methacholine challenge may have a limited therapeutic impact in subjects with isolated cough:* Cough is a common respiratory symptom and can signify underlying asthma. Methacholine challenge has been part of some diagnostic algorithms for subjects with cough. Our experience is that cough is a common reason for referral for a methacholine challenge. Two of the common causes of cough are so-called *cough-variant asthma* (cough as the only symptomatic manifestation of asthma with variable airflow obstruction and AHR) and *eosinophilic bronchitis* (cough as a manifestation of airway eosinophilia with no variable airflow obstruction and no AHR). In subjects with cough-variant asthma, a positive methacholine challenge provides useful physiologic information; however, it has been shown not to predict a positive response to asthma therapy. In subjects with eosinophilic bronchitis, the methacholine challenge will be negative and importantly this does not predict nonresponse to asthma therapy, that is, inhaled corticosteroids (ICS). One can use such data to argue that for subjects with isolated cough, alternate diagnostic strategies might be indicated (e.g., induced sputum inflammatory cell analysis) or, alternatively, one could recommend a diagnostic trial of ICS (or oral corticosteroid).

4. *Deep TLC inhalations during methacholine challenge can cause false-negative results:* This concern and caveat has been outlined previously in this chapter. It is important to recall as one of the interpretative caveats that the dosimeter method when performed as outlined by the ATS may produce false-negative results. While this has not been critically investigated, it may be more likely to occur in subjects whose asthma is treated and is well controlled and may be less of a problem before treatment has commenced (i.e., before diagnosis). However, it is important to remember that in laboratories where TLC inhalations are used for methacholine administration, there may be unacceptably frequent false-negative challenges.

5. *A positive methacholine challenge (AHR) is not synonymous with asthma:* One common area of misinterpretation of the

methacholine challenge that we have seen is that clinicians have frequently considered that a positive methacholine challenge is synonymous with asthma. There are, however, many reasons other than asthma for a (false) positive methacholine test including a significant proportion of normal asymptomatic nonasthmatic subjects, a sizable proportion of subjects with rhinitis but no asthma, and subjects with other lung diseases, particularly COPD. We have also noted that at least occasionally this has been extended so that the arbitrary definitions of mild, moderate, and severe AHR have been inappropriately equated with mild to moderate and severe asthma. Nothing could be further from the truth. Most subjects with borderline or mild AHR (PC_{20} 1 to 16 mg/mL) actually have no asthma whatsoever. Most subjects with moderate to marked AHR (PC_{20} < 1 mg/mL) have only mild asthma. Subjects with moderate or severe asthma will rarely be seen in the diagnostic methacholine challenge laboratory as the test is not necessary to confirm the diagnosis. We have found the problem of equating positive methacholine challenge with asthma and equating severity of AHR with severity of asthma to be a particular problem in areas where asthma is (rightly or wrongly) considered to be an exclusion for participation. The test has been used for the armed forces, police forces, and SCUBA diving assessment. For exclusion from such activities, it would be more appropriate to use one of the indirect challenges.

6. *Remember to consider medication effects:* It is important when performing and interpreting methacholine challenges to recall which medications used acutely and which medications used chronically may have effects on the methacholine response. The inadvertent use of some of the acute medications is likely one explanation for the occasional false-negative challenge. Antimuscarinic drugs, although not widely used in the treatment of asthma, are the most potent inhibitors of the methacholine response. Short-acting and long-acting anticholinergic bronchodilators must be withheld for a surprisingly long duration, at least 8 and 48 hours (or possibly longer), respectively, before a methacholine challenge. It is likely that anticholinergic effects of other drugs (e.g., older antihistamines, phenothiazines, tricyclic and tetracycline antidepressants) may occasionally suppress the methacholine response and this must be kept in mind. The functional antagonists, particularly inhaled beta$_2$-agonists, also can inhibit methacholine challenge. The duration of efficacy of the long-acting drugs can approach or exceed 24 hours and it is appropriate to withhold these for at least this duration. By contrast, the anti-inflammatory drugs (e.g., ICS) have no immediate effect on the methacholine challenge. Their regular use will cause a slight improvement in methacholine challenge; however, the methacholine test will not normalize unless and until the patient becomes completely asymptomatic. Interestingly, we have seen this as an issue of confusion and controversy. We have evaluated patients on large doses of (often many) asthma medications and patients who historically probably do not have asthma whose methacholine tests were negative despite persistent symptoms. The disbelieving clinician and patient have been known to state that the reason for the negative methacholine challenge in this symptomatic patient, who in their opinion clearly does have asthma, is the corticosteroid

treatment. It is important then to remember that specific (anticholinergic) and functional (beta$_2$-agonist) antagonists can cause negative challenges, whereas corticosteroids (in subjects who are still symptomatic) do not.

7. *There is a significant range of* borderline *values:* It is important to recall that the methacholine PC_{20} has a day-to-day variability of at least ± one doubling concentration. This is considered to be primarily a measurement imprecision rather than true variability. For this reason, as well as the lack of a sharp demarcation between normal and asthmatic, there is a borderline range of results between 4 and 16 mg/mL (Table 9-2). Unfortunately, this is precisely the range into which many of the non-negative diagnostic methacholine challenges fall. Results of a borderline AHR (and even mild AHR) challenge must be interpreted with caution using both the pretest probability and, if available, the similarity (or lack thereof) of methacholine-induced symptoms to naturally occurring symptoms.

8. *True false-negative tests:* There are relatively few instances of false-negative methacholine challenges; however, it is important to recall these in interpreting the tests. It is possible to produce allergen-induced asthma in patients with normal methacholine challenges with a high exposure; the same is true for asthma due to occupational sensitizers. Thus, occasional false-negative tests can occur not only out of season but also very early in the allergen season in a seasonal allergic asthmatic individual or very early in occupational exposure in a subject who has occupational asthma. These are probably infrequent clinical occurrences but do occur. It is also possible to see subjects with exercise-induced bronchoconstriction (EIB) who have negative methacholine challenges, which is more likely to be an issue in high-performance elite athletes (see "Indirect Challenges—Who and When") or in children.

Interpretation

A simple interpretation algorithm is outlined in Table 9-3. Briefly, and considering the caveats noted above, a methacholine PC_{20} higher than 16 excludes with reasonable certainty current symptomatic asthma while a PC_{20} less than 1 mg/mL is close to diagnostic of current asthma. PC_{20} values between 1 and 16 will signify a variable likelihood of asthma depending on the pretest probability (i.e., the characteristics of the symptoms) as well as how closely the methacholine-induced

Table 9-3
METHACHOLINE TEST* INTERPRETATION

PC_{20}	Interpretation
> 16 mg/mL	Current asthma very unlikely
1–16 mg/mL	Likelihood of (current) asthma varies depending on pretest probability and similarity of methacholine-induced Sx to natural Sx
< 1 mg/mL	Current asthma very likely

*Tidal breathing and other non-TLC inhalation methods only

symptoms mimic or do not mimic the symptoms for which the test was ordered.

Who and When?

Who, then, should be referred for a methacholine challenge? And when should the challenge be done (Table 9-4)? The ideal subject and timing for a methacholine challenge would be a patient who has chest symptoms, particularly one or more of breathlessness, wheeze, or chest tightness, and yet whose lung function, particularly expiratory flow rates, is within the normal range including less than 12% improvement in FEV_1 following administration of an inhaled beta$_2$-agonist. The *when* of the test should be at a time when symptoms are clinically current, i.e., within the last few days, certainly within the last week.

A second less common situation is the patient with work-related respiratory symptoms in whom methacholine challenges can provide clinically useful data regarding the possibility of occupational asthma. First and foremost, occupational asthma is an area where compensation and legal issues make it imperative that asthma must be confirmed objectively. Second, one can use the (occupational) inflammation-induced changes in methacholine PC_{20} as a surrogate to indicate exposure to a sensitizer. Serial methacholine challenges demonstrating a significant (probably at least three doubling concentrations or eightfold) fall in PC_{20} on exposure and/or equivalent improvement in PC_{20} upon environmental control, particularly if reproducible, provide fairly strong evidence supporting exposure to an occupational sensitizer. Finally, the methacholine challenge can be of value in determining success of environmental control and eventual disability/impairment in subjects with occupational asthma.

Some investigators have suggested that methacholine challenges may be a useful way to monitor asthma treatment. Asthma therapy directed at maximizing improvement in AHR has been shown to be more effective than that monitored by conventional guideline measures (symptoms and FEV_1). At the moment, this is exclusively a research tool; however, in the occasional patient this might provide useful additional data.

There are a number of clinical situations in which methacholine challenge might not be considered the challenge of choice. This would include, first, in subjects with an isolated symptom of cough where methacholine challenge results are of limited therapeutic value. Induced sputum or perhaps other surrogate measures of airway inflammation (exhaled nitric oxide) might provide better guidance for treatment. Second, exclusion of subjects from the armed forces, police forces, SCUBA diving, and so forth would be more appropriately accomplished using an indirect challenge (exercise, EVH). Likewise, subjects with EIB only with high-performance exercise may well be better served by an indirect challenge (exercise or EVH). However, in this setting, a methacholine challenge can be a useful screen. Finally, subjects with reduced airflow obstruction who might have COPD, or COPD plus asthma, are not ideal candidates for a methacholine challenge because of the difficulty interpreting the result in the face of reduced baseline airway caliber.

INDIRECT CHALLENGES

Definition

Indirect challenges provoke bronchoconstriction *indirectly* via one or more intermediate pathways. Frequently, release of inflammatory cell mediators is considered to be the intermediate pathway. In fact, some have chosen to define indirect stimuli based on their capacity to release mast cell and other inflammatory cell mediators; consequently, bronchoconstriction induced by these can be inhibited by a single dose of cromones (sodium cromoglycate, nedocromil), drugs that have no effect on the direct challenges. All of the *physical* stimuli, which include exercise, cold air, hyperventilation, nonisotonic (hypertonic, hypotonic) aerosols, and inhaled particulate irritants, are indirect. A number of chemical stimuli including AMP, propranolol, bradykinins, tachykinins, and more recently mannitol are also indirect. Mannitol is an *osmotic* stimulus and may be more similar to the physical stimuli. In addition, all of the sensitizing stimuli (allergen, occupational) are indirect.

One of the features of indirect challenges that differentiates them from direct challenges (Table 9-5) is that the

Table 9-4		
WHO? WHEN? AND WHO NOT?		
Who	**When**	**Why**
Current asthma Sx (wheeze, tight, SOB) Normal FEV$_1$	Sx current	(1) High NPV to rule out asthma (2) Where positive provides physiologic rationale for Rx
Occupational asthma	At work and away from work	(1) Need to confirm asthma objectively (2) Δ PC$_{20}$ ≥ 3 doubling concs highly suggests a sensitiser
Monitoring asthma Rx	On and off Rx	Mainly research at this point
Who not	**Why not**	**Alternative**
Cough	Poor predictor of response to Rx	(1) Sputum eosinophils (2) Diagnostic ICS trial
Armed Forces SCUBA diving	Too sensitive	Indirect (EVH, mannitol)
EIB especially elite athletes (and possibly children)	(1) False negatives occur (2) Too sensitive re permission to use beta$_2$-agonists	Indirect (EVH, mannitol)

Table 9-5
DIRECT VERSUS INDIRECT CHALLENGES

	Direct	Indirect
Dose of stimulus needed	Low	High
Sensitivity and negative predictive value	High*	Low
Specificity and positive predictive value	Low to fair†	High
Correlation with eosinophils	++	++++
Response to anti-inflammatory Rx	++	++++
Inhibition by single-dose cromone	–	+++
Example	Methacholine	Exercise, EVH
Availability	High	Exercise-medium Others low

–, nil; + to ++++, low to high correlation.
*With non-TLC methacholine methods
†Depends on pretest probability

indirect challenges require a relatively high dose of the stimulus to provoke bronchoconstriction. When compared to the top concentration of methacholine in the diagnostic lab (16 mg/mL), AMP with the same diagnostic administration system is taken up to a concentration of 200 or 400 mg/mL. Other differences between direct and indirect challenges outlined in Table 9-5 will be discussed as follows.

Since naturally occurring asthma relates more to exposure to agents that provoke bronchoconstriction indirectly, it was hypothesized that indirect airway responsiveness should be both more specific for asthma and should correlate better with current asthma activity and current asthma inflammation. Numerous investigations have supported this. Indirect challenges are much more specific for asthma. One could argue that a positive exercise test, appropriately done and defined, is virtually diagnostic of asthma (i.e., EIB). The indirect challenges show better correlation than methacholine PC_{20} with airway eosinophils; this has been best documented for AMP. AMP challenge improves more with anti-inflammatory treatment (ICS, environmental control) compared to methacholine. As would be anticipated, a diagnostic test with the high level of specificity and positive predictive value of the indirect challenge will naturally have a low sensitivity and a low negative predictive value. Therefore, it is important to understand that the indirect challenges provide different and complementary data to the methacholine challenge.

Indirect Challenges—Who and When

Currently, our understanding of the applicability and availability of indirect challenges is in its infancy (or perhaps early childhood). This is partly compounded by lack of approval of any of the chemical stimuli for human use in North America. Consequently, the current position of AMP or mannitol challenges is that of only a research tool. Thus, we are limited to exercise, EVH, and hypertonic saline as the currently available indirect challenges.

1. *Exercise, EVH:* Exercise is probably the bronchoprovocation challenge with the longest history. It is also a common naturally occurring stimulus that provokes bronchoconstriction and symptoms in subjects with asthma. An appropriately designed test (several minutes of near maximal physical activity) will provoke bronchoconstriction primarily due to drying of the airway (osmotic) in many subjects with asthma. Fairly sophisticated technology is required to do exercise tests and some subjects with additional medical problems are unable to do exercise. The EVH challenge is easier technically, can be performed in virtually any patient, and has been recommended as a superior and easier challenge to use when looking for EIB. The indications for EVH testing (i.e., the *who*) would include first subjects with exercise-induced respiratory symptoms and a negative methacholine test, and, second, subjects who desire admission to the armed forces, police forces, permission to get a SCUBA diving license, and so forth. The EVH test is much more specific and avoids the overly high sensitivity of the methacholine challenge. It is also practical in that the EVH test mimics exercise, which is the primary concern regarding participation in such activities. Third, EVH or exercise testing would be the initial test recommended when assessing athletes for high performance competition. There are two somewhat related issues regarding elite athletes. The first is providing confirmation that the subject has EIB and is thus allowed to use inhaled beta$_2$-agonist, a restricted agent that requires objective documentation for Olympic and other athletes to use. The second, of course, is to confirm a diagnosis of EIB in a subpopulation of individuals who have a significant prevalence of false-negative methacholine challenges. (It is possible that children with EIB fall into this category as well.)

2. *Hypertonic saline:* The hypertonic saline challenge is not widely used in North America. It is an example of a highly specific and relatively insensitive indirect challenge. Individuals inhale increasing amounts of hypertonic saline (increasing hypertonicity, increasing duration) from a high-output ultrasonic nebulizer. Many patients find the challenge a bit uncomfortable. Hypertonic saline is also used for sputum induction to assess the level of sputum eosinophils. When looking at only sputum inflammatory cells, a bronchodilator is usually administered before the hypertonic saline inhalation. One of the advantages of the hypertonic challenge, therefore, is that it can be used as a single challenge with a dual purpose, first to measure

the (indirect) airway responsiveness and, second, to induce sputum for eosinophil assay.

3. *AMP:* The AMP challenge is not currently approved in North America. A doubling dose-response curve can be obtained using methods analogous to methacholine challenge. Higher doses are required. The improved relationship between airway inflammation and inflammatory/anti-inflammatory events suggest that this might be the ideal challenge used to monitor asthma therapy if indeed research concludes that there is some large advantage to monitoring asthma control and asthma therapy with bronchoprovocation tests.

4. *Mannitol challenge:* The new dry powder mannitol challenge involves inhalation of doubling doses of this osmotic alcohol-sugar using dry powder capsule inhaler. The result is a very simple and portable indirect challenge, which compares well to exercise and EVH. Large-scale comparisons with methacholine have yet to be reported. Administration by deep inhalation will add to its diagnostic specificity. The mannitol challenge shows potential to be an easy replacement for exercise EVH and possibly AMP.

CONCLUSION

Bronchoprovocation challenges are useful in the clinical evaluation of subjects with asthma or suspected asthma. The highly sensitive methacholine challenge, a direct challenge, is particularly valuable in excluding current asthma when it is negative. When positive, particularly in subjects with high pretest probability, the test provides a physiologic rationale for trials of asthma therapy. Indirect challenges on the other hand are highly specific and poorly sensitive. Their precise role remains to be determined. However, they are probably the ideal challenge for accessing patients who wish to get into the armed forces, police forces, and to SCUBA dive, and also the ideal challenges to use for high-performance elite athletes. Where indicated, they would also be the ideal challenge used to monitor therapy/environmental control.

Acknowledgment

The author thanks Jacquie Bramley for assisting in the preparation of this manuscript.

SUGGESTED READING

Anderson SD, Argyros GJ, Magnussen H, et al: Provocation by eucapnic voluntary hyperpnoea to identify exercise induced bronchoconstriction. Br J Sports Med 2001;35:344–347.

Cockcroft DW, Davis BE, Todd DC, et al: Methacholine challenge: comparison of two methods. Chest 2005;127:839–844.

Crapo RO, Casaburi R, Coates AL, et al: Guidelines for methacholine and exercise challenge testing-1999. Am J Respir Crit Care Med 2000;161:309–329.

Hargreave FE, Ryan G, Thomson NC, et al: Bronchial responsiveness to histamine or methacholine in asthma: measurement and clinical significance. J Allergy Clin Immunol 1981;68:347–355.

Hargreave FE, Dolovich J, O'Byrne PM, et al: The origin of airway hyperresponsiveness. J Allergy Clin Immunol 1986;78:825–832.

Holzer K, Anderson SD, Chan HK, et al: Mannitol as a challenge test to identify exercise-induced bronchoconstriction in elite athletes. Am J Respir Crit Care Med 2003;167:534–537.

Irwin RS, French CT, Smyrnios NA, et al: Interpretation of positive results of a methacholine inhalation challenge and 1 week of inhaled bronchodilator use in diagnosing and treating cough-variant asthma. Arch Intern Med 1997;157:1981–1987.

Joos GF, O'Connor B, Anderson SD, et al: Indirect airway challenges. Eur Respir J 2003;21:1050–1068.

Perrin B, Lagier F, L'Archeveque J, et al: Occupational asthma: validity of monitoring of peak expiratory flow rates and non-allergic bronchial responsiveness as compared to specific inhalation challenge. Eur Respir J 1992;5:40–48.

van den Berge M, Polosa R, Kerstjens HA, et al: The role of endogenous and exogenous AMP in asthma and chronic obstructive pulmonary disease. J Allergy Clin Immunol 2004;114:737–746.

Allergy Skin Tests: Use and Interpretation

Larry W. Williams

- Skin testing to aeroallergens in asthmatic individuals provides information with several uses:

- The nonatopic asthmatic individual is identified, so that unhelpful environmental interventions may be avoided, and clinical time more fruitfully spent on issues such as medication adherence.

- The patient with sensitivity to important indoor allergens, especially dust mite, animals, and cockroach, is identified. In these patients, allergen avoidance may lead to improvement of asthma, as may allergen immunotherapy. These patients are also likely to respond to anti-immunoglobulin E therapy if response to controllers is suboptimal.

- The patient with sensitivity to seasonal allergens (pollens and outdoor molds) may be detected. Patients with clearly pollen-induced asthma are relatively uncommon, but skin testing is useful to determine if seasonal symptoms indeed might be pollen or mold associated. For these patients, limited avoidance procedures may be considered. If there is concomitant allergic rhinitis not responding to pharmacotherapy, immunotherapy will reduce nasal (and potentially pulmonary) symptoms.

RATIONALE FOR SKIN TESTING IN ASTHMA

Immediate hypersensitivity skin testing is a simple clinical technique to determine if a patient has specific immunoglobulin E (IgE) to allergens. As many as 85% of children and young adults with asthma are atopic and will have specific IgE to at least some allergens. Skin testing provides a quick and inexpensive means to determine which allergens may be involved in the continuation of asthma symptoms. Among wheezy children younger than about 4 years, the prevalence of atopy is lower, but in this group skin testing has additional value as a prognostic factor favoring resolution of wheezing in those with negative tests. Among elderly asthmatic individuals the prevalence of atopy is also reduced, but as in all age groups, the results are useful for selecting those for whom allergen controls would be helpful.

Multiple lines of evidence suggest the importance of allergy to inhaled allergens in the pathogenesis of asthma. Examples of such evidence include:

- Newborn infants who go home into households with high levels of dust mite allergen are more likely to have asthma at 11 years of age than infants entering households with little dust mite allergen.[1]

- Children and adults with dust mite sensitivity and household exposure to dust mite have improvement in asthma when removed for several weeks to a domicile with low mite levels (reviewed in Platts-Mills[2]).

- Emergency room visits and asthma deaths increase when there are spikes in *Alternaria* spore counts in outdoor air.

- Cat-sensitized asthmatic individuals may develop wheezing within minutes of entering a home where there are cats.

- Children with cockroach sensitivity living in homes with high levels of cockroach allergen have greater asthma morbidity than similarly exposed, nonsensitized children or sensitized but nonexposed children.

- Patients with IgE to perennial allergens who have moderate or severe asthma uncontrolled by inhaled corticosteroids are improved by therapy with monoclonal anti-IgE (omalizumab).

The evaluation of occupational asthma is aided by skin testing. A number of syndromes of occupational asthma involve IgE-mediated reactions to inhaled allergens; examples include rodent (mouse) sensitivity in laboratory workers and domestic animal sensitivity among veterinary workers.

Skin testing is also used to identify allergens for inclusion in allergen immunotherapy. Immunotherapy is more easily shown to be effective in allergic rhinitis than in asthma, but a recent meta-analysis is also favorable for immunotherapy in asthma.[3] In addition, concurrent allergic rhinitis may require immunotherapy for control.

TECHNIQUES OF SKIN TESTING

Two basic approaches to skin testing exist: epicutaneous and intracutaneous. The most common methods of epicutaneous testing are the prick and prick-puncture techniques, with several other techniques also in use. Intracutaneous testing is performed by intradermal injection. Both methods depend on presentation of allergen to allergen-specific IgE bound to IgE receptors on the surface of mast cells resident in the skin. If a sufficient number of IgE-receptor units bind the allergen, the receptors are aggregated on the cell surface and a signaling pathway triggered that leads to the release of preformed mediators and the synthesis and release of other mediators. Vasoactive mediators are responsible for the erythema and swelling at the skin test site. Histamine, the most prevalent of these mediators by weight, causes itching at the skin test site, along with local vasodilation and capillary leak, which produce a transient wheal. Even in the very sensitive patient, appropriately chosen prick skin tests rarely cause a systemic reaction because only tiny amounts of allergen are needed at the test site.

The probability of systemic reaction to an intradermal skin test is higher, but still not prohibitively common.

Prick Skin Test Techniques

Prick testing as originally described employed a straight surgical skin closure needle or a hypodermic needle. A drop of allergen extract was placed on the skin and a very superficial prick made through it. Modern prick testing devices have replaced needles in routine practice for reasons of safety and convenience. Figure 10-1 shows the geometry of testing with a modern prick device. The operator holds the device at an angle of approximately 45 degrees to the skin and advances the tip downward until it just makes contact with the skin; then the point is swung upward from the skin, with minimal to no pressure on the skin. The simultaneous lateral and upward movements of the pricking motion transmits a small lateral and upward force to the skin at the point of the device, producing a very tiny prick on the surface. Such a lesion is estimated to allow approximately 0.1 nanoliter (10^{-10} L) of the allergen solution to pass below the epidermal basement membrane. A visible scratch on the surface of the skin is not necessary, and in fact is not desired. Such a scratch is poorly reproducible and, especially in the dermatographic patient, it may induce a nonspecific wheal and flare. In the past, various forms of scarifiers were used in skin testing to produce a visible scratch to which an allergen solution could be applied. Because of the nonspecific response in many patients, scratch testing as formerly practiced has been almost entirely abandoned. Figure 10-2 demonstrates the wheal and flare that can be produced on dermatographic skin with minimal pressure and stroking with a blunt pointer.

Present-day prick testing devices are inexpensive, easy to use, and disposable. They typically have one or more sharp points on the end of a 3- to 4-cm plastic rod. Examples of such devices are shown in Figure 10-3 with a straight needle for comparison. The points of the bifurcated and multipoint devices are short (1 to 2 mm), preventing deep penetration of the skin even if the prick is accidentally applied with inappropriate pressure. In addition, the multipointed tip retains a tiny drop of allergen extract when dipped into a well of the solution. Because the loaded device simultaneously deposits the allergen solution at the site and makes the skin prick, application time is reduced compared to needle prick techniques. In addition, since only a very small drop of extract is left on

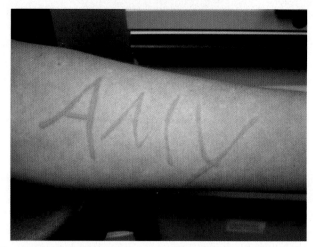

Figure 10-2 Dermatographism. Gentle pressure on very dermatographic skin yields an obvious wheal and flare in the following minutes. This individual wrote her name on her arm with the cap of a pen.

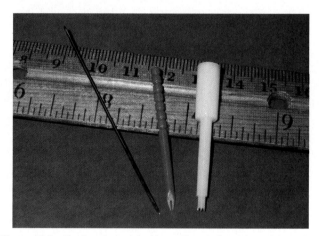

Figure 10-3 Devices for prick skin testing. Left to right: straight surgical needle, bifurcated disposable needle, multipoint disposable device.

the skin, the patient does not have to be prone for testing on the back. A separate pricking device is used for each allergen tested. This technique is quick, relatively painless, and can be used without much anxiety even in very young children.

Prick skin test techniques that avoid pressure to the skin are less prone to false positives or the problem of a nonspecific wheal with the negative control. Even the nondermatographic subject is likely to have some wheal and flare to a negative control (saline) when sufficient pressure is applied as the prick is made. Some dermatographic subjects will have small wheals of 2 to 4 mm at the site of negative control tests even with good technique with no pressure. This response does not invalidate the testing but does require that the interpretation of all wheals be made relative to the negative control. For most purposes, a wheal at least 2 to 3 mm larger than the negative control wheal is considered to be a positive. Scoring of skin tests is greatly simplified when gentle technique is used and there is no wheal at the negative control site.

A second commonly used epicutaneous testing method is the prick-puncture technique. Similarly to prick testing, prick-puncture technique uses a plastic rod to administer the allergen solution and create the skin lesion in a single motion. Unlike prick testing, the puncture technique uses simple

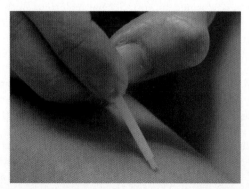

Figure 10-1 Close-up of prick skin testing on the forearm. The tip of the prick device is about to contact the skin at a roughly 45-degree angle. The points on the end of the device carry a small drop of an allergen solution.

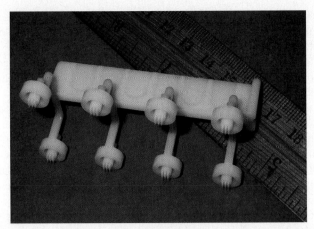

Figure 10-4 Multiple test device for prick skin testing. Multiheaded prick-puncture device viewed from inferior and lateral aspect. Each of the eight multipointed heads can carry a different allergen extract.

downward pressure to create a small puncture in the epidermis. Commonly used prick-puncture devices have from one to nine points that retain an allergen drop and can be applied individually as described above. Up to 10 devices may be fitted to a carrier that allows multiple puncture tests to be administered simultaneously (Fig. 10-4). Some operators value the ability to administer the tests in rapid fashion, but several caveats are necessary with this form of testing. First, because pressure is needed to consistently produce a skin puncture with the device, difficulty with interpretation will occur in dermatographic patients. Secondly, our experience has been that these devices are more uncomfortable than gently applied prick tests. In small children, if more than one set of eight tests need to be applied, cooperation for the second and subsequent sets may be lost. Last, if the skin surface being tested is not relatively flat, the pressure applied at the sites may be variable (or even absent) leading to false positives or false negatives. As with prick testing, positives are usually defined as tests with a wheal 2 to 3 mm greater than the negative control. A fair percentage of subjects tested with this technique will have a palpable wheal at the negative control site.

A last epicutaneous method employs a plastic rod with two or four symmetrically arranged points loaded with allergen as for prick testing. However, rather than being advanced to the skin at a 45-degree angle, the device is held at 90 degrees to the skin and advanced to touch the skin. While gentle pressure is applied, the device is rotated between the thumb and forefinger to create a small circular scratch (diameter of about 2 to 3 mm, depending on the device). This technique very often produces a wheal at the negative control site and is more uncomfortable than other methods. It is much less commonly used.

Techniques of Intradermal Testing

Intradermal testing is more labor intensive, and, as will be discussed below, less likely to be helpful in the evaluation of asthma. A 25- to 27-gauge needle on a 1-mL syringe is loaded with approximately 0.02 to 0.03 mL of allergen extract. The needle is advanced into (but not through) the skin at a very shallow angle with the bevel up. A small skin bleb is raised

by injecting most or all of the syringe contents. Care must be taken that there is not an air bubble in the syringe or needle. Compared to prick testing, a much more dilute solution of allergen must be used since the amount deposited in the skin is obviously greater, a factor responsible for the more frequent occurrence of systemic reactions with this technique. Since there is a physical injection into the skin, there is usually a wheal at the negative control site, and the skin test reaction must be scored in relation to the negative. Wheals induced by this technique are generally much larger than those induced by prick technique. A positive is usually read if the wheal is at least 10 mm larger than the negative control.

REAGENTS FOR SKIN TESTING

Reagents for skin testing are available from several commercial suppliers. Careful matching of the allergen extract, concentration, and technique is necessary for safety and validity. For asthmatic individuals, skin testing to aeroallergens is reasonable, but testing to foods is unlikely to yield useful results. Commonly tested indoor allergens with proven relation to asthma include the house-dust mite (*Dermatophagoides* spp.), cat, dog, and cockroach. Several molds may be important, including *Alternaria*, *Aspergillus*, *Cladosporium*, and *Hormodendrum*. For prick testing, undiluted stock extract in 50% glycerin is usually used. Compared to simple aqueous extracts lacking glycerin, glycerinated reagents have a long shelf life if refrigerated when not in use. The conventions used for describing the concentrations of these materials are often confusing to nonallergists. A few extracts, mostly grasses, are standardized, with the allergenic potency expressed in reference to the skin test responses of a panel of very sensitive subjects tested with the material. Such materials are usually sold at 10,000 BAU (biologic allergy units) per mL. For reagents where standardization has not been accomplished, the concentration is usually expressed as a ratio of the weight of starting allergen to extracting buffer. An extract of ragweed, for example, might be labeled as 1:10, meaning that 10 g of purified ragweed pollen was incubated in 100 mL of buffered saline in the initial step for preparation of the extract. A few extracts will be labeled with the microgram content of a single major allergen present in the extract. For example, a dust mite extract might be labeled with content in micrograms of Der p 1, one of the major allergenic proteins of the dust mite. Because the amount of allergen deposited beneath the epidermis with prick testing is so low, it is safe to perform prick testing with the concentrated stock solution as purchased. Intradermal tests are typically done with a 1:1000 dilution in saline of the stock material. Intradermal testing with the stock solution is likely to induce nonspecific false positives at least partially due to the glycerin, or to cause a systemic reaction because of the use of such a large amount of allergen. If dilutions of 1:10 or 1:100 of the stock solution are used, some of the wheals induced will be due to the irritant nature of the higher protein content rather than to specific triggering by allergen-specific IgE.

COMPARATIVE VALUE OF PRICK AND INTRADERMAL TESTS

The value of routine intradermal skin tests in asthmatic individuals is controversial. Skin tests by any technique are not simple "yes/no" predictors for the occurrence of clinically significant reactions when the lower airway (or any other tissue) is exposed to the allergen. Skin tests obviously challenge mast cells in the skin rather than mast cells in any other particular organ. Not surprisingly, the predictive value of tests in the skin is variable, and in some settings quite poor. Determination of the sensitivity, specificity, and predictive values for skin tests requires a gold standard test for comparison (and for predictive values, knowledge also of the disease prevalence). In the setting of food allergy, the gold standard is the placebo-controlled, double-blind, oral food challenge, a practical test that is reflective of real world exposures associated with disease. For nasal allergy, challenge by nasal instillation of pollen or pollen extract can be used, but such a nasal challenge is limited by uncertainty over the amount of allergen that would reflect real world exposure and the time frame over which that exposure should occur. For asthma, the analogous test is bronchial challenge with a nebulized solution of the allergen. Even more so than with nasal challenge, there is uncertainty as to the maximum amount of allergen that should be inhaled and tolerated before the allergen is judged irrelevant to the patient's disease.

Other challenges to the airway have been used. Some investigators have simultaneously exposed the upper and lower airways either in an exposure chamber or with a facial mask covering the nose, mouth, and possibly the eyes. These methods have potential to better replicate typical routes and levels of exposure but still may only be useful for determining immediate response to relatively large amounts of allergen, as opposed to ongoing low-level exposure. It is unclear whether low-level, chronic exposures to aeroallergen may be involved in the maintenance of airway inflammation in asthma. A further difficulty of all the challenge techniques (except food challenge) is that they are limited to investigational settings.

The multiple issues cited above prevent investigators from assuming that a bronchial allergen challenge is the gold standard test with which to compare skin tests.

The models of food allergy and nasal challenge may offer some guidance in understanding the predictive value of skin tests for lower airway symptoms. For food allergy there is good evidence that the prick skin test is clinically useful to discriminate patients at high versus low risk of reaction when the tested food is eaten. Intradermal testing in those who are prick-test negative does not identify patients who will react on food challenge and is thus not indicated.[4] A study of nasal challenge with timothy grass pollen has discriminated between the value of prick and intradermal tests. Patients with symptoms of seasonal rhinitis and a positive prick test reacted to relatively small amounts of intranasally administered pollen.[5] Among subjects with a history of seasonal rhinitis but a negative prick skin test there was no difference in reactivity on nasal challenge between those who were positive or negative on an intradermal skin test. Both groups required far more pollen to induce nasal symptoms on challenge than did the prick-positive group (Fig. 10-5). Subjects with no history of nasal symptoms and no positive skin tests tolerated more pollen than the other three groups. Intradermal testing did not demonstrate a group of patients with increased nasal sensitivity that had been negative on prick testing; therefore, for this pollen, there was no additional information obtained by intradermal skin testing. The study also suggests that there are people with nonallergic nasal symptoms who have nonspecific (possibly irritant) reactions to pollen instillation at high doses of pollen. Nasal sensitivity to irritant effects could result from underlying inflammation of a nonallergic nature (such as in the syndrome of nonallergic rhinitis with eosinophilia). Another study of allergic rhinitis used nasal provocation to identify allergic and nonallergic patients before skin tests. There was

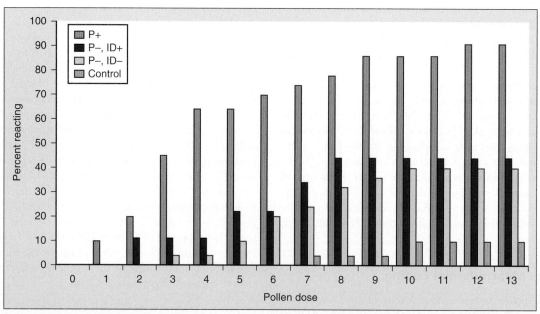

Figure 10-5 Nasal challenges with grass pollen. The bars show cumulative positive nasal challenge at each dose of timothy grass pollen. Dose 1 is 50 pollen grains. Subsequent doses are serial threefold increases. Dose 13 is 885,350 grains. The P+ group is statistically different from the other three groups. The ID+ and ID− groups do not significantly differ from each other. Control, nonallergic subjects; ID+, positive intradermal test; ID−, negative intradermal test; P+, positive prick test to timothy. P−, negative test. *(Data from Nelson HS, Oppenheimer J, Buchmeier A, et al: An assessment of the role of intradermal skin testing in the diagnosis of clinically relevant allergy to timothy grass. J Allergy Clin Immunol 1996;97:1193–1201.)*

no improvement in recognition of true positives when carefully performed intradermal end-point titration testing was compared to simple prick testing.[6]

Data for bronchial allergen challenge is more complicated. All the data regarding bronchoprovocation are limited by the uncertainty of the significance when increasing amounts of allergen are administered. Some authors have attempted to control for this issue by determining doses of inhaled allergen that are tolerated by nonallergic, nonasthmatic subjects.[7] With this caveat, several observations on bronchoprovocation and skin tests are well supported.

The probability of bronchial sensitivity (by bronchoprovocation) increases with increasing size of the wheal produced by prick testing. The probability of bronchial sensitivity varies inversely with the concentration of antigen required to induce a positive intradermal skin test (Table 10-1). Prick skin tests with a wheal greater than 9 mm were associated with a 50% probability of positive bronchoprovocation. Intradermal skin tests at a 1:1000 dilution yielded 27% positive on bronchoprovocation, increasing to 61% positive among those with a positive test at 1:10000 dilution, a rate similar to prick test positives with a large wheal.

Given the similar predictive values of very dilute intradermal tests and strongly positive prick tests, it would be reasonable to prefer the simpler prick test unless the intradermal test identified challenge-positive individuals who would have been labeled as negative by the prick test. As seen above, such patients do not appear to be identified in studies of food allergy or rhinitis. The published bronchoprovocation studies do not adequately address whether intradermal tests identify such patients; however, a strong case against routine intradermal testing comes from a study using a cat allergen exposure chamber.[8] Subjects in the study were exposed to cats in a small room that housed two cats. Subjects remained in the exposure chamber for up to several hours while nasal and eye symptoms, pulmonary symptoms, and lung function were monitored. No subjects who were prick-negative but intradermal-positive developed significant symptoms or a decrease in forced expiratory volume in 1 second (FEV_1). The authors conclude that the intradermal test added no information about clinical cat sensitivity.

The data above lead to the conclusion that intradermal testing for aeroallergens in asthmatic individuals is not routinely necessary. The value of intradermal testing to aeroallergens remains hypothetical at best, since a group of subjects with provable allergic disease who are identified only by this technique has not been found. For a patient with a very suggestive history for asthma symptoms related to a particular allergen, but a negative prick skin test, intradermal testing might be justified, but only at a relatively dilute concentration of the specific allergen in question.

SKIN TEST SCORING

Skin tests are scored by a variety of methods. In North America, simple, semiquantitative scoring based on the size of wheal produced by the allergen is commonly used. Table 10-2 shows a typical scoring method for prick skin tests, but there is no standard definition for the scoring grades. To avoid the variability in such scoring systems and to make transfer of data between practices more understandable, it is preferable to record the actual wheal size (and possibly the flare size) for each test, rather than a score. Other rational methods exist. For example, a common Scandinavian system compares the wheal induced by allergen to the wheal size of the histamine control. In this scheme, wheals less than 25% the size of the histamine wheal are considered negative.

SKIN TEST REAGENTS

A large number of allergen extracts are available for clinical use; however, only a limited number are likely to be useful in the evaluation of asthma. Screening with the common species of dust mite (*Dermatophagoides farinae* and *D. pteronyssinus*) is important because subjects in all but very arid regions will have exposure. Recent housing surveys show that essentially all homes in the United States have measurable amounts of cat and dog allergens in the vacuumed house dust. Cockroach allergen is not limited to the inner city, as cockroach allergen can be detected in about 20% of homes in the mid-Atlantic region where no cockroaches are reported by the occupants. Many homes contain common mold spores either produced in the home or infiltrating from outdoor air. Screening with several mold species is reasonable, including some or all of *Alternaria*, *Aspergillus*, *Cladosporium*, and *Hormodendrum*, and possibly others. If windows are opened in temperate weather, pollen allergens may be found in the household dust. Individuals with seasonal asthma symptoms related to pollens

Table 10-1
SKIN TESTS AND BRONCHIAL CHALLENGE

	% Positive on Bronchial Challenge
Prick Skin Test (Stock Solution) Wheal	
>9 mm	50
5–9 mm	35
2–5 mm	25
<2 mm	3
Intradermal Skin Testing Dilution	
Positive at 10^{-5} dilution	61
Positive at 10^{-4} dilution	35
Positive at 10^{-3} dilution	27
Negative at 10^{-3} dilution	4

Wheal size in prick testing and dilution at which a positive occurs in ID testing is related to probability of positive bronchoprovocation.
Adapted from Spector S, Farr R: Bronchial inhalation challenge with antigens. J Allergy Clin Immunol 1979;64:580–586.

Table 10-2
SKIN TEST SCORING

Score	Mean Diameter of Wheal (mm)	Flare (Erythema)
0	0	Absent
1+	0	Present
2+	≤3	Present
3+	3-5	Present
4+	>5	Present

The presence of erythema and a palpable wheal at the test site determine the test score. The positive and negative controls are also scored.

are difficult to demonstrate; however, poor control of allergic rhinitis may worsen asthma control, suggesting that testing for common regional pollens of grasses, weeds, and trees is of value. The timing of pollen seasons and selection of the regionally appropriate pollens are beyond the scope of this discussion but are well covered in standard texts.[9] Generally, fewer than 30 allergens would be needed for initial screening of an asthmatic individual for inhalant allergy.

IN VITRO TESTS FOR ALLERGY

Skin testing detects IgE bound to the mast cell surface. Very small but measurable amounts of allergen-specific IgE can also be detected in the serum. The original technique to measure allergen-specific IgE, called the RAST (radioallergosorbent test), is the model from which newer methods have developed. The tests all depend on binding of a specific allergen mixture to a solid carrier to which serum can be applied. Allergen-specific IgE in the serum then binds to the allergen on the solid phase. The bound IgE is detected by an antihuman IgE coupled to a signaling system. In the original RAST test, the signal was radioiodine (^{125}I) bound to the antihuman IgE; in newer tests signaling is usually via enzymatic production of a colored or fluorescent molecule that can be detected by photometry.

Commercial kits for measurement of specific IgE to a large number of allergens are available. Unfortunately the manufacturers of these methods do not use a consistent system to report results. In addition, not all systems can reliably report gravimetric results, i.e., ng of specific IgE per volume of serum. The original RAST system compared the analyzed serum to a control serum that exhibited little allergen binding and arbitrarily assigned increasingly high allergen binding to "class" results from I to V. More recent testing systems provide results in International Units (or ng) of allergen-specific IgE per milliliter. As specific IgE to an aeroallergen increases, there is increasing probability that the allergen is clinically significant, but values associated with defined predictive values are not known because challenge data correlated to the test results are not available. For comparison, for food allergens, using oral food challenge as the gold standard, the food-specific IgE that is clearly diagnostic of food allergy varies widely among common food allergens. As examples, in children an IgE to egg of 6 kU/L (determined by the Phadia "CAP" system) is 95% predictive of reaction on challenge, but for wheat, a CAP value at the upper limit of the range (100 kU/L) does not reach more than about 75% predictive value for reaction on challenge. For older in vitro tests or newer tests reported in class ranges, food IgE values of class II and below are generally predictive of a negative food challenge, although such RAST results are formally positive compared to negative controls. Similar data for aeroallergens are not available, but it appears that in vitro tests are useful if not over-interpreted. As a useful rule of thumb, positive results greater than about 3 kU/L (or class III) are much more likely to be associated with clinically significant allergen sensitivity than lower values.

UNPROVEN TECHNIQUES

Over the years, numerous tests have been proposed to diagnose allergic sensitization. A number have never been proven to aid in the management of asthma but continue to be used by some practitioners.

Intradermal end-point titration has been advocated as a means of determining the degree of sensitivity of a patient to an allergen. The technique uses serial intradermal skin tests of an allergen mixture, usually beginning at a quite dilute concentration (e.g., $\sim 10^{-5}$ of the stock solution) to which the skin test is negative, and proceeds through a series of more concentrated solutions to the first concentration that produces a clear-cut positive reaction. There are two clinical situations where this form of skin testing has been adequately validated to warrant clinical use: testing for allergy to insect venom and to some antibiotics. Some proponents of serial intradermal testing to aeroallergens believe that the end point so determined may allow them to identify a safe starting dose for immunotherapy. This starting dose may indeed be safe, but the cost of titration to multiple allergens probably outweighs any savings from starting immunotherapy at a higher initial dose. In addition, the discomfort of intradermal testing makes this method poorly tolerable, if not abusive, for small children.

An extension of end-point titration testing is called the provocation-neutralization technique. According to practitioners of this method, the most dilute concentration of allergen that causes a wheal clearly distinguishable from the negative control will have unique properties when administered orally to the patient: the intradermal provoking dose will be neutralizing when given by mouth. The neutralizing dose is then prescribed to be taken for relief of symptoms or given prior to exposure to prevent symptoms. Since the dilute solution produces only a local wheal when injected in a skin area of approximately 15 mm^2, administration of a fraction of a milliliter of the same solution to a much larger surface in the mouth and gut is very unlikely to produce symptoms. Thus the orally administered dose is safe, but there is no proof of any immediate protective effect. Any perceived benefit is almost certainly a placebo response.

IgG RAST tests are widely available. This test is analogous to the IgE RAST with the substitution of an antihuman IgG for the antihuman IgE. There are a few situations where serum IgG specific for an aeroallergen has clinical relevance. For instance in occupational exposure to *Aspergillus*, high titers of IgG anti-*Aspergillus* can help identify patients who have hypersensitivity pneumonitis related to the mold. When such antibodies are measured in analysis of subjective symptoms such as fatigue, headache, or cognitive difficulties, the results do not have a proven relation to any disease, and are more likely to hinder than promote accurate evaluation of the problem.

Other unusual practices sometimes promoted for analysis of allergy include electrodermal testing and applied kinesiology.[9] New methods for the purported diagnosis and management of allergy and asthma continue to emerge. The practitioner must be alert to the evidence (if any) supporting the use of new methods.

SUMMARY

Skin testing, particularly prick testing, can be a useful technique to establish the presence of atopy and to guide environmental controls that can benefit patients. Referral to an allergy specialist is recommended if skin testing is considered. However, there is still significant variability in the skin techniques and interpretation. Several national societies are evaluating this issue in hopes of providing consistent guidelines.

The absence of atopy in the form of negative skin testing is also valuable, so that focus on medication adherence and other contributing factors that may exacerbate asthma can be considered.

REFERENCES

1. Sporik R, Holgate ST, Platts-Mills TA, Cogswell JJ: Exposure to house-dust mite allergen (Der p I) and the development of asthma in childhood. A prospective study. N Engl J Med 1990;323:502–507.
2. Platts-Mills TA: Allergen avoidance. J Allergy Clin Immunol 2004;113:388–391.
3. Abramson MJ, Puy RM, Weiner JM: Allergen immunotherapy for asthma. Cochrane Database Syst Rev 2003;(4):CD001186.
4. Bock S, Buckley J, Holst A, May C: Proper use of skin tests with food extracts in diagnosis of food hypersensitivity. Clin Allergy 1978;8:559–564.
5. Nelson HS, Oppenheimer J, Buchmeier A, et al: An assessment of the role of intradermal skin testing in the diagnosis of clinically relevant allergy to timothy grass. J Allergy Clin Immunol 1996;97:1193–1201.
6. Gungor A, Houser SM, Aquino BF, et al: A comparison of skin endpoint titration and skin-prick testing in the diagnosis of allergic rhinitis. Ear Nose Throat J 2004;83:54–60.
7. Aas K: The Bronchial Provocation Test. Springfield, IL, Charles C Thomas, 1975.
8. Wood RA, Phipatanakul W, Hamilton RG, Eggleston PA: A comparison of skin prick tests, intradermal skin tests, and RASTs in the diagnosis of cat allergy. J Allergy Clin Immunol 1999;103:773–779.
9. Adkinson NF, Yunginger JW, Busse WW, et al (eds): Middleton's Allergy: Principles and Practice. Philadelphia, Mosby, 2003.

Noninvasive Tests, Exhaled Nitric Oxide, and Exhaled Breath Condensate—Do They Help Diagnose Asthma?

Glenn J. Whelan and Phillip E. Silkoff

CLINICAL PEARLS

- The fractional concentration of exhaled nitric oxide (FE_{NO}) is steadily becoming an accepted method to aid in the diagnosis and treatment of asthma. The term "inflammometer" has been used to describe FE_{NO}'s utility in assessing airway inflammation.

- The normal range for FE_{NO} is less than 20 parts per billion (ppb) and 20 to 30 ppb is often seen in steroid-naïve patients with asthma. However, the range is large and higher values have been noted.

- Nasal NO is considered to be a contaminant, as concentrations are orders of magnitude greater and are measured in parts per million (ppm). FE_{NO} collected from the lung contaminated with nasal NO will result in erroneous data. Collection of FE_{NO} needs to be performed in such a manner that will not allow for such nasal contamination (positive pressure with velum closure).

- The method of FE_{NO} collection and analysis is well described in the 2005 ATS/ERS recommendations for FE_{NO} collection. One of the more important things to keep in mind is the flow rate at which the patient will exhale. Flow rate will greatly influence the results from the FE_{NO} analyzer. Generally, the greater the flow rate (e.g., 0.25 L/sec), the lower the FE_{NO} result, and the converse for a lower flow rate (0.05 L/sec). Because of the patient controlling the pressure of exhaled air, this will cause velum closure. With velum closure, nasal NO will be minimized and not contaminate the sample.

- Exhaled nitric oxide (eNO) can be elevated in several conditions other than asthma, including bronchiectasis and upper respiratory infections. Cystic fibrosis, sarcoidosis, vocal cord dysfunction, and chronic obstructive pulmonary disease do not classically demonstrate elevation in eNO.

- FE_{NO} will decrease in response to corticosteroid treatment. FE_{NO} is very sensitive to corticosteroids, in that it will rapidly fall and rise with the initiation and discontinuation of corticosteroids, respectively.

Asthma is a syndrome with various underlying etiologies and clinical presentations. Asthma may present in an obvious and not so obvious manner. Because of the heterogeneous nature of asthma, there is no one clinical test that can accurately diagnose the disease with complete confidence. The hallmark of clinical diagnosis is based on asthma symptoms accompanied by lung function testing (e.g., spirometry), and in some cases methacholine challenge. However these clinical tests do not directly measure the amount of inflammation that is occurring locally in the lung that drives disease manifestations. Over

the past 2 decades, asthma has been recognized as a disease of inflammation, and therefore several tests have been developed to characterize the type and degree of inflammation in its diagnosis and treatment course. These tests include induced sputum for investigation of inflammatory cell types (e.g., including eosinophils and mediators). However, these tests do not come without inconvenience or invasiveness, which may make the patient reticent to undergo such testing, and may also put the patient at risk for adverse events such as bronchospasm. Furthermore, these tests do not provide immediate data; the results must be analyzed in a laboratory and reported before a clinician can make an interpretation.

Over the past decade, the fractional concentration of exhaled nitric oxide (FE_{NO}) has been extensively studied as a marker of inflammation in the lung. Although there is still much to discover about FE_{NO} and lung inflammation in asthma, it is steadily becoming an accepted method to aid in the diagnosing and treatment of asthma. The term "inflammometer" has been used to describe FE_{NO}'s utility in assessing airway inflammation. The assessment of FE_{NO} is a convenient and noninvasive method for directly assessing inflammation in the lung in a "real-time" manner.

Another method for assessing lung inflammation is by use of exhaled breath condensates (EBC). The fluid phase of exhaled breath, which is a biological fluid, contains mediators that partially originate in the lung. This is also noninvasive, but is far behind the sophistication of FE_{NO} in research and clinical application. EBC will be briefly discussed at the end of this chapter.

This chapter covers the physiology and pathophysiology of FE_{NO}, its use in asthma diagnosis, clinical ranges of FE_{NO} concentrations, methods of collection, detection, guidance in pharmacotherapy, and limitations of the use of FE_{NO} in asthma.

FE_{NO}

Physiology/Pathophysiology

The discovery of nitric oxide (NO), an important physiologic mediator, with physiologic action originally attributed to an unidentified "endothelial relaxing factor," dates back to the 1980s. Further detection of NO in exhaled breath of healthy and asthmatic individuals was elucidated in the early 1990s. NO is produced in discrete concentrations in the healthy human airway where it is important in physiologic functions such as maintaining airway patency. Conversely, in the asthmatic lung, NO is overproduced, both contributing to and formed during airway inflammation. NO, a reactive species, may directly contribute to oxidative stress, as do reactive oxygen species (including peroxynitrite).

NO is formed by the transformation of L-arginine to L-citrulline via nitric oxide synthase (NOS), as well as several cofactors including NADPH, O_2, Ca^{2+}, and calmodulin. NOS is currently observed in three isoforms. Two are constitutive (nNOS, NOS1; eNOS, NOS3); these consistently produce NO in very small amounts (picomoles) and diffuse locally for physiologic effect. The constitutive enzymes are calcium dependent, and steroid resistant. NOS2, or iNOS, is an inducible form, in response to pro-inflammatory cytokines, which is calcium independent, and responsive to corticosteroids. iNOS is produced continually in amounts thousands of times greater (nanomoles) than the constitutive isoforms. iNOS has been observed to originate from several sources including airway epithelium, vascular endothelium, and inflammatory cells (eosinophils). It was originally thought that iNOS was the sole contributor to increasing FE_{NO} in asthma; however, there has been increasing evidence that the constitutive NOS enzymes may be up-regulated in asthma.

Analysis

Nitric oxide analyzers used to measure FE_{NO} have evolved with much sophistication over the past 10 years. As of May 2003, the Aerocrine exhaled nitric oxide monitoring system NIOX was granted clinical approval by the US Food and Drug Administration (for ages 4 to 65 years). The analyzers in current use do not measure NO directly, but rather by a chemiluminescent reaction with ozone. NO is drawn into a chamber and is combined with ozone. The reaction then yields NO_2, O_2, and a photon, which is captured by the photomultiplier tube that analyzes and reports a proportional value of NO. Future monitors in early clinical testing phases will be much smaller, portable, and likely use a different method of NO detection (e.g., protein-binding or laser).

Measurement

CLINICALLY MEANINGFUL FE_{NO} CONCENTRATION RANGES

FE_{NO} is measured in parts per billion (ppb) in asthmatic patients. Although there are currently no clearly established cut-off points at which a patient would be considered asthmatic based on the level of FE_{NO}, it has been generally considered that 20 to 30 ppb in the steroid-naïve patient is indicative of inflammation. These are normal data published, and "normal levels" show considerable variability (e.g., FE_{NO} concentrations have been observed greater than 400 ppb). Individual data for FE_{NO} may be more meaningful, analogous to a "personal best" level for peak expiratory flow measures. Nasal NO is considered to be a contaminant, as concentrations are orders of magnitude greater and are measured in parts per million (ppm). FE_{NO} collected from the lung contaminated with nasal NO will result in erroneous data. Collection of FE_{NO} needs to be performed in such a manner that will not allow for such nasal contamination (positive pressure with velum closure).

The system of the interface between the patient and the nitric oxide analyzer is set up in a manner that allows for real-time analysis, with a biofeedback to assist in "coaching" the patient. Real-time analysis allows for repeat attempts, if necessary.

The method of FE_{NO} collection and analysis is well described in the 2005 American Thoracic Society/European Respiratory Society (ATS/ERS) recommendations for FE_{NO} collection. One of the more important things to keep in mind is the flow rate at which the patient will exhale. Flow rate will greatly influence the results from the FE_{NO} analyzer. Generally, the greater the flow rate (e.g., 0.25 L/sec), the lower the FE_{NO} result, and the converse for a lower flow rate (0.05 L/sec). Because of the patient controlling the pressure of exhaled air (5 to 20 cm H_2O), this will cause velum closure. With velum closure, nasal NO will be minimized and not contaminate the sample.

OFFLINE COLLECTION OF FE_{NO}

A key advantage of online FE_{NO} is the immediate data provided. However, there may be instances in both the clinical and research realm in which a "live" acquisition of FE_{NO} may be either inconvenient to the patient or the patient is unable to perform sufficient technique (e.g., sleeping or intubated patients or young children). Therefore, the clinician may be able to obtain the patient's FE_{NO} while offline and analyze the exhalate at a later time. Offline collection has demonstrated equivalency and reproducibility to the online collection of FE_{NO}. Collection methods are described in the ATS/ERS guidelines.

FACTORS AFFECTING FE_{NO} (INTERPRETATION)

Several factors can affect FE_{NO} results and interpretation. The circumstances described below must be applied in the differential diagnosis of asthma, as clinical presentation with incongruent FE_{NO} results may be indicative of a diagnosis other than asthma.

Neutrophilic Asthma

Asthma is often presented as an atopic disease that is largely mediated by eosinophils, Th2 lymphocytes, and mast cells. FE_{NO} is strongly correlated with eosinophilic asthma, as is shown by a strong correlation with sputum eosinophils. It has been observed that in asthmatic patients with more severe disease, neutrophils tend to have more involvement. In an interesting study done by Jatakanon and colleagues,[1] 55 asthmatic patients were grouped according to severity, and compared with 12 healthy controls. Eosinophils, eosinophilic markers (eosinophil cationic protein [ECP], interleukin 5 [IL-5]), and neutrophils with neutrophilic markers (myeloperoxidase, IL-8) were obtained by induced sputum. FE_{NO} was also recorded (0.083 to 0.1 L/sec). Because of the patients' asthma severity, moderate and severe persistent asthmatic patients were on concomitant inhaled corticosteroid therapy, and this may likely have confounded results. Nevertheless, neutrophils appeared to increase according to severity, in that mild asthmatics were similar to healthy controls, but severe asthmatic patients had a greater total neutrophil count compared with healthy controls ($P < .001$) and mildly asthmatic individuals ($P < .01$) (Table 11-1). Interestingly, FE_{NO} in asthmatic patients was significantly greater than healthy controls, but did not increase according to disease severity (controls: 7.9 ppb, mildly asthmatic individuals: 24 ppb [$P < .001$], moderately asthmatic patients: 12 ppb [$P < .05$], and severely asthmatic patients: 19 ppb [$P < .001$]). This is likely due to the concomitant administration of inhaled corticosteroids (ICSs), as FE_{NO} is sensitive to corticosteroid therapy (discussed in more detail later in the chapter). These

Table 11-1
SPUTUM CHARACTERISTICS OF PARTICIPANTS WHO WERE HEALTHY CONTROLS OR MILD, MODERATE, OR SEVERELY ASTHMATIC

Characteristic	Normal	Mild Asthma	Moderate Asthma	Severe Asthma
Volume, mL	2.9 (2.5–3.2)	2.9 (2.2–3.6)	2.6 (1.9–3.2)	2.7 (2.1–3.5)
TIC, × 10^6/mL	0.67 (0.46–1.03)	1.10 (0.54–2.14)	1.36 (0.54–2.14)	1.87 (1.31–5.42)[†,‡]
Tmac, × 10^6/mL	0.43 (0.26–0.76)	0.66 (0.35–1.10)	0.55 (0.27–1.57)	0.53 (0.42–0.81)
Tneu, × 10^6/mL	0.22 (0.11–0.34)	0.25 (0.20–0.71)	0.64 (0.32–1.02)	1.20 (0.55–2.61)[§,∥]
Teos, × 10^6/mL	0 (0–0)	0.03 (0.01–0.09)[¶]	0 (0–0.06)	0.04 (0–0.33)[**]
Tsq, × 10^6/mL	0.20 (0.14–0.32)	0.18 (0.10–0.31)	0.17 (0.10–0.30)	0.20 (0.07–0.27)
Macrophages, %	71.7 (57.8–78.6)	58.3 (47.7–66.1)[**]	49.9 (40.2–62.4)	33.1 (11.6–57.8)[‡,§]
Neutrophils, %	27.7 (20.6–42.2)	35.4 (29.8–46.1)	48.9 (37.1–57.6)	53.0 (38.4–73.5)[‡,**]
Eosinophils, %	0.0 (0.0–0.1)	4.2 (1.9–8.0)[††,‡‡]	0.5 (0–2.6)	4.5 (0.3–11.4)[§]
Lymphocytes, %	0.2 (0.0–0.3)	0.2 (0.0–0.3)	0.0 (0.0–0.6)	0.0 (0.0–0.3)
Squamous epithelium, %	22.5 (17.4–32.2)	18.8 (8.2–29.1)	13.9 (7.9–34.1)	6.1 (2.5–46.1)
ECP, ng/mL	7.3 (0–24)	60.7 (29.6–163.6)[†]	32.5 (7.5–84.5)	163.6 (90.2–717)[‡,‡‡]
IL-8, ng/mL	0.3 (0.2–0.6)	1.5 (0.4–2.6)	1.9 (1.5–2.7)[*]	3.6 (2.3–5.8)[§,∥]
MPO, ng/mL	0 (0–2.5)	4.6 (0–23.2)	15.7 (4.2–32.4)[∥]	26.0 (16.8–38.5)[‡,§]

ECP, eosinophil cationic protein; IL-8, interleukin-8; MPO, mycloperoxidase; Teos, total eosinophil count; TIC, total inflammatory cell count; Tmac, total macrophage count; Tneu, total neutrophil count; Tsq, total squamous epithelial cell count.
*Data shown as medians with 25–75 percentiles shown in parentheses.
[†]P <.01 compared with normal.
[‡]P <.05 compared with mild asthma.
[§]P < .001 compared with normal.
[∥]P < .01 compared with mild asthma.
[¶]P < .01 compared with normal.
[**]P < .05 compared with normal.
[††]P < .001 compared with normal.
[‡‡]P < .05 compared with moderate asthma.
[§§]P < .01 compared with moderate asthma.
Data from Jatakanon A, Uasuf C, Maziak W, et al: Neutrophilic inflammation in severe persistent asthma. Am J Respir Crit Care Med 1999;160:1532–1539.

results suggest that neutrophils are more involved in severe asthma and are possibly insensitive to corticosteroid therapy; thus FE_{NO} does not provide as a favorable biomarker for neutrophil-associated inflammation.

Chronic Obstructive Pulmonary Disease (COPD)

Similar to neutrophil-associated asthma, COPD is an inflammatory disease that has significant neutrophil involvement. COPD presenting with fixed airflow obstruction may demonstrate components of asthma, and the differential may be observed with the use of FE_{NO}. Fabbri and associates[2] studied a group of patients who were previously diagnosed with COPD (and fixed airflow obstruction), with the application of several tests including high-resolution computed tomography, pulmonary function testing, a burst of oral corticosteroids, bronchial hyperresponsiveness challenges, skin prick tests, induced sputum, white blood cell counts, and FE_{NO} tests. A subset of participants underwent bronchoscopy with bronchoalveolar lavage, and bronchial biopsy. FE_{NO} was significantly different in patients with asthma versus those with COPD (37.5 ± 9.2 versus 11.1 ± 1.7 ppb, respectively, P < .01). This was also similar to sputum eosinophils (8.5% versus 1.25%, P < .01) (Fig. 11-1). Furthermore, eosinophils recovered from the lamina propria were significantly different between patients with asthma versus COPD (50 versus 5 cells/mm², respectively, P < .01), CD4+ ratio (218 versus 109 cells/mm², respectively, P < .05). Differences were observed in carbon monoxide diffusing capacity (DLCO), change in forced expiratory volume in 1 second (FEV_1) in response to albuterol and a 15-day course

of prednisone. There were no significant differences in age, FEV_1, FEV_1/forced vital capacity (FVC) ratio, or bronchial hyperresponsiveness between patients with a history of asthma or COPD, demonstrating significant fixed airflow obstruction.

Bronchiectasis and Cystic Fibrosis (CF)

Bronchiectasis is a serious condition that involves chronic inflammation along with structural changes in the bronchi, and especially bronchioles. Bronchiectasis has many etiologies, is a heterogeneous disease (diffuse versus focal, columnar versus varicose versus cystic, lobular location, and so forth), and is still under much investigation for understanding its natural course. Bronchiectasis is, however, associated commonly with cystic fibrosis and pulmonary infections (gram negative and mycobacterial).

Kharitonov and co-workers[3] observed a difference in patients with bronchiectasis (n = 39) when compared with healthy controls (n = 79). Participants were diagnosed with bronchiectasis if they had a history of chronic cough or sputum production, and followed up with either a chest radiograph or computed tomography. Participants with bronchiectasis were ruled out for CF (sweat test), primary ciliary dyskinesia, and allergic bronchopulmonary aspergillosis. Furthermore, there was a subset of bronchiectatic participants who were on concomitant ICS. FE_{NO} was measured via chemiluminescence at 0.25 L/sec. Bronchiectatic participants not on concomitant ICS had an elevated FE_{NO} (285 ± 49 ppb) when compared with participants on ICS with bronchiectasis (88 ± 13.4 ppb, P < .01) (Fig. 11-2). Participants on ICS did not differ from healthy controls (89 ± 2.7 ppb).

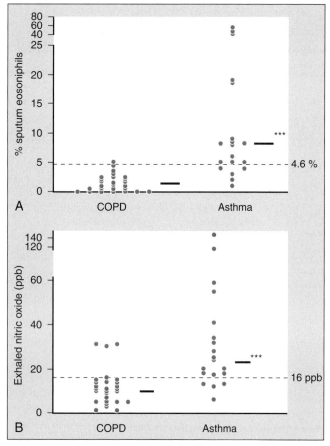

Figure 11-1 Percent sputum eosinophils (A) and concentration of exhaled NO (B) in patients with fixed airflow obstruction and a history of either asthma or COPD. The *horizontal solid bars* indicate the median value for each group. The best cut-off points to discriminate between the two groups are 4.6% sputum eosinophils (**A**) and 16 ppb exhaled NO (**B**). Asterisks indicate a significant difference ($P < .01$) between patients with a history of asthma and patients with a history of COPD. *(Data from Fabbri LM, Romagnoli M, Corbetta L, et al: Differences in airway inflammation in patients with fixed airflow obstruction due to asthma or chronic obstructive pulmonary disease. Am J Respir Crit Care Med 2003;167:418–424.)*

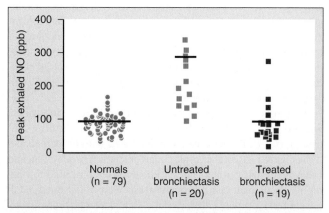

Figure 11-2 FE$_{NO}$ in bronchiectatic participants who were treated with ICS (*pink squares*) and those who were not treated with ICS (*blue squares*) were compared with healthy controls (*orange circles*). Bronchiectatic participants on concomitant ICS had FE$_{NO}$ values lower than untreated participants ($P < .01$), but were similar when compared with healthy controls. *(Data from Kharitonov SA, Wells AU, O'Connor BJ, et al: Elevated levels of exhaled nitric oxide in bronchiectasis. Am J Respir Crit Care Med 1995;151:889–893.)*

On the contrary, patients with CF and bronchiectasis do not demonstrate appreciable differences in FE$_{NO}$ when compared with healthy controls. Possible explanations as to why FE$_{NO}$ was not increased in the face of this inflammatory disease is suggested that as FE$_{NO}$ is primarily affected by the viscous secretions in that NO is unable to diffuse across, NO is absorbed by the pulmonary circulation, and/or the NO may react to form NO2, NO3, or peroxynitrite. This serves as an example of how multiple pulmonary disease states can present with difficulty in interpreting FE$_{NO}$ results.

Upper Respiratory Tract Infections

Upper respiratory tract infections (URTI) can substantially increase FE$_{NO}$. The mechanism suspected in this case is likely due to several inflammatory mediators in response to infection (tumor necrosis factor alpha [TNFα], IL-1β, interferon gamma [INFγ], and nuclear factor kappa beta [NF-κβ]) are all involved in the upregulation of iNOS (NOS2). This was keenly observed in 18 adult participants in the study of Kharitonov and colleagues.[4] These participants demonstrated signs and symptoms of URTI and were compared with 72 healthy controls. During infection, participants had an FE$_{NO}$ of 315 ± 57 ppb, compared with after recovery (3 weeks after infection, 87 ± 9 ppb) and healthy controls (88 ± 3 ppb, $P < .001$). There was no change in lung function parameters in these participants (>90% predicted for both FEV$_1$ and FVC). These results may confound the asthmatic patient, while a URTI will likely cause an asthma exacerbation; it is important to interview the recovering patient, as FE$_{NO}$ may be elevated by artifact, giving the impression of poorly controlled asthma.

Vocal Cord Dysfunction

Vocal cord dysfunction (VCD) is an elusive and complex syndrome of laryngeal spasms associated with either physical stimuli (e.g., smoke, perfume) or emotional stress, and is frequently mistaken for asthma. Patients will present with (severe) inspiratory wheeze, but usually normal pulse oximetry. Patients with VCD (without concomitant asthma) are generally unresponsive to asthma medications and are commonly diagnosed as steroid-resistant asthmatic patients. In pure VCD, because of the lack of inflammation from the respiratory tract, FE$_{NO}$ will not be elevated. This was demonstrated by Peters and associates,[5] who measured FE$_{NO}$ in healthy controls (9.7 ± 1.0 ppb), acute asthmatic patients (15.8 ± 0.9 ppb), stable asthmatic patients (13.5 ± 1.5 ppb), and patients with VCD (8.0 ± 3.5 ppb). Asthmatic patients, both acute and stable, were significantly different from control participants ($P < .001$), whereas the participants with VCD were not significantly different from healthy controls. FE$_{NO}$ is particularly useful in the diagnosis of VCD versus asthma, as demonstrated here; FE$_{NO}$ is not increased in patients with VCD. However, it should be noted that asthmatic patients do occasionally present with VCD.

Sarcoidosis

Sarcoidosis is a complex disease involving granulomatous lesions in several organ systems including the lungs. There is significant airway inflammation involved in sarcoidosis, with Th1 and Th1-relevant cytokines. Sarcoidosis of purely pulmonary involvement may initially present with asthma-like symptoms and is responsive to corticosteroid treatment. Studies do not demonstrate significant differences in FE_{NO} between patients with and without sarcoidosis. FE_{NO} differences begin to surface when atopy is observed as a concomitant condition.

Other Factors

Other diseases that affect FE_{NO} include primary ciliary dyskinesia (lower than normal), primary biliary cirrhosis (increased), and heart failure (lower than normal), to name a few. Other factors that affect FE_{NO} include cigarette smoking (lower), exercise (increase or decrease), age (in children, FE_{NO} tends to increase as age increases), and food that is high in nitrates or arginine (increase). It is suggested to avoid activities that may affect measurement at least 1 hour before FE_{NO} analysis. These are some examples that demonstrate several factors that may confound the interpretation of FE_{NO}. Although these add to the complexity of interpretation, this does not lessen the value of FE_{NO} measurement.

CLINICAL APPLICATION OF FE_{NO} IN ASTHMA

Diagnosis

FE_{NO} AS A CLINICAL TOOL: COMPARISON WITH OTHER CLINICAL DIAGNOSTIC TOOLS

FE_{NO} may be considered the first effective noninvasive "inflammometer." It is an important distinction from other clinical diagnostic tools such as spirometry. There is a disconnect between FE_{NO} and FEV_1, FVC, which has led to scrutiny of its clinical utility, as it is not usually seen that lung function and FE_{NO} have a direct correlation. However the same argument is used for FE_{NO}'s utility; otherwise, there would be no purpose in measuring it. It has been suggested that FE_{NO} is a more rapid responder to changes in the status of the disease. Furthermore, the discordance between FE_{NO} and spirometric parameters lends to the idea that asthma is a heterogeneous disease. There are multiple publications in the current literature that provide sufficient data to support the diagnosis of asthma by use of FE_{NO}.

Persistent asthma of a mild nature is relatively difficult to diagnose because in conventional asthma models, abnormal airway physiology is expected. However in mild persistent asthmatic individuals, low levels of inflammation persisting may not provide for accurate clinical diagnosis, demonstrating normal lung function (>90% predicted FEV_1, FVC). Clinicians must rely on self-described patient history, which is not always completely reliable. Smith and co-workers[6] compared FE_{NO} to other traditional methods of diagnosing asthma in 47 pediatric and adult patients (8 to 75 years) who were previously undiagnosed with asthma. The study consisted of three visits that were 2 weeks apart, with a steroid "burst" given between weeks 2 and 3. Seventeen were diagnosed with asthma: 12 with mild, 4 with moderate, 1 with severe according to Global Initiative for Asthma (GINA) guidelines. The remaining 30 patients did not have asthma. There were significant differences between asthmatic and nonasthmatic individuals in regard to FE_{NO}, FEV_1% predicted, bronchodilator

reversibility, FEV_1/FVC ratio, sputum eosinophils, and sputum neutrophils. The authors continued on to analyze the predictive value of each parameter. Using a cut-off of 20 ppb, FE_{NO} demonstrated a predictive value (88% sensitivity, 79% specificity) comparable to that of sputum eosinophils higher than 3% (86% sensitivity, 88% specificity), as seen in the provided receiver operating characteristic (ROC; Fig. 11-3). This contrasts to FEV_1 less than 90% predicted (35% sensitivity, 93% specificity) and FEV_1/FVC ratio less than 80% (47% sensitivity, 80% specificity). Because of the high values provided in comparing to traditional determinants, the authors concluded that FE_{NO} was superior in ability to diagnose persistent asthma of a mild nature. FE_{NO} (performed at a flow rate of 0.25 L/sec) has shown to be as good as bronchial hyperresponsiveness challenges with methacholine and adenosine 5'-monophosphate (AMP) for the diagnosis of asthma.

Dupont and colleagues[7] sought to determine the diagnostic utility of FE_{NO} in 240 patients who had symptoms suggestive of obstructive airway disease. A respiratory physician examined the patients for asthma. The physician was blinded to the results of their FE_{NO} tests but was able to use other conventional clinical diagnostic criteria. One hundred sixty participants were diagnosed with asthma, and 80 were not. Among the 80 participants who did not have asthma, the most common alternative diagnoses were postnasal drip (n = 29), chronic cough (n = 15), chronic bronchitis (n = 12), and gastroesophageal reflux disease (GERD) (n = 7). FE_{NO} was measured with a flow rate of 0.2 L/min. In the asthmatic group FE_{NO} was 25 ppb, versus 11 ppb in the nonasthmatic group (P < .001). By use of ROC curves, the investigators concluded that the FE_{NO} cut-off point for diagnosis of asthma was greater than 13 ppb, with a sensitivity of 85% and specificity

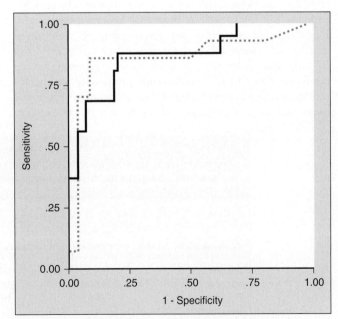

Figure 11-3 Receiver operator characteristic (ROC) curve demonstrating the sensitivities and specificities for FE_{NO} (*solid line*) and sputum eosinophils. With a cut-off of 20 ppb, FE_{NO} has a sensitivity of 88% and specificity of 76%, while sputum eosinophils, at >3% have a sensitivity of 86% and specificity of 88% for asthma diagnosis. (*Data from Smith AD, Cowan JO, Filsell S: Diagnosing asthma comparisons between exhaled nitric oxide measurements and conventional tests. Am J Respir Crit Care Med 2004;169:473–478.*)

of 80%. We must remind the reader that flow rates greatly affect FE_{NO} values; therefore, a greater FE_{NO} value would be suspected (25 to 30 ppb) by use of 0.05 L/sec, compared to the 0.2 L/sec used in this study.

Some asthmatic individuals present solely with chronic cough. Chatkin and colleagues[8] used FE_{NO} to make the distinction of patients with chronic cough with and without asthma. The study compared wheezing asthmatic patients to controls and patients with chronic cough (n = 105). The participants in the chronic cough group (average duration of chronic cough was 53 weeks) were subsequently examined by an experienced respiratory physician to determine which participants had cough-variant asthma and those who did not. The physician was blinded to the results of the FE_{NO} tests. FE_{NO} was measured at 0.045 L/sec, while participants exhaled at a resistance of 20 mm Hg. The results are displayed in Table 11-2. Controls, wheezing asthmatic patients, nonasthmatic patients with cough, and patients with asthma and predominantly cough had FE_{NO} concentrations of 28.3, 69.0, 16.7, and 75.0 ppb, respectively. Because of the poor positive-predictive value (60%) of these results, the authors suggest that this test may be of more value when ruling out asthma. This also suggests that using FE_{NO} should not be used as the sole diagnostic test for asthma.

EOSINOPHILIC INFLAMMATION

As stated previously, asthma is largely characterized by eosinophilic inflammation, which correlates with bronchial responsiveness. Eosinophilic inflammation in asthma is largely responsive to corticosteroid treatment. As mentioned previously, more severe asthmatics may present with neutrophil-involved inflammation, making treatment difficult. FE_{NO} is also associated with eosinophilic inflammation, and has been compared to serum eosinophilic cationic protein (SECP) as well as bronchial hyperresponsiveness. Piacentini and associates[9] set out to compare these three markers of eosinophilic inflammation (including FEV_1) in 57 asthmatic children, 63% of whom were receiving low to moderate doses of ICS (fluticasone propionate and beclomethasone dipropionate) for at least 6 months. FE_{NO} was measured by chemiluminescence, in which values were

obtained at the end of exhalation, said to represent the alveolar concentration of NO. Comparing ICS use (~7.5 ppb) to no ICS use (~15.7 ppb), FE_{NO} was the only parameter to distinguish between treatments ($P = .0024$). Interestingly, bronchial hyperresponsiveness was higher in patients who were on concurrent ICS versus those who were not (but did not reach statistical significance). Additionally SECP did not change with the treatment of ICS. Throughout the study population, FEV_1 correlated negatively with FE_{NO} ($r = -0.35$, $P < .01$), while in the ICS treated group, FE_{NO} also had a negative correlation with FEV_1 ($r = -0.426$, $P < .012$). In the participants not on ICS, a negative correlation was observed between PC_{20} and SECP ($r = -0.581$, $P = .0011$). Because FEV_1 was higher than 95% in both groups, FE_{NO} is able to differentiate between patients who are and are not taking ICS, lending to the observation that although a child appears to have normal lung function, unchecked inflammation may be ongoing and setting the stage for worsening asthma later in life. Notably, the study took place in the Italian Alps (1756 meters in altitude).

A subset of patients with eosinophilic bronchitis (EB) tend to be middle-aged, and present with a dry cough that is responsive to corticosteroid treatment but do not otherwise present with symptoms of asthma per se. The immunopathology of EB is still under debate, as some have reported an association with mast cells, while others have not observed mast cell infiltration into the airway smooth muscle. In these patients, a close correlation exists between eosinophils, eosinophil markers (MBP), and FE_{NO}. This suggests FE_{NO} is strongly associated with eosinophilic inflammation. However, it is difficult to make the distinction between EB and asthma based on cells and cellular markers, as there is likely a different component of inflammation in asthma. This may add limitation to the utility of FE_{NO}.

FE_{NO} AND SEVERE ASTHMA

Severe airflow obstruction, high peak flow variability, persistent wheezing, frequent hospitalizations, intubations, and high doses of inhaled corticosteroid usage with frequent bursts of oral corticosteroids are hallmarks of severe asthma. Severe

---

Table 11-2
PATIENT CHARACTERISTICS SHOWING DIFFERENCES BETWEEN HEALTHY CONTROLS, PATIENTS WITH CHRONIC COUGH (NONASTHMATIC AND ASTHMATIC), AND WHEEZING ASTHMATIC PATIENTS

Characteristic	Healthy Controls	Chronic Cough Nonasthmatic	Chronic Cough Asthmatic	Wheezing Asthmatics
Sex, M/F	8/15	9/21	2/6	13/31
Age, yr (± SD)	38 (8)	47 (15)	41 (12)	38 (14)
FE_{NO}, ppb	28.3	16.7	75.0	69.0
Skin test				
Atopic	0	14	8	44
Nonatopic	23	13	0	0
Not performed	0	3	0	0
FEV_1, % predicted (± SD)	94 (6)	92 (5)	93 (6)	74 (8)

Patients' characteristics and median exhaled nitric oxide levels in the studied groups.
Data from Chatkin JM, Ansarin K, Silkoff PE: Exhaled nitric oxide as a noninvasive assessment of chronic cough. Am J Respir Crit Care Med 1999;159:1810–1813.

asthma is also characterized as refractory asthma, in that regardless of patients using high doses of ICS in addition to oral/systemic corticosteroids, they remain poorly controlled, and are thus deemed as steroid insensitive (SI) or steroid resistant (SR). Steroid insensitivity/resistance has several etiologies, ranging from genetic to acquired. Much is unknown about this subtype of severe asthma, and much research has been dedicated to understanding the nature of SI/SR.

Other subtypes of severe asthma are described by either the presence or lack of eosinophils in the airway (EOS+ and EOS−, respectively). Silkoff and co-workers[10] set to determine if the use of FE_{NO} (measured at 0.05 L/sec) will aid in the identification of the EOS− subtype of severe asthma compared to bronchoscopy. Participants who completed all measures included 20 participants with severe asthma, 15 subjects with mild to moderate asthma, and 17 healthy controls included in the study. Figure 11-4 shows the differences in FE_{NO} among all groups. On the whole, severe asthmatic patients did not demonstrate a significant difference from other asthmatic patients or healthy controls; however, delineation between EOS+ and EOS− signifies the heterogeneity in FE_{NO} production between these two types of severe asthma (and may be predictor of steroid responsiveness). FE_{NO} showed a positive correlation with the results of tissue eosinophils from bronchoscopy (r = 0.54, P = .007), as well as tissue lymphocytes (r = 0.40, P = .003), and tissue mast cells (r = 0.44, P = .05). ROC analysis found 56% sensitivity and 100% specificity for identification of EOS+ subtype FE_{NO} asthmatic patients who had a FE_{NO} level above 72.9 ppb. These results are suggestive of FE_{NO} being able to detect EOS+ severe asthmatics, who are likely to have more severe exacerbations. The authors suggested that the reason why FE_{NO} was unable to distinguish between asthma severities may be because of a small sample size in each group, as well as concomitant corticosteroid use.

ASTHMA REMISSION

Along with substantial variability seen with asthma, remission may also play a role in the pathogenesis of asthma. Remission is usually observed in late childhood and adolescence. FE_{NO} has been investigated in the prediction of relapse in children who have undergone remission from asthma. Pijnenburg and colleagues[11] enrolled 40 children (6 to 18 years) who had been symptom free for 6 months while on low-dose ICS. Children on leukotriene modifiers were not eligible. Study participants underwent a 2-week run-in period, after which, if they were still symptom free, they underwent a 26-week medication-free period and were observed for asthma relapse. Lung function was measured, as well as FE_{NO} (0.05 L/sec) throughout the study period. Thirty-seven children completed the study, nine of which experienced a relapse in asthma, the majority of which relapsed between weeks 4 and 12. Figure 11-5 shows FE_{NO} results in those who did and did not relapse arranged according to time points after stopping their ICS. After 4 weeks stopping ICS, FE_{NO} was greater in children who relapsed (35.3 ppb) versus those who did not (15.7 ppb, P = .009). ROC analysis gives 71% sensitivity and 93% specificity in the ability of a FE_{NO} level of 49 ppb to accurately predict a relapse. Symptom scores and lung function tests were unable to predict asthma relapse. This study demonstrates the predictive ability of FE_{NO} compared to other conventional measures.

Van den Toorn and associates[12] investigated an older age group (adolescents aged 18 to 25 years), who had been in clinical remission from asthma for at least 1 year. Twenty-one participants in clinical remission were compared to

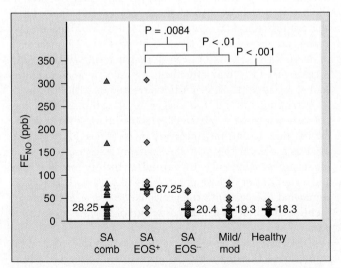

Figure 11-4 Chart showing the differences in FE_{NO} between severe asthmatic individuals (SA), mild/moderate asthmatic individuals, and healthy controls. Severe asthmatic individuals do not show a significant difference between the other groups until the group is divided up into those that are eosinophil positive (EOS+) and eosinophil negative (EOS−); corresponding P values are shown in the chart. *(Data from Silkoff PE, Lent AM, Busacker AA, et al: Exhaled nitric oxide identifies the persistent eosinophilic phenotype in severe refractory asthma. J Allergy Clin Immunol 2005;116:1249–1255.)*

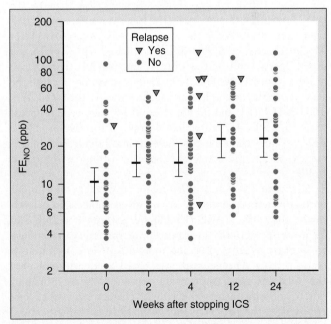

Figure 11-5 FE_{NO} values in patients with and without an asthma relapse. For each period (0–2, 2–4, 4–12, and 12–24 weeks) patients were classified according to whether they relapsed or not in the period indicated. FE_{NO} values were obtained at the start of each period. For patients without a relapse, geometric mean FE_{NO} and 95% confidence intervals are given. The x-axis depicts number of weeks after withdrawal of ICS. One patient relapsed in the first period (0–2 weeks), one between 2 and 4 weeks, six between 4 and 12 weeks, and one after 12 weeks. *(Data from Pijnenburg MW, Hofhuis W, Hop WC, et al: Exhaled nitric oxide predicts asthma relapse in children with clinical asthma remission. Thorax 2005;60:215–218.)*

21 with current asthma and 18 healthy controls. Duration of remission ranged from 1 to 12 years (average 5 years). FE_{NO}, bronchial hyperresponsiveness (BHR) (by methacholine and AMP challenges), and $FEV_1\%$ were measured in each group. Participants in remission and with asthma both had FE_{NO} levels greater than healthy controls (14, 22, and 1 ppb, respectively; $P < .001$), but were not significantly different from each other. The authors report a trend for a lower FE_{NO} level in those who have been in remission longer. Both BHR tests demonstrated significant differences between each study population. The results of this study suggest that FE_{NO} may be a more sensitive marker of underlying unchecked inflammation as compared to methacholine or AMP challenges. This study should be repeated with a larger sample size to determine if there is a relationship with lower FE_{NO} levels and duration of remission. This would give a more precise inflammatory picture.

FE_{NO} Response to Medications

As discussed above, FE_{NO} will decrease in response to corticosteroid treatment. In fact, FE_{NO} is very sensitive to corticosteroids, in that it will rapidly fall and rise with the initiation and discontinuation of corticosteroids, respectively. Therefore FE_{NO} may be a very useful tool in the treatment of asthma.

Clinical response to a short course (burst) of oral corticosteroids may be used to diagnose asthma. In a study by Smith and co-workers[13] participants with respiratory symptoms were enrolled to determine the effect of fluticasone on lung function as well as FE_{NO}. Fifty-two participants (14 to 71 years) completed the study; 27 were diagnosed with asthma. FE_{NO} was delineated into three categories: less than 15, 15 to 47, and more than 47 ppb. The highest number of participants were diagnosed in the more than 47 ppb category (15 of 17 participants, 88%, $P < .001$), compared with 7 of 18 and 5 of 17 participants in the 15 to 47 ppb and less than 15 ppb groups, respectively. This is especially interesting, because the $FEV_1\%$ (±SD) predicted at baseline was 101.4% (13.3%), 100.8% (14.8%), and 90.9% (12.6%) for each category (less than 15, 15 to 47, more than 47 ppb, respectively). These $FEV_1\%$ values could be considered nonasthmatic, and in this case, were less predictive of diagnosing asthma as compared to FE_{NO}.

Response to anti-inflammatory medication comes with substantial variability in any given subject. In a landmark study, the CARE (Childhood Asthma Research and Education) Network[14] investigated the variability in response to fluticasone propionate and montelukast in children aged 6 to 17 years. The network attempted to identify not only the variability associated with response to these medications, but to identify factors that would characterize which circumstances the patient would respond to each medication. Children were included if they had mild-moderate asthma, no ICS use in the previous 4 weeks, and no leukotriene modifying drugs in the previous 2 weeks from randomization. This was a randomized, cross-over, double-blind, double-dummy trial in which patients would receive fluticasone propionate by Diskus at 100 μg twice daily plus placebo, or montelukast once daily with age-appropriate dosing plus placebo, for 8 weeks, and were then crossed over for another 8 weeks. The primary outcome was a change in $FEV_1\%$ (7.5%) to define

response to a treatment. Several other parameters were investigated, including FE_{NO}. Overall, in regards to response as defined by a greater than 7.5% increase in $FEV_1\%$, participants responded to neither medication (55%), fluticasone alone (23%), both medications (17%), and montelukast alone (5%). Participants with a higher baseline FE_{NO} (54 ppb) had a better response to fluticasone propionate, along with blood eosinophil counts, ECP, IgE levels, lower prebronchodilator $FEV_1\%$ and FEV_1/FEV, and methacholine values, compared to neither medication. According to this study, accounting for interpatient variability, FE_{NO} plays a role in the predictive response to fluticasone, but not montelukast.

A goal in the treatment of asthma is to use the lowest titratable dose with optimal disease control. FE_{NO} may be useful in this capacity. Smith and colleagues[15] demonstrated optimal dose titration with FE_{NO} when compared to conventional guidelines. One hundred ten persistent asthmatic participants (average age 44.8 years) were enrolled and initiated on fluticasone propionate 750 μg per day for 4 weeks. At 4 weeks, participants were randomized to be treated according to conventional guidelines (Global Initiative for Asthma [GINA]), which were measurements of symptoms, bronchodilator use, peak flow variability, and spirometry), or by measure of FE_{NO} (considered uncontrolled if more than 15 ppb; measured at 0.25 L/sec). During the study, participants were assessed every 4 weeks, and the ICS dose was titrated by 250 μg per day upwards (maximum of 1000 μg/day) or downwards according to GINA guidelines or FE_{NO}, until optimal control was achieved. The study was conducted in two phases: Phase I was to achieve optimal control, and Phase II was to monitor over the course of twelve months to determine control (with dose changes allowed). At the end of the first phase (optimization), the fluticasone propionate dose in the FE_{NO} group was 292 μg per day, while the dose in the conventional group was 567 μg per day ($P = .003$). At the end of the second phase (monitoring), the fluticasone propionate dose in the FE_{NO} group was 370 μg per day, while the dose in the conventional group was 641 μg per day ($P = .003$). FE_{NO} was not different between the FE_{NO} and conventional groups at the end of phase I (8.2 versus 6.5 ppb, $P = .10$) or the end of phase II (8.6 versus 7.6, $P = .29$). The results of this study suggest that FE_{NO} may effectively be used alone as a clinical tool to monitor efficacy of asthma treatment with ICS.

Extending beyond the diagnosis of asthma, FE_{NO} has been shown to be a relatively effective marker for predicting response to anti-inflammatory medications. FE_{NO} may be used as a clinical tool to follow patient response to asthma medications, adherence to anti-inflammatory medications, and a monitor of disease progression/remission. This section somewhat overlaps with the previous section, as in the aforementioned studies inhaled corticosteroids were an integral part.

Corticosteroids provide the prime example of a dose response relationship with FE_{NO}. Jones and colleagues[16] conducted a study in 65 participants (19 to 64 years) who were previously controlled with ICS. Participants discontinued their therapy until loss of control was observed, at which point, they received prednisone 20 mg for 2 days. They were then randomized to receive placebo, 50, 100, 200, or 500 μg per day of beclomethasone dipropionate over the course of 8 weeks. FE_{NO} (measured at 0.25 L/sec), lung function, and methacholine challenge were measured throughout the study. FE_{NO} demonstrated a significant and linear response when observing changes between week 1 and the end of treatment ($P = .015$), as did FEV_1 ($P = .006$). However, the authors observed a favorable change in FE_{NO} at the end of week 1 ($P < .05$), but not in FEV_1. This suggests a more rapid response is observed in FE_{NO} compared to lung function when initiating ICS treatment, and expectedly, FE_{NO} will also react rapidly when ICS therapy is discontinued.

Early studies with omalizumab in the treatment of asthma have demonstrated decreases in FE_{NO}. Likewise, similar results have been observed with leukotriene receptor antagonists (LTRAs); however, there is variation in the literature. FE_{NO} is not influenced by inhaled beta-2 adrenoreceptor agonists (both long- and short-acting), theophylline, or mast cell stabilizers.

EXHALED BREATH CONDENSATE

In light of the desire for noninvasive markers of inflammation or disease progression, exhaled breath condensate (EBC) is a more recent advent in pulmonary research. There are many similarities between EBC and FE_{NO}, but they are different in many ways. EBC contains many soluble volatile and nonvolatile substances. These include hydrogen peroxide, nitrogen oxides (including nitrotyrosine and nitrosothiols), adenosine, arachadonic acid metabolites (including leukotrienes, thromboxanes, and prostaglandins), 8-isoprostane, aldehydes, ammonia, cytokines, and DNA, to name a few (pH is also frequently measured). Additionally, there are several commercial and custom-made EBC collection devices. As expected, with the magnitude of substances in EBC, variability and validity in detection are of key concern. The ATS and ERS have formed a task force in an attempt to begin standardization of this method of detection of inflammation.

In collecting EBC, briefly, an apparatus is set up so that the patient may perform tidal breathing for approximately 10 minutes to yield 1 to 2 mL of EBC. The inspired air will come from a room-temperature nonpolluted source. Because the circuit is cold in order to produce condensate, if the inspired air were to originate from the same circuit, then the patient may be subject to cold-air induced bronchospasm, altering the desired results. The expired air must be cooled to form a condensate, which is then collected and analyzed. The analysis method of the chemicals acquired depends on the chemical/protein in question. The EBC sample must be readily handled and stored properly, as leaving the sample at room temperature will contaminate it, allow for volatile gases to escape, or allow unstable chemicals/proteins to degrade, rendering the sample useless.

Leukotrienes are involved with both asthma airway inflammation and bronchoconstriction, which makes them attractive candidates for EBC analysis. Carraro and associates[17] set out to examine EBC (cysteinyl leukotrienes [Cys-LT]), LTB_4, ammonia, FE_{NO}, and lung function in asthmatic children with and without exercise-induced bronchospasm (EIB). A second aim of the study was to determine in children with EIB if there was a change in EBC after a 3-day course of montelukast. Nineteen asthmatic children and 14 healthy control children participated. EBC was collected over 15 minutes of tidal breathing, without a nose clip, and participants were instructed to swallow periodically. FE_{NO} was measured with the Niox system at 0.05 L/sec. Cys-LT and LTB_4 were measured via enzyme immunoassay. EBC and FE_{NO} were performed before and after a 20-minute exercise challenge (treadmill), while spirometry was performed during the exercise challenge. Eleven children were determined as having EIB (>12% loss in FEV_1), nine of which were able to undergo the 3-day challenge with montelukast. At baseline, EBC Cys-LTs in EIB asthmatic individuals were greater than non-EIB asthmatic individuals (42.2 versus 11.7 pg/mL, respectively, $P < .05$) and healthy control participants (5.8 pg/mL, $P < .001$). There was no statistical difference between non-EIB asthmatic individuals and healthy controls. Three days of montelukast therapy allowed for a 32% decrease in EBC Cys-LTs, but due to the variability in the results, did not achieve statistical significance ($P = .098$). EBC Cys-LTs did significantly correlate with postexercise drop in FEV_1 ($r = 0.7$, $P < 5.1$).

Asthmatic individuals had a greater concentration of FE_{NO} compared to nonasthmatic individuals (57.5 ppb [EIB], 29.5 ppb [non-EIB], 8.8 ppb [controls]; $P < .001$); however, montelukast did not significantly change baseline FE_{NO} concentrations. There was no difference between any of the groups for baseline FEV_1 values. However in the EIB group, forced expiratory flow between 25% and 75% of vital capacity (FEF_{25-75}) was lower when compared to the non-EIB or healthy control groups ($P < .05$). FE_{NO} did correlate significantly with postexercise drop in FEV_1 ($r = 0.5$, $P < .05$).

The results of the above study lend support to a possible clinical application for the utility of EBC in the diagnosis and treatment of asthma. This chapter discussed the applications of FE_{NO} in the diagnosis and treatment of asthma, as well as serving as an introduction to EBC research and application. As the diagnosis and characterization of asthma evolve, so will the diagnostic tools. FE_{NO} and EBC are two nascent modalities that will allow for more convenient and less invasive diagnosis and clinical monitoring of asthma. Because of the complex nature of asthma, it is unreasonable to expect a single diagnostic test to be able to make a solid diagnosis. However, the future of FE_{NO} and EBC will probably see detection devices that are smaller, more compact, more accurate, and less expensive (perhaps disposable) than current technology. This is an exciting time, as we are witnessing the foundation of noninvasive "inflammometers," which will likely prove to be very useful in the diagnosis, treatment, and monitoring of asthma.

REFERENCES

1. Jatakanon A, Uasuf C, Maziak W, et al: Neutrophilic inflammation in severe persistent asthma. Am J Respir Crit Care Med 1999;160:1532–1539.
2. Fabbri LM, Romagnoli M, Corbetta L, et al: Differences in airway inflammation in patients with fixed airflow obstruction due to asthma or chronic obstructive pulmonary disease. Am J Respir Crit Care Med 2003;167:418–424.
3. Kharitonov SA, Wells AU, O'Connor BJ, et al: Elevated levels of exhaled nitric oxide in bronchiectasis. Am J Respir Crit Care Med 1995;151:889–893.

4. Kharitonov SA, Yates D, Barnes PJ: Increased nitric oxide in exhaled air of normal human subjects with upper respiratory tract infections. Eur Respir J 1995;8:295–297.
5. Peters EJ, Hatley TK, Crater SE, et al: Sinus computed tomography scan and markers of inflammation in vocal cord dysfunction and asthma. Ann Allergy Asthma Immunol 2003;90:316–322.
6. Smith AD, Cowan JO, Filsell S: Diagnosing asthma comparisons between exhaled nitric oxide measurements and conventional tests. Am J Respir Crit Care Med 2004;169:473–478.
7. Dupont LJ, Demedts MG, Verleden GM: Prospective evaluation of the validity of exhaled nitric oxide for the diagnosis of asthma. Chest 2003;123:751–756.
8. Chatkin JM, Ansarin K, Silkoff PE: Exhaled nitric oxide as a noninvasive assessment of chronic cough. Am J Respir Crit Care Med 1999;159:1810–1813.
9. Piacentini GL, Bodini A, Costella S, et al: Exhaled nitric oxide, serum ECP and airway responsiveness in mild asthmatic children. Eur Respir J 2000;15:839–843.
10. Silkoff PE, Lent AM, Busacker AA, et al: Exhaled nitric oxide identifies the persistent eosinophilic phenotype in severe refractory asthma. J Allergy Clin Immunol 2005;116:1249–1255.
11. Pijnenburg MW, Hofhuis W, Hop WC, et al: Exhaled nitric oxide predicts asthma relapse in children with clinical asthma remission. Thorax 2005;60:215–218.
12. van den Toorn LM, Prins JB, Overbeek SE, et al: Adolescents in clinical remission of atopic asthma have elevated exhaled nitric oxide levels and bronchial hyperresponsiveness. Am J Respir Crit Care Med 2000;162:953–957.
13. Smith AD, Cowan JO, Brassett KP, et al: Exhaled nitric oxide: a predictor of steroid response. Am J Respir Crit Care Med 2005;172:453–459.
14. Szefler SJ, Phillips BR, Martinez FD, et al: Characterization of within-subject responses to fluticasone and montelukast in childhood asthma. J Allergy Clin Immunol 2005;115:233–242.
15. Smith AD, Cowan JO, Brassett KP, et al: Use of exhaled nitric oxide measurements to guide treatment in chronic asthma. N Engl J Med 2005;352:2163–2173.
16. Jones SL, Herbison P, Cowan JO, et al: Exhaled NO and assessment of anti-inflammatory effects of inhaled steroid: dose-response relationship. Eur Respir J 2002;20:601–608.
17. Carraro S, Corradi M, Zanconato S, et al: Exhaled breath condensate cysteinyl leukotrienes are increased in children with exercise-induced bronchoconstriction. J Allergy Clin Immunol 2005;115:764–770.

Invasive Tests: Bronchoalveolar Lavage and Biopsy: The Scope of the Scope

Anandhi T. Murugan and William J. Calhoun

In the early 1970s the advent of the fiber-optic bronchoscope and use of BAL (bronchoalveolar lavage) in obtaining cellular and soluble materials from airway for in vitro analysis was a major breakthrough in pulmonary research (Fig. 12-1). However, these techniques were not broadly used in the study of asthma until the 1980s because of concern for safety and potential risks of airway constriction and clinical compromise in patients with airway hyperresponsiveness. Since then, accumulating evidence regarding the safety of bronchoscope and associated techniques (BAL, bronchial biopsy, and bronchoprovocation) in adults and children with asthma has encouraged research using these techniques. These studies have provided important insights into the immunopathogenesis, pharmacodynamics, and therapeutics of asthma. Indeed, most current concepts of asthma have been derived from bronchoscopic studies of asthmatic individuals. Hence, clinicians caring for asthmatic individuals should have a thorough understanding of the utility, techniques, limitations and implications of these procedures.

DEFINITIONS

Bronchoscopy is an invasive procedure in which a flexible bronchoscope is inserted into the airways through nose, mouth, endotracheal tube, or tracheostomy to visualize the tracheobronchial tree). BAL involves instilling fluid into a wedged bronchoscope and recovering the cells and soluble substances lining the medium and small airways and alveoli. These materials closely reflect the in vivo milieu. Bronchial washings, in contrast, sample larger airways and have more limited utility, and are principally used for diagnosis of infectious diseases. Bronchial brushings from trachea and bronchi

harvest epithelial cells, which can be cultured for ex vivo studies. Endobronchial and transbronchial biopsies with histology, immuno-histochemical staining, and in situ hybridization techniques provide valuable information regarding cellular and chemical mediators involved in airway inflammation and remodeling. Segmental allergen challenge (SAC) allows localized and controlled bronchoprovocation with a small amount of antigen to detect allergic inflammation and sensitization. Further, it permits quantification of inflammation without causing generalized bronchoconstriction. SAC has helped to differentiate the pathogenesis of atopy with and without asthma, and asthma with and without atopy (Fig. 12-2).

NATURAL HISTORY

Allergic asthma is a complex disease process. Antigen exposure triggers biphasic response in most allergic asthma patients, consisting of early and late asthmatic responses (Fig. 12-3). The early asthmatic response (EAR) occurs within minutes after allergen exposure and lasts for 2 to 3 hours. EAR is characterized by mucosal edema and bronchospasm, mediated through release of vasoactive and bronchospastic mediators like histamine, tryptase, and cysteinyl leukotrienes. In contrast, the late asthmatic response (LAR) occurs 6 to 8 hours after exposure to the inciting agent and lasts for 24 to 72 hours. LAR is characterized by early recruitment of neutrophils, followed by brisk influx of activated eosinophils and helper T lymphocytes, particularly those of Th2 phenotype. These Th2 lymphocytes produce interleukin 4 (IL-4), IL-5, granulocyte-macrophage colony-stimulating factor (GM-CSF), and other cytokines, resulting in amplified allergic inflammation and airway hyperresponsiveness (AHR) (Fig. 12-4).

Persistence of inflammation may lead to subepithelial fibrosis of the airway walls causing progressive irreversible airflow limitation. This process of structural change of the airway is called "remodeling." Remodeling may differ with respect to severity of asthma and presence or absence of atopy, but in general the degree of remodeling bears only a loose relationship to asthma severity. Definitive data do not exist about the mechanisms of remodeling, but intriguing studies suggest that AHR is the best physiologic correlate of remodeling. Confirmatory evidence regarding whether early recognition and treatment of asthma might prevent progressive loss of lung function is lacking, both in adults and in children.

STRENGTHS

The major strength of bronchoscopic evaluation of airways is the recovery of biological samples in the form of cellular and soluble materials from medium and small airways and alveolar

	1880	1900	1960	1970	1980	1990	2000	2005
Gustav Killian	Rigid bronchoscopy →							
Chevalier Jackson		Bronchoalveolar débridement →						
Shigeto Ikeda			Fiberoptic bronchoscopy →					
Reynolds and Newball				Bronchoalveolar lavage →				
Shigeto Ikeda					Video bronchoscope →			
PJ Godard						BAL in asthma patients →		
CE Brightling							Cytokine analysis →	
G Cox								Thermoplasty →

Figure 12-1 History and advancements in bronchoscopic techniques.

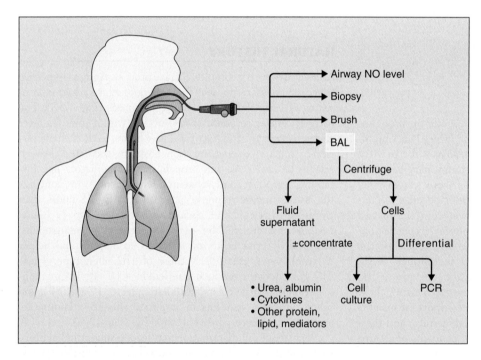

Figure 12-2 Specimen procurement through bronchoscopy. *(From Kavuru MS, Dweik RA, Thomassen MJ: Role of bronchoscopy in asthma research. Clin Chest Med 1999;20:153–189.)*

spaces (Tables 12-1 to 12-3). These procedures can be safely performed in healthy subjects, and in patients with mild and moderate forms of reactive airway disease. Until the advent of the flexible bronchoscope, most airway and lung specimens used for scientific study were acquired from autopsies of patients who succumbed to fatal asthma. Information obtained through studies involving bronchoscope has tremendously added to our knowledge pool on the nature of the specific inflammatory pathways that underlie asthma pathobiology.

COMPLICATIONS

Bronchoscopy and associated techniques are relatively safe procedures in mild and moderate asthmatic individuals. Complications include adverse effects of medications used

before and during the bronchoscopic procedure, hypoxemia, hypercarbia, wheezing, increased airway resistance, hypotension, laryngospasm, bradycardia, or other vagally mediated phenomena. Mechanical complications such as pneumothorax and hemoptysis occur more commonly following biopsies. Infection hazard for health care workers or other patients and death, although rare, are potential complications.

BRONCHOALVEOLAR LAVAGE

Technique

The technical aspects of BAL have been extensively investigated for more than 2 decades regarding the specific lavage sites to enhance yield, volume of aliquots, dwell time, and correlation with brushings and biopsy. The 4- to 8-mm

Figure 12-3   Risk factors for asthma.

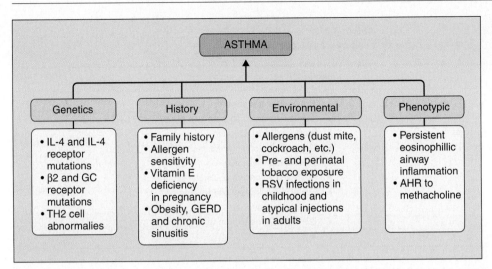

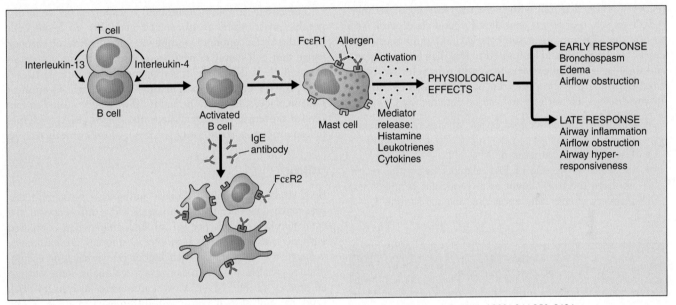

Figure 12-4   Early and late asthmatic response. *(Adapted from Busse WW, Lemanske RF Jr: Asthma. N Engl J Med 2001;344:350–362.)*

bronchoscope is wedged at the level of fourth- to sixth-generation bronchus. At this level, BAL will sample 1% to 3% of total lung volume. Fluid recovery and therefore total cell count tend to be high in the right middle lobe, and hence that site is commonly employed. Alternatively, the lingula on the left or anterior segment of the upper lobe may be acceptable. Sterile normal saline warmed to a temperature of 37° C is preferred in asthma patients to increase recovery and to avoid thermally induced bronchoconstriction. Aliquots of 20 to 60 mL are instilled through the working channel and generally recovered by gentle hand aspiration. Some investigators use wall suction, but this technique is associated with microtrauma to airways and spuriously high total protein values, and admixture of red blood cells. A small dwell time or periodic deep breathing techniques are recommended by various investigators to enhance cell recovery. Fluid

Table 12-1	
INDICATIONS FOR BRONCHOSCOPY IN ASTHMA	
Research	**Clinical**
• **Descriptive analysis:** Cytologic and histologic specimen procurement. • **Mechanism:** To study airway physiology and pathogenesis and participation of various mediators and cytokines. • **Therapeutic effects:** Pharmacodynamics of medications and other interventions.	• **Diagnostic:** Rarely used clinically. Asthma may be ruled out by documenting absence of thickened Lamina reticularis. • **Therapeutic:** Thermoplasty.
Adapted from Kavuru MS, Dweik RA, Thomassen MJ: Role of bronchoscopy in asthma research. Clin Chest Med 1999;20:153–189.	

Table 12-2
CONTRAINDICATIONS FOR BRONCHOSCOPY IN ASTHMA

Absolute	Relative
• Lack of consent from the patient. • Uncooperative patient. • Lack of adequate facilities to care for emergencies. • Inability to adequately oxygenate during the procedure. • Anaphylaxis to local anesthetic. • Status asthmaticus. • Uncorrected bleeding diathesis (biopsy).	• FEV_1 < 60% of predicted. • Severe refractory hypoxemia or any degree of hypercarbia. • Bronchodilator dependence. • Upper respiratory infection in past 4 wks. • Exacerbation in past 2 wks. • Unstable hemodynamic status. • Unstable cardiovascular disease • Uremia (biopsy). • Pulmonary hypertension (biopsy). • Age > 60 years.

Adapted from Kavuru MS, Dweik RA, Thomassen MJ: Role of bronchoscopy in asthma research. Clin Chest Med 1999; 20:153–189.

recovery is noted to fall with increasing severity of asthma. A 50% to 80% recovery is considered a good yield, with 70% to 80% being common in subjects without pulmonary diseases. The lavage should be limited to less than four segments and total lavage volume of less than 480 mL. Selective bronchial sampling may be preferred over BAL while studying airway diseases like asthma and can be obtained by

- Small volume unwedged lavage of airways (bronchial wash),
- Use of balloon catheter, or
- Fractional processing of BAL aliquots (using the recovery from the first aliquot as a "bronchial sample," and recovery of later aliquots as the "alveolar sample").

The lavage sample is stored and transported on ice in disposable plasticware or siliconized glassware to avoid cells adhering to the container. Samples are usually filtered through gauze and cell count is performed using a hemocytometer. The sample is then centrifuged or membrane filtered to isolate cells for cytologic examination with Wright-Giemsa or Papanicolaou staining. Supernatant fluid can be stored or frozen for protein analysis by radioimmunoassay (RIA), enzyme-linked immunosorbent assay (ELISA), or other methods.

Utility

BAL studies of stable asthmatic individuals with mild disease have generally shown no significant difference in the total number of cells per mL of BAL fluid when compared with normal volunteers. However eosinophil predominance is suggestive of asthma, with higher percentages of eosinophils associated with active or severe asthma in some but not all studies (Table 12-4). Flow cytometric analysis of BAL fluid has not shown consistent differences in CD4, CD8, or the ratio as can be seen in interstitial lung disease (ILD). The majority of the mediators currently thought to have a significant role in the pathophysiology of asthma (e.g., IL-1, IL-2, IL-4, IL-5, IL-6, IL-10, IL-13, GM-CSF, tumor necrosis factor alpha [TNF-a], intercellular adhesion molecule 1 [ICAM-1]) were identified by invasive studies using bronchoscopy and BAL. Also, similar studies evaluating the effects of various therapeutics like steroids, cromolyn sodium, and beta-agonists have enhanced our understanding of how

Table 12-3
PROCEDURE MONITORING

A. Preprocedure evaluation
- Medical history and physical examination
- Spirometry
- Pulse oximetry
- Assessment of bronchial hyperresponsiveness (optional)
- CBC, Coagulation tests for biopsy
- IgE and screening chemistry (optional)
- Premedications: Beta-agonists, atropine, and anxiolytic (optional)

B. During the procedure
- Continuous monitoring of oximetry, blood pressure and EKG
- Monitoring and recording of subject symptoms, and total doses of medications given
- Intravenous catheter (optional)
- Supplemental oxygen
- Topical lidocaine (max dose less than 400 mg)

C. Postprocedure
- Pulse oximetry monitoring
- Observe until return of gag reflex
- Expect low-grade fever, sore throat, mild nose bleed, drop in peak flow
- Assessment of clinical status (heart, lung, and level of alertness)
- Discharge instructions with follow-up appointment and contact telephone number

Adapted from Jarjour NN, Peters SP, Djukanovic R, et al: Investigative use of bronchoscopy in asthma. Am J Respir Crit Care Med 1998;157:692–697.

Table 12-4
CELLULAR COMPONENTS OF BAL

Component	Healthy Volunteers	Stable Asthma	After SAC
Total cell count, × 10^4 cells/mL)	5.8–26.9	4.4–26	8–12
Macrophages, %	86–95	58–94	85–92
Lymphocytes, %	6–12	5–19	5–7
Neutrophils, %	1–3	0–4	0.08
Eosinophils, %	0–1	0–8	0–1.7

Adapted from Kavuru MS, Dweik RA, Thomassen MJ: Role of bronchoscopy in asthma research. Clin Chest Med 1999; 20:153–189.

specific mediators and cellular inflammation are modulated by therapeutic agents, encouraging new drug developments.

Limitations

The cellular and mediator characterizations of asthmatic airways through BAL have failed to show consistent correlation with clinical severity. One area of controversy is how mediators should be quantified and reported. Using quantification in terms of absolute μg per mL of BAL fluid lacks standardization from laboratory to laboratory, and therefore makes comparisons between laboratories more difficult. Further, as the disease state changes, and volume recovery changes, it can be difficult to interpret even serial evaluation in the same subject. These limitations are commonly mitigated by the use of careful control subjects studied by the same laboratory or by meticulous protocol definition and execution as has been done in the U.S. Severe Asthma Research Program [SARP].

The utility of BAL to differentiate asthma and chronic obstructive pulmonary disease (COPD) was extensively studied in the past. More recently, the pathological characterization of asthma and COPD was based on predominance of eosinophils, CD4+ lymphocytes, and Th-2 cytokines in asthmatic individuals. Predominance of neutrophils, CD8+ lymphocytes, and macrophages in COPD patients has been questioned, fueling the debate of Dutch versus British hypotheses regarding the origin of obstructive lung diseases.

Safety

Medications used before and during the bronchoscopic procedure can cause adverse effects like hypotension, respiratory depression, anaphylaxis, and cardiac rhythm abnormality. Topical use of lidocaine is limited to 400 mg by National Institutes of Health (NIH) guidelines. However, other studies have suggested that higher doses, closer to 600 mg or 9 mg/kg, are acceptable. Lidocaine overdose may produce central nervous system (CNS) symptoms such as light-headedness, headache, dysarthria, tinnitus, sedation, perioral numbness, and tingling. Postbronchoscopy fever may occur as frequently as 1 in 4 patients and can be associated with headache, chest pain, and myalgias. It spontaneously resolves within 24 to 48 hours, and is mitigated by nonsteroidal anti-inflammatory agents. Possible release of proinflammatory cytokines in response to the procedure has been implicated as the cause of fever, as true pneumonia is rare. However, BAL does not cause sustained airway inflammation or obstruction. Cough is a very commonly occurring complication, which in most cases is self-limiting. Administering adequate local anesthesia can alleviate the symptom. Wheezing is seen more commonly among severe asthmatic individuals. Hypoxemia rarely requires termination of procedure. Supplemental oxygen is used invariably to prevent hypoxia, especially in asthma patients.

BRONCHIAL BRUSHING

Technique

A sheathed bronchial brush (5 mm) is advanced through the working channel of the bronchoscope. Under bronchoscopic guidance, the brush is advanced out of the sheath to the selected subsegmental bronchi. After specimen is collected by gentle strokes, the brush is withdrawn into the sheath and removed. Some investigators recommend that the brush be left protruding while the whole bronchoscope is withdrawn to reduce cell loss in the working channel and increase yield of viable cells; however, utmost care needs to be practiced to avoid contamination from upper airways. Bronchial brushing is usually limited to 1 to 2 segments per procedure and 2 to 4 brushes per segment, but this is somewhat variable depending on the study design and hypothesis posed.

Smears are prepared by rolling the brush over a glass slide in circular movements and immediately fixed with 4% ethanol to avoid excessive air-drying and preserve cellular morphology. Cell cultures are prepared by agitating the brush suspending cells into collagen medium enhanced with epidermal growth factors and other supplements. Cell recovery is about 3 million with 50% to 80% viability.

Utility

Bronchial brushing provides fresh single epithelial cells that are unobtainable through BAL or biopsies. Epithelium was originally thought to be a physical barrier forming the first line of defense against airborne pathogens. Bronchial brushes and cell cultures from harvested cells have showed the inflammatory role of epithelial cells in asthma pathogenesis and variation in response to bronchodilators. Bronchial epithelial cells from asthmatic individuals exhibit structural and functional differences from healthy subjects, like cytokeratin profiles, augmented release of anti-inflammatory mediators (IL-6, prostaglandin E2 [PGE2], epidermal growth factor [EGF], 15-hydroxyeicosatetraenoic acid [15-HETE], faster doubling time, and increased susceptibility to apoptosis.

Limitations

Bronchial brushings yield only epithelial cells with contamination from some inflammatory cells and viability is introduced by different specimen procuring and processing techniques. Epithelial cell cultures are models to study various mechanisms ex vivo. However, results from these experiments must be interpreted with caution, because ex vivo systems differ greatly from in vivo cellular responses to stimuli due to lack of communication with other compartments and neural and humoral feedbacks. However, samples from well-characterized asthmatic and healthy control subjects can provide valuable information regarding mechanisms of cellular behavior and/or gene and protein expression. Placing this information in the correct clinical context of the complex asthmatic airway remains challenging.

Safety

Bronchial brushing is a very safe procedure. Minor bleeding is common, particularly with aggressive brushing technique, but the amount is quite small and easily controllable, either by suction or, rarely, by use of local epinephrine.

BRONCHIAL BIOPSY

Technique

The quality of biopsy specimens depends on the technicality of sample procurement and processing. Usually one to eight

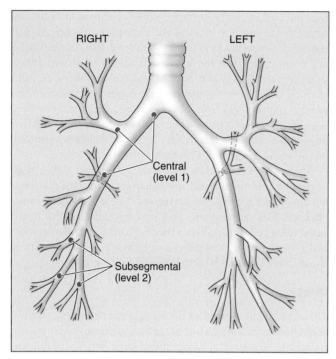

Figure 12-5 Bronchial biopsy sites. *(Adapted from Jeffery PK, Wardlaw AJ, Nelson FC, et al: Bronchial biopsies in asthma. An ultrastructural, quantitative study and correlation with hyperreactivity. Am Rev Respir Dis 1989;140:1745–1753.)*

from the proximal and distal lung are not pooled. Samples are then readily processed by snap-freezing, or fixation with 4% paraformaldehyde and paraffin embedding as indicated by the proposed analysis. Paraffin embedding preserves morphology and frozen sections are preferred for fluorescent in-situ hybridization (FISH) and most immunohistochemistry. The inflammatory cellular infiltration of bronchial epithelium and lamina propria is assessed by computerized image analysis, and expressed as cells per unit area, or per length of basement membrane.

Utility

Bronchial biopsies have been used in asthma research since late 1970s. Biopsies provide morphological information on various anatomical compartments of airways, such as epithelium, basement membrane, submucosa, and smooth muscle. Tissue components are evaluated by light microscopy, electron microscopy, immunohistochemical stains, FISH, or polymerase chain reaction (PCR) for mRNA expression for cytokines and adhesion molecules.

Much information on airway structure has been learned through the use of bronchial biopsies obtained via bronchoscopy. Bronchial biopsies have shown eosinophilic infiltration brought on by cytokines from activated T lymphocytes as the histological hallmark of symptomatic asthma. Healthy subjects have intact epithelium and lack cellular infiltrates in submucosa. In contrast, asthma patients show evidence of epithelial shedding, goblet cell hyperplasia, thickened lamina reticularis, and submucosal eosinophilic and lymphocytic infiltration. Thickened basement membrane due to increased collagen deposition in the reticular layers and proliferation of myofibroblasts is the hallmark of airway remodeling (Fig. 12-6). Of note, this collagen is not Type IV basement membrane collagen, but rather Types I, III, and V, suggesting that remodeling incorporates some aspects of the fibrotic or healing response.

Rarely, it may be helpful to obtain a bronchial biopsy from a patient suspected of having asthma. In situations where the diagnosis is unclear and the clinical data are contradictory, evidence of eosinophilic inflammation and airway wall remodeling (see later in chapter) can support the diagnosis of asthma. In contrast, the absence of airway wall remodeling may help to exclude the diagnosis of asthma.

bronchial biopsies are obtained from the same lung under direct bronchoscopic vision, using cupped or alligator forceps inserted through the working channel of the bronchoscope. The segmental and subsegmental carina of the lower lobe basal bronchi are the preferred and most commonly employed site (Fig. 12-5). Care should be taken to avoid previous biopsy sites, because biopsy may leave small scars. When combined with BAL, BAL is almost always performed before biopsy to avoid contamination of BAL with blood from the biopsy site.

Samples are usually pooled because most studies have failed to detect immunohistologic differences at different ciliated airway levels reached by the bronchoscope directly without fluoroscopic guidance—generally the second- to fourth-generation airways; significant differences in airway histology are seen between the terminal and respiratory bronchioles and samples obtained more proximally and thus samples

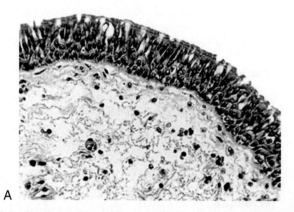

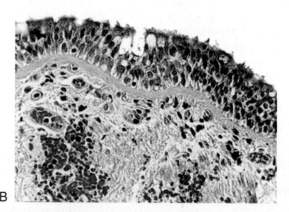

Figure 12-6 Specimen of bronchial mucosa from a subject without asthma (A) and a subject with asthma (B). Note the thickened subepithelial basement membrane beneath the epithelial layer and the increased cellularity in the subject with asthma (**stained blue**). These findings are not seen in the normal biopsy. *(From Busse WW, Lemanske RF Jr: Asthma. N Engl J Med 2001;344:350–362.)*

Asthmatic airways show increased granulation of mast cells and high-affinity IgE receptor-bearing cells. Steroids and other anti-inflammatory interventions have been shown to reduce T-cell and eosinophil infiltration of the lamina propria. Also increased is the expression of IL-4, IL-5, endothelin, eotaxin, and ICAM-1; these studies of protein and mRNA expression have added to the understanding of pathogenesis of asthma. Biopsy specimens are used in studying the mucosal nerves and neuropeptides shedding light as to the function of neural circuits in causing bronchospasm. A recent study suggests a possible pathologic classification of steroid-dependent refractory asthma based on histology as eosinophil-predominant (eosinophilic phenotype) and eosinophil-deficient (neutrophilic phenotype) subgroups. However, clinical and pathophysiologic differences among these subgroups remain to be studied; such a study is currently under way as part of the U.S. SARP.

Limitations

The quality of the biopsies is limited by the number of samples obtained, technical skills of the bronchoscopist and pathologist, and to a great extent by the disease process. Studies using bronchial biopsies to quantify inflammation are limited by normal anatomic variability, patchy focal inflammation, sample size, number of biopsy specimens, and quantification of cellular infiltrate. Studies evaluating the variability and reproducibility of data obtained from BAL of asthmatic individuals suggest a sample size of 8 to 25 subjects to study individual cell types and 13 to 48 subjects per arm in parallel design drug studies to establish adequate statistical power. But, interestingly, many studies are conducted on smaller numbers of patients and equivocal results in such studies may just reflect Type II statistical errors. Consequently, it is important to evaluate bronchial biopsy studies for size, reproducibility, and replication.

Safety

Endo- and transbronchial biopsies increase the overall complication rates associated with bronchoscopy from 0.12% to 2.7%, increasing the procedure-related mortality rate from 0.04% to 0.12%. Two major complications of bronchoscopic biopsies are pneumothorax and bleeding. Pneumothorax occurs in 1% to 4% of the study population, virtually exclusively with transbronchial biopsies. Use of fluoroscopy for transbronchial biopsies has been shown to reduce the incidence of pneumothorax significantly. Routine postprocedure radiologic evaluation is not recommended if definitive postoperative fluoroscopy can be accomplished. Acute onset of chest pain or shortness of breath following bronchoscopic biopsies should raise concern and be aggressively evaluated.

Significant hemorrhage (>25 mL) occurs in 5% to 9% of patients undergoing biopsies. The risk is increased in uremic patients with BUN (blood urea nitrogen) more than 30 mg/dL or creatinine more than 3 mg/dL to 45%. No particular coagulopathy is associated with increased risk; however caution is advised in patients with platelet count less than 50,000. History of excessive bleeding related to previous surgical procedures has been found to be the best predictor of bleeding following bronchial biopsies. Routine testing of prothrombin time (PT), activated prothrombin time (APTT), and bleeding time is not warranted as they do not have significant predictability of clinically significant bleeding complications.

Bronchoscopic biopsy-related hypoxemia and bronchospasm as measured by peak flow have been shown to be similar in asthmatic individuals and healthy subjects. Further maximum fall in peak flow occurs when biopsy is combined with BAL rather than with biopsy alone.

Ethical questions have been raised because of the increased risk of complications in studies involving volunteers who may not directly benefit from these studies. Accordingly, all such studies must be conducted under the supervision of a well-informed institutional review board.

SEGMENTAL ALLERGEN CHALLENGE

Technique

Various triggers have been used in the past for SAC, including cold air, aerosolized hyper- or hypotonic saline, or aerosolized or soluble antigen. Allergic stimuli are preferred in such investigations because they activate both early-phase (mediator-rich) and late-phase (inflammatory) responses. To perform SAC, the subject must have allergic skin test reactivity to at least one allergen. The specific allergen dosage to be used in SAC is obtained by

- End-point skin titration (EPST) method, one fourth of the dose required to produce a 4 × 4-mm skin wheal,
- A standard constant dose, or
- A fraction (5% to 20%) of antigen-PD_{20} (dose of antigen required to reduce FEV_1 by 20% during the early phase of whole lung antigen challenge).

Each of these approaches has merit, and the relative advantages are not clinically important.

Utility

Segmental allergen challenge in mildly asthmatic individuals provides real-time simulation of the disease process in a controlled situation and is a powerful tool in evaluating allergen-induced airway inflammation. This technique overcomes the limitations of aerosolized allergen challenge by precisely controlling the allergen dosing, delivery to smaller airways, and determining the temporal sequence of inflammatory mediator influx in relation to the exacerbating factor. The degree of inflammation and reactiveness is reasonably localized. One major advantage of SAC is the ability to obtain control samples from the same patient, at the same time point, from a different segment. Studies using SAC have shown that

- SAC produces EAR and LAR in atopic asthma patients but not in nonatopic asthmatic individuals or in healthy control subjects.
- EAR is marked by influx of histamine, prostaglandins, leukotrienes and thromboxane and by vascular protein leak, and relative paucity of cellular reaction.
- EAR is associated with low T cells, low CD4/CD8 ratio in BAL fluid (Table 12-5), possibly modulated by inflammatory cellular adhesion molecules.
- Cellular influx with neutrophil predominance occurs within 6 to 8 hours of allergen exposure.

Table 12-5
CELLULAR INFLAMMATION KINETICS IN ASTHMATICS FOLLOWING SAC

BAL FLUID CELLULAR CHARACTERISTICS*

Time	Parameter	Saline	Low Antigen Dose	Medium Antigen Dose	High Antigen Dose
5 minutes	Cells × $10^{6\dagger}$	11.0 (7.3–17.8)	8.2 (6.0–16.2)	12.3 (9.0–18.1)	12.2 (7.1–15.3)
	AM, %	92.0 (84.5–94.8)	90.7 (81.3–94.5)	90.3 (80.7–93.7)	85.0 (76.0–95.1)
	LYM, %	5.0 (4.0–8.0)	5.3 (3.0–7.8)	5.0 (3.0–10.3)	7.0 (2.8–14.8)
	NEU, %	0.0 (0.0–1.8)	0.8 (0.0–1.0)	0.5 (0.0–1.0)	0.3 (0.0–1.0)
	EOS, %	0.0 (0.0–1.5)	1.0 (0.0–1.8)	0.5 (0.0–4.0)	1.7 (0.0–6.8)
48 hours	Cells × $10^{6\dagger}$	13.2 (12.1–23.9)	21.0 (15.3–37.2)§	29.2 (18.6–36.9)§	43.8 (21.5–86.1)§
	AM, %‡	84.0 (74.8–90.7)§	77.7 (67.7–86.6)§	67.0 (58.0–78.0)§	48.0 (27.4–69.3) §
	LYM, %	9.0 (2.8–11.8)	6.0 (2.1–10.5)	6.0 (3.0–10.0)	5.0 (3.3–9.2)
	NEU, %	4.0 (0.7–7.7)§	5.0 (2.4–9.5)§	4.0 (1.3–6.7)§	4.0 (1.2–11.0)§
	EOS, %‡	1.3 (0.4–3.8)§	4.0 (3.0–10.8)§	17.7 (4.0–34.3)§	36.0 (16.8–54.3)§

AM, Alveolar macrophages; EOS, eosinophils; LYM, lymphocytes; NEU, neutrophils.
*Data are expressed as medians with 25%–75% interquartiles shown in parentheses.
†Total BAL cells.
‡$p < .05$, Kruskal-Wallis analysis of variance (effect of antigen dose).
§$p < .05$, Wilcoxon's test (5 min versus 48 hr).

BAL-SOLUBLE MEDIATORS*

Time	Parameter	Saline	Low Antigen Dose	Medium Antigen Dose	High Antigen Dose
5 minutes	Volume, mL†	75.0 (53.3–79.5)	73.0 (45.0–82.5)	68.5 (60.0–77.0)	67.0 (55.8–73.8)
	Total protein, µg/mL	100 (85–134)	92 (70–116)	95 (80–129)	120 (75–147)
	Histamine, pg/mL‡	110 (74–256)	386 (188–522)$^\parallel$	245 (92–1,125)$^\parallel$	948 (259–1,965)$^\parallel$
	IL-5, pg/mL	0.0 (0.0–0.0)	ND¶	ND	ND
	GM-CSF, pg/mL	0.5 (0.0–1.0)	ND	ND	ND
48 hours	Volume, mL†	70.0 (60.8–73.3)	74.0 (67.8–81.8)	73.0 (63.0–77.0)	68.5 (58.0–74.0)
	Total protein, µg/mL§	174 (131–200)$^\parallel$	173 (142–262)$^\parallel$	216 (155–364)$^\parallel$	324 (216–449)$^\parallel$
	Histamine, pg/mL	60 (40–110)	96 (82–260)	133 (108–222)	270 (111–518)
	IL-5, pg/mL‡	0.3 (0.0–1.3)	2.7 (1.0–9.4)	5.0 (1.5–21.7)	24.7 (8.6–34.3)
	GM-CSF, pg/mL	0.7 (0.0–1.1)	0.7 (0.0–0.9)	1.0 (0.7–1.3)	1.0 (0.3–2.9)

*Data are expressed as medians with 25%–75% interquartiles shown in parentheses.
†Volume of BAL fluid recovered (120 mL injected).
‡$p < 0.0001$, Kruskal-Wallis analysis of variance.
§$p < 0.05$, Kruskal-Wallis analysis of variance.
∥$p < 0.05$, Wilcoxon's test (5 min versus 48 hr).
¶Not done.
From Jarjour NN, Calhoun WJ, Kelly EA, et al: The immediate and late allergic response to segmental bronchopulmonary provocation in asthma. Am J Respir Crit Care Med 1997;155:1515–1521.

- Eosinophilic inflammation that marks LAR has been observed as early as 24 to 48 hours postexposure, which lasts for 10 to 15 days. The T-cell infiltrate is of helper T cells, enriched for those of the Th2 phenotype (IL-4, IL-5 secreting) (Figs. 12-7 and 12-8).

SAC has been a significant advancement in drug development. Pharmacologic attenuation of LAR following allergen challenge supports the role of IgE antibodies and LT-D receptor antagonists in asthma therapy.

Limitations

Care should be taken when extrapolating SAC findings to acute asthma exacerbations caused by viral infections and nonatopic asthma. Studies conducted using SAC are limited due to lack of physiological data and safety concerns in severe asthma patients, and they raise ethical questions. Response to SAC is inherently heterogeneous even in the same individual

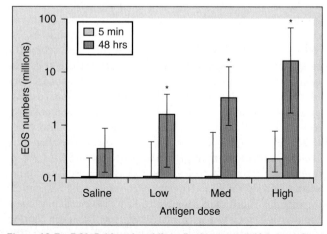

Figure 12-7 BAL fluid eosinophils at 5 minutes and 48 hours after SAC. *(Data from Jarjour NN, Calhoun WJ, Kelly EA, et al: The immediate and late allergic response to segmental bronchopulmonary provocation in asthma. Am J Respir Crit Care Med 1997;155:1515–1521.)*

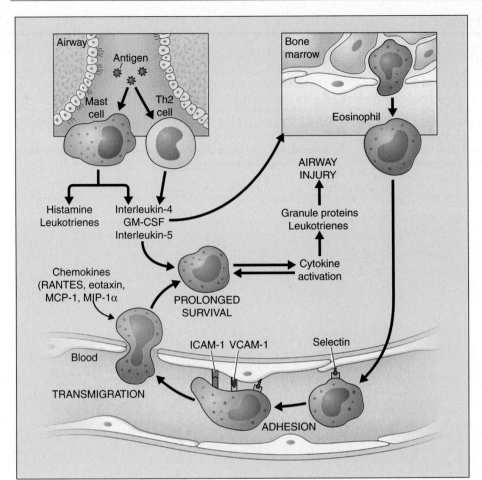

Figure 12-8 Inflammatory pathways. *(Adapted from Busse WW, Lemanske RF Jr: Asthma. N Engl J Med 2001;344:350–362.)*

when repeated over time because of variations in segmental location, endobronchial dosing, and bioavailability. Given the heterogeneity in the airway response and individual variations, studies of the effects of interventions should be replicated and interpreted with caution.

Safety

SAC is usually well tolerated. The most common complications associated with SAC are cough and wheeze. Studies show that FEV_1 (forced expiratory volume in 1 second) may decrease by 10% to 35%, 2 hours after SAC, and returns to baseline by 24 hrs. When combined with BAL and endobronchial biopsies, the fall in FEV_1 is greater and prolonged. The rare occurrence of hypoxia is usually mild and resolves rapidly with supplemental oxygen. Basic precautionary measures followed for bronchoscopy and BAL are generally sufficient to ensure the safety of volunteers undergoing SAC.

BRONCHIAL THERMOPLASTY

Proliferation (hyperplasia) and hypertrophy of airway smooth muscles are important parts of airway remodeling in chronic asthma. The correlation between airway smooth muscle mass and asthma severity has led to the invention of a novel therapy aiming to reduce the ability of smooth muscles to contract, called *bronchial thermoplasty* (BT). BT is performed by controlled radiofrequency ablation of smooth muscles in airway walls from central bronchi down to airways of 3 mm in diameter, which results in a

low-grade thermal injury to the airway that resolves with involution of smooth muscle. This study reported clinically significant and persistent reduction in AHR after BT for as long as 2 years, but no change in spirometric measurements. Although promising, further safety data and follow-up studies assessing efficacy and long-term complications are required.

ETHICAL ISSUES

Invasive research studies of the airway in asthma are relatively safe, but there is risk of both minor (relatively common) and significant (uncommon) complications. Accordingly, it is essential to perform invasive investigations of asthma only in the context of carefully reviewed protocols that have been subject to rigorous review by an institutional review board. In some settings, such as in pediatric studies, the use of invasive techniques for research purposes is often limited to those subjects who require bronchoscopy for a clinical indication.

The use of invasive procedures for clinical diagnosis and management of asthma is not common, because the diagnosis of asthma generally rests on a compatible history, coupled with either a physiologic bronchodilator response, or a positive provocative challenge to an agent such as methacholine. However, in selected situations, invasive assessment of the airway may provide important clinical information that aids in the diagnosis and management of a specific patient. In these cases, medical ethics demand that the physician make the best informed judgment regarding risk and benefit for that specific patient.

SUGGESTED READING

Balzar S, Wenzel SE, Chu HW: Transbronchial biopsy as a tool to evaluate small airways in asthma. Eur Respir J 2002;20:254–259.

Bousquet J, Jeffery PK, Busse WW, et al: Asthma. From bronchoconstriction to airways inflammation and remodeling. Am J Respir Crit Care Med 2000;161:1720–1745.

Busse WW, Lemanske RF Jr: Asthma. N Engl J Med 2001;344:350–362.

Cox G, Miller JD, McWilliams A, et al: Bronchial thermoplasty for asthma. Am J Respir Crit Care Med 2006;173:965–969.

Elston WJ, Whittaker AJ, Khan LN, et al: Safety of research bronchoscopy, biopsy and bronchoalveolar lavage in asthma. Eur Respir J 2004;24:375–377.

Jarjour NN, Calhoun WJ, Kelly EA, et al: The immediate and late allergic response to segmental bronchopulmonary provocation in asthma. Am J Respir Crit Care Med 1997;155:1515–1521.

Jeffery PK, Wardlaw AJ, Nelson FC, et al: Bronchial biopsies in asthma. An ultrastructural, quantitative study and correlation with hyperreactivity. Am Rev Respir Dis 1989;140:1745–1753.

Kavuru MS, Dweik RA, Thomassen MJ: Role of bronchoscopy in asthma research. Clin Chest Med 1999;20:153–189.

Moore WC, Peters SP: Severe asthma: an overview. J Allergy Clin Immunol 2006;117:487–494.

Reynolds HY: Use of bronchoalveolar lavage in humans—past necessity and future imperative. Lung 2000;178:271–293.

ASSESSMENT

Clinical Assessment of Asthma

Peter G. Gibson

Asthma is a multicomponent illness that is chronic and subject to periodic exacerbations. Airway inflammation and airway hyperresponsiveness are key pathophysiological components of asthma that lead to variable airflow obstruction; an increased sensitivity of the airways to environmental triggers; and episodic symptoms of wheeze, cough, and dyspnea. This chapter deals with the clinical assessment of asthma and complements other sections that address the assessment of the pathophysiologic components such as airway hyperresponsiveness (see Chapter 9) and inflammation (see Chapter 16).

The clinical assessment of asthma requires periodic evaluation of each of the components outlined in Table 13-1. Clinical assessment should be regular and planned, as this forms the basis of clinical care, including successful pharmacotherapy. Regular clinical assessment is necessary to identify the appropriateness of therapy and the person's response to treatment.

Each clinic visit should include an assessment of asthma control, together with an assessment of asthma self-management skills and the use and appropriateness of treatment. When asthma is uncontrolled or problems develop, additional assessment of relevant triggers and specific problems is required.

This chapter describes the assessment of the person with asthma during a routine clinic visit, and then moves on to clinical assessment in special situations such as an asthma exacerbation, rhinitis, upper airway disorders, dysfunctional breathing, and pregnancy.

ASSESSMENT DURING ROUTINE CLINIC VISITS

Asthma Control

The clinical assessment of asthma requires evaluation of several domains that include symptoms, rescue bronchodilator use, lung functions, and asthma exacerbations. These domains are then assessed collectively as *asthma control*.

SYMPTOMS

The typical symptoms experienced by people with asthma include dyspnea, wheeze, cough, and chest tightness. Symptoms in asthma exhibit variability, which can be characterized by assessing the timing and pattern of the symptoms (Table 13-2). The types of symptoms experienced in asthma are not specific for the condition, its control, or its severity. It is necessary to assess the timing and pattern of symptoms as well, to better assess asthma. Several symptom pattern combinations emerge as particularly useful when assessing asthma. These are

- Nocturnal asthma symptoms
- Asthma symptoms on waking
- Activity limitation because of asthma symptoms

The validation for these symptom patterns in asthma is derived from several sources. These include likely symptom mechanisms (Table 13-3), expert opinion (Fig. 13-1), and the ability to detect deteriorating asthma (Fig. 13-2). Studies of nocturnal asthma show that the development of nocturnal waking due to asthma is associated with a deterioration of eosinophilic airway inflammation and airway hyperresponsiveness. Since inflammation and hyperresponsiveness are key pathophysiologic features of asthma, this provides a mechanistic explanation for the importance of nocturnal waking in asthma (see Table 13-3). When a panel of international

Table 13-1
CLINICAL ASSESSMENT DOMAINS IN ASTHMA CARE

Asthma Control
Symptoms
Lung function
Exacerbations

Asthma Skills
Inhalation technique
Knowledge
Self-monitoring
Adherence
Written action plan

Asthma Treatment
Compare with guideline recommendations
Is there overtreatment or undertreatment?

Asthma Triggers
Are triggers identified and avoided where possible?

Problems
Are there additional problems?

Table 13-2
ASSESSMENT OF ASTHMA SYMPTOMS

Symptom Type
Dyspnea
Wheeze
Cough
Chest tightness
Symptom Pattern
Response to triggers
Response to treatment
Intensity
Frequency
Symptom Timing
Nocturnal
On waking
With exercise

Table 13-3	
MECHANISMS OF ASTHMA SYMPTOMS	
Cough	Stimulation of irritant receptors, bronchoconstriction
Wheeze	Bronchoconstriction
Chest tightness	Small airway narrowing, gas trapping
Dyspnea	Increased work of breathing
Nocturnal	Inflammation, bronchial hyperresponsiveness

asthma exacerbation. Daytime symptoms had a false-positive rate of 30% (see Fig. 13-2).

These symptoms can be assessed by clinical history, the use of a symptom diary, or a multidimensional asthma control questionnaire (http://www.qoltech.co.uk/Asthma1.htm#acq)[1] (see Chapter 15). Whatever technique is used, it is important to specifically assess several symptom patterns, rather than relying solely on a global question (e.g., How is your asthma?) to accurately assess asthma.

SYMPTOM PERCEPTION

People with asthma vary in their awareness of symptoms. This can be influenced by several factors, including environmental circumstances, the rate of change of symptoms, psychosocial factors, and the duration of symptomatic episodes. People with reduced awareness of symptoms are now a well-recognized group that may be at risk of more severe exacerbations. The reduced awareness can be due to denial or chronic poor asthma control with persistent symptoms that leads to sensory adaptation to the provoking stimulus. An indicator of poor perception is finding significant airflow obstruction in a person who reports few symptoms. People with poor perception of asthma symptoms need to be given additional measures to help identify deteriorating asthma such as regular monitoring of peak expiratory flow (PEF).

Perception within an individual can vary over time, and can be modified by treatment. For example, symptom perception was found to improve after inhaled corticosteroid therapy.

RELIEVER MEDICATION USE

People with asthma use fast-acting bronchodilators to relieve asthma symptoms. Monitoring this use is an important part of the clinical assessment of asthma. Important aspects to monitor are the frequency of bronchodilator use, the response of symptoms to bronchodilators, and the duration of that response. Deteriorating asthma control is associated with increasing frequency of bronchodilator use, a shorter duration of effect, and incomplete relief of symptoms. When assessing bronchodilator use, it is usual to assess the frequency of use over the preceding week. Use of a reliever for symptom management on two or more occasions per week is an indication of poor asthma control.

Recording occasions of use (rather than number of inhalations) allows for individuals who may use less (e.g., one puff) or more (e.g., three or four puffs) bronchodilator

experts were asked to rate the usefulness and importance of various symptom combinations in the clinical assessment of asthma, more than 90% rated nocturnal waking as very important, followed by exercise limitation, morning waking, dyspnea, and wheeze[1] (see Fig. 13-1). These symptom ratings formed the basis for an asthma control questionnaire.

An additional use of symptom assessment in asthma is the detection of deteriorating asthma. The ability of symptoms to accurately detect an exacerbation is another way of examining the validity of various symptom patterns. In a study of more than 400 asthma exacerbations,[2] the false-positive rate of symptoms was examined, that is, where the symptom developed, but this was not followed by an exacerbation. This analysis showed that nocturnal waking had the lowest false-positive rate (<10%), and was therefore highly specific for an

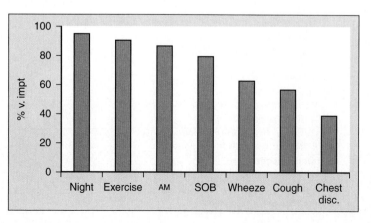

Figure 13-1 Relative importance of symptom patterns in asthma as evaluated by international experts. The graph shows the percentage of clinical experts rating the symptom as very important in the clinical assessment of asthma. *(Data from Juniper EF, O'Byrne PM, Guyatt GH, et al: Development and validation of a questionnaire to measure asthma control. Eur Respir J 1999;14:902–907.)*

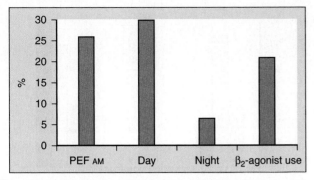

Figure 13-2 Symptoms and asthma exacerbations. The false-positive rate (symptoms but no exacerbations) in detecting asthma exacerbations is shown. PEF AM, morning peak expiratory flow. *(Data from Tattersfield AE, Postma DS, Barnes PJ, et al: Exacerbations of asthma: a descriptive study of 425 severe exacerbations. The FACET International Study Group. Am J Respir Crit Care Med 1999;160:594–599.)*

for symptom management. When using occasions of bronchodilator use to assess control, it is important to monitor that required for symptom management, and not that used routinely for maintenance pharmacotherapy.

PHYSICAL EXAMINATION

While physical examination is of limited value in the routine assessment of stable asthma, during an acute exacerbation the physical examination is very important. Physical examination in stable asthma can often be normal because of the variable nature of the disease. Wheezing is the most typical abnormal physical finding, but has limited specificity and sensitivity for asthma.

During an acute exacerbation, physical examination forms an essential part of the assessment of the severity of the exacerbation, and this is used to guide therapy and monitor its effect (see Chapter 22). Careful observation can give a rapid and accurate assessment of the severity of airflow limitation in acute asthma. Impaired level of consciousness, the extent to which dyspnea limits speech, the use of accessory muscles, and tachycardia each indicate severe airflow obstruction.

LUNG FUNCTION

Variable expiratory airflow obstruction is a defining physiological characteristic of asthma, and measurement of this characteristic forms an essential part of the clinical assessment of asthma. This can be assessed by measurement of the response in FEV_1 (forced expiratory volume in 1 second) to bronchodilator (bronchodilator responsiveness), measurement of the fall in FEV_1 to a provoking stimulus (airway hyperresponsiveness), or assessment of peak expiratory flow variability (diurnal variability). Reduction or elimination of lung function variability is a goal of asthma treatment.

It is recommended that lung function be assessed at each clinic visit by measurement of spirometry. This allows identification of airflow limitation, which may be present in the absence of symptoms in people who have adapted to persistent asthma and have "poor perception." There are published recommendations for the technique and equipment to be used in office spirometry (www.thoracic.org). The values obtained need to be compared to published reference values, with account taken for variations in spirometry that occur with age, gender, height, and ethnic background. The information obtained from spirometry is complementary to that obtained

from symptom assessment. Spirometry has good reproducibility when performed according to guidelines. Repeatability is within 5%, and a change is clinically significant when it is greater than 10%.[3]

ASTHMA CONTROL

The composite assessment of symptoms, rescue bronchodilator requirements, and lung function is termed *asthma control*. This is increasingly seen as a more useful form of clinical assessment of asthma since it allows an integration of the many and variable components of asthma both within and between individuals. Symptoms are assessed in terms of their pattern (daytime, nighttime, morning wakening) and frequency. Any nighttime wakening from asthma is considered to represent inadequate control, whereas daytime symptoms twice or more per week represent poor control. In addition, the need for rescue bronchodilator treatment, reduced lung function, and exacerbation frequency are also included in an assessment of asthma control. Poor control is characterized by rescue bronchodilator treatment needed twice or more per week, lung function reduced to below 80% of personal best values, and any exacerbation occurring in the past year. Asthma control can be assessed by direct questioning of these components or the use of a questionnaire, of which several are available.

ASTHMA EXACERBATIONS

Asthma is subject to periodic exacerbations in response to a variety of triggers. These events represent deterioration in asthma that is outside the person's usual day-to-day asthma variation. Severe exacerbations of asthma require medical assessment and intervention to prevent progressive deterioration. These exacerbations are recognized by the need for oral corticosteroids and medical assessment either as an unscheduled doctor's visit, emergency room attendance, or hospitalization. Infrequently, intensive care admission may be required. A person with more than one severe exacerbation in a 12-month period is considered to have uncontrolled asthma. At each asthma review it is important to enquire about recent exacerbations. This forms part of the assessment of asthma control, and also provides an opportunity to investigate and reinforce early recognition and treatment of deteriorating asthma by the patient. In addition, the health care professional should establish whether treatment of exacerbations has been effective and, if not, work with the person with asthma to develop an effective treatment plan for asthma exacerbations.

Asthma Skills

A range of asthma management skills can be used by people with asthma to reduce exacerbations and improve quality of life. Assessment of these skills (see Table 13-1) can correct deficiencies and reinforce correct self-management practices.

INHALATION DEVICE TECHNIQUE

The delivery of therapy by inhalation forms the basis of asthma therapy, since it gives the best efficacy to side-effect ratio. Successful inhaled therapy depends on using adequate inhalation device technique and, consequently, assessment of inhaler device technique should be performed regularly in people with asthma. The components of this assessment include selecting an appropriate inhalation device for a person with asthma, instructing them in its use, and periodically assessing the adequacy of their inhalation device technique.

Device Selection

The range of available device-medication combinations is large. Pictorial charts are available to illustrate this range and assist in device recognition. There are several considerations to the decision of which device is suitable for a particular individual. These address key domains such as the following:

- Cost and availability of the device
- Ability of the person to prepare the device for use
- Adequacy of the inspiratory effort
- Ability to coordinate actuation and inspiration
- Ability to learn and perform the noncrucial steps involved in inhaler device use, such as shaking before use, breath-hold, and slow, deep inspiration.

The cost and availability of particular devices reflect local regulatory and reimbursement schedules, and the practitioner needs to be familiar with the local availability. Each device requires specific preparation, and the ability to do this is crucial for efficacy. For example, physical limitations from arthritis such as reduced joint mobility, joint pain, and muscle weakness can reduce the ability to press a pressurized metered-dose inhaler (pMDI), which requires the thumb and index finger to exert pressure while in a fully extended position. Several devices, such as dry powder inhalers (DPIs) and breath-actuated inhalers require adequate inspiratory flow for use, generally more than 30 L/min. If this cannot be achieved, then device use is impaired. Coordination of the actuation with inspiratory effort is a crucial step with pMDI use. Inability to do this is one of the most common limitations to effective pMDI use. This, like the other steps, needs to be specifically taught and directly observed to ensure adequate pMDI use (Table 13-4).

Device Technique

Each inhaler device has a specific correct technique that consists of device preparation, crucial steps for drug delivery, and noncrucial steps for drug delivery. If one of the crucial steps is not followed, then lung deposition is minimal. Correct technique with the noncrucial steps can enhance lung deposition. These steps need to be taught and assessed periodically to ensure ongoing adequate device use. If a person cannot be taught correct technique with one device, then selection of an alternate device is required (see Table 13-4).

Inhalation Device Polypharmacy

The number of inhalation devices available for use in asthma is continually increasing. Whereas this allows for greater choice,

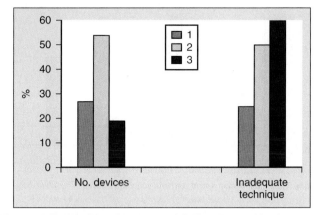

Figure 13-3 Number of devices used (*left*) and rate of inadequate inhaler technique (*right*) among adults with persistent asthma. (Data from McDonald VM, Gibson PG: Inhalation-device polypharmacy in asthma. Med J Aust 2005;182:250–251.)

it also creates a problem unique to aerosol therapy, namely the use of several different devices by the same person, a situation termed *inhalation device polypharmacy*. In one survey, most people (73%) used more than one type of delivery device for their asthma therapy[4] (Fig. 13-3). Commonly this was a pressurized metered dose inhaler for their short-acting bronchodilator, and a dry powder inhaler for their controller medication. As increasing numbers of devices were used, the rate of incorrect inhaler technique increased, and when three or more devices were used, more than 60% of patients had a crucial flaw in technique with one device such that lung delivery would be negligible. Consequently, in addition to assessing device technique, it is important to minimize the number of devices prescribed for and used by people with asthma. This places a significant burden on health care professionals to be competent with the use and assessment of several different devices. For an asthma expert, proficiency with all locally available devices is a reasonable goal. However, for a practitioner managing a wide range of conditions, this may not be achievable, and one approach is to choose a single pressurized inhaler (with spacer) and a single dry powder device and become proficient in the prescription, use, and assessment of these devices.

KNOWLEDGE

Knowledge of asthma and its treatment is generally considered an essential prerequisite for successful therapy. Improving knowledge alone is not sufficient to improve health outcomes, but having a good understanding of what asthma is and how it is treated enables better adherence to the treatment plan. In studies of adherence, poor knowledge is often found to be a contributor to poor adherence. Asthma knowledge can be assessed in several ways, including direct questioning, and by validated questionnaire. The key domains to cover in asthma knowledge assessment are listed in Table 13-5.

SELF-MONITORING

Asthma exacerbations are a major cause of morbidity for people with asthma. Because of the episodic nature of asthma, all people with asthma are at risk of an asthma exacerbation. Most (>80%) asthma exacerbations involve a gradual deterioration over several days, which means there is an opportunity to detect and treat the exacerbation early in order to limit its severity. The early detection and treatment of an

Table 13-4
OVERCOMING PROBLEMS WITH INHALER DEVICE SELECTION

Problem	Solution
Impaired device actuation	Add adaptor to inhaler
Impaired coordination of inspiration and actuation	Breath actuated MDI, DPI, pMDI and spacer
Reduced inspiratory effort	pMDI with spacer

Table 13-5
ASTHMA KNOWLEDGE DOMAINS

- Symptoms of asthma
- Asthma control: understanding, monitoring
- Asthma triggers
- Asthma treatments
- Symptoms of deteriorating asthma
- Advice about how and when to seek medical attention

asthma exacerbation can be facilitated by self-monitoring and a written treatment plan that instructs the person when and how to increase treatment. When this approach is used in the context of an asthma self-management education program, then there is a significant reduction in hospitalizations for asthma, emergency room visits for asthma, unscheduled doctor visits, and episodes of nocturnal asthma.

People with asthma can monitor symptoms and/or lung function. In randomized trials, written action plans based on symptom monitoring give similar beneficial results to plans based on PEF monitoring. Lung function parameters that can be monitored using portable devices include PEF and spirometry. Sustained compliance with PEF monitoring is difficult to achieve and, consequently, periodic monitoring is recommended.

PEF Monitoring

The portability and ease of use of modern PEF meters make them suitable for home monitoring by people with asthma on a day-to-day basis. They provide an objective measure of airflow obstruction in asthma. However, as the measurement is limited to a single point on the flow-volume curve (Fig. 13-4), the results are not interchangeable with other measures such as FEV_1. PEF can underestimate the degree of airflow obstruction in some settings, such as when there is worsening gas trapping. This limits their utility as discriminatory measures between

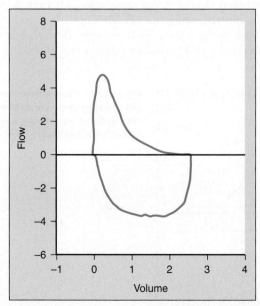

Figure 13-4 Flow-volume curve in asthma showing reduction of expiratory airflow.

patients, but PEF monitoring with comparison of results within an individual remains useful. This represents a further argument for comparing results with the person's personal best values.

PEF measures are effort dependent and careful instruction in PEF technique is required. PEF variability can be assessed in several ways:

- Amplitude as a percentage of the mean: the difference between the maximum and minimum each day is expressed as a percentage of the mean value.
- Minimum morning prebronchodilator PEF, as a percentage of the recent best, termed *min%max*.
- PEF with and without the addition of bronchodilator response.

The advantages of the min%max method are that only a single daily recording is required, and the measure correlates well with airway hyperresponsiveness.

Further developments in PEF monitoring have seen the application of statistical process control (SPC) methods to the interpretation of PEF charts. SPC methods are widely used in the manufacturing industry where strict product control is required, and early detection of any product variation is needed. When applied to asthma, this method carefully identifies action points based on the inherent variability of the person's PEF, and can be shown to be more useful than preset action points. It requires some math, but provides a superior result.

Despite the availability and technical simplicity of the measurement tools and the advances in interpretation, adherence to PEF recording remains an ongoing limitation of the use of PEF monitoring. To minimize this, guidelines recommend monitoring in several defined situations. These include confirming the diagnosis of asthma, improving asthma control, identifying environmental asthma triggers, evaluating treatment needs, assessing control in people with poor symptom perception, and monitoring asthma in people with near-fatal attacks or difficult to control asthma.

When using PEF monitoring to confirm the diagnosis of asthma, an improvement in PEF of 60 L/min or more after bronchodilator suggests a diagnosis of asthma. The severity of asthma can also be graded by measuring baseline airflow obstruction and diurnal PEF variability. When measures are made twice daily, before and after bronchodilator, for a 14-day period, then the degree of PEF variability can be graded to indicate asthma severity. The upper normal limit of variability is 8% when measured in this way.

A variety of electronic spirometers are available for assessment of asthma. The American Thoracic Society has published recommended performance criteria for electronic spirometers. In addition, the electronic monitoring device needs to be durable, easy to use, easy to instruct the patient in use, and able to be integrated into an asthma action plan, and must have adequate technical support available.

ADHERENCE

Assessing adherence to therapy and use of the written action plan forms a key part of the clinical assessment of asthma. Methods of assessment include direct questioning and the use of dose counters. Direct questioning needs to be conducted in a nonjudgmental fashion, with the aim of forming a partnership with the patient that will facilitate good adherence. The limitation of direct questioning is the lack of objective validation of the response; however, a response that affirms nonadherence can be believed, and forms the starting point of an investigation of the causes of nonadherence and ways to reduce it.

Many inhalation devices can be fitted or manufactured with a dose counter. Dose counters are useful to alert both the patient and the clinician to nonadherence, and also to alert the patient when the inhaler is close to empty and it is necessary to refill the prescription. Some of the newer noninvasive markers of inflammation are also suitable for assessing adherence. The finding of increased eosinophilic inflammation in a person prescribed inhaled corticosteroid therapy can be due to nonadherence.

WRITTEN ASTHMA ACTION PLAN

A written asthma action plan is a key part of an asthma self-management education program that allows the early detection and treatment of an exacerbation. The key components of an asthma action plan are:

- When to increase treatment
- How to increase treatment
- How long to remain on the increased treatment
- When to call for help

Action plans can take several forms and are described in more detail in Chapter 51. The use of the action plan should be assessed at each visit by direct questioning. People with asthma frequently alter their prescribed action plan, and it is important to regularly discuss and modify the plan to achieve concordance with the person regarding the acceptance and use of the written asthma action plan.

CLINICAL ASSESSMENT IN SPECIAL SITUATIONS

Acute Asthma

Asthma exacerbations can be severe and life-threatening, requiring rapid assessment and treatment. Once the diagnosis of an acute exacerbation is made, then assessment of symptoms and physical examination forms a key part of the severity assessment and monitoring the response to treatment. The degree of respiratory distress can be assessed by the ability of

the person to talk in full sentences, phrases, or words only. Observation gives important information on the acute severity when is it directed to assessment of the following factors:

- Alertness
- Respiratory rate
- Accessory muscle use

During an acute exacerbation, agitation indicates moderate or severe disease; however, when a respiratory arrest is imminent, then drowsiness or confusion develops. The use of accessory muscles such as retraction of the sternocleidomastoid occurs with increasing severity of airflow obstruction, and indicates at least moderate airflow obstruction with an FEV_1 less than $1.5\,L$ in an adult. Additional factors that can be assessed are the degree of tachycardia, pulsus paradoxus, airflow obstruction, and an assessment of oxygenation.

Certain additional factors in the clinical history indicate an increased risk of asthma death. These are

- History of near-fatal asthma
- History of intubation for asthma
- Recent hospitalization/emergency care visit
- Current or recent oral corticosteroid use
- Excessive rapid-acting β-agonist use
- History of psychiatric or psychosocial problems
- Use of sedatives, illicit drugs
- History of noncompliance with medications or plans

Rhinitis and Upper Airway Disorders

Rhinitis frequently complicates asthma and can be responsible for troublesome symptoms. Additional complications are sinusitis and nasal polyposis. Specific questioning can identify the presence of nasal symptoms and differentiate these from asthma symptoms. Active nasal disease can also be associated with uncontrolled asthma, and therefore the identification and treatment of rhinitis is important in symptom control.

Vocal cord dysfunction (VCD) can mimic asthma or occur in association with asthma. VCD represents paradoxical vocal cord closure during inspiration. This can be recognized by direct visualization via fiber-optic laryngoscopy, or a reduction in the inspiratory limb of the flow-volume curve (Fig. 13-5). In VCD without asthma, the expiratory limb

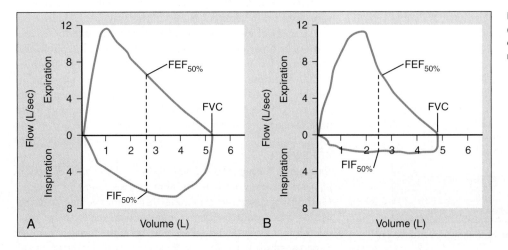

Figure 13-5 Flow-volume curve in **(A)** a healthy person and **(B)** vocal cord dysfunction, showing a severe reduction of inspiratory flow.

of the flow volume curve is usually normal. Several features help differentiate VCD from asthma:

- In VCD, the dyspnea typically occurs with inspiration.
- The "tightness" reported is usually at the level of the jugular notch.
- There is a poor response to bronchodilator.

In addition, other symptoms help localize the problem to the larynx, such as intermittent hoarseness, marked coughing, and triggering of symptoms by vocal stress (singing, shouting, voice projection).

Dysfunctional breathing refers to episodic asthma-like symptoms in people without objective evidence of asthma, with an erratic breathing pattern, in whom specific "breath-focused" therapy improves or resolves symptoms.[5] In primary care, up to 30% of people with apparent asthma may have this problem.

Surgery

Surgery represents a potentially high risk for people with asthma. Respiratory complications include bronchospasm, asthma exacerbation, lower respiratory tract infection, and atelectasis. The type of surgery (e.g., abdominal surgery) may limit the ability to use an inhaler adequately, and result in inappropriate omission of maintenance asthma therapy. Conversely, use of oral corticosteroid can limit wound healing and compromise the surgical outcome. Before, during, and after surgery people with asthma require an assessment of asthma control, asthma skills, and asthma treatment as described above. This assessment then needs to be integrated with the demands of surgery and an appropriate management plan developed. For example, a person having abdominal surgery will have reduced inspiratory effort. They may need to change their maintenance therapy to a pMDI-spacer using tidal breathing, as shown in Table 13-4. This change will involve education of the patient and health care staff on the correct use of the new device.

Gastroesophageal Reflux

Gastroesophageal reflux disease (GERD) and asthma frequently coexist, and each condition may adversely affect the other. It is important to assess GERD in people with asthma, especially in asthma that is not well controlled. Some asthma treatments, such as theophylline, may worsen GERD. GERD with proximal regurgitation may cause respiratory symptoms including cough and inspiratory dyspnea, which can be mistaken for poor asthma control. Identification and treatment of this will improve overall symptom control.

Occupational Asthma

Assessment of the workplace and the potential for occupational exposure is an important part of the assessment of asthma. Occupational exposures may cause airway irritation and worsen symptoms in a person with preexisting asthma. Similarly, exposure to sensitizing agents may induce asthma and early identification of this is needed to obtain good long-term outcomes. Assessment of occupational asthma requires

knowledge of potential occupational sensitizers, and the likely occupations in which these are encountered. The clinical assessment requires that several distinct questions be addressed:

1. Does the person have asthma confirmed by objective evidence?
2. Is the person exposed to a known occupational sensitizer?
3. What is the temporal relationship between exposure and change in asthma status?

Specific challenge with the suspected provoking agent can confirm diagnosis but is available only in specialized centers, and other approaches are required for routine care. For high molecular weight occupational sensitizers, the use of nonspecific bronchial provocation test, to address question 1, and skin prick tests together with measurement of specific IgE in serum represents an alternative to specific provocation challenge. For low molecular weight sensitizers, a combination of nonspecific bronchial provocation test with skin prick test has excellent sensitivity when compared to specific inhalation challenge.

INTEGRATED CLINICAL ASSESSMENT

The outcome of a systematic clinical assessment is to integrate the findings and use them to plan future management. When symptom control is acceptable and skills are optimal, then treatment can be assessed and consideration given to reduction in maintenance therapy. During dose reduction, symptoms are monitored to indicate when the minimum maintenance dose has been reached. When symptom control is suboptimal, then several issues need to be addressed (Table 13-6). Asthma self-management skills need to be assessed and optimized, triggers need to be assessed and managed, and then if poor control persists, treatment can be modified. It can be seen that the clinical assessment of the person with asthma is an iterative process that continues over time, involving the domains of asthma symptom control, skills, triggers, and therapy (Fig. 13-6). Failure to address skills and triggers and only focusing on treatment puts the patient at risk of overtreatment, while failure to adequately assess symptom control puts the patient at risk of undertreatment. A standardized composite assessment form is shown in Figure 13-7.

Table 13-6
WHAT TO DO WHEN THERE IS POOR CONTROL

Assess and Correct Skills
Inhaler technique
Adherence
Understanding and use of action plan
Assess and Manage Triggers
Allergens
Rhinitis
Gastroesophageal reflux
Review Medication
Optimize inhaled corticosteroid dose
Step up treatment category according to guidelines

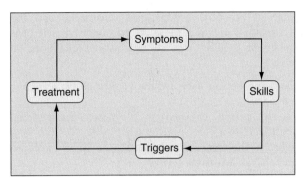

Figure 13-6   Iterative asthma care.

Date: Record Number:
Name:
Address:
DOB:

Dear Dr
Mr/Mrs/Ms_____was referred to the Asthma Management Service and has
attended _____ visits. The areas which could benefit from ongoing review are indicated below.

CURRENT ASTHMA MEDICATIONS: {describe}

CURRENT ASTHMA CONTROL:
β₂ use _____times per day/week;
night waking with asthma symptoms _____times/week;
morning waking with asthma symptoms _____times/week
PEAK FLOW: PRE _____AM _____PM (Predicted _____)
POST_____ AM _____PM

ASTHMA SKILLS: Inadequate **(I)** Adequate **(A)** Optimal **(O)** Not applicable **(NA)**

INHALER TECHNIQUE:
Device: MDI (puffer) Spacer Turbuhaler Accuhaler Handihaler Other _____

SELF MONITORING: (Ability to record peak flow and symptoms) PEF/SYMPTOMS

ACTION PLAN:
When to increase treatment:
How to increase treatment: (see attached plan)
For how long:
When to see doctor:

SMOKING HISTORY: YES/NO
OTHER RELEVANT PROBLEMS:

We have suggested **FOLLOW UP** with

Yours sincerely,

Respiratory Specialist   **Educator**

Figure 13-7   Standardized Asthma Assessment Form. *(Copyright Asthma Management Service, John Hunter Hospital, Newcastle, Australia. Reprinted with permission.)*

REFERENCES

1. Juniper EF, O'Byrne PM, Guyatt GH, Ferrie PJ, King DR: Development and validation of a questionnaire to measure asthma control. Eur Respir J 1999;14:902–907.
2. Tattersfield AE, Postma DS, Barnes PJ, et al: Exacerbations of asthma: a descriptive study of 425 severe exacerbations. The FACET International Study Group. Am J Respir Crit Care Med 1999;160:594–599.
3. American Thoracic Society: Standardization of spirometry, 1994 update. Am J Respir Crit Care Med 1995;152:1107–1136.
4. McDonald VM, Gibson PG: Inhalation-device polypharmacy in asthma. Med J Aust 2005;182:250–251.
5. Thomas M, McKinley RK, Freeman E, et al: Breathing retraining for dysfunctional breathing in asthma: a randomized controlled trial. Thorax 2003;58:110–115.

How Do You Classify Asthma by Severity?

James E. Fish

CLINICAL PEARLS

- Asthma severity may be defined by the intensity of therapy required for maintenance of long-term control.

- Regardless of disease severity, day-to-day control can vary over time.

- Patients with mild severity can still experience serious or even life-threatening exacerbations.

- Current approaches to defining asthma severity are limited because of poor correlations between different measures of disease activity.

- Further work is needed to define better end points to measure severity and control.

- Experience suggests that for most patients, severity does not progress over time.

Asthma is a chronic disorder characterized by a relatively persistent underlying level of pathophysiologic abnormality that may be interrupted by periods of worsening of symptoms and lung function. Asthma *severity* describes the relatively persistent degree of abnormality of the disorder that, from a clinical standpoint, is reflected by the intensity of treatment required to maintain control of symptoms and lung function over an extended period of time. The term disease *control*, in contrast, refers to the level of disease activity at any given point in time and as such reflects the effectiveness of current therapy. Accordingly, asthma *severity* and asthma *control* should be viewed as related but distinct ways to describe the clinical status of the patient (Box 14-1).[1] Hence, a patient with mild severity as measured over an extended time interval can have intervening periods of poor control, including episodes that require intensive treatment or even hospitalization. Conversely, a patient with severe asthma may be well controlled, albeit on multiple medications at high doses. Features of asthma control are discussed in greater detail in Chapter 15.

In general, defining the level of severity in an asthmatic patient is useful for characterizing the burden of disease on a more long-term basis and for identifying treatment needs for chronic maintenance therapy. Classifying a patient by severity is also of value in predicting outcomes, particularly the risk of future events such as loss of control, exacerbations, or hospitalization. Clinical investigations also take advantage of severity classifications in order to define the population of interest.

APPROACHES TO CLASSIFY ASTHMA SEVERITY

Classifications of severity from mild to severe have been published in two widely accepted clinical practice guidelines. Both guidelines reflect the opinions of recognized asthma experts in the United States and Europe. The Global Initiative for Asthma (GINA) and the National Asthma Education and Prevention Program (NAEPP) guidelines define asthma as being intermittent or persistent in nature based on frequency of symptoms.[2,3] Both guidelines classify persistent asthma as mild, moderate, or severe using similar criteria based on daytime and nighttime symptoms and pulmonary function tests. Recent NAEPP guidelines have added rescue beta-agonist use as an additional criterion for determining severity. Differences between the NAEPP and GINA classification algorithms are largely related to a higher level of impairment required for moderate and severe asthma in the NAEPP guidelines. Although it is often assumed that intermittent asthma is mild in nature, it should be noted that patients with infrequent symptoms and relatively normal pulmonary function may still experience serious or even life-threatening episodes under unusual circumstances.

Both the GINA and NAEPP guidelines classify asthma severity based on symptoms and pulmonary function prior to initiation of therapy as illustrated in Tables 14-1 and 14-2. This approach to classifying severity provides a useful framework for estimating the intensity of therapy that is likely to be required to achieve control of symptoms in patients who are newly diagnosed with asthma. However, practitioners frequently encounter patients who already carry a diagnosis of asthma and are already on asthma medications. Failure to account for medication use when assessing severity in these patients can lead to an underestimate of severity and, as a corollary, an overestimate of the prevalence of mild asthma. To address this problem, both guidelines attempt to classify

BOX 14-1 Defining Asthma Severity

- Asthma *severity* describes the relatively persistent degree of pathophysiologic abnormality that is reflected by the intensity of treatment required to maintain control of symptoms and lung function over an extended period of time.
- Asthma *control* refers to the level of disease activity at any given point in time and reflects the effectiveness of current therapy.
- Asthma severity and asthma control are related but distinct ways to describe the clinical status of the patient.

Table 14-1
NAEPP CLASSIFICATION OF ASTHMA SEVERITY BEFORE TREATMENT IN ADULTS AND YOUTHS 12 YEARS AND OLDER*

Component of Severity	Intermittent	Persistent		
		Mild	Moderate	Severe
Symptoms	≤2 days/week	>2 days per week but not daily	Daily	Throughout the day
Nighttime awakenings	≤2 ×/month	3–4 ×/month	>1×/week but not nightly	Often 7×/week
Short acting beta-agonist use for symptoms	≤2 days/week	>2 days per week but not >1×/day	Daily	Several times per day
Interference with normal activity	None	Minor limitation	Some limitation	Extremely limited
Pulmonary function	Normal FEV_1 between exacerbations; $FEV_1 \geq 80\%$ predicted; FEV_1/FVC normal	$FEV_1 < 80\%$ predicted; FEV_1/FVC normal	$FEV_1 \geq 60\%$ but $< 80\%$ predicted; FEV_1/FVC reduced $\geq 5\%$	$FEV_1 < 60\%$; FEV_1/FVC reduced $> 5\%$
Exacerbations (consider frequency and severity)	0–1 per year	>2 per year		

*Severity level is determined in accordance with the worst impairment category; for classification in children younger than 12 years of age, see Chapter 20.

severity by taking into account current medication use and the response to such therapy. For example, using the NAEPP guidelines (Table 14-3), a patient taking a low dose of an inhaled corticosteroid with a short-acting beta$_2$-agonist for rescue and who has minor symptoms only once weekly, has fewer than 3 nights with symptoms per month, and has relatively normal pulmonary function, would be considered to be well controlled and responsive to an appropriate level of therapy for mild persistent asthma. In contrast, a patient taking the same regimen but who experiences daily symptoms and who has pulmonary function between 60% and 80% of their predicted normal values would require a more intensive regimen, one more specifically tailored to a patient with moderate persistent asthma.

Table 14-2
GINA CLASSIFICATION OF ASTHMA SEVERITY BEFORE TREATMENT

Step	Indications
Step 1 Intermittent	Indications Symptoms < once/week Brief exacerbations Nocturnal symptoms ≤ 2 ×/month $FEV_1/PEF \geq 80\%$ PEF/FEV_1 variability < 20%
Step 2 Mild persistent	Symptoms > once/week; < once/day Exacerbations may affect activity/sleep Nocturnal symptoms > 2 ×/month $FEV_1/PEF \geq 80\%$ PEF/FEV_1 variability 20%–30%
Step 3 Moderate persistent	Symptoms > once/week; < once/day Exacerbations may affect activity/sleep Nocturnal symptoms > 1×/week FEV_1/PEF 60%–80% PEF/FEV_1 variability > 30%
Step 4 Severe persistent	Symptoms daily Frequent exacerbations Frequent nocturnal symptoms Limitation of physical activities $FEV_1/PEF \geq 60\%$ PEF/FEV_1 variability > 30%

In addition to the severity definitions offered in the guidelines cited above, other groups have taken alternative approaches to defining severe asthma in an attempt to gain a better understanding of this phenotype. These groups include investigators associated with the National Heart, Lung, and Blood Institute Severe Asthma Research Program, the European Network for Understanding Mechanisms of Severe Asthma, and the Epidemiology and Natural History of Asthma: Outcomes and Treatment Regimens (TENOR) Trial.[4-6] Information derived from these investigations suggests that a classification strategy that includes measures of health care use may more accurately identify severe asthma patients than a strategy based on symptoms, lung function, and medication use alone.

FACTORS AFFECTING ASTHMA SEVERITY

Although asthma severity may be viewed as an inherent property of the disease process, a number of factors may play a role in determining severity. Many of these factors not only determine asthma severity, but they play also a significant role as comorbid conditions that warrant medical intervention in their own right (Box 14-2).

Obesity

An association between asthma and obesity has been recognized, but the nature of the association remains controversial. Asthma and obesity are both highly prevalent chronic conditions; hence, it is not surprising that a link between the two conditions has been considered. Most cross-sectional studies indicate that asthma prevalence is increased in children as well as adults who are obese. Whether this association implies a causal relationship is the subject of debate. It has been argued that asthmatic individuals tend to become obese because of a more sedentary lifestyle, although this argument has been refuted by longitudinal data showing that obesity often predates the incidence of asthma. Most epidemiologic studies indicate that the association between obesity and asthma is particularly strong in women.

Table 14-3
NAEPP SEVERITY CLASSIFICATION AFTER TREATMENT

Lowest Level of Treatment to Maintain Control	Severity			
	Intermittent	Mild Persistent	Moderate Persistent	Severe Persistent
Steps	1	2	3–4	5–6

Levels of treatment are defined by the following in adults and youths 12 years and older*:
Step 1: Short-acting beta-agonists
Step 2: Low-dose inhaled corticosteroids
Step 3: Low-dose inhaled corticosteroids plus long-acting beta-agonist; or, medium dose inhaled corticosteroids
Step 4: Medium-dose inhaled corticosteroids plus long-acting beta-agonist
Step 5: High-dose inhaled corticosteroids plus long-acting beta-agonist
Step 6: High-dose inhaled corticosteroids plus long-acting beta-agonist plus oral corticosteroids
*For treatment in children younger than 12 years, see Chapter 20.

BOX 14-2 Determinants of Asthma Severity

- Obesity
- Gastroesophageal reflux
- Environmental exposure
- Corticosteroid insensitivity
- Sinusitis
- Aspirin sensitivity
- Genetic

The thesis that asthma severity is influenced by obesity is supported by studies demonstrating improvement in symptoms and lung function after weight loss and by studies showing an association between disease severity and body mass index. In contrast, others have failed to confirm such associations, and still others have shown that the severity of asthma exacerbations requiring emergency room treatment did not differ between obese and nonobese patients. Because obesity by itself can cause a reduction in lung function with attendant symptoms of wheeze and dyspnea, finding proof that obesity affects the inherent severity of asthma is fraught with difficulty. Nevertheless, most studies suggest that obesity as a comorbid condition exaggerates symptoms and that weight loss has beneficial effects as measured by symptoms and medication use.

Gastroesophageal Reflux

A number of sources have cited an association between gastroesophageal reflux (GER) and difficult-to-treat asthma. Up to 60% of asthmatic adults have been reported to demonstrate acid reflux by pH monitoring or other imaging techniques. Although numerous studies have shown a high prevalence of GER in asthma, a high prevalence by itself does not imply a causal relationship to severe asthma. In fact, data supporting a causal link are confounded by problems related to the accuracy of the diagnosis of asthma as well as the diagnosis of GER. Reflux or aspiration of gastric contents, by itself, can trigger wheeze and cough and thus mimic asthma. Because few published studies have provided objective evidence supporting an asthma diagnosis, it is possible that many so-called asthma patients were incorrectly diagnosed as having asthma on the basis of symptoms that could be attributed to GER itself.

The role of GER in asthma and as a determinant of asthma severity is perhaps best elucidated by an analysis of the effect of GER therapy on asthma. Although the literature suggests an association, few studies have focused on patients with severe asthma and many lacked adequate documentation of an asthma diagnosis or lacked appropriate controls. The link between asthma and GER is discussed in further detail in Chapter 39.

Environmental Exposure

To the extent that avoidance of environmental triggers of asthma can prevent exacerbations, reduce the need for drug treatment, and decrease use of emergency facilities, environmental factors appear to play a significant role in determining asthma control and severity. The relative importance of different indoor allergens as determinants of asthma severity may vary in different populations. For example, cockroach allergen but not dust mite exposure has been shown to be associated with greater morbidity and severity in asthmatic children living in an inner-city environment, whereas dander exposure may be a relatively more important determinant of morbidity among suburban and rural dwellers. Exposure to occupational allergens, on the other hand, has been associated with severe asthma in patients with adult-onset asthma but not in patients with childhood-onset asthma. Whether low-intensity exposure to environmental allergens and other substances can contribute to longer-term, subclinical airway inflammation and progression of asthma severity is unknown. However, the thesis that chronic exposure to asthmogenic substances can lead to disease progression is supported by studies showing that patients with occupational asthma due to low molecular weight chemicals can either experience remission or progression of their disease depending on the duration of exposure before removal from the workplace.

Corticosteroid Insensitivity

Although inhaled corticosteroids have proven benefits in the management of most patients with asthma, an appreciable number of patients, estimated at 5% to 25% of the total population, demonstrate a diminished response to these agents. This phenomenon of "steroid insensitivity" reflects what is recognized as the inherent variability of treatment responses among individuals. This variability is seen with virtually all medications and it is estimated that 70% to 80% of the variability has a genetic basis. The mechanisms underlying steroid insensitivity in asthma have been attributed to a variety of molecular and inflammatory processes as well as alterations in the glucocorticoid receptor. Although in some patients the use of very high doses of corticosteroids can overcome the diminished responsiveness, the risks of systemic side effects at these doses become an important clinical consideration. A large multicenter and multinational study demonstrated that as many as 25% to 30% of subjects fail to achieve good control of asthma despite the use of high-dose inhaled corticosteroids, indicating that steroid insensitivity may be an important determinant of asthma severity.[7]

Sinusitis

A link between asthma and rhinosinusitis has been recognized for many years. Whether rhinosinusitis in some way contributes to asthma severity, however, remains somewhat controversial. The prevalence of rhinosinusitis has been reported to be comparable in patients with mild to moderate asthma and those with severe asthma. On the other hand, severity of sinus involvement as measured by computed tomography (CT) scans has been found to correlate with asthma severity, suggesting a relationship between the two entities. Some studies have reported that patients with both sinusitis and asthma were more likely to be oral corticosteroid-dependent, more likely to have nasal polyps, and more likely to have aspirin sensitivity. One of the more persuasive arguments for a relationship between severity of rhinosinusitis and severity of asthma is the reported benefit of treating sinus disease on asthma management. A number of studies have demonstrated that treatment of sinusitis with antibiotics leads to improvement in asthma symptoms as well as improvement in pulmonary function. Although there is an abundance of evidence indicating that sinusitis plays an important role in asthma, particularly severe or difficult-to-treat asthma, most of the literature describing this role is derived from either subjective observations or studies lacking proper controls or adequate study design. Therefore, further attempts to better understand the pathobiology and management of rhinosinusitis and their effects on asthma severity would be of value.

Aspirin Sensitivity

Aspirin-induced asthma is a clinical syndrome characterized by chronic rhinosinusitis and asthma precipitated by ingestion of aspirin and other nonsteroidal anti-inflammatory drugs. The syndrome is also frequently associated with nasal polyposis. The condition usually manifests in the third or fourth decade of life and appears to occur more frequently in females. It is estimated that approximately 5% to 20% of all asthmatic individuals have aspirin sensitivity. The majority of patients with aspirin sensitivity have moderate to severe asthma that often requires intervention with systemic corticosteroids. Various surveys indicate that 40% to 50% of patients require chronic oral corticosteroids to maintain control. The airways of aspirin-sensitive patients demonstrate intense eosinophilic

inflammation, although it is unclear whether the inflammatory reaction differs from that seen in non–aspirin sensitive asthmatic individuals and why the underlying asthma in these patients is more difficult to control.

Genetic

It is generally accepted that asthma is an inherited disorder with a complex polygenic pathogenesis. Using candidate gene approaches and genome screening strategies, a number of genes and chromosome regions associated with asthma susceptibility have been identified. Few studies, however, have focused on genetic mutations that determine asthma severity. Part of the problem again is the lack of a single clear end point by which severity can be measured and distinct phenotypes of asthma severity can be defined. To the extent that asthma severity can be defined by an individual's response to treatment, pharmacogenetic studies of mutations in genes associated with the treatment response appear promising. Recent studies have shown that polymorphisms of the beta$_2$-adrenergic receptor gene may be associated with poor outcomes with respect to pulmonary function, while other studies currently under way are exploring genes associated with the response to other forms of treatment, such as corticosteroids and leukotriene modifiers.

LIMITATIONS IN DEFINING ASTHMA SEVERITY

The use of published schemes for classifying asthma severity is not without limitations. For example, reliance on patient-reported symptoms depends on the accuracy of patient recall, which may vary widely within the population. Clinical experience tells us that a patient may not recall having experienced significant morbidity several weeks earlier if their current level of control is perceived as adequate. Moreover, an abundance of studies have shown discordance between patient-reported symptoms and lung function measurements, suggesting that these different end points may reflect distinctly different aspects of the disease.[8,9] There are many examples in which asthma therapy had no appreciable effect on pulmonary function over time and yet had a significant salutary effect on morbidity as measured by exacerbations requiring oral corticosteroids, symptom-free days, resource use, and airway reactivity. Although peak expiratory flow (PEF) has been recommended as a useful tool for monitoring control, studies have shown PEF to be a poor predictor of symptoms as well as impending exacerbations. These observations suggest that pulmonary function tests have limitations with respect to assessing severity as well as control. The poor correlation between symptoms and pulmonary function applies not only to information obtained at a single point in time, but also to longitudinal observations, as either end point category is a weak predictor of change in the other with therapy over time.

Attempts to define other measures that might better reflect disease severity are under development. For example, different instruments are being developed to measure asthma severity and asthma control as distinct properties of the disease. Recent studies have shown, however, that these instruments are incapable of distinguishing between severity and control because they largely measure the same parameter, symptom frequency. Certain validated instruments designed to measure asthma control, such as the Asthma Control Test and the Asthma Control Questionnaire, are capable of predicting future utilization of health care services. Thus, if asthma severity can be defined by the risk of future adverse outcomes, these instruments may prove to be of value as additional measures of severity. The role of quality of life questionnaires in assessing asthma severity remains unclear, although studies have shown that the different elements used by treatment guidelines to assign severity, such as symptoms, lung function, and rescue beta-agonist use, do not predict health-related quality of life at any level of severity.

Recognizing the limitations of conventional lung function measurements as an objective surrogate for patient-reported symptoms or other measures of disease control and quality of life, there has been considerable interest in exploring alternative objective markers that might reflect disease severity. Much of this has focused on markers of airway inflammation. Airway eosinophilia, in particular, has been an attractive target, since it is generally viewed as the most characteristic feature of asthmatic inflammation. Although some studies have reported quantitative associations between eosinophil numbers in airway biopsies and clinical severity, the large variability between individual patients and among different levels of severity limits the specificity of this approach. Moreover, biopsy studies in patients with severe asthma in adults and children have identified patient phenotypes in which neutrophils were the predominant inflammatory cell type or where evidence of inflammation was altogether lacking. Other biopsy studies have indicated that the severe asthma phenotype is associated with increased airway smooth muscle or with enhanced collagen synthetic activity of airway fibroblasts. Although these are potentially important findings, these investigations typically involve small numbers of subjects and are too preliminary to have clinical application.

The use of induced sputum, a far less invasive approach as compared to endobronchial biopsy, has also been evaluated with inconclusive results. In one study, it was shown that adjustment of inhaled corticosteroids to maintain sputum eosinophils to 3% or less of total cells resulted in fewer exacerbations and less oral corticosteroid use than treatment adjusted in accordance with symptoms, pulmonary function, and rescue beta-agonist use. However, at the end of treatment, conventional measures of severity such as symptoms, lung function, rescue beta-agonist use, and health-related quality of life did not differ between treatment groups. These findings suggest that sputum eosinophilia may be of value in predicting risk of future events and to this extent may have a potential role in defining asthma severity.

The fraction of nitric oxide in exhaled breath (eNO), another marker of airway inflammation, has also been shown to correlate with severity in patients who demonstrate high levels of airway eosinophilia and airway hyperresponsiveness to methacholine. Exhaled NO levels have been used to adjust inhaled corticosteroid dosages in patients with mild to moderate asthma, and it has been shown that eNO-guided adjustments can result in clinical control comparable to conventional guideline-based adjustments but at significantly lower inhaled corticosteroid doses. These findings suggest that eNO levels may bear some relationship to disease severity and control, but further investigations are needed to examine the sensitivity and specificity of this measurement as a means to distinguish between different levels of asthma severity.

The use of these surrogate markers of airway inflammation to assess asthma severity is currently limited by significant hurdles related to technical as well as cost considerations. However, newer technological advances are likely to lead to more widespread testing in controlled clinical trials and thus to a better understanding of their utility in assessing asthma severity and control.

There may be weak correlations between or among different clinical end points, but no single measure appears to provide a comprehensive assessment of asthma severity or control. On the surface, the use of a composite end point that takes into account multiple aspects of asthma severity and control would seem to be an ideal approach to address this problem. However, choosing the right end points and deciding how to weigh such measures in a composite end point is likely to be a formidable research task in its own right. Indeed, given the heterogeneity of asthma phenotypes, a uniform composite end point may not be suitable for all. Rather, to properly grade asthma severity and control, it is possible that different composite end points composed of a variety of end points and weightings may be needed for different patient populations.

DOES SEVERITY CHANGE OVER TIME?

Whereas most chronic diseases tend to worsen over time, there is a common perception that asthma becomes more severe with longer duration of disease. Support for this conventional view of the natural history of asthma is lacking, however. Some epidemiologic studies have suggested that there is an accelerated decline in FEV_1 (forced expiratory volume in 1 second) over time in asthmatic individuals as compared with individuals who are not asthmatic, although this finding has been challenged in other studies. From my own perspective, the decline in FEV_1 between asthmatic and nonasthmatic individuals appears to be more parallel than divergent when cigarette smokers are excluded from the analysis. Clinical experience indicates that many patients diagnosed with mild asthma at an early age will continue to have mild asthma throughout their lives and the same is true for severe asthma. This is supported by long-term longitudinal data in a population of asthmatic individuals followed from age 7 to 42 years.[10] Patients with the worst symptoms and lung function at age 7 were the patients with the worst symptoms and lung function at age 42. Those with the mildest changes as youngsters continued to be mild as adults. These findings suggest that the severity of asthma may be determined very early in life, a thesis supported by an increasing amount of data.

It is important to note, however, that asthma control may vary significantly over the course of time. Accordingly, asthma severity may also appear to vary significantly over time if severity is assessed by evaluating symptoms, lung function, and rescue beta-agonist use at a single point in time. Discrete assessments at a single point in time may lead to over- or underestimation of severity. New tools that are designed to evaluate disease control over longer time intervals will better serve the goal of accurately defining asthma severity.

SEVERITY PHENOTYPES

The extremes of severity, that is, severe and mild persistent asthma, present unique challenges to the clinician. These challenges range from how we define these extremes of severity to how we should best manage these different phenotypes of severity.

Severe Phenotype

Although severe asthma represents less than 10% of the asthmatic population, those with severe asthma manifest most of the morbidity of the disease and consume the overwhelming portion of health care use and economic costs. Because of its relative importance in this regard, there has been much interest in defining the clinical characteristics, pathogenesis, and natural history of severe asthma. Confounding this effort is the ongoing problem of defining severe asthma. In addition to the definitions in the NAEPP and GINA guidelines, other definitions have been described in large multicenter investigations of severe asthma in the United States and Europe.[4,6] These initiatives have expanded the definition of severe asthma to include the use of high-dose inhaled corticosteroids, periodic or continuous use of oral corticosteroids, and increased health care utilization despite this aggressive therapy. What has emerged from these studies is the understanding that patients with severe asthma by any definition are a heterogeneous group with multiple phenotypes based on age, duration of disease, response to corticosteroids, sensitivity to aspirin, persistent airflow obstruction, and the presence or absence of eosinophilic inflammation. Most studies show that there is a gender shift in severe asthma with age: Severe asthma is more prevalent in males in childhood and more prevalent in females in adulthood. Some investigators have shown that disease severity as measured by lung function in patients whose onset of disease occurred in childhood appears related to disease duration. By contrast, in patients with adult-onset asthma, disease severity appears unrelated to disease duration. Additionally, patients with adult-onset asthma have been shown to have persistent airway eosinophilia despite treatment with corticosteroids, but they tended to have lower immunoglobulin E (IgE) levels and fewer positive allergen skin tests compared with patients with severe asthma whose onset occurred in childhood.

These findings indicate that severe asthma is not a single nosologic entity, but rather a syndrome comprising multiple disorders that have common clinical manifestations but their own distinct, perhaps overlapping, etiologic or pathogenetic mechanisms. Current efforts in large prospective studies in severe asthma are likely to improve our understanding of the pathogenesis and natural history of different phenotypes and provide a better approach to individualize current and future therapies. Such studies may also help to better identify the patient with severe asthma.

Severe asthma may be defined as the persistence of symptoms despite the use of high-dose inhaled corticosteroids. Before applying such a definition, it is important to be certain that the lack of an apparent response to corticosteroids is not due to other factors, such as failure to adhere to the prescribed medication regimen. Nonadherence is a common problem among asthmatic patients and practicing physicians should remain aware of this issue. Severe asthma can also be misdiagnosed in patients who present with symptoms that mimic asthma but who in fact have another diagnosis.

The most common conditions to consider in the differential diagnosis of asthma include other forms of chronic airway disease, particularly chronic obstructive pulmonary disease (COPD). Difficulties in diagnosis arise from the fact that COPD not only mimics asthma in clinical presentation, but may also coexist with asthma as a comorbid condition. Further diagnostic problems arise from the fact that a component of irreversible airway obstruction may prevail in asthmatic patients, and a significant proportion of smokers meeting diagnostic criteria for COPD experience episodic bronchospasm with cough, wheezing and dyspnea. Moreover, such episodes are often improved clinically as well as physiologically by bronchodilator or corticosteroid medications.

Laryngeal dysfunction masquerading as asthma is another condition frequently misdiagnosed as severe or even life-threatening asthma. In vocal cord dysfunction syndrome, the vocal cords adduct during inspiration, leaving a narrowed air passage. Patients with this syndrome typically present with acute episodes of dyspnea and wheezing that are seemingly out of proportion to what is expected based on lung function measured between episodes. Patients may present with stridor and use of accessory muscles of respiration. In my experience, hoarseness or a "barking" cough is often a prelude to an acute episode. Patients with this syndrome may often be intubated and they are frequently treated with high-dose systemic steroids for long periods of time. This unusual condition is discussed in greater detail in Chapter 38.

Mild Phenotype

The prevalence of mild persistent asthma has been difficult to ascertain for a number of reasons. First, many patients with mild disease, particularly those who have no perceived limitations on activity or lifestyle, fail to recognize a health problem and have never been diagnosed with asthma. Still others may fall outside the health care system because they may self-medicate with over-the-counter drugs. Estimating the prevalence of mild asthma in children is even more difficult because of problems in correctly diagnosing asthma in children with recurrent pulmonary infections. Patients with mild asthma also exhibit a substantial degree of variability insofar as they tend to shift from meeting criteria for mild persistent asthma to meeting criteria for moderate persistent or even mild intermittent over time. This is in contrast to patients with severe asthma who are more likely to meet criteria for severe disease over a sustained period of time. For these reasons, few clinical trials have been able to recruit large numbers of patients meeting criteria for mild asthma. Instead, most published trials have expanded symptom and lung function criteria to include patients with mild as well as moderate persistent asthma. Because there is little information on patients with mild asthma as a distinct group, treatment recommendations for this group remain controversial. In particular, the role of long-acting beta-agonists in patients who are adequately controlled on low-dose inhaled corticosteroids alone is a topic of current debate. Other studies have questioned the need for long-term inhaled corticosteroids to maintain pulmonary function, although it is generally recognized that low-dose inhaled corticosteroids can prevent exacerbations and afford better control of symptoms than alternative therapies. More information is needed to better understand the natural history of mild asthma as well as to define the best approaches to treatment.

SUMMARY

Asthma severity describes the relatively persistent underlying level of pathophysiologic abnormality present that is reflected by the intensity of treatment required to maintain control of symptoms and lung function over an extended period of time. Asthma control, in contrast, is a reflection of the effectiveness of current therapy. Although the relationship between asthma severity and asthma control largely rests with how well a patient responds to treatment, both are useful descriptors of the clinical state of the patient. Severity classifications are of value in characterizing the burden of disease on a long-term basis, for identifying treatment needs for chronic maintenance therapy, and for predicting outcomes, particularly

the risk of future events such as loss of control, exacerbations, or hospitalization.

Although there are established guidelines for defining asthma severity, such approaches have limitations because of the heterogeneity of the disease and lack of correlation between many different end points that reflect distinct but important aspects of the clinical status of the patient. Further approaches taking into account health care utilization in the definition of asthma severity are likely to improve our ability to identify patients at the severe end of the severity spectrum.

Further reflection on how we define asthma severity and the complex relationship between severity and control will be an important step in making evidence-based guidelines more practicable and effective for health care providers. Refining the ways in which we are able to characterize the burden of disease will not only improve our ability to identify more appropriate long-term treatment needs but it will also place a much needed focus on day-to-day control and how it is best achieved.

REFERENCES

1. Stoloff SW, Boushey HA: Severity, control and responsiveness in asthma. J Allergy Clin Immunol 2006;117:544–548.
2. Global Initiative for Asthma: Global strategy for asthma management and prevention. NHLBI/WHO Workshop Report (Publication No. 02-3659). Bethesda, MD, Department of Health and Human Services, 2002.
3. National Asthma Education and Prevention Program: Expert Panel Report 3. Guidelines for the Diagnosis and Management of Asthma. Bethesda, MD, NIH, Publication Number 08-5846. U.S. Department of Health and Human Services, National Institutes of Health, National Heart, Lung, and Blood Institute, October 2007.
4. American Thoracic Society: Proceedings of the ATS Workshop on Refractory Asthma: current understanding, recommendations, and unanswered questions. Am J Respir Crit Care Med 2000;162:2341–2351.
5. Miller MK, Johnson C, Miller DP, et al: Severity assessment in asthma: an evolving concept. J Allergy Clin Immunol 2005;116:990–995.
6. The ENFUMOSA Study Group: The ENFUMOSA cross-sectional European multicentre study of the clinical phenotype of chronic severe asthma. Eur Respir J 2003;22:470–477.
7. Bateman ED, Boushey HA, Bousquet J, et al: Can guideline-defined asthma control be achieved? The Gaining Optimal Asthma Control study. Am J Respir Crit Care Med 2004;170:836–844.
8. Colice GL, Burgt JV, Song J, et al: Categorizing asthma severity. Am J Respir Crit Care Med 1999;160:1962–1967.
9. Fuhlbrigge AL: Asthma severity and asthma control: symptoms, pulmonary function, and inflammatory markers. Curr Opin Pulm Med 2004;10:1–6.
10. Phelan PD, Robertson CF, Olinsky A: The Melbourne Asthma Study: 1964–1999. J Allergy Clin Immunol 2002;109:189–94.

Asthma Control

Anne L. Fuhlbrigge and Aaron Deykin

The care of patients with asthma should encompass the principles of chronic disease management including periodic assessment of the activity of the disease, goal (outcome) orientation, individualization of therapy, and monitoring of response to that therapy. Asthma severity and asthma control are two important domains used in the assessment and monitoring of disease. Although the individual parameters by which we define them overlap significantly, important distinctions between asthma severity and asthma control exist.

Asthma severity has traditionally defined the intrinsic/physiologic level of disease activity. It is the baseline characteristic of an individual and although it may change, it will do so more slowly over time. As discussed in the previous chapter in more depth, according to the guidelines for the diagnosis and management of asthma, the assessment of severity is determined by the subjective report of current daytime and nighttime symptoms as well as the objective assessment of lung function. The National Asthma Education and Prevention Program Expert Panel Report 3 (NAEPP EPR3) Guidelines highlight that the accurate assessment of the severity of disease can only be done before initiation of treatment.[1] After initiation of appropriate intervention, including education, environmental control, and pharmacotherapy, many of the parameters used to describe severity may be absent or significantly changed.

The concept of asthma control has been introduced to better describe the status of disease in the presence of intervention. Asthma control can change rapidly in response to triggers or therapy and although it is partially determined by the underlying severity of disease, it also incorporates the adequacy of intervention or treatment.

The interplay between asthma severity, asthma control, and the management of disease is illustrated in Figure 15-1. Asthma severity is a determinant of asthma control; however, medical management can modify the impact of the underlying severity on the level of control. Once a patient has been started on therapy, asthma control should be the focus of periodic monitoring. Asthma control can be seen as the short-term assessment of the adequacy of a treatment and can help to inform whether further intervention or adjustment is needed.

THE GOALS OF ASTHMA THERAPY

An important point in linking asthma severity and asthma control is that the goals of therapy are identical for all levels of asthma severity. Any treatment plan needs to be tailored to the specific needs and circumstances of a given patient, but the overall goal is the same for all individuals: to achieve well-controlled asthma. Therefore, to accurately monitor asthma control we have to understand the goals of therapy.

The recommendations for the treatment of asthma are organized around four components of effective asthma management: (1) the use of objective measures of lung function to aid to assess asthma severity and monitor the course of therapy, (2) environmental control measures to avoid or eliminate factors that precipitate symptoms or exacerbations, (3) pharmacologic therapy, and (4) patient education that fosters a partnership among the patients and his or her family and health care providers. The four components serve as a starting point to help clinicians and patients make appropriate decisions regarding asthma management. Based on these

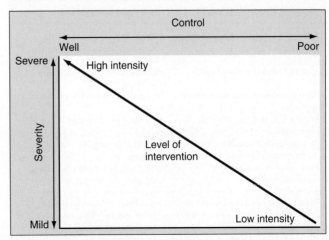

Figure 15-1 Interplay of asthma severity and asthma control.

components, the goals of therapy for asthma have been clearly outlined (Table 15-1). We should be able to prevent troublesome symptoms and recurrent exacerbations, and maintain normal or near normal lung function and activity levels while minimizing side effects. The patient in conjunction with his or her health care provider should discuss the goals for asthma therapy to make sure they meet the patient's and family's expectations and satisfaction for asthma care.

However, many studies have demonstrated that the goals of therapy are not routinely achieved for the majority of subjects with asthma. Some of the difficulty in achieving these goals may be a tendency to overestimate the level of control in many patients. An important component in the clinical assessment of asthma begins with inquiry into symptoms. Yet, variation in the pattern of asthma symptoms reported by persons with asthma can influence the assessment of asthma (Fig. 15-2). Among a population of children with current asthma, less than one third of children report daytime symptoms, nighttime awakenings, and activity limitation simultaneously.[2] Just over a third report two of the three symptom components, while an additional third report only a single symptom component over a 4-week period. Accurate assessment of asthma status requires a combination of parameters and may depend on which parameters are used. Common measures of asthma morbidity are not interchangeable.

This is further illustrated by a study examining how the assessment of asthma burden changes depending on which measures are used.[3] Among a general population of persons with asthma, the burden of disease was divided into three components: (1) self-report of symptoms (both daytime and nighttime) over the preceding 4 weeks (short-term burden), (2) report of symptoms and exacerbations assessed over a longer (12-month) period (long-term burden), or (3) report of the functional impact of disease including activity limitation. It then assessed how the combination of factors influenced the assessment of disease. Figure 15-3 demonstrates how the overall distribution of burden shifts with the incorporation of each additional component of asthma burden.

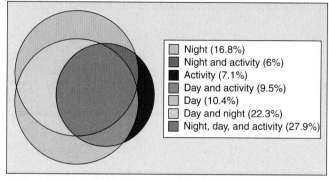

Figure 15-2 **Variability in symptom pattern—the distribution of type and pattern of asthma symptoms among children reporting symptoms in the preceding 4 weeks (N=537).** Each area defines the proportion of children reporting the combination of symptoms outlined in the accompanying legend; for example, 16.9% reported nighttime symptoms only, while 27.9% of children reported concurrent symptoms in each of the three categories. (*Data from Fuhlbrigge AL, Guilbert T, Spahn J, et al: The influence of variation in type and pattern of symptoms on assessment in pediatric asthma. Pediatrics 2006;118:619–625.*)

Thse data highlight the unique information captured by each of the components of asthma symptom burden (short-term symptoms versus long-term symptoms or activity limitation [functional impact]). Assessment of the adequacy of therapy based only on symptoms over the preceding 4 weeks should be expected to give a different estimate of the overall burden of disease than one that incorporates long-term symptoms and/or activity limitation. Importantly, incorporation of a component that focuses on activity limitation has the greatest impact on the distribution of symptom burden.

Finally, it has been shown that the conventional clinical outcomes routinely used in defining asthma severity and asthma control can be separated into four independent components (factors). In addition to asthma-related quality of life, daytime symptoms, nighttime symptoms, and measures of airway caliber are important separate factors.[4] This suggests the need for objective measures, such as pulmonary function, in the diagnosis and monitoring of individuals with asthma, and the NAEPP EPR3 Guidelines, which recommend spirometry for diagnosing and assessing the severity of asthma in order to make "appropriate therapeutic recommendations."[1]

However, because a universally accepted, comprehensive asthma assessment tool is lacking, there is significant variation in the approach to assessing asthma control in current clinical practice. In the sections that follow, we review various asthma assessment techniques, highlighting their areas of strength as well as their clinical applicability.

MARKERS OF LUNG FUNCTION

Spirometry

Spirometry assesses airway caliber by measuring the volume of gas exhaled and the rate of exhalation during a forced maximal expiratory maneuver. To perform spirometry, the patient is seated and is instructed to completely fill his or her lungs. When the patient cannot inhale any additional air, he or she is urged to immediately exhale as forcefully and as completely as possible into the spirometer, which records the total volume of air exhaled (the forced vital capacity, FVC) and the

Table 15-1
GOALS OF THERAPY AND RELATIONSHIP TO WELL-CONTROLLED ASTHMA

Goals of Asthma Therapy	Well-Controlled Asthma
Prevent chronic and troublesome symptoms	Asthma symptoms and rescue bronchodilator use twice a week or less
Maintain normal activity levels	No limitations on exercise, work, or school
Prevent recurrent exacerbations of asthma	Infrequent exacerbations
Maintain (near-) normal pulmonary function	Normal or personal best PEF or FEV$_1$
Provide optimal pharmacotherapy with minimal or no adverse effects	No nighttime or early morning awakening
Meet patients' and families' expectations	Well-controlled asthma by patient and physician assessment

Based on National Asthma Education and Prevention Program: Expert Panel Report 3 (EPR3): Guidelines for the Diagnosis and Management of Asthma (Pub. No. 08-4051). Washington, DC, U.S. Department of Health and Human Services, Public Health Service, National Institutes of Health, National Heart, Lung, and Blood Institute, 2007.

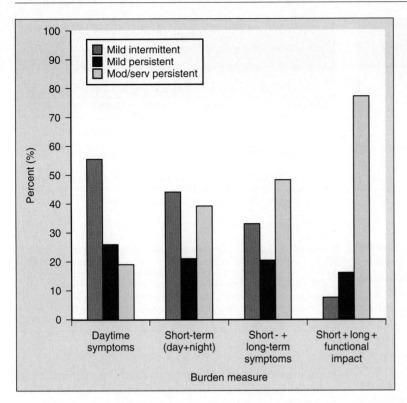

Figure 15-3 **Distribution of asthma burden.** Proportion of individuals classified as having mild intermittent, mild persistent, or moderate/severe persistent disease stratified by the individual component measures of asthma burden: (1) daytime symptoms, (2) short-term symptoms burden (day + night), (3) short- + long-term symptoms, and (4) global symptom burden (short-term [day + night] + long-term + functional impact). (*Data from Fuhlbrigge AL, Guilbert T, Spahn J, et al: The influence of variation in type and pattern of symptoms on assessment in pediatric asthma. Pediatrics 2006;118:619–625.*)

quantity exhaled in the first second of exhalation (the forced expired volume in 1 second, FEV_1). In addition to reporting these volumes and comparing them to normal values based on the patient's age, sex, height, and race, most spirometers also produce a graphical output of the expiratory volume versus the instantaneous flow rate, called a flow-volume loop (Fig. 15-4). Because spirometry is dependent on adequate cooperation and effort from the patient, it is necessary to examine the numerical and graphical data to ensure that they are of sufficient quality for clinical use (Table 15-2). In addition to achieving familiarity with the features of adequate spirometry, clinicians using this technique in asthma need to have an adequate understanding of basic interpretation strategies before applying the results for clinical decision-making purposes.

The FEV_1 is the most frequently used spirometrically determined quantity used to assess asthma control. Because this measure is objective and noninvasive, many experts have previously promoted the widespread use of spirometry in clinical practice to guide asthma care. Studies have demonstrated that in asthma the risk of a future asthma attack is increased in those with lower FEV_1 measures as compared with patients with more preserved lung function. However, other studies have suggested that in an individual patient, there is poor correlation between FEV_1 and asthma symptoms. Further, many studies have shown that the effects of asthma medications on FEV_1 do not necessarily correspond to the effects of these medicines on other important clinical aspects of asthma such as symptoms, exacerbations, and quality of life.[5]

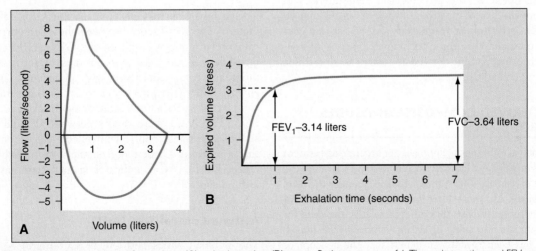

Figure 15-4 **Flow-volume loops.** Normal flow-volume (**A**) and volume-time (**B**) curves. Both curves are useful. The expiratory time and FEV_1 can be easily visualized from the volume-time curve and the peak flow visualized from the flow-volume curve. In this individual the FEV_1 is 3.14 L and the FVC is 3.64 L as illustrated.

Table 15-2
CRITERIA FOR A TECHNICALLY ACCEPTABLE FVC MANEUVER

- Explosive exhalation as evidenced by
  - a smooth, brisk upstroke on the flow-volume loop
  - a sharp peak on the flow volume loop
- Complete exhalation as evidenced by
  - zero flow on the flow-volume loop at end-exhalation
  - a plateau on the volume-time curve
  - expiratory time of at least 6 seconds
- Lack of artifact from the upper airway obstruction or cough as suggested by a smooth descending limb of the flow-volume loop

Table 15-3
INDIVIDUAL COMPONENTS OF ASTHMA CONTROL INSTRUMENTS

Parameter	Assessment Instrument			
	NAEPP	ACQ	ATAQ	ACT
Symptom frequency				
Day	X	X		X
Nocturnal	X	X	X	X
Activity limitation	X	X	X	X
Rescue medication	X	X	X	X
Pulmonary function	FEV_1 or PEF	FEV_1		
Self-perception of control			X	
				X
Symptom severity rating	X	X		
Time frame	Last week and last month	Last week	Last 4 weeks and last year	Last 4 weeks

ACQ, Asthma Control Questionnaire; ACT, Asthma Control Test; ATAQ, Asthma Therapy Assessment Questionnaire; FEV_1, forced expiratory volume in 1 second; GINA, Global Initiative for Asthma; NAEPP, National Asthma Education and Prevention Program; PEF, peak expiratory flow.

Peak Expiratory Flow Rate (PEFR)

Like FEV_1, measurement of PEFR with a hand-held meter provides an objective measure of airway caliber. However, unlike spirometry, the patient can perform the maneuver at home or at work, which facilitates measurement of airflow on a daily basis. In this regard, PEFR monitoring has the capacity to provide the clinician with information not only about the severity of airflow obstruction, but also about the degree of variability of obstruction in an individual patient, which may reflect disease instability. While in asthmatic patients the AM-PM variability is usually 10% or less, individuals with asthma demonstrate increased diurnal variability that further increases during periods of loss of control. For example, one study demonstrated that over 30% of patients requiring hospitalization for asthma had AM-PM peak flow changes of 50%.

While these considerations make PEFR monitoring in clinical practice theoretically attractive, it must be noted that most patients are not sufficiently compliant with regular measurements to be helpful. In addition, certain PEFR meters may not provide consistently accurate results (as compared to more formal measures of PEFR by a spirometer), and further potential for error exists due to poor measurement technique, which can occur in the unmonitored home setting. In light of these limitations and lack of specific data to the contrary, it is not clear that PERF adds information regarding asthma control above that which can be obtained by soliciting patient reports of symptoms or need for rescue medications.

In sum, while the objective measurement of airflow obstruction through spirometry or PEFR measurements provides an assessment of the physiological consequences of asthma, it appears clear that neither of these tools, when used alone, is sufficiently robust to quantify overall asthma control. We recommend that these techniques be used in conjunction with other patient-derived measures to determine asthma control and adjust therapy.

PATIENT-DERIVED COMPOSITE MEASURES OF CONTROL

The importance of a composite approach for accurate assessment of the level of impairment has been highlighted and has led to the development of validated instruments to help quantify the level of asthma control. Although differences in the exact content of the various instruments exist, they all acknowledge the need for a composite approach to assessing asthma control (Table 15-3). However, it has been recently proposed that the concept of asthma control should be divided into two dimensions: current

impairment or discomfort and future risk.[6] Current impairment is defined by the level of symptoms, functional impairment, and level of obstruction.

The available instruments focus on quantifying this first dimension, current impairment.

Asthma Therapy Assessment Questionnaire (ATAQ)

The Asthma Therapy Assessment Questionnaire (ATAQ), developed by Vollmer and colleagues,[7] has been validated. Significant associations between ATAQ score and health care use and quality of life have been demonstrated. The instrument is short and easy to use; it contains a set of four control problems (yes/no) with a point given for each positive response. The total score ranges from 0 to 4 with more points indicating more control problems (poorer control). A pediatric version of the instrument has been developed for use in children.

Asthma Control Questionnaire (ACQ)

The Asthma Control Questionnaire (ACQ) has also been validated.[8] The ACQ score has been shown to correlate with a measure of control based on the GINA/NIH criteria. This instrument includes six questions on symptoms, activity limitation and $beta_2$-agonist use, with an optional assessment on airway caliber (total questions = 7). Each question is scored from 0 to 6 with the total score being the average of the questions. The ACQ score ranges between 0 (well controlled) and 6 (extremely poorly controlled). Recent studies show that a score of 1.5 or more on the 7-item Asthma Control Questionnaire (ACQ) indicates that a patient has inadequate asthma control.

Asthma Control Test (ACT)

The Asthma Control Test (ACT) is a 5-item (see Table 15-3) self-administered survey.[9] Each question is scored from 1 to 5, with the total score being the sum of all questions. The range of the total score can be from 5 to 25. Recent analysis shows that when a cut-off point of 19 was used to distinguish poorly controlled asthma, the ACT had a reasonable sensitivity and specificity when compared with a specialist assessment of the level of control. Similar to the ATAQ, a pediatric version has recently been developed for use in children.

Health-related Quality of Life

Many clinicians also recognize a role for formal assessment of health-related quality of life (HRQOL) in clinical management of asthma. The existing measures of asthma control, lung function, and markers of inflammation do not tell us about the functional impairments and how they impact patients with asthma in their everyday lives. One of the goals of asthma therapy is to meet patients' and families' expectations and needs. To do this we need to ensure that the functional impairments that are important to the patient are addressed and patient well-being is included in the management goals. While several validated instruments for the assessment of asthma health-related quality of life are available and widely used in the research setting, the routine use of HRQOL in clinical practice is in its infancy. Studies are needed to examine whether its inclusion in patient management, independent from assessment of asthma control, is worthwhile and beneficial. When the independent factors contributing to asthma health status are examined, HRQOL is independent from daytime and nighttime symptoms and measures of airway caliber.

DOMAIN OF ASTHMA CONTROL: RISK

As discussed, the current instruments outlined in the previous section (ACT, ATAQ, ACQ) focus on quantifying the dimension of current impairment. The assessment of the second dimension, future risk, is more difficult. Yet a great deal of effort has been directed at identifying surrogate markers of future risk with several markers of inflammation such as induced sputum eosinophilia or exhaled nitric oxide (NO) considered as tools for the assessment of asthma; each may provide additional guidance in monitoring patients with asthma.

Novel Biological Markers

Airway inflammation in asthma is associated with hyperresponsiveness to external stimuli, an increased percentage of eosinophils measured in induced sputum, and elevated concentration of NO in exhaled gas. Because of the improved understanding of the central role of airway inflammation in propagating the clinical manifestations of asthma and the need to identify objective measures of asthma control, there has been increasing interest in applying these markers as assessments of asthma control.[10]

Airway Hyperresponsiveness

Airway hyperresponsiveness is most frequently quantified by bronchial provocation testing in which the concentration of a smooth muscle agonist, such as methacholine, needed to

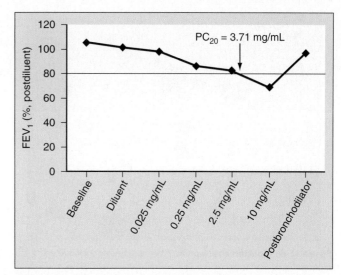

Figure 15-5 FEV$_1$ during methacholine challenge and calculation of PC$_{20}$. A sample graphical output of a methacholine bronchial challenge test demonstrating progressive reductions in FEV$_1$ and calculation of the PC$_{20}$.

reduce the FEV$_1$ by 20% (the methacholine PC$_{20}$) is determined (Fig. 15-5). Bronchial provocation testing is available in many hospital-based pulmonary function–testing laboratories and in some specialty outpatient practices. While many common asthma medications reduce hyperresponsiveness, the correlation between the effects of medication on this measure and their effects on asthma symptoms and need for rescue medication is inconsistent. Although one study has demonstrated improved asthma outcomes in patients whose inhaled corticosteroids were adjusted to suppress symptoms and optimize lung function in addition to the suppression of hyperresponsiveness as compared with patients whose care was titrated to symptoms and lung function alone, these improved outcomes occurred in the context of considerably higher doses of inhaled corticosteroids.[11] Thus, from this study we cannot determine if a measure of hyperresponsiveness (methacholine PC$_{20}$, in this case) improved asthma outcomes by specifically targeting patients who needed additional therapy or by serving as a nonspecific mechanism through which higher doses of inhaled corticosteroids could be applied.

Sputum Eosinophils

Quantification of eosinophils in sputum induced by the inhalation of hypertonic saline has been frequently used for research purposes (Fig. 15-6). The technique involves pretreating the patient with high-dose inhaled bronchodilators followed by 12 minutes of breathing through a circuit attached to a high-output ultrasonic nebulizer filled with 3% saline. Every 2 minutes during inhalation, the patient clears his or her mouth of saliva and then expectorates in a specimen container. Lung function (either PEFR or FEV$_1$) is monitored and compared to pre-inhalation baseline for safety purposes. Following the nebulization period, most experts recommend administration of additional bronchodilators and serial pulmonary function monitoring to ensure the patient's lung function returns to baseline. A total of at least 1 mL of sputum is needed for effective processing and quantification.

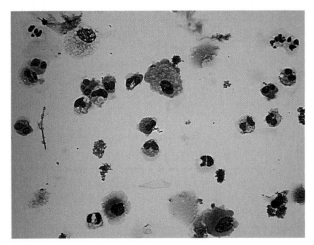

Figure 15-6   Sputum eosinophils. A hematoxylin and eosin stained specimen of induced sputum from a patient with asthma. Multiple eosinophils with red-purple staining are present. (*Photomicrograph kindly provided by Ms. Jane Liu and Dr. John Fahy.*)

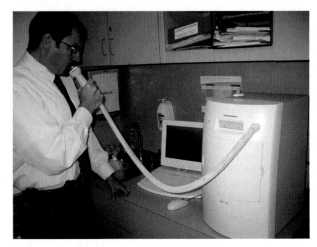

Figure 15-7   Performing eNO measurements. One of the authors performing exhaled NO measurements in an office setting.

Like airway hyperresponsiveness, this measure is elevated in those with asthma as compared with those who do not have asthma, is frequently higher during periods of clinical instability, and responds to the application of asthma therapies to a variable degree. Importantly, recent evidence suggests that in moderate to severe asthma, adjustment of inhaled corticosteroids on the basis of sputum eosinophils alone results in fewer asthma exacerbations than care guided by usual clinical criteria without an increase in the overall dose of inhaled corticosteroid applied.[12] While these results suggest that assessment of sputum cellularity may provide important information about asthma control, this technique requires specialized training and considerable laboratory and personnel resources. Further, the induction procedure may cause significant bronchospasm and approximately 15% of asthmatic individuals cannot produce a suitable specimen.

Exhaled Nitric Oxide

Nitric oxide is produced in the airway epithelium, nerves, and vasculature, as well as by infiltrating inflammatory cells. Asthmatic individuals have higher levels of exhaled NO as compared with healthy subjects, and these levels may rise further during exacerbations. Anti-inflammatory treatments such as corticosteroids, leukotriene receptor agonists (LTRAs), and anti–immunoglobulin E (IgE) reduce NO values in asthma. Measurement of exhaled NO is considerably less cumbersome than bronchoprovocation testing or sputum induction. Although the currently available equipment needed for this technique is large and costly, these machines can be accommodated in most clinical settings (Fig. 15-7). Notably, more portable and economical devices are being developed. A recent trial demonstrated that assessment of asthma control and subsequent adjustment of inhaled steroids by exhaled NO measurements was associated with similar outcomes as medication adjustment on the basis of symptoms and lung function.[13] While the NO-based strategy resulted in the use of 40% lower doses of inhaled corticosteroids (ICSs), it is not clear if this difference reflects optimal individualization of medications in the NO group or overtreatment in the con-

trol group. Future studies are needed to determine the appropriate role of exhaled NO monitoring for the assessment of asthma control.

CONSIDERATIONS IN POORLY CONTROLLED ASTHMA

Despite appropriate medical care, up to 90% of patients being treated for asthma do not achieve adequate asthma control as reflected by continued symptoms or reduced lung function. While in some of these individuals continued symptoms may reflect asthma that is resistant to medical therapy, practitioners should consider other factors when expectations for asthma control are consistently not achieved.

First, it is critical to confirm that the patient's symptoms are, in fact, related to asthma. Other diseases such as congestive heart failure, gastroesophageal reflux disease, vocal cord dysfunction, chronic obstructive pulmonary disease (COPD), or central airway obstruction (due to a foreign body or tumor) can mimic the symptoms and lung function findings of asthma. Allergic bronchopulmonary aspergillosis (ABPA) (see Chapter 43) may worsen lung function and symptoms in patients with asthma or other airway diseases and should be considered, especially in a patient who initially achieves control, but then deteriorates over time. Additionally, anxiety or other psychiatric conditions may present as intractable dyspnea or cough. In children or young adults, occult cystic fibrosis may be misdiagnosed as asthma and should be considered. Importantly, many of these conditions may coexist with true asthma, presenting additional clinical challenges. With patients in whom adequate asthma control cannot be achieved, it is reasonable to reevaluate the history and examination, focusing on excluding alternate diagnoses. Depending on the clinical context, chest radiography, reexamination or repetition of pulmonary function testing, video laryngoscopy, or 24-hour esophageal pH monitoring may be helpful (Table 15-4).

A second important cause of poor asthma control is nonadherence to medical therapy (see Chapter 50). Many studies have shown that patients may use no more than 50% of the inhaled corticosteroid doses prescribed. Although the factors leading to such poor adherence are variable across

Table 15-4
CONSIDERATIONS IN POORLY CONTROLLED ASTHMA

Consideration	Evaluation
Alternate or concomitant diagnosis	
COPD	CXR, lung volumes, DLCO
CHF	CXR, echocardiogram
GERD	Trial or therapy, 24-hour pH monitor
Bronchiectasis	CT scan of chest
ABPA	Sputum culture, serum IgE, CBC, serum precipitins
Vocal cord dysfunction	Laryngoscopy
Central airway obstruction	CT scan of neck/chest
Anxiety	Trial of therapy, psychiatric evaluation
Medical nonadherence	Review of pharmacy records
Poorly responsive asthma	Trial of alternate therapy followed by maximally intensified therapy

ABPA, Allergic bronchopulmonary aspergillosis; CHF, congestive heart failure; COPD, chronic obstructive pulmonary disease; CT, computed tomography; CXR, chest X-ray; DLCO diffusing capacity of the lung for carbon monoxide; GERD, gastroesophageal reflux disease.

individuals, a limited understanding of the chronic nature of asthma, fear of medication side effects, and the cost of medications are common considerations. While it can be difficult to document nonadherence, computerized pharmacy records may be helpful in those being treated in a closed health care system. Unfortunately, as difficult as it is to document, the treatment of nonadherence is equally challenging. In patients who are nonadherent with outpatient oral corticosteroids, intramuscular administration of triamcinolone may be therapeutic and diagnostic. Otherwise, continued attempts at counseling, education, and encouragement may be helpful for patients in whom poor adherence is suspected.

Patients with inadequate asthma control despite exclusion of alternate (or concomitant) diagnoses and nonadherence may have asthma that is not responsive to the therapeutic agents being applied. While inhaled corticosteroids are considered as first-line controller agents, the response to these agents, as well as all asthma therapies, is heterogeneous across individuals. Studies have demonstrated that in terms of lung function improvements, up to 60% of patients may not respond to inhaled corticosteroids. Thus, it is reasonable to consider addition (or substitution) of other classes of controller medications for ICS in patients who do not achieve asthma control with these agents alone. Further, within an individual, some elements of asthma control, such as symptoms or frequency of exacerbations, may improve with a given therapy, while other measures, such as lung function, fail to respond accordingly. In this regard, a comprehensive assessment of several asthma control parameters and the relative importance of these parameters for the patient is appropriate before determining that overall control is unacceptable. Finally, as discussed, we have to ensure we are routinely assessing asthma using a composite measure.

PITFALLS AND CONTROVERSIES

Asthma Severity versus Asthma Control

Asthma is a complex clinical syndrome characterized by episodic escalations in disease activity above a usual baseline.

Although practitioners may use severity and control interchangeably, the terms refer to distinct clinical aspects of the disease. *Severity* most appropriately describes the intensity of the disease and, to an extent, the degree to which the baseline disease burden affects the patient. In contrast, the term *control* has been introduced (in the NAEPP EPR3 Guidelines) to better describe the status of disease in the presence of intervention. It is important for practitioners to understand and consider the distinction between severity (the essential intensity of the disease) and control (the short-term assessment of the adequacy of a given patient's treatment and whether further intervention or adjustment is needed) as they manage patients with asthma. The care of patients with asthma should encompass the principles of chronic disease management including periodic assessment of the activity of the disease, goal (outcome) orientation, individualization of therapy, and then monitoring of response to that therapy.

Predictors of Therapeutic or Untoward Responses

The response to asthma medications is heterogeneous across individuals, asthma outcomes, and specific therapies. For example, a given patient may respond, in terms of lung function, to ICS and not to an LTRA, but may experience improved symptoms with an LTRA and not an ICS. In this regard, techniques to "predict" which therapies are likely to be beneficial or deleterious for which patients will be helpful. Although this field is still evolving, studies appear to demonstrate that asthmatic individuals with high levels of exhaled NO or sputum eosinophils are more likely to realize lung function benefits from ICS, and those with high levels of eosinophils may additionally be at risk for future exacerbations if they do not receive ICS.

It is likely that the variable manifestations of asthma and the heterogeneous treatment responses result, in part, from genetic factors. In this regard, there is increasing evidence that individuals with specific polymorphisms in the gene encoding the beta-agonist receptor may have reduced beneficial responses (or even deleterious effects) when regularly using these agents. However, in light of the significant logistical and financial barriers involved, coupled with the uncertain clinical benefits, incorporating marker assessments and genetic testing into routine asthma management remains controversial at the current time.

WHAT INSTRUMENTS TO USE?

We have outlined several validated measures for assessing asthma control. No comparison between the existing measures has been performed and the similarities between the instruments outweigh their differences. However, the role of these instruments in the routine assessment of patients in daily practice is just beginning to be formally evaluated. The challenge to the assessment and monitoring of asthma is how assessing the level of asthma control (current impairment), relates to changes in asthma therapy, and how regular assessment impacts the second dimension of control: that of future risk. The assessment of future risk is more difficult, yet, similar to the assessment of current impairment, no single measure of disease status will likely provide a direct estimate of future morbidity such as exacerbations or loss of lung function.

HOW MUCH CONTROL IS "ENOUGH"?

While most practitioners can agree that limitations to activity, bothersome symptoms, and risk of exacerbations or death are all components of asthma control that should be adequately addressed through therapy, there is significant controversy regarding the minimal level of disease that is acceptable. Although many recognize that a given level of symptoms or limitation may be acceptable to a particular patient, or at least may not justify, for that patient, additional medical interven-tion, some argue that even in patients such as this therapy should be escalated with the goal of elimination of all disease manifestations if possible. This line of reasoning is based on the frequent observation that patients minimize symptoms and accommodate to chronic limitations to their activities. In this regard, such patients may not fully appreciate the degree to which their disease and their quality of life could be improved by additional therapy. Given the improved understanding of the long-term toxicities of higher-dose ICS and lack of con-vincing evidence that chronic application of asthma therapies changes the natural history of this condition, the mandate for recommending complete control of asthma, regardless of patient preferences, remains controversial.

REFERENCES

1. National Asthma Education and Prevention Program: Expert Panel Report 3 (EPR3): Guidelines for the Diagnosis and Management of Asthma (Pub. No. 08-4051). Bethesda, MD, U.S. Department of Health and Human Services, Public Health Service, National Institutes of Health, National Heart, Lung, and Blood Institute, 2007.
2. Fuhlbrigge AL, Guilbert T, Spahn J, et al: The influence of variation in type and pattern of symptoms on assessment in pediatric asthma. Pediatrics 2006;118:619–625.
3. Fuhlbrigge AL, Adams RJ, Guilbert TW, et al: The burden of asthma in the United States: level and distribution are dependent on interpretation of the National Asthma Education and Prevention Program Guidelines. Am J Respir Crit Care Med 2002;166(8):1044–1049.
4. Juniper EF, Wisniewski ME, Cox FM, et al: Relationship between quality of life and clinical status in asthma: a factor analysis. Eur Respir J 2004;23(2):287–291.
5. Lazarus SC, Boushey HA, Fahy JV, et al: Long-acting beta2-agonist monotherapy vs continued therapy with inhaled corticosteroids in patients with persistent asthma: a randomized controlled trial. JAMA 2001;285(20):2583–2593.
6. Stoloff SW, Boushey HA: Severity, control, and responsiveness in asthma. J Allergy Clin Immunol 2006;117(3):544–548.
7. Vollmer WM, Markson LE, O'Connor E, et al: Association of asthma control with health care utilization and quality of life. Am J Respir Crit Care Med 1999;160(5 Pt 1):1647–1652.
8. Juniper EF, O'Byrne PM, Guyatt GH, et al: Development and validation of a questionnaire to measure asthma control. Eur Respir J 1999;14:902–907.
9. Nathan RA, Sorkness CA, Kosinski M, et al: Development of the asthma control test: a survey for assessing asthma control. J Allergy Clin Immunol 2004;113(1):59–65.
10. Deykin A: Biomarker-driven care in asthma: are we there? J Allergy Clin Immunol 2006;118(3):565–568.
11. Sont JK, Willems LN, Bel EH, et al: Clinical control and histopathologic outcome of asthma when using airway hyperresponsiveness as an additional guide to long-term treatment. The AMPUL Study Group. Am J Respir Crit Care Med 1999;159(4 Pt 1):1043–1051.
12. Green RH, Brightling CE, Woltmann G, et al: Analysis of induced sputum in adults with asthma: identification of subgroup with isolated sputum neutrophilia and poor response to inhaled corticosteroids. Thorax. 2002;57(10):875–879.
13. Smith AD, Cowan JO, Brassett KP, et al: Use of exhaled nitric oxide measurements to guide treatment in chronic asthma. N Engl J Med 2005;352(21):2163–2173.

Assessment of Airway Inflammation

John G. McCartney and Nizar N. Jarjour

CLINICAL PEARLS

- Identify underlying inflammatory processes related to asthma.
- Understand the role of bronchoscopy and bronchoalveolar lavage in the evaluation of asthma.
- Consider issues regarding safety and patient selection for research protocols.
- Recognize the contribution of segmental allergen challenge as a research protocol.
- Identify noninvasive techniques of assessment of airway inflammation.

The earliest description of asthma is credited to Aretaeus of Cappadocia, second century BC, who detailed "attacks" of asthma potentially leading to suffocation. In 1764, Watson described the postmortem examination of a 28-year-old male with enormous distension of the lungs and an inability to decompress with intense pressure.[1] In 1921, Huber and Koessler described autopsy findings of patients who suffered fatal asthma exacerbations including glandular hyperplasia, smooth muscle hypertrophy, abundant secretions, bronchial wall thickening, and airway inflammation with prominent eosinophilia.[2] Over the past 3 decades the presence and contribution of airway inflammation has been recognized in patients whose conditions ranged from mild, intermittent symptoms to fatal asthma.

It is now appreciated that this process involves multiple cells including eosinophils, macrophages, mast cells, lymphocytes, neutrophils, cytokines, and other mediators. While initial studies were based on autopsies of patients who died with or from asthma, direct assessment of airway inflammation became more feasible with the development of fiber-optic bronchoscopy allowing safe retrieval of lower airway samples, including bronchoalveolar fluid, brushings, and bronchial tissue, for in vivo analysis. Demonstrating the persistence of airway inflammation, even in patients with mild or asymptomatic asthma led to a greater emphasis on regular use of anti-inflammatory agents in asthma. Bronchial biopsies in adults and children with asthma have also revealed changes of airway remodeling in early stages of the disease. In addition, the use of segmental allergen challenge has further advanced our understanding of the inflammatory response to allergic stimulation in atopic subjects with and without asthma.

Adding to the insight provided by bronchoscopy, techniques for noninvasive monitoring of airway inflammation continue to advance. The potential to reliably assess inflammation through induced sputum, exhaled breath condensate, or exhaled nitric oxide shows promise for both research and clinical applications, especially in patients with severe asthma where the potential for side effects may preclude bronchoscopy. This chapter focuses on the techniques currently available for assessment of airway inflammation, with particular emphasis on patient selection and safety.

BRONCHOSCOPY

Interest in accessing the lower airway for clinical and research purposes has existed for multiple generations. In the early 1970s, Ikeda and colleagues developed a flexible instrument, the fiberoptic bronchoscope, dramatically increasing the ability to sample the bronchial tissues.[3] In 1974, Reynolds described the technique of "bronchial" (bronchoalveolar) lavage providing washings of the alveolar surface, to recover respiratory cells and secretions for evaluation of cell functions, microbiological studies, and protein analysis.[4]

The incorporation of fiber-optic bronchoscopy and bronchoalveolar lavage as tools in asthma research developed cautiously over the next decade. There are clear advantages for sampling airway specimens in patients demonstrating the full spectrum of asthma severity, rather than sampling obtained through postmortem examinations of those who died from acute severe attacks. These benefits needed to be considered in the context of potential complications from using invasive techniques. Through early studies in both healthy and mild asthma subjects, the safety of fiber-optic bronchoscopy and bronchoalveolar lavage (BAL) was established and these techniques have become accepted as research tools. Studies using BAL fluid have shown increased numbers and activation of inflammatory cells and higher levels of pro-inflammatory mediators in asthma compared with healthy controls (Fig. 16-1). Multiple mediators and cytokines have been detected through analysis of BAL fluid including interleukins, leukotrienes, prostaglandins, tryptase, soluble adhesion molecules, and histamine. In addition, fiber-optic bronchoscopy and BAL fluid have been used to evaluate the effectiveness of established and new asthma therapies, expanding our knowledge of the inflammatory process associated with asthma.

There is no standard technique to performing fiberoptic bronchoscopy or BAL collection across research groups. Typically, the bronchoscope is inserted through the nares or the mouth after light sedation and topical anesthesia of the nose and upper airway. The bronchoscope is wedged in a segmental or subsegmental bronchus. Sterile fluid is then introduced through the bronchoscope in aliquots of 20 to 60 mL. The fluid is typically warmed to body temperature

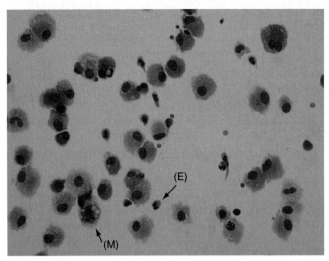

Figure 16-1   Smear of BAL showing eosinophils (E) and macrophages (M). (Magnification ×20).

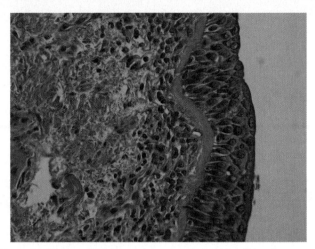

Figure 16-2   Bronchial biopsy from a patient with mild asthma. (Hematoxylin and eosin, magnification ×20).

to avoid thermally induced bronchoconstriction. The effluent is recovered using intermittent suction. The total volume of fluid instilled during the bronchoalveolar lavage procedure may range from 100 to 400 mL. In healthy subjects, and those with mild disease, a recovery of 80% of the fluid is expected; however, a recovery of 50% or less is not uncommon in patients with moderate to severe disease. While periodic deep breathing may increase the yield of effluent, this can also lead to fluid leakage, stimulating cough.[5]

There is also no universally accepted method of processing BAL specimens or reporting the findings. Typically, the cellular component is removed by centrifugation and cell count (total cells or cells/mL) and differential are obtained. Proteins, immunoglobulins, cytokines, and other substances are usually analyzed in the supernatant and reported using "per mL of BAL fluid."

Endobronchial brushings obtained during fiber-optic bronchoscopy provide bronchial epithelial cells for in vitro studies of their function and gene expression. Endobronchial biopsies can be obtained using a small alligator or cup forceps. This technique has allowed detailed descriptions of the morphology of asthmatic airways and samples for immunohistochemical staining of inflammatory cells within the various epithelial and submucosal layers (Fig. 16-2). Further studies of endobronchial biopsy specimens evaluating in situ hybridization of cytokine production and gene activation have led to a deeper understanding of the inflammatory cascade involved in asthma. Last, there is evolving interest in transbronchial biopsy specimens obtained during research bronchoscopies. These parenchymal samples allow direct examination of the small airways. Experience using this technique for research purposes is still limited; however, it could prove to be a useful research tool in asthma because it samples the small airways that are thought to be critically important in asthma pathogenesis.

BRONCHOPROVOCATION

Bronchoprovocation is a tool to test airway hyperresponsiveness in asthma. It can be done with nonspecific agents (e.g., methacholine) or specific allergens. In allergic patients, inhalation of a relevant allergen provokes airway obstruction and inflammation with significant eosinophilia. Asthma subjects typically respond at a much lower dose compared with allergic subjects without asthma. Inhaled allergen challenges allow for determination of lung function response including early and late responses, but these challenges have some drawbacks. In particular, the amount of allergen actually delivered to the lower airways and the specific location of allergen deposition cannot be determined in these studies. Segmental allergen challenge, which involves deposition of an antigen via bronchoscope wedged in a lung segment, overcomes these limitations by inoculating specific bronchial segments allowing for more precise dosing and localization. Bronchoscopy and BAL per se do not evoke a generalized inflammatory response. Multiple segments can be challenged with varying antigen concentrations, or with instillation of an antiasthma drug in one segment and placebo in another, allowing dose-response studies or examination of the antiallergic effect of a given medication. Antigen is typically delivered in volumes of 5 to 20 mL with doses targeting a certain degree of airway obstruction, or based on the response to inhaled allergen challenge or skin-testing titration methods. Allergen is inserted through the bronchoscope in a wedged position to avoid spillage and contamination of other bronchial segments. Follow-up examinations with BAL, brushings, or endobronchial biopsies can then be from minutes to days after antigen instillation.[5] Using this technique, BAL analysis has demonstrated the release of mast cell mediators immediately after allergen challenge, a neutrophil predominance within hours of challenge, and eosinophil infiltration that peaks 2 to 3 days and lasts up to 2 weeks or longer after the challenge. This technique has proven to be a powerful tool in the assessment of both the early and late phases of allergic inflammation.

BRONCHOSCOPY IN CHILDREN

Research bronchoscopy, which is well accepted in adults with asthma, was more recently extended to children with asthma. Fiber-optic bronchoscopy is a commonly used technique in assessing airway diseases in children including recurrent pulmonary infections, stridor, and foreign body manipulations.

The use of BAL in children as a research tool has provided significant insight into patterns of inflammation associated with asthma, infantile wheezing, chronic cough, and other allergic diseases across various age groups. Stevenson and colleagues showed increased BAL eosinophilia in children with atopic asthma compared to children with virus-associated wheezing.[6] Bronchoscopy has gradually been incorporated into some of the research studies of children with asthma. Bronchial biopsies in young asthmatic individuals have shown early changes of airway remodeling suggesting that these subclinical abnormalities are not simply the result of long-standing poorly controlled airway inflammation in adults with asthma. More recent studies have linked rhinoviral infection of the lower airways to persistent respiratory symptoms following upper respiratory tract infections.

BRONCHOSCOPY SAFETY

The appropriate selection of research participants, either those with asthma or other airway diseases or healthy subjects, is crucial for subject safety and data integrity. While there are multiple studies documenting the safety of these procedures in clinical and research settings, these procedures can be associated with serious adverse outcomes, including asthma exacerbations, fever, infections, bleeding, and even death. Early research bronchoscopy studies were performed in patients with mild asthma and showed that this procedure could be performed safely with minimal side effects. In 1985, the first National Institutes of Health workshop on safety of bronchoscopy and BAL suggested that these procedures can be performed in subjects with mild asthma with minimal risk.[7] Since that report, there has been significant increase in clinical experience with the use of bronchoscopy in patients with asthma and other airway diseases with varying degrees of severity. These studies demonstrated the safety of bronchoscopy in patients with mild to moderate asthma provided that appropriate attention is paid to patient selection, preparation, pre- and postprocedure administration of bronchodilators, monitoring with continuous pulse oximetry monitoring, and supplemental oxygen delivery. As comfort levels with the use of these techniques increased, investigators gradually included asthma patients with more severe disease in their research studies. Initial guidelines suggested a relative contraindication in patients with an FEV_1 (forced expiratory volume in 1 second) of less than 60% for research bronchoscopy. However, recently patients with more severe disease have been included in research studies, provided additional monitoring and safeguards are incorporated.[8]

One source of potential risk while performing bronchoscopy is the use of sedation and topical anesthetics. Whether given orally, intravenously, or via intramuscular injection, sedation is used to provide comfort, but should be targeted to the patient's status and specific study to avoid unnecessary side effects and complications. Although not a Food and Drug Administration (FDA)-approved route of administration, topical anesthesia with direct instillation of lidocaine into the airways is commonly used during bronchoscopy. Most research centers have adopted a total dose of 600 mg (or 9 mg/kg) as an upper limit per procedure. Generally, one should aim to minimize sedation and anesthetic while avoiding discomfort to study subjects.

NONINVASIVE TECHNIQUES

Although the role of invasive methods for assessing airway inflammation has evolved, there has also been significant interest in the development of noninvasive techniques in clinical and research protocols. Noninvasive techniques allow for expanded subject eligibility to include patients with more severe disease and during acute exacerbations in whom bronchoscopy is less well tolerated. In addition, these techniques provide increased accessibility in ambulatory settings due to fewer monitoring and equipment requirements. Last, given the noninvasive nature of these techniques, subjects are more likely to accept serial examinations for continued evaluations.

Induced Sputum

Sputum production is a common complaint in patients with inflammatory disorders of the airways, like asthma, cystic fibrosis, and chronic obstructive pulmonary disease (COPD). Clinically, sputum collection for evaluation of pulmonary infections is widely used. The routine use of sputum for analysis of inflammatory markers is limited by variability in methods for sample collection and processing. Sputum induction is accomplished by administration of either normal or hypertonic saline via nebulization. Subjects are typically treated with short-acting beta-agonists before sputum induction to reduce the chances for bronchoconstriction. Monitoring of pulmonary functions during sputum induction is also recommended, either with periodic spirometry or peak flow measurements. If the patient's oxygenation is marginal before initiation of the protocol, continuous monitoring with pulse oximetry should also be considered.

Sputum expectoration requires cooperation between the person obtaining the sample and the subject. Generally, the subject is asked to fast for 4 hours before sputum induction to reduce concerns over nausea and emesis; brush teeth immediately before collection to reduce oropharyngeal contamination; and rinse mouth with water immediately before collection and dry oral membranes with tissues.[9]

The predominant inflammatory cell present in sputum is the neutrophil. Increased sputum eosinophilia is seen in asthmatic individuals compared with healthy subjects (Fig. 16-3). Sputum eosinophilia in steroid-naïve asthmatic individuals is generally suggestive of a steroid-responsive process, and a marked reduction in eosinophil counts is typically observed after treatment with corticosteroids. Some studies have targeted sputum eosinophil levels to adjust inhaled corticosteroid dose with significant reductions in asthma exacerbations and improvement in lung functions. In these studies, patients without eosinophilia were able to reduce the dose of inhaled steroid without deterioration in lung function.[10,11]

A second population of subjects with asthma, either experienced or naïve to corticosteroid therapy, have significantly higher levels of neutrophils in their sputum. These subjects are less responsive to corticosteroid therapy compared with patients with an eosinophilic predominance. For patients without eosinophilia, alternate therapies may need to be considered. In asthma and other airway diseases, such as COPD and chronic cough, analysis of induced sputum may prove

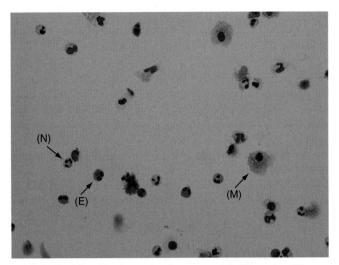

Figure 16-3 Induced sputum showing neutrophils (N), eosinophils (E), and a macrophage (M). (Gram stain, ×20 magnification).

to be a useful clinical tool in the assessment of underlying inflammation as part of the disease process and monitoring of therapeutic responses.[12]

Exhaled Nitric Oxide

Nitric oxide is present in many tissues and organ systems throughout the body including the respiratory tree, typically present at higher concentrations in the sinuses and nasopharynx relative to the lower airways. Nitric oxide is involved in multiple regulatory functions, including bronchial and vascular tone. Its presence as a marker of underlying inflammation in asthma has been investigated for more than 2 decades after initial studies demonstrated higher levels of exhaled nitric oxide in subjects with asthma and other allergic diseases compared with healthy controls. More importantly, similar to the presence of eosinophilia in induced sputum, an elevated concentration of nitric oxide has been shown to predict responsiveness to inhaled corticosteroids and levels of exhaled nitric oxide decline with the addition of this therapy. Exhaled nitric oxide shows promise as a marker in the diagnosis of asthma and as a surveillance parameter in those subjects with established disease.[13] The potential of exhaled nitric oxide to predict exacerbations of asthma was recently examined and levels were found to be elevated before the fall in lung function or the development of clinical symptoms of asthma exacerbations.[15] While there is need for standardized normal ranges to account for possible differences in age, sex, and ethnicity, this modality shows significant potential.[14]

There are two primary methods for collecting exhaled nitric oxide for both clinical and research protocols. An "offline" technique uses the collection of exhaled breath in a specialized reservoir that allows for storage and subsequent analysis of the nitric oxide content. "Online" nitric oxide techniques use continuous sampling and quantification during exhalation for dynamic measurements and flow analysis. "Offline" techniques allow for collections at remote locations to the analyzer, but the benefits of "online" measurements include the ability for real-time analysis and comparisons between individual breaths. Multiple factors may affect the actual collection and quantification of exhaled nitric oxide, including ambient nitric oxide levels, nasopharyngeal contamination, smoking status, and airway infections. Ingestion of certain foods and beverages, particularly those containing nitrates, can also alter exhaled nitric oxide levels. Therefore, patients are asked to take nothing by mouth for 1 hour before sample collection. Medications can also affect exhaled nitric oxide levels, particularly those that affect airway caliber and nitric oxide production including the leukotriene modifiers. Exhaled nitric oxide levels are a very sensitive indication of inhaled corticosteroid use and could be used to "spot check" patients' compliance with their controller anti-inflammatory therapy. With standardization of protocols to determine exhaled nitric oxide levels, this test has the potential for monitoring airway inflammation in patients with asthma to determine disease control and adherence to inhaled corticosteroid therapy.

Exhaled Breath Condensate

Another method of assessment of airway inflammation in asthma and other allergic and nonallergic airway diseases involves the collection of aerosolized airway fluid and volatile compounds. This fluid is collected as exhaled breath passes through a condensing apparatus and contains a mixture of water vapor and both nonvolatile and volatile compounds. The nonvolatile compounds include various cytokines, surfactants, ions, lipids, and serotonin. The volatile compounds include ethanol, ammonia, and hydrogen peroxide. The collected material can also be analyzed for pH.

The source of exhaled breath condensate (EBC) remains somewhat controversial. One theory suggests that EBC is produced by turbulent flow, primarily in the larger airways where cartilaginous rings can alter airflow. Others suggest that EBC is generated from the opening of closed respiratory bronchioles and alveoli during inspiration. The actual source of EBC is likely a combination of these sources. Exhaled breath is passed through a condenser where droplets of airway lining fluid collect on a cooled surface. Various research centers use different "home-made" devices for collection and cooling of the exhaled breath. There are also several commercial devices available for EBC collection.

Similar to exhaled nitric oxide analysis, there are no standardized normal ranges with relation to age, sex, or ethnicity for EBC. Fluid analysis for hydrogen peroxide, leukotrienes, and cytokines in bronchiectasis, cystic fibrosis, COPD, acute respiratory distress syndrome (ARDS), and other illnesses has been reported.[16] One particular area of interest has been the change in pH of EBC during acute asthma exacerbations. Hunt and colleagues have demonstrated the acidification of exhaled breath condensate in acute asthma exacerbations compared to normal controls and normalization following the addition of inhaled corticosteroids.[15] Neutralizing the pH with nebulization of a bicarbonate solution has also been proposed as a therapeutic measure in those with demonstrated acidity of EBC. Serial sampling of exhaled breath condensate may ultimately allow monitoring of therapeutic effects of anti-inflammatory medicines and possibly even compliance with prescribed regimens.

SUMMARY

Understanding of the underlying inflammatory process in asthma and other pulmonary diseases continues to evolve.

It is now appreciated that airway inflammation plays an important role in the pathophysiology of asthma and other lung disease. The ability to safely and efficiently evaluate airway inflammation in a standardized protocol has significantly expanded the knowledge of these various conditions. There are now several modalities available for both clinical and research protocols to assess and monitor the inflammatory cascade (Table 16-1). Bronchoscopy, bronchial biopsy, bronchoalveolar lavage, and segmental allergen challenge have enhanced our understanding of the role of airway inflammation in asthma. The role for noninvasive technology to provide similar information continues to expand. With improvements in noninvasive techniques, the potential to apply these modalities for both diagnosis and monitoring in clinical and research settings is promising. Standardized protocols and reference ranges are still needed, but these noninvasive techniques may ultimately allow the routine application of these modalities to outpatient settings for patient assessment and directing treatment decisions.

Table 16-1
MONITORING AIRWAY INFLAMMATION IN ASTHMA

Method	Measurement	Limitation
Induced sputum	Eosinophils	Standardization of technique Patient cooperation
Flexible bronchoscopy	Eosinophils	Invasive modality Technical expertise
Exhaled nitric oxide	Nitric oxide levels	Cost of equipment
Exhaled breath condensate	pH	Standardization of collection

REFERENCES

1. Siegel S: History of asthma deaths from antiquity. J Allergy Clin Immunol 1987;80:458–462.
2. Huber HL, Koessler KK: The pathology of bronchial asthma. Arch Intern Med 1922;30:689–760.
3. Ikeda S: Flexible bronchofibroscope. Ann Otol Rhinol Laryngol 1970;79:916–919.
4. Reynolds HY, Newball HH: Analysis of protein and respiratory cells obtained from human lungs by bronchial lavage. J Lab Clin Med 1974;84:559–573.
5. Jarjour NN, Peters S, Calhoun WJ, Djukanovic R: Investigative use of bronchoscopy in patients with asthma. Am J Respir Crit Care Med 1998;157:692–697.
6. Stevenson EC, Turner G, Heaney LG, et al: Bronchoalveolar lavage findings suggest two different forms of childhood asthma. Clin Exp Allergy 1997;27:991–994.
7. Goldstein RA, Hurd SS: Summary and recommendations of a workshop on the investigative use of fiberoptic bronchoscopy and bronchoalveolar lavage in individuals with asthma. J Allergy Clin Immunol 1985;76:145–147.
8. Busse WW, Wanner A, Adams K, et al: Investigative bronchoprovocation and bronchoscopy in airway diseases. Am J Respir Crit Care Med 2005;172:807–816.
9. Paggiaro PL: Sputum induction. Eur Respir J 2002;20S37:3S–8S.
10. Green RH, Brightling CE, McKenna S, et al: Asthma exacerbations and sputum eosinophil counts: A randomized controlled trial. Lancet 2002;360:1715–1721.
11. Jatakanon A, Lim S, Barnes PJ: Changes in sputum eosinophils predict loss of asthma control. Am J Respir Crit Care Med 2000;161:64–72.
12. Brightling CE: Clinical applications of induced sputum. Chest 2006;129:1344–1348.
13. ATS/ERS Recommendations for standardized procedures for the online and offline measurement of exhaled lower respiratory nitric oxide and nasal nitric oxide, 2005. Am J Respir Crit Care Med 2005;171:912–930.
14. Taylor DR: Nitric oxide as a clinical guide for asthma management. J Allergy Clin Immunol 2006;117(2):259–262.
15. Hunt JF, Fang K, Malik R, et al: Endogenous airway acidification. Implications for asthma pathophysiology. Am J Respir Crit Care Med 2000;161:694–699.

Asthma Triggers: What Really Matters?

Patrick H. Win and Iftikhar Hussain

- Clinicians must take time to carefully identify potential asthma triggers at the time of initial evaluation and at each follow-up visit to minimize unnecessary morbidity from asthma.

- Just as asthma phenotypes vary among patients, so too do their specific triggers. Thus, care must be individualized and reviewed regularly as triggers can change over time. New-onset, uncontrolled asthma may be a sign of a new asthma trigger previously not identified.

- After asthma triggers are identified and confirmed with testing (if necessary), every effort should be made to avoid or eliminate these specific triggers of asthma symptoms (with the exception of exercise).

- Opportunities to minimize infectious triggers must always be taken. This should include influenza and pneumococcal vaccinations.

In the preceding chapters, authors have discussed the various important aspects of the clinical asthma assessment. As is the case with assessing level of control, severity, and inflammation, identifying triggers for asthma is an integral part of the initial evaluation of newly diagnosed asthmatic individuals. Furthermore, reviewing potential asthma triggers at each follow-up visit helps educate asthma patients. This education is a preventative first step in identifying and modifying risk factors that are responsible for poor quality of life, unnecessary morbidity, and mortality. In this, the final chapter of Section III, we will review our current concepts of asthma triggers and their role in the assessment and management of asthma. We hope to organize the classification of asthma triggers, and provide quick reference tables to simplify the initial assessment and follow-up management of asthmatics. By the end of this chapter, you will be "armed" with the information to rapidly assess, educate, and intervene upon the asthma triggers that really matter.

What is an asthma trigger? Asthma triggers are any condition or stimuli that cause inflammation or hyperresponsiveness of the airways that result in the symptoms of asthma: wheezing, shortness of breath, chest tightness, and/or coughing. Given the heterogeneity of asthma phenotypes, it is important to understand that triggers will vary among patients. So focusing on the relevant triggers for each patient is of utmost importance. While some asthmatic individuals are atopic, others are not. Accordingly, while allergen avoidance may vastly help the so-called "extrinsic" asthmatic individual by preventing morbidity and exacerbations, exposure to aeroallergens may

not be detrimental to the nonatopic, "intrinsic" asthmatic individual (Box 17-1). Furthermore, even within the group of atopic asthmatic individuals, some will be sensitized to seasonal allergens (trees, grasses, or weeds), while others will be triggered by perennial allergens (cat, dog, or dust mites). Given we have little, precious time at every patient encounter, it is imperative that we have a systematic approach to assessing and intervening upon asthma triggers targeted to the individual patient (Box 17-2). Accordingly, asthma triggers can be conveniently placed into groups by etiology: allergens, irritants, medications, weather changes, infections, emotions, gastroesophageal reflux, foods, and exercise (Table 17-1).

In genetically predisposed individuals, allergen exposure may lead to sensitization resulting in the formation of allergen-specific immunoglobulin E (IgE) by B lymphocytes. This process of allergen sensitization is uncommon within the first year of life, as formation of IgE to specific aeroallergens does not commonly occur before the age of 2 to 3. In these individuals, the combination of allergen sensitization to common aeroallergens (Table 17-2) and reexposure to these allergens can trigger symptoms of asthma. Subsequent allergen exposure through the respiratory tract results in T_H2-type lymphocyte recruitment, mast cell activation through IgE, and

BOX 17-1 Definitions

Aeroallergen: Any airborne substance that can result in an IgE-mediated allergic response. Typically these include tree, grass, and weed pollen; mold spores; and perennial allergens like cat and dog dander, dust mite, and cockroach.

Asthma trigger: Any condition or stimuli that cause inflammation or hyperresponsiveness of the airways that results in wheezing, shortness of breath, chest tightness, and/or coughing.

Atopy: The genetic predisposition to develop any of the classic allergic diseases (atopic dermatitis, allergic rhinitis, and asthma). Atopy involves the capacity to produce specific-IgE in response to common environmental allergens such as house-dust mites, foods, and tree and grass pollen.

Irritant: Any substance, chemical, or physical factor that triggers asthma symptoms by nonspecific mechanisms resulting in increased bronchial hyperreactivity. Examples include smoke and cold air.

Samter's Triad: A medical condition consisting of asthma, aspirin sensitivity, and nasal polyposis. This triad is typically identified in patients in their 20s and 30s and may not include other atopic diseases. It is also commonly known as aspirin-sensitive asthma, aspirin triad, and aspirin-induced asthma and rhinitis (AIAR).

BOX 17-2 Assessment

1. Review the patient's history of asthma and past episodes of exacerbation, with care taken to identify potential asthma triggers
2. Confirm potential allergic triggers
   a. Epicutaneous skin testing
   b. Intradermal skin testing
   c. Radioallergosorbent testing (in vitro)
3. Review patient's environment
4. Review patient's exposures
5. Review comorbid conditions
6. Review medications

Table 17-1
COMMON ASTHMA TRIGGERS

Allergens (seasonal and perennial aeroallergens)

Nonallergic irritants (smoke, strong odors from chemicals, air pollutants, occupational exposures [Chapter 42])

Medications (beta-blockers, nonsteroidal anti-inflammatory drugs)

Weather changes (changes in temperature and humidity)

Infections (sinusitis or viral infections)

Emotions (laughing, crying)

Reflux

Food (food allergy and food additives)

Exercise

Table 17-2
AEROALLERGENS THAT TRIGGER ASTHMA

Seasonal
Pollens
1. Trees (ash, birch, maple, oak, walnut, others)
2. Grasses (timothy, Kentucky blue grass, Bermuda, others)
3. Weeds (ragweed, pigweed, cocklebur, lamb's quarters, others)

Perennial
House-dust mite (*Dermatophagoides pteronyssinus* and *Dermatophagoides farinae*)
Animal (cat, dog, guinea pig, horse, hamster, mouse, others)
Cockroach (*Blattella germanica, Periplaneta americana, Blattella orientalis*)

Seasonal and Perennial
Molds (Alternaria, Aspergillus, Cladosporium, others)

whole pollen grains are quite large, plants can extrude allergen-containing particles that are less than 10 μm in size through the pores in their outer covering. This relatively small size likely facilitates entry into the lower airways, and results in the aforementioned allergic cascade with subsequent inflammation. The presence and time of release of these airborne allergens vary according to location and climate. Generally speaking, tree pollen is released first, in the springtime; grasses come later in the spring and early summer; and weed pollen arrives in late summer and early fall lasting until the first frost. Accordingly, pollen-allergic patients can have significant asthma exacerbations during their specific pollen season or seasons. Exposure to seasonal pollens is classically

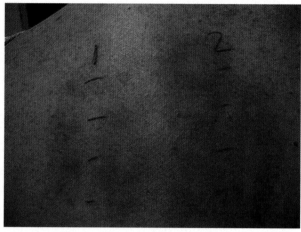

Figure 17-1 Epicutaneous skin testing (using an 8-headed multitest device) in a middle-aged asthmatic individual revealed sensitivities to multiple trees (labeled "1") and grasses (labeled "2"). Notice the negative saline control in the right-upper corner of panel 2 and the negative reaction to red maple in the left-lower position of panel 1. (*Courtesy of Patrick H. Win, MD.*)

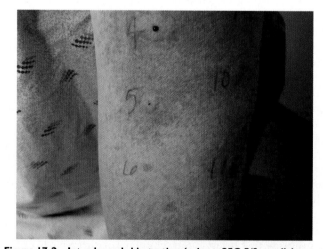

Figure 17-2 Intradermal skin testing (using a 25G 5/8 needle) to weeds on a young asthmatic male who reported itchy, watery eyes, nasal congestion, and worsening shortness of breath and wheeze in the fall. After epicutaneous skin testing revealed only minimal sensitivities to trees and grasses, intradermal skin testing (more sensitive) revealed strong cutaneous reactions to multiple weeds. With the patient's history of worsening symptoms in the fall, this testing provided a better explanation for his worsening seasonal symptoms. Although the patient displayed multiple positive intradermal tests, he was clearly not allergic to lamb's quarters (labeled "6"). (*Courtesy of Patrick H. Win, MD.*)

eosinophil influx. The ensuing inflammation from this milieu of cells and cellular mediators is thought to be responsible for not only acute asthma exacerbations, but also chronic inflammation. Allergen sensitivity is commonly diagnosed by a combination of history and positive epicutaneous skin (Fig. 17-1) and/or intradermal testing (Fig. 17-2), and in some cases, in vitro testing such as allergen-specific radioallergosorbent testing or newer technologies. After the diagnosis is made, health care providers should strive to identify the allergic triggers of asthma, treat comorbid underlying disease (e.g., rhinitis) with appropriate medications, and implement environmental controls to eliminate or minimize exposure to these factors.

Seasonal allergens from trees, grasses, and weeds are predominantly derived from air/wind-borne pollen. Even though considered an outdoor exposure, with peak outdoor pollen concentrations occurring in the morning. Unfortunately, during the grass pollen season, pollen can be found indoors at high levels in bedding, furniture, and carpeting. This is facilitated by leaving home windows open and using window and attic fans to cool the inside environment.

To minimize morbidity, asthma patients should be educated about their specific pollen sensitivities and corresponding "high-risk" seasons, as avoidance is the best way for patients to reduce risk of asthma flare. Decreasing exposure and, in turn, asthma exacerbations can be facilitated by remaining indoors, closing windows, avoiding the use of cooling fans, and using car and home air-conditioning as much as possible. This is particularly important in the early morning, the time of peak airborne pollen concentration. Early morning outdoor exercise should be strictly avoided, as the combination of peak pollen counts and cardiovascular exercise with increased oxygen demand, increased respiratory rate, and larger tidal volumes can be a dangerous combination. Recognizing that complete avoidance is not always feasible, using locally available pollen counts to help inform patients of potential high-exposure days can be quite helpful in reducing allergen exposure.

Perennial allergens that trigger asthma include domesticated animals, house-dust mites, and cockroaches. Cat and dog exposures are among the most common causes of perennial asthma triggers; however, all warm-blooded feathered or furry animals, including hamsters, rabbits, guinea pigs, and birds can produce allergen. Exposure to these allergens, in turn, may induce IgE-mediated reactions and asthma exacerbations. Pet allergens are ubiquitous in our environment as 30% to 40% of American homes have pets, and even trace amounts of cat or dog allergen can be found in virtually any home (>90%, even in homes without cats or dogs). Acute symptoms may develop in cat- or dog-sensitive asthmatic patients within minutes after entering a home where these animals reside.

Cat allergen, mainly *Fel d* 1, is a 17-kDa heterodimer comprising two disulfide-linked peptide chains. *Fel d* 1 is produced in the sebaceous glands and is typically spread via contact with cat saliva, dander, and urine. Common allergens are present in all breeds of cat (including lions, tigers, and hairless cats), but males produce more allergen than females. Cat allergen can be very small (<3 to 4 μm), and the distribution in the household air at any time is highly variable. Cat allergen is also very light and sticky, so it becomes airborne easily and can accumulate on household furniture, carpeting, and walls. These unique characteristics allow it to remain suspended in the air for long periods and to be inhaled deeply into the lungs, possibly accounting for its greater potential to trigger asthma symptoms than other aeroallergens. The level of cat allergen that is required to induce asthma symptoms is not well defined, so strict avoidance and proper cleaning after an animal has been removed from the household are key to preventing morbidity. Cat allergen levels drop slowly after animal removal, so brief trials of cat avoidance are useless. In fact, it takes approximately 5 months for cat allergen to drop to levels similar to those found in homes without cats, and 4 to 6 months after the animal has been removed for asthma patients to achieve any improvement in symptoms. Unfortunately, the clothes of cat owners constitute the vehicle of passive transport of *Fel d* 1 to cat-free environments, so recontamination to some extent is unavoidable.

In contrast to cat allergen, where the major antigenic component has been identified, dog allergen appears to be more heterogeneous, containing many varied allergens (primarily *Can f* 1 and *Can f* 2). Contrary to popular belief, it is impossible to generalize certain dog breeds as either "nonallergenic" or "hypoallergenic." In fact, all dogs have common allergens, but there may be differences in an individual's response to a particular dog breed or possibly even an individual dog of a specific breed. Despite this, even though many patients claim that "My pet has never bothered me," patients are notoriously poor at perceiving asthma symptoms when they have chronic, continuous exposure to allergens to which they have become sensitized. This is likely due to, at least in part, their emotional attachment to their animal.

The best "treatment" for all animal allergies is strict avoidance, including removal of the animal that is triggering symptoms of asthma from the home. When animal removal is not possible, confining the pet to carpet-free areas, outside the bedroom, may be beneficial. These measures, combined with the use of a HEPA (high-efficiency particulate air) or electrostatic air filter may provide additional benefit in "light" allergen removal (e.g., cat and dog allergen). Weekly or biweekly washing of pets, by a family member or individual other than the asthmatic patient, may also help to decrease allergen exposure and symptoms. Interestingly, dog, but not cat, ownership during infancy has been shown to reduce the development of allergic sensitization, and absolute number of pets, and not the type of furred pet, might also reduce future risk.

The two species of house-dust mite, *Dermatophagoides pteronyssinus* and *Dermatophagoides farinae*, are the most important mite allergens in North America. House-dust mites are microscopic (approximately 0.3 mm long), sightless, eight-legged acarids that feed on sloughed human skin. The most allergenic parts of the house-dust mite are its body parts and fecal matter. One ounce of house dust can contain approximately 40,000 dust mites. Thus a bed, a common site of house dust mites, may contain approximately 2 million dust mites. In contrast to pet allergy, dust mite–sensitive asthmatic patients are rarely aware of symptoms immediately, even when levels of dust mite allergen in a home are high. Studies indicate that the critical level of house-dust mites that poses a risk factor for asthma ranges from 100 to 500 mites per gram of house dust (about 2 to 10 μg of *Der p* 1), while acutely ill mite-sensitive asthmatic patients usually reside in homes with more than 500 mites per gram of house dust (>10 μg of *Der p* 1).

House-dust mite levels vary with humidity, temperature, season, and type of home furnishings. The most important factor influencing growth of house-dust mites is humidity. Asthmatic patients who are mite-sensitive and live in environments with suitable sites for mite growth (e.g., wall-to-wall or bedroom carpeting and upholstered or overstuffed furniture) are at greater risk in more humid climates. House-dust mites optimally reproduce in bedding and carpeting where the relative humidity in the home is higher than 50%. Accordingly, improper setting of the central air humidifier (commonly part of a home's central heating and air-conditioning unit) may worsen asthma control; while dehumidifiers set to keep humidity levels lower than 50% may be beneficial in reducing asthma symptoms from house-dust mite exposure. Although using other environmental control measures to minimize dust mite exposure are generally endorsed by allergists as a preventative first step to reduce asthma flares, studies examining their use are conflicting and have provided much controversy. Some studies using relatively basic dust mite control measures have shown no effect on asthma symptoms or reduction in mite growth; whereas other studies that use methods of extensive cleaning and dust mite proofing (e.g., mattress and pillow covers) to minimize mite exposure have been associated with a reduction in asthmatic symptoms, medication use, and morbidity. Furthermore, some studies have shown that patients exposed to lower levels of house-dust mites not only have decreased asthma symptoms and medication use, but also have improvement in nonspecific bronchial hyperresponsiveness. Having said this, the Cochrane Library meta-analysis on house-dust mite control measures for asthma, including 49 trials that examined the use of physical, chemical, and combination methods to reduce house-dust mite exposure, showed no benefit/effect on frequently reported outcomes (AM peak flow, asthma symptom scores, and medication use). The reviewers mention that many of the trials included in this analysis were of poor quality, making their conclusions difficult to interpret. If environmental control measures are suggested, the bedroom is the most important room to target, as most of our day in the home (approximately 8 to 10 hours during the night for sleep) is spent there. Other areas of the home, such as the living or family room that contains overstuffed furniture or carpeting, must be considered as potential sites of significant house-dust mite exposure. Proposed environmental controls to be considered include replacing wall-to-wall carpeting with hardwood or vinyl flooring, encasing bedding in dust-mite impermeable material, frequent dusting (with mask or by an unaffected individual), replacing upholstered/overstuffed furniture with leather furniture, replacing fabric curtains with blinds, washing bedding weekly in hot water (60°C or 130°F), washing and high-heat drying or freezing of stuffed toys, reducing humidity to less than 50%, frequent vacuuming (with HEPA filter and double-thickness bags) by an individual not sensitive to dust mites (or with mask), and using acaricides and/or tannic acid to mitigate house-dust mite infestation.

Cockroach has also been identified as a major allergen capable of triggering asthma exacerbations. The ability of cockroach allergen to stimulate the formation of specific IgE antibodies has been demonstrated by end point skin test titration and radioallergosorbent testing. Furthermore, a causal relationship between bronchospasm and sensitivity to cockroach allergen has been proved in bronchial provocation studies. Positive skin tests to cockroach allergen are reportedly present in 20% to 53% of allergic patients and as high as 49% to 61% of asthmatic patients. Although there are about 50 species of cockroaches that live in the United States, only 3 have been shown to induce allergen-specific IgE: the American, German, and Asian/Oriental cockroaches. Cockroach allergen usually is found in kitchen cabinets and kitchen floor dust, as they usually hide out in cabinets and behind refrigerators. A study in urban asthmatic patients has shown that cockroach sensitivity may be as important a risk factor for inner-city asthmatic individuals as house-dust mite allergy. Because elimination of cockroach infestation requires aggressive, repeated extermination efforts with irritant chemicals (deltamethrin powder or cypermethrin), it is best performed by professional exterminators. Cockroach baits and gels (fipronil and hydramethylnon) can be purchased at local superstores. These are generally safer and relatively nontoxic to mammals (pets and children), but may not be as effective in cases of severe infestation. Other partially effective measures include restricting havens by caulking and sealing cracks in plaster work and flooring, controlling dampness, reducing the availability of food, and restricting access to the dwelling (sealing sources of entry around doors).

Molds and fungi are aeroallergens that can trigger significant asthma symptoms in both a seasonal and perennial fashion. Unlike pollens, molds have ill-defined seasonal peaks and nadirs for airborne mold spore levels. Only in the northernmost areas of the United States are there consistent seasonal increases in mold counts. In this region, mold counts increase starting in May or June and decrease by October or November, having peaked in July or August. In the South, airborne molds are present throughout the winter, with a peak in summer or early fall. Clinically, molds are divided into two groups: outdoor and indoor.

The two most common outdoor molds are *Alternaria* and *Cladosporium*. Other common outdoor molds include *Fusarium*, *Spondylocladium*, and *Helminthosporium*. These outdoor or field molds grow in soil, on plants, and in decaying vegetation such as cut grass or raked leaves. Mold levels are affected by temperature, wind, rainfall, and humidity. Rain or high humidity levels will lower mold spore counts temporarily, but afterwards, counts rise rapidly. Generally, a late summer–autumn peak is seen for common fungal spores.

Similar to the aforementioned avoidance measures for pollen-sensitive asthmatic individuals, asthma symptoms from exposure to mold spores may be minimized by staying indoors as much as possible (especially during peak spore concentrations) and keeping home and automobile windows closed. The importance of minimizing mold exposure in mold-sensitive asthmatic individuals cannot be overemphasized. It is clear, from the observation of "New Orleans asthma" and other recently described cases of mold-induced asthma, that inhalation of large quantities of mold spores can produce severe, life-threatening asthma exacerbations in mold-sensitive patients. Although it is unclear what etiological factors are responsible for these cases of severe mold-sensitive asthma flares, it is hypothesized that because mold spores are smaller than pollen, they are more likely to enter and inflame the lower airways.

The two most important indoor molds are *Aspergillus* and *Penicillium* (also known as mildew). The amount of indoor mold in any dwelling depends on several important factors: age and composition of the structure, type of heating and cooling system, and use of humidifiers. Dark and humid (often poorly ventilated) basements are ideal sites for mold growth. The next most common sites of mold growth are the bathroom and the kitchen. In tropical and subtropical climates, fungi may grow on the walls of the house as a result of water seepage and humidity. To avoid this, the walls can be tiled or cleaned as necessary. Home heating, cooling, and humidification systems are also potential sources of fungal growth, although air-conditioning generally reduces indoor humidity and hence discourages mold growth. Most fungal spores in an indoor environment are nonviable spores that will be found in house-dust reservoirs such as carpeting, bedding, and furniture. Implementing the same precautions used to reduce levels of dust mites is the best way to eliminate mold spores from the home. Levels of viable indoor mold spores can be reduced by removing or cleaning mold-laden objects. Levels may also be reduced by use of dehumidifiers (set humidity level < 50%) in the basement and air-conditioners in the bedroom or family room. Air-conditioners and dehumidifiers reduce humidity and filter large fungal spores, lowering the mold and yeast count indoors, although their benefit in reducing asthma symptoms is controversial. Home humidifiers should be used with caution and cleaned frequently because of the potential for mold and *Actinomyces* growth. Bathrooms and kitchens should be well ventilated. Electronic air filters also lower the level of mold spores within a dwelling. When the major source of molds within a home is a wet or damp cellar, the basement should be kept free of carpeting, immediately dried out after a rainstorm, and, whenever possible, protected with a drain tile and sump pump.

Nonallergenic indoor triggers (Table 17-3) of asthmatic symptoms are a heterogeneous group of irritants that affect bronchial hyperreactivity in a non-IgE–dependent fashion. As with all other asthma triggers, each should be identified and meticulously eliminated or avoided. Active and passive tobacco cigarette smoke, consisting of very small, light particles that remain airborne for long periods, is a high-risk trigger for all asthmatic individuals. Studies have demonstrated that children may be at increased risk of developing asthma and allergic sensitization when exposed to passive smoke. Other studies in children show worsening asthma symptom severity, higher medication requirements, more frequent emergency department visits, and increased airway responsiveness when exposed to passive maternal tobacco smoke. Active cigarette smoking not only has direct, deleterious effects on the lung parenchyma, it also reduces the efficacy of inhaled and systemic corticosteroids. Thus, smoking cessation must be a primary objective for the patient, friends, and family members of asthmatic patients. Other forms of smoke, such as that of wood-burning stoves, also have negative effects on the lower respiratory tract. Additional airborne irritants, fumes, and strong odors (e.g., chalk dust, talcum powder, paint fumes, insecticides, household cleaning sprays, polishes, cooking oil fumes, perfumes, and cosmetics) may initiate or exacerbate asthmatic symptoms in some patients. Other indoor pollutants include carbon monoxide, formaldehyde, nitric oxide,

nitrogen oxides, and bacterial endotoxin. In all of these cases, adequate ventilation plays a pivotal role in successful prevention of asthma symptoms, as air stagnation has been shown to be a surrogate marker for the accumulation of indoor pollutants. Other important preventative avoidance measures include household cleaning and proper maintenance of gas appliances.

Nonallergic outdoor irritants (see Table 17-3) that trigger asthma are also exceedingly common and important to identify and eliminate. Studies have implicated several outdoor pollutants as potential triggers of asthma symptoms. Air pollutants such as ozone, nitrogen oxides, acidic aerosols, and particulate matter can lead to asthma symptoms and frank exacerbations. Other important outdoor asthma triggers include exposure to vehicle traffic (especially diesel exhaust), which might exacerbate preexisting allergic conditions by enhancing airway responses to allergen, a potential compounding effect. On occasion, weather and atmospheric conditions create brief periods of intense air pollution in a defined geographic area. At these and other times and in areas of high outdoor pollution, patients with asthma should avoid unnecessary outdoor physical activity (especially exercise) and try to stay indoors in a clean environment. As with pollen and aeroallergens, air-conditioning and filters may be helpful in preventing unnecessary morbidity. When working outdoors in polluted areas is unavoidable, taking a preventative, short-acting inhaled bronchodilator beforehand may prevent acute asthma symptoms. If prolonged outdoor polluted conditions are likely to persist, it is a good idea to tell patients to leave the polluted area before mild symptoms spiral into an acute asthma flare.

Hundreds of substances have been identified as occupational irritants or allergens that can trigger asthma symptoms. One can access a fairly comprehensive list of potential occupational asthma triggers at http://asmanet.com. An overview of these triggers and occupational asthma is covered in Chapter 42. Levels of exposure above which sensitization occurs have been proposed for many chemicals, so primary prevention is possible with proper precautionary measures. However, once a patient has been sensitized, the level of exposure necessary to induce symptoms may be very low, and resulting exacerbations may become progressively severe on reexposure. Attempts to reduce occupational exposure have been successful, especially in the industrial setting, where potent sensitizers have been replaced by less allergenic or sensitizing substances. For example, primary prevention of latex allergy has been very successful. This has been accomplished by producing powder-free, lower allergen-content gloves. In cases where prevention is not possible, the early identification of occupational sensitizers and the removal of affected patients from these environments are critical to the successful management of occupational asthma.

Numerous medications (Table 17-4) have been implicated in triggering asthma symptoms. The most common offenders include nonsteroidal anti-inflammatory drugs (NSAIDs) and β-blockers. Approximately 5% to 10% of adult asthmatic patients will have an acute worsening of asthma symptoms after ingesting NSAIDs. Samters Triad or "the aspirin triad" can be identified in some adult asthmatic patients. The response to aspirin or other NSAIDs typically begins within

Table 17-3
NONALLERGIC IRRITANTS THAT TRIGGER ASTHMA

Indoor
Smoke (tobacco, wood-burning stove)
Strong odors (perfumes and cosmetics)
Particulates (chalk dust, talcum powder)
Fumes (household cleaning products, insecticides, paints, chemicals, cooking)
Outdoor
Smoke (wood/tree, refuse and chemical fires)
Exhaust (diesel fumes)
Other (ozone, chemicals)

Table 17-4
MEDICATIONS AND AGENTS THAT TRIGGER ASTHMA

ACE-inhibitors	Nebulized medications
Aldesleukin (IL-2)	(beclomethasone, pentamidine,
Amiodarone	propellants)
Beta-agonists (paradoxical)	Nonsteroidal anti-inflammatory
Beta-blockers (systemic	drugs
and ocular)	Nitrofurantoin
Dipyridamole	Propafenone
Ergots	Protamine
Hydrocortisone	Radio-contrast media
Illicit drugs (cocaine and heroin)	Vinblastine (+ mitomycin)

an hour of aspirin ingestion and may be associated with profound rhinorrhea, lacrimation, and, potentially, severe bronchospasm. Patients sensitive to aspirin usually are reactive to all other NSAIDs (e.g., ibuprofen, naproxen), and variations in the frequency and severity of adverse responses appear to depend on the potency of each drug within this class of compounds to inhibit the activity of the COX-1 enzyme. Sensitivity to NSAIDs is not IgE-mediated and involves the modulation of eicosanoid production. NSAIDs likely act by reducing the formation of prostaglandins that help maintain normal airway function while increasing the formation of asthma-provoking eicosanoids, including hydroxyeicosatetraenoic acids and cysteinyl leukotrienes. Thus, if aspirin-sensitive asthmatic individuals require treatment with an NSAID, the use of a selective COX-2 inhibitor is a viable treatment option, especially when combined with an inhibitor of leukotriene synthesis or leukotriene receptor antagonist. In addition, there is evidence that mast cell activation occurs, and its mediators can be detected in nasal secretions during an episode of aspirin-induced asthma. This syndrome should be of concern in any asthmatic patient with nasal polyposis, chronic sinusitis, and eosinophilia, although nasal polyposis and sinusitis may precede the onset of recognized NSAID-sensitivity by years. β-Blockers administered either orally or via eye drops (for hypertension or glaucoma, respectively) may exacerbate asthma symptoms via bronchospasm. As a general rule, these medications should be not be used by asthmatic individuals, as other classes of drugs may be used to successfully treat these underlying comorbidities. If β-blockers are used, close medical supervision is essential to prevent unnecessary morbidity. As is the case with all of the aforementioned asthma triggers, avoidance is the treatment of choice.

Weather and atmospheric changes also commonly trigger asthma symptoms. Classically, cold dry air can induce bronchoconstriction in asthmatic individuals. Atmospheric conditions that typically trigger asthma symptoms include changes in temperature and humidity, barometric pressure, or gusts of wind. Perhaps of greater importance than these changes are the effects these atmospheric changes have on seasonal and perennial allergens. For example, pollen and mold counts have seasonal patterns and release of these allergens is highly dependent upon "proper" environmental conditions to allow successful release and plant pollination/procreation. As aforementioned, it is well recognized that exposure to molds or pollens during a particular season can induce asthmatic attacks in sensitized (allergic) individuals, so any atmospheric change (seasonal change or sudden gust of wind) that increases exposure to these allergens is potentially detrimental to allergen-sensitized asthmatic individuals. Furthermore, with seasonal changes (particularly the fall and winter) also comes an increased exposure to viruses like rhinovirus and influenza that commonly precipitate asthma attacks.

Respiratory viral and bacterial infections (Table 17-5) are a major cause of morbidity and mortality in people with asthma. Respiratory viruses trigger acute exacerbation of asthma in children and adults. These infections frequently result in outpatient visits and hospitalizations. Additionally, these infections make asthmatic individuals more sensitive to other asthma triggers. Typical respiratory tract infections that cause airway inflammation and trigger asthma include the "common cold" and flu, bronchitis, ear infections, sinusitis, and pneumonia. Asthma attacks that occur in conjunction with an upper or lower respiratory tract infection may be more severe than exacerbations that occur without concomitant infection.

The most common respiratory viruses are the rhinovirus ("common cold" virus), respiratory syncytial virus (RSV), and certain influenza viruses. These viruses are present in most patients hospitalized with life-threatening asthma exacerbations and acute non–life-threatening asthma flares. Asthmatic individuals are not more susceptible to upper respiratory tract rhinovirus infections than healthy, nonasthmatic individuals, but they do suffer more severe consequences of lower respiratory tract infections. Recent epidemiologic studies suggest that viruses provoke asthma attacks by additive or synergistic interactions with allergens or irritants like air pollutants. An impaired antiviral immunity to rhinovirus may

Table 17-5
COMMON INFECTIONS THAT TRIGGER ASTHMA

*Viruses (**bold** is most common respiratory clinical presentation)*
Rhinovirus (1–100+ serotypes; causes "**common cold**," bronchitis and bronchiolitis)
Coronavirus (2299E and OC43 serotypes; causes "**common cold**")
Influenza (A, B, and C serotypes; causes "common cold," **pneumonia** and bronchitis)
Parainfluenza (1, 2, 3, and 4 serotypes; causes "common cold," **laryngotracheobronchitis**, and bronchiolitis)
Respiratory syncytial virus (A and B serotypes; causes "common cold," pneumonia, bronchitis, and **bronchiolitis**)
Adenovirus (1–4 serotypes; causes "common cold," **pneumonia**, bronchitis and bronchiolitis)
Metapneumovirus (**bronchiolitis**)
Bacteria
Streptococcus pneumoniae (sinusitis and pneumonia)
Haemophilus influenzae and *parainfluenzae* (sinusitis and pneumonia)
Moraxella catarrhalis (sinusitis and pneumonia)
Staphylococcus aureus (pneumonia)
Klebsiella pneumoniae (pneumonia)
Atypical (*Chlamydia pneumoniae* and *Mycoplasma pneumoniae* causing pneumonia)

lead to impaired viral clearance and, in turn, prolonged symptoms. Viral respiratory tract infections exacerbate asthma by recruiting T_H2-type cells into the lungs. Currently, we have no specific antiviral strategies for preventing the exacerbation of asthma by respiratory viral infection; however, clinical trials of potential antiviral agents are ongoing. Indirect prevention strategies focus on reducing overall airway inflammation to reduce the severity of the host response to respiratory viral infections.

Although many bacterial infections are known to cause asthma exacerbations in susceptible individuals, recent attention has been focused on lower respiratory tract infections with atypical bacteria. *Mycoplasma pneumoniae* and *Chlamydia pneumoniae* are thought to be common triggers of asthma. Whether these bacteria are the inciting agents for the onset of disease or acute exacerbations has yet to be definitively determined; however, there are also data supporting the notion that infection with atypical bacteria may be a contributing factor to difficult-to-treat asthma.

Strenuous physical exercise can also trigger asthma attacks. Exercise can cause asthma symptoms to flare, especially when asthma is not well controlled. Mouth breathing; exercising in cold, dry air; or prolonged, strenuous activities such as medium- to long-distance running can increase the likelihood of exercise-induced bronchospasm—an obstruction of transient airflow that usually occurs 5 to 15 minutes after the onset of physical exertion. Although exercise can trigger asthma in certain people, it is one trigger that should not be avoided. Exercise strengthens the cardiovascular system and may lessen the sensitivity to asthma triggers. To minimize the effects of this trigger, asthmatic individuals should start any new exercise regime slowly, gradually building strength and endurance, and warm up gradually at the beginning of each exercise session. Avoiding exercise outdoors in extremely cold weather or during peak pollen seasons is also a prudent measure.

Asthma and gastroesophageal reflux disease (GERD) are common medical conditions that often coexist. Studies have shown conflicting results on whether lower esophageal acidification can act as a trigger for asthma. In fact, asthma might precipitate GERD symptoms; thus, a temporal association between the two does not establish that GERD triggers asthma. Randomized trials investigating different treatment modalities for GERD in asthma have been conducted to determine whether treatment of GERD improves asthma symptoms and outcomes. A meta-analysis of randomized controlled trials concluded that therapy for GERD, including acid-suppressive treatment with a proton-pump or histamine-2 receptor antagonists, does not consistently improve lung function, asthma symptoms, nocturnal asthma, or lessen the use of asthma medications. Littner and colleagues showed that in adult patients with moderate-to-severe persistent asthma and symptoms of acid reflux, treatment with 30 mg of lansoprazole twice daily for 24 weeks did not improve asthma symptoms, pulmonary function, or reduce albuterol use. However, this dose significantly reduced asthma exacerbations and improved quality of life, particularly in those patients receiving more than one asthma-controller medication. With all of this being considered, untreated GERD

symptoms may affect airway reactivity in patients with asthma. Thus, treating patients for symptoms of GERD with concomitant asthma has become standard practice and should be considered.

Exposure to food allergens and additives (see Fig. 17-3) can cause a variety of symptoms. It is widely believed that allergic reactions to foods are common asthma triggers, but definitive evidence to support this concept is lacking. Despite this lack of data, some asthmatic individuals report worsening asthma symptoms after ingesting specific foods and food additives. Food additives that have been implicated include salicylates, food preservatives, monosodium glutamate, and some food-coloring agents. Sodium metabisulfite, a preservative in many beverages (including beer and wine) and foods, is thought to release sufficient sulfur dioxide to provoke bronchoconstriction. For some people, eating a particular food (common culprits include milk, eggs, peanuts, tree nuts, soy, wheat, fish, and shellfish) can trigger asthma symptoms. This constellation of food sensitivity and worsening asthma symptoms tends to correlate with a more severe course of disease. Patients with food allergies and underlying asthma experience more severe reactions to food allergens than do patients without asthma, because their reactions are more likely to involve life-threatening respiratory symptoms.

Allergic reactions that involve respiratory symptoms are almost always more severe than reactions that do not involve the

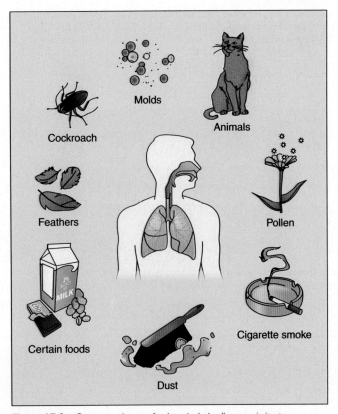

Figure 17-3 Common triggers of asthma include allergens, irritants, gastroesophageal reflux disease, medications, weather changes, viral and bacterial infections, emotion stressors, foods and food additives, and physical exercise.

respiratory tract. Particularly susceptible food-sensitive asthmatic individuals have been reported to react to merely inhalation without ingestion; however, isolated symptoms of rhinitis or asthma without concomitant cutaneous or gastrointestinal symptoms are rare. Nevertheless, if any type of food triggers an asthma attack, the best treatment is strict avoidance.

Although asthma is not a psychological condition, emotional or nervous stress can trigger asthma symptoms. Stress alone cannot provoke asthma; however, if accompanied by anxiety, stress can cause fatigue, potentiating coughing, shortness of breath, and wheezing. A strong feeling or emotional behavior, such as laughing or crying, may trigger asthma symptoms because of the accompanying change in breathing patterns. As with any other chronic health condition, proper rest, nutrition, and exercise are important to overall well-being and can help in managing asthma.

Effective control of asthma depends on identification and alleviation of exacerbating factors. Triggers of asthma frequently include ongoing exposure to allergens and irritants, medications, weather and atmospheric changes, upper and lower respiratory tract infections, uncontrolled gastroesophageal reflux disease, foods and food additives, and emotional stress and anxiety (Fig. 17-3). It is of paramount importance to recognize contributing factors early, and eliminate exposure to prevent unnecessary morbidity and mortality. A key theme to this chapter has been avoidance, which in many cases is quite difficult; but by following a systematic method for identifying and removing potential triggers from the asthmatic individual's environment, the goal of optimum asthma control can be accomplished with a combined, concerted effort on the part of the physician and patient.

SUGGESTED READING

Algorithm for the diagnosis and management of asthma: a practice parameter update. Ann Allergy Asthma Immunol 1998;81:415–420.

Attaining optimal asthma control: a practice parameter. J Allergy Clin Immunol 2005;116(5):S3–11.

Global Initiative for Asthma (GINA): Global strategy for asthma management and prevention (NIH Publication No. 02-3659). Bethesda, MD, National Institutes of Health, National Heart, Lung, and Blood Institute, 1995. Issued January, 1995 (updated 2002) Management Segment (Chapter 7): Updated 2005 from the 2004 document.

Gøtzsche PC, Johansen HK, Schmidt LM, et al: House dust mite control measures for asthma. Cochrane Database Syst Rev 2004;(4):CD001187.

Lemanske R, Busse W: Asthma: factors underlying inception, exacerbation, and disease progression. J Allergy Clin Immunol 2006;117:S456–461.

Littner M, Leung F, Ballard E, et al: Effects of 24 weeks of lansoprazole therapy on asthma symptoms, exacerbations, quality of life, and pulmonary function in adult asthmatic patients with acid reflux symptoms. Chest 2005;128(3):1128–1135.

Murray CS, Poletti G, Kebadze T, et al: Study of modifiable risk factors for asthma exacerbations: virus infection and allergen exposure increase the risk of asthma hospital admissions in children. Thorax 2006;61(5):376–82. [Epub 2005 Dec 29.]

Practice parameter for the diagnosis and management of asthma. J Allergy Clin Immunol 1995;96:S707–780.

MANAGEMENT

The Goals for Asthma Management: Short and Long Term

Ravi Aysola and Mario Castro

- The goal of asthma treatment is to minimize symptoms and exacerbations, minimize medication side effects, and optimize lung function.
- Patients' understanding of their disease and ability to recognize symptoms is fundamental to achieving control.
- Regular objective monitoring of pulmonary function is helpful to assess degree of airflow obstruction.
- Use of composite measures of asthma control is a useful and practical way of achieving patient and provider goals of asthma management.

Multiple expert panels including the National Asthma Education and Prevention Program (NAEPP)[1] and Global Initiative for Asthma (GINA)[2] have published goals of asthma management along with guidelines regarding assessment of asthma severity and suitable pharmacotherapy (see Chapter 19). A comprehensive approach starting with accurate diagnosis and assessment of asthma severity, followed by treatment with appropriate medications, is central to achieving the guideline-defined goals. This chapter is focused on clarifying the goals of asthma management, which can then be used as a starting point and reference framework for ongoing care of the patient with asthma.

The goal of asthma treatment is to minimize symptoms and exacerbations, minimize medication side effects, and optimize lung function (Tables 18-1 and 18-2). To achieve these goals, patients and providers need to have a coordinated approach toward assessing asthma control, severity, and defining goals of treatment along with a management plan to achieve those goals. Open communication between patients and providers is central to developing and maintaining an effective treatment regimen. Clinicians need to address patients' expectations and concerns regarding therapy, including potential side effects from medications, as well as the need for patient self-monitoring and regular follow-up.

IMPAIRMENT—PREVENT SYMPTOMS

Patients' understanding of their disease as well as their ability to recognize symptoms is fundamental to appropriate assessment of disease control and severity (Table 18-3). Appropriate assessment and monitoring of asthma includes monitoring the two domains—current impairment and future risk. *Impairment* refers to the frequency and intensity of symptoms and functional limitations the patient is experiencing or has recently experienced. Patients and their families need to be educated

regarding the symptoms of asthma and the different types of medications that are used for treatment. The appropriate use of long-term controller medications, such as inhaled corticosteroids (ICSs) and long-acting beta-agonists (LABAs), versus the use of short-term reliever medications, such as short-acting beta-agonists (SABAs), should be clearly explained. Patients and their families should also learn to identify factors that trigger asthma attacks and exacerbations. The first step toward achieving asthma control is accurately defining severity. Asthma *control* refers to the degree to which asthma manifestations (symptoms, functional impairments, risk of untoward events) are minimized, and the adequacy of treatment, while *severity* concerns the underlying intensity of the disease process.

Patients often underestimate disease severity and overestimate control. The Asthma in America survey[3] found that over

Table 18-1
SHORT-TERM VERSUS LONG-TERM MEASURES OF ASTHMA CONTROL

Short-term Measures	Long-term Measures
Symptoms (daytime/nocturnal)	Exacerbations/need for oral corticosteroids
Beta-agonist use	Missed school/work
Lung function (PEF, FEV_1, PC_{20})	Longitudinal lung function
Airway inflammation (sputum, exhaled breath condensate, nitric oxide)	Hospitalizations/Emergency Department visits
Composite measures (questionnaires)	Health care costs
	Quality of life
	Airway remodeling
	Mortality

Table 18-2
GOAL OF ASTHMA THERAPY: ACHIEVE CONTROL

Reduce Impairment
Prevent chronic and troublesome symptoms
Require infrequent use of inhaled SABAs (≤2 days/week)
Maintain (near) "normal" pulmonary function
Maintain normal activity levels
Meet patients' expectations of, and satisfaction with, asthma care
Reduce Risk
Prevent recurrent exacerbations
Minimize need for emergency department visits or hospitalizations
Prevent progressive loss of lung function
Provide optimal pharmacotherapy, with minimal or no adverse effects

NAEPP, National Asthma Education and Prevention Program; SABAs, short-acting beta₂-agonists. Available at http://www.nhlbi.nih.gov/guidelines/asthma/epr3/resource.pdf.

Table 18-3
THE NATIONAL ASTHMA EDUCATION AND PREVENTION PROGRAM RECOMMENDS MONITORING SIX AREAS WHEN ASSESSING ASTHMA CONTROL

Signs and symptoms of asthma
Pulmonary function including spirometry and PEF
Quality of life and functional status
Medications (adherence and potential side effects from medication)
Exacerbations and hospitalizations
Patient-provider communication and patient satisfaction
Monitoring asthma control with biomarkers (requires further evaluation)

a 4-week period, 61% of patients in the survey whose level of symptoms classified them as having moderate persistent asthma actually considered their asthma to be "well controlled" or "completely controlled." Additionally, over the 4-week study period, 32% of patients who had symptomatic severe persistent asthma actually considered their asthma to be "well controlled" or "completely controlled." This finding is not unique to the U.S. population as demonstrated in the AIR survey, a worldwide extension of the initial Asthma in America survey that involved 11,000 patients in 29 countries. The authors again found significant disparity between patients' reported symptoms and their perception of asthma control. Specifically, 32% to 49% of patients reporting severe symptoms and 39% to 70% reporting moderate symptoms categorized their current level of asthma control to be "well" or "complete." The discrepancy between self-reported symptoms and self-assessment of asthma control may reflect patients' inability to recognize symptoms, tolerance of symptoms, or limited expectations regarding the benefits of treatment (Fig. 18-1).

To obtain a complete picture of asthma severity and control, providers need to monitor six areas of patients' asthma symptoms, lung function, quality of life, medication use and side effects from medications, exacerbations and healthcare utilization, and patient-provider communication and satisfaction (see Table 18-3). Provider assessments of asthma status should focus on specific questions regarding symptoms of coughing, wheezing, shortness of breath, and chest tightness, particularly the presence of these symptoms at night. Patient records of self-monitoring, including symptom diaries and peak expiratory flow (PEF) records, should be reviewed periodically. A seventh area, monitoring asthma control with minimally invasive biomarkers, such as exhaled nitric oxide or sputum eosinophils, is of interest but requires further evaluation before they can be recommended for routine asthma care (see Chapter 11).

RISK—PREVENT EXACERBATIONS

Risk refers to the likelihood of asthma exacerbations, progressive decline in lung function, or risk of adverse effects from medications. Specific questions regarding increased use of SABAs and need for systemic corticosteroids, as well as unscheduled urgent care or emergency department visits, help the clinician assess disease activity. The frequency, duration and severity of exacerbations should be detailed along with documentation of precipitating factors and the type of treatments instituted, especially the need for hospitalization, intensive care unit (ICU) admission, and/or intubation.

Inappropriate assessment of asthma severity hampers care. Several studies have found limited use of long-term controller medications, specifically ICS, when they were indicated, and excessive use of SABAs. Adams and associates,[4] in a U.S. national population survey based on self-reported information, found that only one fourth to one third of persons

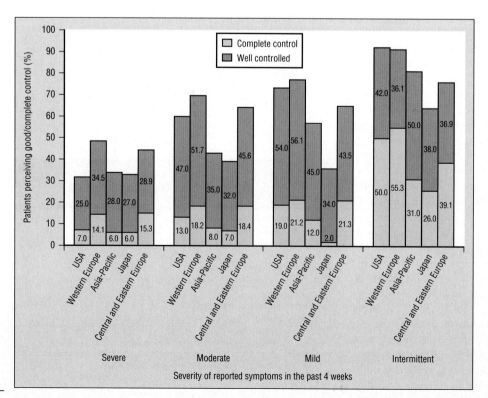

Figure 18-1 AIR survey of self-reported symptoms and self-assessment of asthma control. The discrepancy between self-reported symptoms and self-assessment of asthma control may reflect patients' inability to recognize symptoms, tolerance of symptoms, or limited expectations regarding the benefits of treatment. *(Data from Asthma in America: a landmark survey. Executive summary. Research Triangle Park, NC: Glaxo Wellcome, 1998.)*

who, according to NAEPP guidelines, should be using anti-inflammatory medications reported using them. In patients who described severe limitations due to asthma, only 26% reported using an anti-inflammatory medication, usually an ICS, and nearly 80% reported current use of a reliever medication (SABA) (Fig. 18-2).

In the United States and worldwide, management of asthma clearly falls short of guideline-defined practices. In an international multicenter survey study involving nearly 11,000 patients in 29 countries (AIR survey), Rabe and co-workers[5] found that asthma significantly limited the normal activities of patients, ranging from 17% in Japan to 68% across Central and Eastern Europe. The study also found that the majority of patients reported frequent use of quick-relief SABA, but limited use of preventive medicines such as ICS. This was noted among patients with varying degrees of asthma severity. These results have led many clinicians to question whether the expert-defined goals are realistic and achievable in general practice and were the impetus behind the Gaining Optimal Asthma Control (GOAL)[6] study.

The GOAL study evaluated whether a systematic approach to assessing and treating asthma could be effective in achieving the guideline-defined asthma control set forth by the expert panels (GINA, NAEPP). The 1-year, stratified, randomized, double-blind, parallel-group study compared the efficacy and safety of individual, predefined, stepwise increases of salmeterol/fluticasone propionate with fluticasone propionate alone in achieving two predefined composite measures of asthma control. The definitions of control were derived from the GINA/NAEPP guidelines and classified as "totally controlled," "well controlled," or "uncontrolled." The composite measures included the following equally weighted asthma outcomes:

- Peak expiratory flow (PEF)
- Rescue medication use
- Symptoms
- Nighttime awakenings
- Exacerbations
- Emergency visits
- Adverse events

After defining the severity of asthma and degree of control, patients were managed according to the GINA guidelines. Asthma control was initially assessed over an 8-week period. Uncontrolled patients were stratified according to the current dose of ICS being used. A subsequent "step-up" phase involved titration of salmeterol/fluticasone propionate (LABA/ICS) or fluticasone propionate (ICS) alone until total control was achieved or the highest dose of study drug was reached.

For all strata, the proportion of patients who achieved "totally controlled" or "well controlled" asthma at the end of phase 1 was greater in the LABA/ICS group compared with the ICS alone group. Control was also achieved significantly faster with the use of LABA/ICS versus ICS alone (Fig. 18-3). The GOAL study demonstrated that in most patients with uncontrolled asthma across a wide range of severities, comprehensive guideline-defined control can be achieved and maintained. Patients who achieved control recorded very low rates of exacerbation and near-maximal health status scores. Even patients who did not attain control as per the study definitions showed

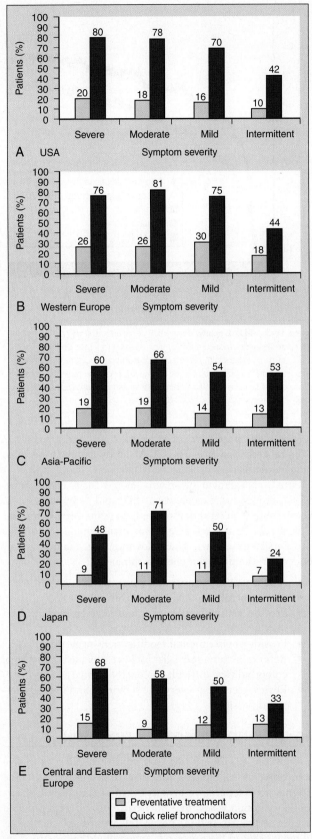

Figure 18-2 AIR survey of corticosteroid (ICS) and short-acting beta-agonist (SABA) use. In patients who described severe limitations due to asthma, only 26% reported using an anti-inflammatory medication, usually an ICS, and nearly 80% reported current use of a reliever medication (SABA). *(Data from Asthma in America: A landmark survey. Executive summary. Research Triangle Park, NC, Glaxo Wellcome, 1998.)*

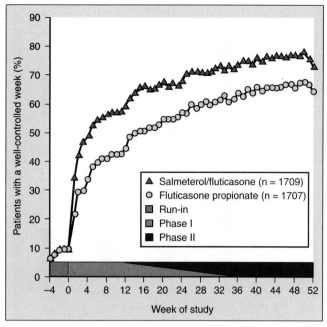

Figure 18-3   GOAL study. Proportion of patients achieving a well-controlled week (noncumulative) over weeks 4 to 52 for all strata combined on treatment with salmeterol/fluticasone or fluticasone propionate. *(Data from Bateman ED, Boushey HA, Bousquet J, et al: Can guideline-defined asthma control be achieved? The Gaining Optimal Asthma ControL Study. Am J Respir Crit Care Med 2004;170:836–844.)*

a considerable improvement in health status and a reduction in the exacerbation rate. The GOAL study demonstrated that guideline-defined control can be achieved.

Initial management of asthma should focus on minimizing symptoms and exacerbations by rapid "stepping-up" of therapy with inhaled and, if needed, systemic corticosteroids. ICSs should be the cornerstone of management in patients with persistent asthma. The following steps summarize key concepts in the management of asthma:

- Assess asthma severity and control first
- Gain control as quickly as possible
- Provide asthma action plan and written management plan
- Provide environmental modification suggestions
- Refer to asthma specialist for severe persistent asthma, comorbidities, difficult-to-control asthma
- Review treatment every 1 to 6 months and reduce therapy if possible

MONITORING PULMONARY FUNCTION

In addition to monitoring symptoms, regular objective monitoring of pulmonary function is necessary, as some patients do not perceive symptoms until the degree of airflow obstruction is severe. Older patients and patients who have experienced severe, near-fatal asthma exacerbations are more likely to have poor perception of airflow obstruction. PEF monitoring with a PEF meter can be a valuable tool in assessing airflow obstruction and can be performed by patients. Patients should be educated on how to appropriately use a peak flow meter and review the technique periodically with their provider to ensure reliable measurements. Patients with moderate to severe asthma and those

with poor perception of disease severity benefit most from regular PEF monitoring. Formal spirometry including measurement of FEV_1 should also be performed at least yearly to assess airflow obstruction and to check the accuracy of recorded PEF. The measurement of PEF should not be used as a substitute for formal spirometry in the initial diagnosis of asthma.

Although there are standardized values for PEF based on age, height, and gender, significant ethnic and racial variations do exist. As a result, patients monitoring their PEF should establish a personal best as a basis for comparison. PEF values less than 80% of a patient's personal best should alert the patient to the need for more frequent monitoring. Guidance regarding the frequency and timing of PEF measurements, as well as instructions regarding medication changes (e.g., starting oral corticosteroids) and notifying providers should be given to patients in the form of a written asthma action plan (see Chapter 51).

COMPOSITE MEASURES OF SYMPTOMS, QUALITY OF LIFE, AND FUNCTIONAL STATUS

The effects of asthma symptoms on an individual's daily activities can help give a more complete picture of overall asthma control. Several questionnaires and comprehensive surveys have been developed to assess the impact of asthma symptoms on a patient's quality of life. The Asthma Symptom Score developed by Castro and colleagues[7] is a questionnaire that patients use to rate each of four symptoms: cough, wheezing, shortness of breath, and nocturnal asthma symptoms. The baseline Asthma Symptom Score was inversely related to the time to exacerbation and was predictive of an asthma exacerbation following ICS withdrawal. The Asthma Symptom Utility Index (ASUI)[8] is a symptom assessment scale developed to measure preference-based outcomes in clinical trials. It is an 11-item index designed to summarize the frequency and severity of five selected asthma-related symptoms and side-effects. The ASUI correlated with FEV_1 (forced expiratory volume in 1 second) percent predicted and FEV_1/FVC (forced vital capacity). The index may also be capable of differentiating patient groups based on asthma severity. The ASUI scores also correlated well with the well-validated Asthma Quality of Life Questionnaire (AQLQ). In addition, the Asthma Control Test (ACT) is a short, simple, patient-based tool that is available for monitoring asthma control (www.asthmacontrol.com). The ACT demonstrates responsiveness to changes in asthma control and lung function. A cutoff score of 19 or less identifies patients with poorly controlled asthma.[9] Last, the Asthma Control Questionnaire (ACQ) is a seven-item questionnaire that has been validated to measure the goals of asthma management. Six of the questions can be self-administered and the Seventh question is FEV_1 percent predicted measured from spirometry. The ACQ is responsive to changes in asthma control. A cutoff value of greater than or equal to 1.5 identifies a patient not well controlled.[10]

Although helpful, many of the quality-of-life surveys are not practical for use in everyday clinical practice, as they are time consuming and need to be administered by a provider. However, providers should focus on key areas when assessing quality of life, including:

- Missed school or work due to asthma
- Reduction in usual activities (including exercise, sports, recreation) due to asthma
- Nocturnal symptoms and disruption of sleep due to asthma

The use of composite measures of asthma control is a useful and practical way of achieving patient and provider goals of asthma management.

MONITORING PATIENT SATISFACTION

The successful management of asthma in the long term depends on maintaining communication between patient and provider, close monitoring of disease activity both by patient and provider, and periodic objective evaluation of asthma control and lung function. Open communication between provider and patient is essential to the effective care and successful self-management of asthma. Patients who understand their disease and the treatments for it are more likely to be adherent to their medical regimen. Patients should be questioned regarding their satisfaction with asthma control and with the quality of their care. Discussions about the expectations of treatment, goals of therapy, and whether those goals are being met should be a part of regular visits.

Once asthma is controlled, defined by using a composite measure that includes subjective and objective patient values as well as objective measures of lung function, therapy should be gradually scaled back. Addition of LABAs or anti-IgE (immunoglobulin E) therapy should be considered in patients not controlled with ICSs alone and to minimize side effects. As demonstrated by the GOAL study, the combination of ICSs and LABAs may allow for reduction in the dose of ICSs and more rapid disease control; however, LABAs should not be used as a substitute for ICS. Leukotriene antagonists (LTAs) may be of value as add-on therapy to SABAs in patients with mild disease and potentially in patients with exercise-induced asthma.

In addition to minimizing symptoms and exacerbations as well as optimizing functional status, long-term goals of managing asthma include minimizing airway inflammation and maintaining normal or near normal lung function. Novel, noninvasive techniques for monitoring airway inflammation are available currently, but are still in early phases of development and standardization. Promising techniques include measuring exhaled NO and exhaled breath condensate, which may complement methods like monitoring sputum eosinophil counts and current physiologic and radiographic assessments. Ultimately, the ability to monitor asthmatic individuals and predict and prevent exacerbations is the goal. Detecting subclinical airway inflammation and effectively treating it may prevent subsequent exacerbations.

Overall, the combination of providing appropriate education; monitoring patient symptoms, lung function, and airway inflammation; preventing exacerbations; and minimizing side effects from therapy will lead to improved long-term asthma management. Addressing these patient- and provider-centered goals of asthma management will lead to greater satisfaction with the care provided and improved outcomes.

REFERENCES

1. National Asthma Education and Prevention Program: Full Report of the Expert Panel: Guidelines for the Diagnosis and Management of Asthma (EPR-3). Bethesda, MD, National Heart, Lung and Blood Institute, 2007.
2. Global Initiative for Asthma (GINA): Global strategy for asthma management and prevention: NHLBI/WHO Workshop Report (Publication No. 02-3659). Bethesda, MD, National Institutes of Health, National Heart, Lung and Blood Institute, 2002 (revised in 2006).
3. Asthma in America: a landmark survey. Executive summary. Research Triangle Park, NC, Glaxo Wellcome, 1998.
4. Adams RJ, Fuhlbrigge A, Guilbert T, et al: Inadequate use of asthma medication in the United States: Results of the Asthma in America national population survey. J Allergy Clin Immunol 2002;110:58–64.
5. Rabe KF, Adachi M, Lai CKW, et al: Worldwide severity and control of asthma in children and adults: The global asthma insights and reality surveys. J Allergy Clin Immunol 2004;114(1):40–47.
6. Bateman ED, Boushey HA, Bousquet J, et al: Can guideline-defined asthma control be achieved? The Gaining Optimal Asthma Control Study. Am J Respir Crit Care Med 2004;170:836–844.
7. Castro M, Bloch SR, Jenkerson MV, et al: Asthma exacerbations after glucocorticoid withdrawal reflect T cell recruitment to the airway. Am J Respir Crit Care Med 2004;169:842–849.
8. Revicki D, Leidy N, Brennan-Diemer F, et al: Integrating patient preferences into health outcomes assessment. The multiattribute asthma symptom utility index. Chest 1998;114:998–1007.
9. Schatz M, Sorkness CA, Li JT, et al: Asthma control test: Reliability, validity, and responsiveness in patients not previously followed by asthma specialists. J Allerg Clin Immunol 2006;117:549–556.
10. Juniper EF, Bousquet J, Abetz L, Bateman ED: Identifying "well-controlled" and "not well-controlled" asthma using the Asthma Control Questionnaire. Respir Med 2006;100:616–621.

The "Asthma Guidelines": What Do the Experts Teach Us?

Sujani Kakumanu and William W. Busse

It is estimated that 300 million people suffer from asthma worldwide with the burden of asthma affecting morbidity, mortality, and cost, both in terms of health care and loss of productivity. Furthermore, global analyses have continued to show that the mortality rate for asthma in the United States has remained stable, despite advances in asthma treatment. To improve asthma diagnosis and management nationwide, the first National Asthma Education and Prevention Program (NAEPP) expert panel convened in 1989 to address asthma as a national public health problem and to translate scientific evidence into standardized clinical practice. By constructing the guidelines, the NAEPP provides recommendations based on the best scientific evidence available, supplementing with expert consensus opinion for areas where sufficient data were unavailable. These efforts were extended globally with the Global Initiative for Asthma (GINA), which further recognized that asthma management must be tailored to the particular needs and resources of individual communities. The goal of both the NAEPP and GINA guidelines is to provide a general evidence-based approach to managing asthma that is comprehensive, specific, and flexible to individual patient and community needs.

The strength of clinical guidelines is their foundation in scientific evidence. Appropriately, recent revisions of both the NAEPP (2007) and the GINA guidelines (2006) have categorized the evidence used to justify recommendations based on study design, methods, study characteristics, and outcomes measured (Table 19-1). Evidence in category A is assigned to randomized, controlled trials that showed a consistent pattern of findings to the population for which the recommendation is made. Category B evidence is from end points of intervention studies that include only a limited number of patients, or post hoc or subgroup analysis. Category C evidence is from outcomes of uncontrolled or nonrandomized trials or observational studies. Category D evidence is constructed from a panel consensus opinion and is based on clinical experience and expert opinion. Category D evidence is reserved for situations in which scientific data are lacking or incomplete. By critically evaluating the evidence and the manner in which the data were obtained, the guidelines continue to emphasize the translation of sound scientific research into medical practice. These recommendations are then categorized into asthma domains pertaining to the pathophysiology of asthma, measures of assessment and monitoring, control of risk factors that exacerbate asthma, pharmacologic therapy, and education.

DEFINITION AND PATHOPHYSIOLOGY

A definition of asthma as a chronic inflammatory disorder with variable degrees of airflow obstruction was developed by the NAEPP at its inception in 1989 and reinforced in subsequent revisions, most recently in 2007. Several factors contribute to this airway obstruction including airway smooth muscle spasm, mucosal edema, mucus hypersecretion, inflammation, and, in susceptible patients, airway remodeling. Many cells are involved in this disease process, including mast cells, eosinophils, neutrophils, epithelial cells, and T lymphocytes with a particular involvement of the Th2 subpopulation. These Th2 lymphocytes release proinflammatory cytokines such as interleukin (IL)-4, IL-5, and IL-13, and chemokines, such as RANTES and eotaxin, that contribute to further inflammatory cell recruitment and airway hyperresponsiveness. Furthermore, the release of other inflammatory mediators such as histamine, cysteinyl leukotrienes, prostaglandin D2, and platelet-activating factor promote bronchospasm and airway edema. In allergic individuals, this inflammation can be provoked by exposure to inhaled antigen (Fig. 19-1). This inflammatory cascade manifests clinically as recurrent episodes of wheezing, shortness of breath, and cough. Variability in the severity and chronicity of disease in individual asthmatic patients most likely stems from varying degrees of airway inflammation. In addition, recent studies have suggested that in certain patients, the disease process changes to involve structural changes within the airway such as collagen deposition and airway smooth muscle hypertrophy, as well as mucus gland and goblet cell hyperplasia (Fig. 19-2). This transition has been termed airway remodeling and is characterized

Table 19-1
DESCRIPTION OF LEVELS OF EVIDENCE USED IN CONSTRUCTING THE NHLBI ASTHMA GUIDELINES

Evidence Category	Sources of Evidence	Definition
A	Randomized controlled trials (RCTs). Rich body of data.	Evidence is from end points of well designed RCTs that provide a consistent pattern of findings in the population for which the recommendation is made. Category A requires substantial numbers of studies involving substantial numbers of participants.
B	Randomized controlled trials (RCTs). Limited body of data.	Evidence is from end points of intervention studies that include only a limited number of patients, post hoc or subgroup analysis of RCTs, or meta-analysis of RCTs. In general, Category B pertains when few randomized trials exist, they are small in size, they were undertaken in a population that differs from the target population of the recommendation, or the results are somewhat inconsistent.
C	Nonrandomized trials. Observational studies.	Evidence is from outcomes of uncontrolled or nonrandomized trials or from observational studies.
D	Panel consensus judgment.	This category is used only in cases where the provision of some guidance was deemed valuable but the clinical literature addressing the subject was insufficient to justify placement in one of the other categories. The panel consensus is based on clinical experience or knowledge that does not meet the above-listed criteria.

From Global Initiative for Asthma (GINA): Global Strategy for Asthma Management and Prevention: NHLBI/WHO Workshop Report (Publication No. 02-3659). Bethesda, MD, National Institutes of Health, National Heart, Lung and Blood Institute, 2002 (Revised in 2006).

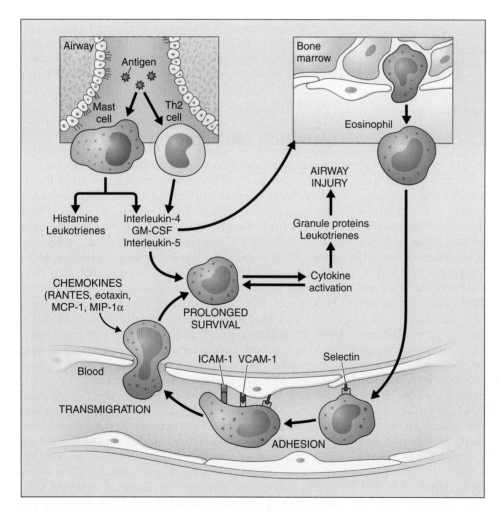

Figure 19-1   Antigen in a sensitized asthma patient interacts with mast cell bound IgE resulting in the release of histamine, cysteinyl leukotrienes, cytokines and chemokines. *(Adapted from Busse WW, Lemanske RF: Asthma. N Engl J Med 2001;344:350–362.)*

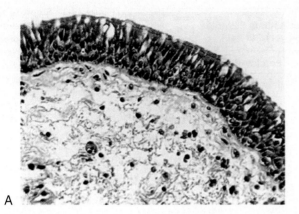
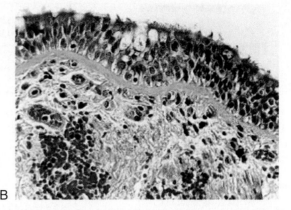

Figure 19-2 Specimen A shows bronchial mucosa from a subject without asthma as compared with specimen B, which is obtained from a patient with mild asthma. The patient with mild asthma shows goblet cell hyperplasia within the epithelial cell lining and a thickened sub basement membrane with collagen deposition and increased cellular infiltrate as compared to specimen A (hematoxylin and eosin stain x 40). *(From Busse WW, Lemanske RF: Asthma. N Engl J Med 2001;344:350–362.)*

by irreversible airflow obstruction as well as decreased responsiveness to glucocorticoid therapy. Recognizing the persistence of airway limitation and the heterogeneity inherent to asthma is crucial both to establishing a diagnosis and determining the severity of illness in asthmatic patients.

COMPONENT I: MEASURES OF ASSESSMENT AND MONITORING: SYMPTOMS, BRONCHODILATOR THERAPY, LUNG FUNCTION, AND ASTHMA ACTION PLANS

The guidelines serve an important purpose not only in their recommendations for therapy but also in providing a framework to evaluate the severity of disease. The current guidelines classify asthma severity based on the presence and frequency of respiratory symptoms, objective measures of lung function, frequency of rescue beta$_2$-agonist use, as well as an assessment of risk. This classification is based on the inherent nature of disease before treatment and is categorized into intermittent, mild persistent, moderate persistent, and severe persistent disease. Furthermore, the most recent revision of the guidelines separate disease assessment by age group as follows: (1) children 0 to 4 years of age, (2) children 5 to 11 years of age, and (3) youths older than 12 years and adults (Figs. 19-3, 19-4, and 19-5). After the onset of treatment, the patient's response to specific medications and continued evaluation of symptoms are important in determining or defining the control of asthma. Impairment of the disease, as defined by clinical symptoms, lung function, and responsiveness to therapy, as well as the risk of future exacerbations, should be monitored by the patient and at each clinic visit. As emphasized in the recent update of the National Guidelines, asthma control is twofold: one that involves management of acute exacerbations and the other focusing on long-term asthma control and preservation of lung function. Given these goals, the guidelines recommend that both the patient and the health care provider assess and reassess the severity of disease on a continual basis and modify treatment accordingly.

Since asthma is a chronic inflammatory disease, ongoing assessments of patient's symptoms and their response to treatment is important in determining asthma severity; this information can then be applied in a stepwise fashion when determining appropriate therapeutic interventions. A patient initially classified

as intermittent, mild persistent, or moderate persistent who continues to have symptoms despite appropriate medical therapy should be reclassified to a higher level of asthma severity, as denoted by the stepwise charts. Similarly, a patient who has achieved asthma control with complete resolution of symptoms for a significant period should attempt a reduction in therapy. If asthma control continues while on reduced therapy, then the patient should be reclassified according to their current treatment and presence of symptoms (Table 19-2). Lung function, as measured by FEV$_1$ (forced expiratory volume in 1 second) and PEF (peak expiratory flow), should be monitored throughout this assessment. A patient without symptoms but with a reduction in FEV$_1$ may not tolerate a reduction of treatment. The guidelines advocate this individualized approach with a stepping-up or stepping-down of therapy, based on the presence and frequency of symptoms, need for bronchodilators, lung function, and number of asthma exacerbations, as a way to optimize asthma control at the most appropriate dose of pharmacologic therapy.

The objective measure of lung function is an integral factor in the assessment of asthma. The FEV$_1$ is the most widely used test of lung function in asthma and has been used both in the construction of stimulus response curves and in bronchodilator testing to determine the presence of airway hyperresponsiveness. In bronchoprovocation testing, such as the methacholine challenge, the reduction of FEV$_1$ by 20% from baseline serves as an index to determine airway hyperresponsiveness, although a positive finding is not specific to asthma. In patients with determined airway hyperresponsiveness, a FEV$_1$ or monitoring for diurnal variations of PEF of greater than or equal to 20% correlates well with airway hyperresponsiveness. FEV$_1$ and PEF are also used in research studies as outcome measurements to determine efficacy of treatment. In this manner, spirometry serves as a measure of the degree of airflow limitation. Determining the pre- and postbronchodilator FEV$_1$, PEF, and FEV$_1$/FVC (forced vital capacity) can further assess the degree of reversibility and the patient's response to beta-agonist therapy. Pulmonary function tests, specifically FEV$_1$, should be performed routinely to follow lung function over time and can also be used to individualize management at home when used in conjunction with PEF values. Although there is no evidence to support the use of asthma action plans based on home lung function monitoring (using peak flow meters) versus clinical assessments,

Components of Severity		Classification of Asthma Severity (Children 0–4 years of age)			
		Intermittent	Persistent		
			Mild	Moderate	Severe
Impairment	Symptoms	≤2 days/week	>2 days/week but not daily	Daily	Throughout the day
	Nighttime awakenings	0	1–2x/month	3–4x/month	>1x/week
	Short-acting beta$_2$-agonist use for symptom control (not prevention of EIB)	≤2 days/week	>2 days/week but not daily	Daily	Several times per day
	Interference with normal activity	None	Minor limitation	Some limitation	Extremely limited
Risk	Exacerbations (consider frequency and severity)	0–1/year	≥2 exacerbations in 6 months requiring oral steroids, or ≥4 wheezing episodes/1 year lasting >1 day AND risk factors for persistent asthma		
			←———— Frequency and severity may fluctuate over time ————→		
			Exacerbations of any severity may occur in patients in any severity category		

Components of Control		Classification of Asthma Control (Children 0–4 years of age)		
		Well Controlled	Not Well Controlled	Very Poorly Controlled
Impairment	Symptoms	≤2 days/week	>2 days/week	Throughout the day
	Nighttime awakenings	1x/month	>1x/month	>1x/week
	Interference with normal activity	None	Some limitation	Extremely limited
	Short-acting beta$_2$-agonist use for symptom control (not prevention of EIB)	≤2 days/week	>2 days/week	Several times per day
Risk	Exacerbations	0–1 per year	2–3 per year	>3 per year
	Treatment-related adverse effects	Medication side effects can vary in intensity from none to very troublesome and worrisome. The level of intensity does not correlate to specific levels of control but should be considered in the overall assessment of risk.		

Figure 19-3 Stepwise approach to asthma diagnosis and management for children 0 to 4 years of age. *(From National Asthma Education and Prevention Program: Full Expert Panel Report 3: Guidelines for the Diagnosis and Management of Asthma (EPR3). Bethesda, MD, National Heart, Lung and Blood Institute, 2007.)*

peak flow meters may be beneficial in patients with moderate to severe asthma to provide an awareness of increased airflow obstruction and, in turn, improve asthma control.

In addition to monitoring symptoms and lung function, several noninvasive markers, most notably exhaled nitric oxide (FE_{NO}), have been introduced to measure the degree of airway inflammation. It is known that exhaled nitric oxide is elevated in patients with asthma and that treatment with inhaled corticosteroids decreases the level of exhaled FE_{NO}. In the future, FE_{NO} may be useful to establish compliance and response to therapy and as a measure used in treatment guidelines. At this time, if FE_{NO} is used, it should be used in conjunction with objective measures of lung function such as spirometry and peak flow monitoring and clinical symptoms. In this manner, it may be used to further establish an accurate, individualized assessment of disease severity and therapy for each patient.

A characteristic feature of asthma is episodic exacerbations that can be provoked by infection, allergen exposure, or inadequate maintenance therapy. An important step in managing exacerbations requires a vigilant monitoring of clinical symptoms and the need for rescue bronchodilators, both by the patient and health practitioner. In the recent revision of asthma guidelines, a risk domain, assessing the number of asthma exacerbations in 1 year, was included as a

Components of Severity		Classification of Asthma Severity (Children 5–11 years of age)			
		Intermittent	Persistent		
			Mild	Moderate	Severe
Impairment	Symptoms	≤2 days/week	>2 days/week but not daily	Daily	Throughout the day
	Nighttime awakenings	≤2x/month	3–4x/month	>1x/week but not nightly	Often 7x/week
	Short-acting beta$_2$-agonist use for symptom control (not prevention of EIB)	≤2 days/week	>2 days/week but not daily	Daily	Several times per day
	Interference with normal activity	None	Minor limitation	Some limitation	Extremely limited
	Lung function	• Normal FEV$_1$ between exacerbations • FEV$_1$ > 80% predicted • FEV$_1$/FVC > 85%	• FEV$_1$ ≥ 80% predicted • FEV$_1$/FVC > 80%	• FEV$_1$ = 60%–80% predicted • FEV$_1$/FVC = 75%–80%	• FEV$_1$ < 60% predicted • FEV$_1$/FVC < 75%
Risk	Exacerbations (consider frequency and severity)	0–2/year >2 in 1 year ——————→ ←—— Frequency and severity may fluctuate over time ——→ for patients in any severity category Relative annual risk of exacerbations may be related to FEV$_1$			

Components of Control		Classification of Asthma Control (Children 5–11 years of age)		
		Well Controlled	Not Well Controlled	Very Poorly Controlled
Impairment	Symptoms	≤2 days/week but not more than once on each day	>2 days/week or multiple times on ≤ 2 days/week	Throughout the day
	Nighttime awakenings	≤1x/month	≥2x/month	≥2x/week
	Interference with normal activity	None	Some limitation	Extremely limited
	Short-acting beta$_2$-agonist use for symptom control (not prevention of EIB)	≤2 days/week	>2 days/week	Several times per day
	Lung function • FEV$_1$ or peak flow • FEV$_1$/FVC	>80% predicted/ personal best >80% predicted	60%–80% predicted/ personal best 75%–80% predicted	<60% predicted/ personal best <75% predicted
Risk	Exacerbations	0–1 per year	2–3 per year	>3 per year
	Reduction in lung growth	Evaluation requires long-term followup.		
	Treatment-related adverse effects	Medication side effects can vary in intensity from none to very troublesome and worrisome. The level of intensity does not correlate to specific levels of control but should be considered in the overall assessment of risk.		

Figure 19-4 Stepwise approach to assessing asthma severity and control for children 5 to 11 years of age. *(From National Asthma Education and Prevention Program: Expert Panel Report 3: Guidelines for the Diagnosis and Management of Asthma (EPR3). Bethesda, MD, National Heart, Lung, and Blood Institute, 2007.)*

Components of Severity		Classification of Asthma Severity (Youths ≥ 12 years of age and adults)			
		Intermittent	Persistent		
			Mild	Moderate	Severe
Impairment Normal FEV₁/FVC: 8–19 yr 85% 20–39 yr 80% 40–59 yr 75% 60–80 yr 70%	Symptoms	≤2 days/week	>2 days/week but not daily	Daily	Throughout the day
	Nighttime awakenings	≤2x/month	3–4x/month	>1x/week but not nightly	Often 7x/week
	Short-acting beta₂-agonist use for symptom control (not prevention of EIB)	≤2 days/week	>2 days/week but not daily	Daily	Several times per day
	Interference with normal activity	None	Minor limitation	Some limitation	Extremely limited
	Lung function	• Normal FEV₁ between exacerbations • FEV₁ > 80% predicted • FEV₁/FVC normal	• FEV₁ < 80% predicted • FEV₁/FVC normal	• FEV₁ > 60% but < 80% predicted • FEV₁/FVC reduced 5%	• FEV₁ < 60% predicted • FEV₁/FVC reduced > 5%
Risk	Exacerbations (consider frequency and severity)	0–2/year >2/year ——————————————————→ ←—— Frequency and severity may fluctuate over time ——→ for patients in any severity category Relative annual risk of exacerbations may be related to FEV₁			

Components of Control		Classification of Asthma Control (Youths ≥ 12 years of age and adults)		
		Well Controlled	Not Well Controlled	Very Poorly Controlled
Impairment	Symptoms	≤2 days/week	>2 days/week	Throughout the day
	Nighttime awakenings	≤2/month	1–3/week	≥4/week
	Interference with normal activity	None	Some limitation	Extremely limited
	Short-acting beta₂-agonist use for symptom control (not prevention of EIB)	≤2 days/week	>2 days/week	Several times per day
	FEV₁ or peak flow	>80% predicted/ personal best	60%–80% predicted/ personal best	<60% predicted/ personal best
	Validated Questionnaires† ATAQ ACQ ACT	 0 ≤0.75 ≥20	 1–2 ≥1.5 16–19	 3–4 N/A ≤15
Risk	Exacerbations	0–1 per year 2–3 per year >3 per year		
	Progressive loss of lung function	Evaluation requires long-term followup care		
	Treatment-related adverse effects	Medication side effects can vary in intensity from none to very troublesome and worrisome. The level of intensity does not correlate to specific levels of control but should be considered in the overall assessment of risk.		

Figure 19-5 Stepwise approach to assessing asthma severity and control for youths older than 12 years and adults. *(From National Asthma Education and Prevention Program: Expert Panel Report 3: Guidelines for the Diagnosis and Management of Asthma (EPR3). Bethesda, MD, National Heart, Lung, and Blood Institute, 2007.)*

Table 19-2
CLASSIFICATION OF ASTHMA SEVERITY AS OUTLINED IN THE 2007 NHLBI GUIDELINES

		Persistent		
	Intermittent	Mild	Moderate	Severe
Lowest level of treatment required to maintain control (See Figures 19-4 and 19-5 for treatment steps)	Step 1	Step 2	Step 3 or 4	Step 5 or 6

From National Asthma Education and Prevention Program: Expert Panel Report 3: Guidelines for the Diagnosis and Management of Asthma: Update on Selected Topics. Bethesda, MD, National Heart, Lung, and Blood Institute, 2002.

measure of severity. Home peak flow monitoring can provide an additional assessment of disease severity. Currently there is no evidence to either support or contest the effectiveness of asthma action plans; however, asthma action plans can provide direction to patients, recommending a step-up of rescue bronchodilators and corticosteroids when needed. Furthermore, if asthma action plans are used, they can educate patients to recognize signs of deterioration and to initiate therapy with rescue bronchodilators and corticosteroids. Asthma action plans can also help patients recognize when to seek medical care. Similarly, asthma patients who require hospitalization should obtain written plans detailing medication use and how to recognize clinical deterioration in the future and potential triggers to exacerbations. Frequent follow-up visits may be required with monitoring of lung function and prevalence of asthma symptoms until complete asthma control is achieved.

COMPONENT II: CONTROL OF FACTORS CONTRIBUTING TO ASTHMA SEVERITY: ATOPY, INFECTIONS, AND ENVIRONMENTAL EXPOSURES

Given that asthma is a chronic inflammatory disorder, recognition of risk factors is important in understanding the pathogenesis and the therapeutic targets for the disease. The inflammation in asthma manifests clinically as recurrent episodes of wheezing, breathlessness, chest tightness, and coughing. Recurrence of symptoms is influenced by host susceptibility to disease as well as environmental influences. Family and population studies have suggested that a genetic predisposition exists for atopic disease. At this time, however, no single gene or group of genes has been identified that code for asthma susceptibility.

Atopy, defined as the presence of immunoglobulin E (IgE)-mediated inflammation in response to environmental allergens, is a strong risk factor for asthma. Longitudinal studies have shown that both allergen sensitization and viral illnesses can influence the development of asthma in susceptible infants. As adults, allergen sensitivity continues to trigger asthma exacerbations. Additional environmental factors, such as occupational exposures and air pollution, can also exacerbate asthma; however, the increased prevalence of asthma in the past 2 decades suggests that this genetic predisposition is influenced by environmental interaction.

Environmental factors, including both allergens and occupational exposures, have been implicated in asthma pathogenesis. Allergen exposure stimulates the production of IgE, sensitizing antibody formation in atopic individuals. In asthma, these IgE antibodies are directed toward environmental allergens, inciting an inflammatory cascade resulting in bronchospasm, mucus production, and airway edema. The presence of IgE antibodies in a susceptible individual is a risk factor for further asthma exacerbations. Although allergen exposure does correlate with allergen sensitization, it is not yet known whether allergen exposure predicts the development of asthma in exposed individuals. However, correlational studies have found that sensitivity to the mold *Alternaria* is a risk factor for severe asthma, whereas indoor allergens such as dust mites, cockroaches, and cats also have also been implicated in provoking asthma exacerbations.

Infections frequently provoke bronchospasm in asthmatic individuals. Although *Mycoplasma* and *Chlamydia* pneumonias have been implicated in asthma pathogenesis, the most frequent triggers of asthma exacerbations are viruses, specifically rhinovirus. The mechanisms by which rhinovirus triggers asthma exacerbations are not well defined but appear to involve both the upper and lower airways, with asthma patients possibly experiencing an altered pro-inflammatory response to viral infection as compared with healthy subjects. The exact mechanism of asthma provocation is unknown but may be multifactorial involving allergen sensitization, allergen exposure, and inflammatory changes in response to viruses as well as defective antiviral activity in some patients.

Occupational and environmental factors play a role in asthma pathogenesis. Occupational exposures can be categorized as sensitizers or irritants, both of which cause inflammatory airway changes leading to airway hyperreactivity. Tobacco smoke is perhaps the most prevalent environmental irritant and is a frequent precipitant of asthma symptoms in both children and adults. Furthermore, exposure to cigarette smoke has been shown to result in decreased lung function and increased symptoms in asthmatic adults. Although a causal link between asthma and smoking has not been established, active smoking is known to contribute to the decline of lung function and may contribute to exacerbations in individuals with asthma.

Other contributing factors in the control of asthma include the presence of rhinitis, sinusitis, gastroesophageal reflux disease, vocal cord dysfunction, and aspirin sensitivity. Use of intranasal corticosteroids, antihistamines, and decongestants and the use of antimicrobials for bacterial sinusitis can improve patency of the upper airway, which has been shown to positively impact asthma symptoms. Similarly, gastroesophageal reflux and vocal cord dysfunction are frequent precipitants of cough in asthma patients; therapy with H_2 blockers, proton pump inhibitors and behavioral modifications can ameliorate symptoms.

The presence of asthma and sensitivity to nonsteroidal anti-inflammatory drugs (NSAIDs) in asthma patients has been well described and can exacerbate symptoms both in the upper and lower airways. Each asthma patient should be queried regarding the effect of aspirin and/or NSAIDs on symptoms of bronchoconstriction, shortness of breath, and cough. In addition, the physical exam and, if needed, diagnostic imaging and procedures should evaluate for the presence of nasal polyps, since the triad of nasal polyps, aspirin sensitivity, and asthma is well described. These patients should be advised to avoid all aspirin and NSAID-containing medicines.

COMPONENT III: PHARMACOLOGICAL THERAPY: INHALED CORTICOSTEROIDS, LONG-ACTING BETA-AGONISTS, LEUKOTRIENE RECEPTOR ANTAGONISTS, ANTI-IGE, AND IMMUNOTHERAPY

The stepwise approach to asthma assessment is not only applicable to diagnosis and assessment of disease severity but is also useful in the treatment and management of individual patients (see Figs. 19-3, 19-4, and 19-5). The cornerstone of therapy in mild or moderate persistent asthma is inhaled corticosteroids, with doses varying from low to high potency (Table 19-3). Current debate exists regarding whether patients with mild persistent asthma require daily inhaled corticosteroids or whether intermittent, directed use is sufficient. Several large randomized controlled trials have investigated inhaled corticosteroids in mild persistent asthma. The Optimal Treatment for Mild Persistent Asthma (OPTIMA) trial was designed to determine the optimal treatment for mild persistent asthma and subsequently found that corticosteroid-naive patients benefited from the daily use of 200 μg of

budesonide. Specifically, these patients showed a 60% reduction in severe exacerbations, as well as a reduction in asthma symptoms, nocturnal awakenings, and bronchodilator use. These results were corroborated by the Inhaled Steroid Treatment as Regular Therapy in Early Asthma (START) trial that investigated the use of 400 μg of budesonide daily in newly diagnosed adult patients with mild persistent asthma; this study showed that patients on daily budesonide had more symptom-free days, fewer courses of systemic corticosteroid, and improved prebronchodilator and postbronchodilator FEV_1 after 1 year of budesonide therapy while also reducing the risk of having a severe asthma exacerbation by half.

More recently, the Improving Asthma Control (IMPACT) trial evaluated whether symptom-initiated use of either 800 μg inhaled budesonide twice daily or alternatively oral prednisone at 0.5 mg/kg/day, for 10 days, in patients previously diagnosed with mild persistent asthma was equal in efficacy to the daily use of inhaled 200 μg budesonide. Patients who intermittently used corticosteroids in high doses as determined by worsening symptoms showed no difference in regards to asthma exacerbations. However, the group using daily budesonide had greater improvements in prebronchodilator FEV_1 and experienced more symptom-free days, decreased sputum eosinophils, and decreased exhaled nitric oxide levels.

What we can conclude from these studies is that while inhaled corticosteroids remain the cornerstone of treatment for mild persistent asthma, a certain subset of patients may tolerate high-dose inhaled corticosteroids only initiated at the onset of worsening symptoms. These patients may attain asthma control without daily inhaled corticosteroid therapy. For all asthma patients, continual assessments should be made to ensure that patients are achieving asthma control, as defined by symptom-free days and elimination of nocturnal awakenings on their current treatment regimens.

Patients with moderate persistent asthma also show improvement with the use of inhaled corticosteroids and those who continue to have symptoms on inhaled corticosteroids show further improvement with the addition of long-acting beta-agonists (LABA). Two large multicenter trials have studied the effect of LABA both in combination with corticosteroids and as monotherapy. Results showed that patients whose asthma was uncontrolled with inhaled corticosteroids alone showed improvement in asthma symptoms, a decreased need for rescue bronchodilators, and improvement of lung function with combination therapy and tolerated a reduction of their inhaled corticosteroid dose by half with the addition of salmeterol. These results were further corroborated by the OPTIMA and the FACET (Formoterol And Corticosteroids Establishing Therapy) trials, both of which investigated the effect of combination therapy with LABA and inhaled corticosteroids and compared the results to the use of inhaled corticosteroids alone. The OPTIMA trial found that combination therapy was superior to inhaled corticosteroid therapy alone in patients whose asthma was uncontrolled on inhaled corticosteroid therapy. Using severe asthma exacerbation and poorly controlled asthma days as the primary outcome variables, the study also found that combination therapy was more effective than doubling the inhaled corticosteroid dose. Similarly, the FACET trial found that the addition of formoterol reduced the rates of asthma exacerbations when used in conjunction

Table 19-3
ESTIMATED EQUIPOTENT DAILY DOSES OF INHALED GLUCOCORTICOSTEROIDS FOR ADULTS*

Drug	Low Daily Dose (μg)	Medium Daily Dose (μg)	High Daily Dose (μg)†*
Beclomethasone dipropionate	200–500	>500–1000	>1000–2000
Budesonide‡	200–400	>400–800	>800–1600
Ciclesonide‡	80–160	>160–320	>320–1280
Flunisolide	500–1000	>1000–2000	>2000
Fluticasone	100–250	>250–500	>500–1000
Mometasone furoate‡	200–400	>400–800	>800–1200
Triamcinolone acetonide	400–1000	>1000–2000	>2000

*Comparisons based on efficacy data
†Patients considered for high daily doses except for short periods should be referred to a specialist for assessment to consider alternative combinations of controllers. Maximum recommended doses are arbitrary but with prolonged use are associated with increased risk of systemic side effects.
‡Approved for once-daily dosing in mild patients.
From Global Initiative for Asthma (GINA): Global Strategy for Asthma Management and Prevention: NHLBI/WHO Workshop Report (Publication No. 02-3659). Bethesda, MD, National Institutes of Health, National Heart, Lung, and Blood Institute, 2002 (revised in 2006).
Notes
• The most important determinant of appropriate dosing is the clinician's judgment of the patient's response to therapy. The clinician must monitor the patient's response in terms of clinical control and adjust the dose accordingly. Once control of asthma is achieved, the dose of medication should be carefully titrated to the **minimum** dose required to maintain control, thus reducing the potential for adverse effects.
• Designation of low, medium, and high doses is provided from manufacturers recommendations where possible. Clear demonstration of dose-response relationships is seldom provided or available. The principle is therefore to establish the minimum effective controlling dose in each patient, as higher doses may not be more effective and are likely to be associated with greater potential for adverse effects.
• As CFC preparations are taken from the market, medication inserts for HFA preparations should be carefully reviewed by the clinician for the equivalent correct dosage.

with inhaled budesonide, both at a low dose of budesonide (100 μg daily) and at a higher dose of budesonide (400 μg), although the higher dose group was associated with a significantly higher FEV_1 than the lower dose group. More recently, the Budesonide/Formoterol Combination Therapy as Both Maintenance and Reliever Medication in Asthma (STAY) trial suggested that the use of combination therapy (formoterol and budesonide), both as a twice a day controller medication and as rescue therapy, can result in fewer severe asthma exacerbations and a concurrent decrease in asthma symptoms with increases in FEV_1 values. These trials provide evidence that the large majority of asthma patients whose disease is uncontrolled with medium dose inhaled corticosteroid will likely benefit from the addition of a LABA. Further research will be needed before evidence-based recommendations advocating combination therapy as rescue medications can be made.

Recent concerns regarding the safety of LABA therapy, specifically the increase of respiratory-related deaths in subpopulations of asthmatic patients, also require further investigation as to precisely which patients may be at increased risk. At this time, however, LABA therapy, in combination with inhaled corticosteroids, remain an effective treatment for most patients with moderate and severe persistent asthma whose disease is uncontrolled on inhaled corticosteroids alone.

Other treatments exist that should be considered under certain situations. Leukotriene modifiers, specifically cysteinyl leukotriene receptor antagonists, may be used as daily controller therapy for mild persistent asthma and as adjunct therapy for moderate persistent and severe persistent asthmatic individuals whose disease is not controlled on medium-dose inhaled corticosteroid therapy. Studies have shown that leukotriene modifiers have a mild anti-inflammatory effect and reduce both symptoms and asthma exacerbations. However, these agents have generally been shown to be less effective on measures of lung function, symptom-free days, and rescue bronchodilator use when compared to inhaled corticosteroids. Nevertheless, leukotriene modifiers have been shown to be effective adjunctive treatment when added to inhaled corticosteroids for adult patients whose asthma is not well controlled on inhaled corticosteroids alone.

Systemic corticosteroids are useful in the treatment of asthma exacerbations and reduce the morbidity of the disease in terms of emergency room visits and need for hospitalizations. However, frequent bursts of corticosteroids are an indication of poor asthma control, and potential adverse side effects such as adrenal insufficiency, weight gain, osteoporosis, and aseptic necrosis further limit its use on a continual basis.

Methylxanthines have been used in oral and parenteral form as a bronchodilator and anti-inflammatory medication, although its use has been limited secondary to significant side effects and drug interactions. A trial of sodium cromoglycate and nedocromil sodium may be initiated in patients with mild persistent asthma and also as prophylactic agents to antagonize early and late phase inflammation that may be triggered by exercise or allergens. However, trials in children have shown that these agents are less effective than corticosteroids as monotherapy in asthma treatment.

Anti-IgE therapy has shown promising results in patients with severe allergic asthma who continue to have symptoms despite optimal therapy on inhaled corticosteroids and β-agonists. Studies have shown that anti-IgE therapy, omalizumab, reduces asthma symptoms, bronchodilator use, exacerbations, and dosage of corticosteroids, but has not always resulted in improvements of lung function. Currently, it largely serves a role in asthma patients in the treatment of severe allergic asthma as adjunctive therapy to inhaled corticosteroids and long-acting beta-agonists.

Clinical trials investigating the effect of subcutaneous immunotherapy have shown some benefit in attaining asthma control and it may be considered in conjunction with beta-agonists and daily controller therapy, such as inhaled corticosteroids. However, given the risk of eliciting an acute allergic reaction with immunotherapy, pharmacological therapy and environmental avoidance should be considered before embarking on long-term immunotherapy.

Antibiotics, although often prescribed for asthma exacerbations, have not been shown to improve selective outcomes. Given a lack of evidence to support the use of antibiotics for acute asthma exacerbations, current guidelines do not advocate the use of antibiotics in this setting. Concerns regarding rising health care cost, emerging bacterial resistance, and lack of efficacy support this recommendation. There are limited data on the effectiveness of antibiotics on coexisting sinusitis, persistent infections, or other situations.

SPECIFIC TREATMENT ISSUES REGARDING CHILDREN

Asthma in children shares similarities with adults in terms of pathophysiology of disease; however, management needs to be tailored to the child's age, drug metabolism, and a desire to minimize effects on growth and development. Furthermore, given that children often metabolize drugs more quickly than adults, doses of oral medication need to be adjusted to establish a therapeutic range. Similar to adults, the severity of asthma should be established according to frequency of symptoms, bronchodilator use, and objective measures of lung function such as FEV_1 and morning PEF values and risk of future exacerbations. Currently, the 2007 guidelines classify severity of asthma and assess asthma control for children 0 to 4 years of age and school-aged children (5 to 11 years of age). Children 12 and older are assessed together with adults. Diagnosis of asthma in young children and infants can be difficult and long-term asthma therapy should be considered after appropriate diagnostic assessment. In all age groups, severity is assessed by frequency and severity of symptoms as well as frequency and severity of exacerbations. Treatment should similarly follow a stepwise approach (see Table 19-2).

Several studies have shown that inhaled corticosteroids are the preferred therapy for children whose symptoms require daily controller therapy. The Childhood Asthma Management Program Research Group (CAMP) trial compared the effects of inhaled budesonide to inhaled nedocromil in children requiring daily controller therapy based on their asthma symptoms and followed these patients over 4 to 6 years. Children on inhaled budesonide had fewer exacerbations, fewer hospitalizations, and improved asthma control as compared with counterparts who received placebo or nedocromil. Furthermore, the CAMP trial showed that although subjects treated with budesonide showed a significant decrease in growth velocity, 1.1 cm less than the mean increase in the placebo group (22.7 versus 23.8 cm, $P = .005$)

in the first year of treatment, this rate of growth decline did not persist. Furthermore, all three treatment groups showed similar growth velocities at the end of the treatment period, which lasted 44 months. Projected final height and bone density were also not affected by inhaled glucocorticoid treatment. These results corroborated previous studies, which reported that children with mild-to-moderate persistent asthma and treated with inhaled budesonide (mean dose 412 μg/day) for an average of 9.2 years showed no decline in attaining their expected adult height.

In terms of the development of cataracts, 1 of 311 children in the budesonide treatment group, who had also received additional systemic steroids during the study, was found to have a minuscule cataract as compared to no cataracts diagnosed in either the placebo or nedocromil treatment group. In the end, treatment with budesonide resulted in decreased asthma exacerbations as indicated by decreased hospitalizations, emergency room visits, and decreased rescue bronchodilator and systemic corticosteroid therapy. This marked improvement in asthma with relatively limited side effects indicates that inhaled corticosteroids are both effective and safe to use as daily controller therapy in children.

The addition of LABA to inhaled corticosteroids has not been widely studied in children. At this time, recommendations to use combination therapy in children with moderate persistent asthma have been made based on favorable data from the adult population, supplemented with expert opinion. Further studies are needed to conclusively determine whether LABAs are the definitive treatment for children with moderate persistent asthma whose disease is uncontrolled on low- to medium-dose inhaled corticosteroids.

Leukotriene modifiers, cromolyn, and sustained release theophylline remain as alternative and adjunctive treatment options for patients with mild, moderate, and severe persistent asthma. Monotherapy with sodium cromoglycate as a daily controller is inferior to inhaled corticosteroids in the relief of asthma symptoms, exacerbations, and lung function. Sustained release theophylline may also be considered in patients with mild persistent asthma as daily controlling therapy; however, its use is limited by its narrow therapeutic window, its rapid metabolism in the pediatric population, and numerous gastrointestinal and central nervous system side effects.

Leukotriene modifiers, because they are delivered orally, remain an attractive option as daily controller therapy in the pediatric population particularly in children under the age of 5. It has been shown to be effective adjunctive therapy to inhaled corticosteroids and beta-agonists in pediatric patients with moderate persistent and severe persistent asthma. At this time no studies exist to indicate that leukotriene modifiers are equal or superior to inhaled corticosteroids as daily controller therapy in patients with moderate or severe persistent asthma. However, they may be a suitable alternative to inhaled corticosteroids in patients with mild persistent asthma.

COMPONENT IV: EDUCATION

The guidelines also provide medical practitioners an evidence-based algorithm to classify and manage asthma patients. Although the guidelines, as supported by the GOAL study, provide an effective way to approach and treat asthmatic patients, they are only as effective as their implementation. Therefore, medical practitioners need to be able to easily access the information as well as the tools needed to monitor and treat asthma as recommended by the guidelines. For example, office spirometry provides an effective and accurate method to monitor lung function while home peak flow monitoring together with clinical symptoms can serve as daily measurement of asthma control. Health care providers as well as the administrative organizations that control health care costs need to participate in the greater availability and accessibility of these tools. Likewise, patient education, when provided by appropriately trained asthma educators, can greatly improve patient technique with complex inhaled medications as well as in the implementation of rescue corticosteroids. In this manner, patients and all levels of health care providers are involved in establishing an integrated and comprehensive method to implement effective asthma disease management. Globally, asthma management may need to be modified in accordance with the availability of local resources, access to inpatient and outpatient health care, and cultural factors.

Patient education not only will improve the delivery of health care but also can improve adherence with medications and other interventions. Although the guidelines provide a framework with which to assess disease severity and determine appropriate management, other tools can facilitate the implementation of guidelines into practice. The Asthma Control Test (ACT), a series of questions that focus on the prevalence and intensity of asthma symptoms and rescue medication use, was recently endorsed by the American Thoracic Society (Fig. 19-6).

GOAL: APPLYING THE GUIDELINES TO CLINICAL PRACTICE

The Gaining Optimal Asthma Control (GOAL) was a multicenter trial designed to determine whether asthma control could be achieved and maintained using the stepwise approach outlined by the asthma guidelines and to determine the consequences of implementing this approach. As compared to prior trials, the GOAL study used asthma control, as defined by the parameters outlined by the guidelines, specifically the presence of asthma symptoms and beta-agonist use, as the primary end points of the study (Table 19-4). Both corticosteroid-naïve patients and patients on low and moderate doses of inhaled corticosteroids were recruited and randomized to receive either fluticasone or combination therapy with fluticasone and salemeterol. There were 3421 patients enrolled for a year. If total control, defined by the complete lack of asthma symptoms, exacerbations, and rescue medication use, was not achieved, the patient underwent a "step-up" of therapy every 12 weeks until total control was achieved or until the maximum dose of treatment was reached. The study showed that totally controlled or well-controlled asthma was achievable if the guideline-based approach was used to determine asthma severity and if therapy was increased if control was not achieved. Furthermore, patients who were treated with fluticasone/ salmeterol combination therapy achieved total asthma control more rapidly and at a lower dose of inhaled corticosteroids than patients treated with fluticasone alone (Fig. 19-7). Response to treatment and the final level of treatment are measures that may

1. In the past 4 weeks, how much of the time did your asthma keep you from getting as much done at work, school, or at home?

All of the time	Most of the time	Some of the time	A little of the time	None of the time
O	O	O	O	O
1	2	3	4	5

2. During the past 4 weeks, how often have you had shortness of breath?

More than once a day	Once a day	3 to 6 times a week	Once or twice a week	Not at all
O	O	O	O	O
1	2	3	4	5

3. During the past 4 weeks, how often did your asthma symptoms (wheezing, coughing, shortness of breath, chest tightness or pain) wake you up at night or earlier than usual in the morning?

4 or more nights a week	2 to 3 nights a week	Once a week	Once or twice	Not at all
O	O	O	O	O
1	2	3	4	5

4. During the past 4 weeks, how often have you used your rescue inhaler or nebulizer medication (such as albuterol)?

3 or more times per day	1 or 2 times per day	2 or 3 times per week	Once a week or less	Not at all
O	O	O	O	O
1	2	3	4	5

5. How would you rate your asthma control during the past 4 weeks?

Not controlled at all	Poorly controlled	Somewhat controlled	Well controlled	Completely controlled
O	O	O	O	O
1	2	3	4	5

Figure 19-6 **Asthma Control Test.** *(From Schatz M, Sorkness CA, Li JT, et al: Asthma Control Test: reliability, validity and responsiveness in patients not previously followed by asthma specialists. J Allergy Clin Immunol 2006;117:549–556.)*

be used to define and determine asthma severity. The GOAL study validates the outcomes advocated by the guidelines as effective measures of control while also showing that totally controlled and well-controlled asthma can be achieved and maintained with the "step-up" approach outlined by the guidelines.

One limitation of the GOAL study is that the study design did not allow for a "stepping down" of therapy in

Table 19-4
DEFINITION OF ASTHMA CONTROL USED IN THE GOAL STUDY BASED ON THE GINA GUIDELINES

	Goals of GINA NIH	Totally Controlled *Each Week All of These Criteria Are Met*	Well Controlled *Each Week 2 or More of These Criteria Are Met*
Daytime symptoms	Minimal (ideally no)	None	≤2 days with symptom score > 1[‡]
Rescue beta$_2$-agonist use	Minimal (ideally no)	None	Use on ≤ 2 days and [≤] 4 occasions/wk
Morning PEF	Near normal	≥80% predicted[†] every day	≥80% predicted[†] every day
Nighttime awakening	Minimal (ideally no)	None	None
Exacerbations*	Minimal (infrequent)	None	None
Emergency visits	No	None	None
Treatment-related adverse events	Minimal	None enforcing change in asthma therapy	None enforcing change in asthma therapy

*Exacerbations were defined as deterioration in asthma requiring treatment with an oral corticosteroid or an emergency department visit or hospitalization.
[†]Predicted PEF was calculated based on the European Community for Steel and Coal standards (40) for patients 18 years and older and on the Polgar standards (41) for patients 12–17 years old.
[‡]Symptom score: 1 was defined as "symptoms for one short period during the day." Overall scale: 0 (none)–5(severe).
GINA, Global Initiative for Asthma; NIH, National Institutes of Health.
Totally and well-controlled asthma were defined by achievement of all of the specified criteria for that week. Totally controlled asthma was achieved if the patient during the 8 consecutive assessment weeks recorded 7 totally controlled weeks and had no exacerbations, emergency room criteria, or medication-related adverse events criteria. Well-controlled asthma was similarly assessed over the 8 weeks. These assessments were for an 8-week period during the double-blind treatment period. Baseline control and control during the open-label phase were assessed over a 4-week period.
Adapted from Bateman ED, Boushey HA, Bousquet J, et al: Can guideline-defined asthma control be achieved? The Gaining OptimaL Control Study. Am J Respir Crit Care Med 2004;170:836–844.

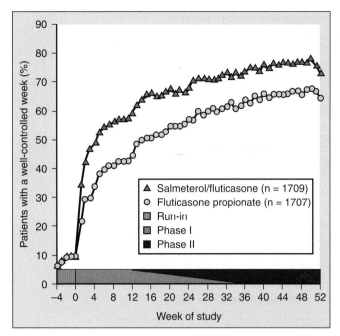

Figure 19-7 GOAL study. Patients with moderate persistent asthma with treatment adjusted according to the GINA guidelines showed that well-controlled asthma could be achieved using a stepwise approach. Furthermore, patients on combination therapy of salmeterol/fluticasone experienced more well-controlled weeks as compared with patients on fluticasone alone *(From Bateman ED, Boushey HA, Bousquet J, et al: Can guideline-defined asthma control be achieved? The Gaining Optimal Asthma ControL Study. Am J Respir Crit Care Med 2004;170:836–844.)*

patients who achieved total control on their current treatment regimen. However, decreasing therapy in patients who have maintained stable lung function and are without symptoms and have no rescue bronchodilator or emergency corticosteroid use is reasonable if these patients are followed closely. In future guidelines, the need and response to therapy may be used to classify disease in individual patients and characterize the severity of asthmatic disease.

CONCLUSION

The asthma guidelines provide both medical practitioners and patients with a framework to assess disease severity and guide management. They further serve as a tool that continually translates scientific evidence into clinical practice, and thereby allows practitioners to base their therapeutic decisions on sound scientific results. It must be remembered that guidelines are a guide, not a rule to asthma management and the key to their success lies in the implementation of sound evidence-based health care to the entire asthma population.

Further information, including the complete GINA guidelines, can be found at www.ginasthma.org, most recently updated in December 2006. The National Asthma Education Prevention Program guidelines are available at http://www.nhlbi.nih.gov/guidelines/asthma with most recent revisions updated in 2007.

SUGGESTED READING

Barnes NC, Miller CJ: Effect of leukotriene receptor antagonist therapy on the risk of asthma exacerbations in patients with mild to moderate asthma: an integrated analysis of zafirlukast trials. Thorax 2000;55:478–483.

Bateman ED, Boushey HA, Bousquet J, et al: Can Guideline-defined asthma control be achieved? The Gaining Optimal Asthma ControL Study. Am J Respir Crit Care Med 2004;170:836–844.

Boushey HA, Sorkness CA, King T, et al: Daily versus as-needed corticosteroids for mild persistent asthma (IMPACT). N Engl J Med 2005;352:1519–1528.

Busse WW, Lemanske RF: Asthma. N Engl J Med 2001; 344:350–362.

The Childhood Asthma Management Program Research Group: Long-term effects of budesonide or nedocromil in children with asthma. N Engl J Med 2000;343:1054–1063.

Gern JE, Brooks D, Meyer P, et al: Bidirectional interactions between viral respiratory illnesses and cytokine responses in the first year of life. J Allergy Clin Immunol 2006;117:72–78.

Gertoft L, Oederson S: Effect of long-term treatment with inhaled budesonide on adult height in children with asthma. N Engl J Med 2000;343:1064–1069.

Global Initiative for Asthma (GINA): Global Strategy for Asthma Management and Prevention: NHLBI/WHO Workshop Report (Publication No. 02–3659). Bethesda, MD, National Institutes of Health, National Heart, Lung, and Blood Institute, 2002 (revised in 2006).

Lazarus SC, Boushey HA, Fahy JV, et al: Long-acting β-2 agonist monotherapy vs. continued therapy with inhaled corticosteroids in patients with persistent asthma (SOCS). JAMA 2001;285:2583–2593.

Lemanske RF, Sorkness CA, Mauger EA, et al: Inhaled corticosteroid reduction and elimination in patients with persistent asthma receiving salmeterol (SLIC). JAMA 2001;285:2594–2603.

National Asthma Education and Prevention Program: Expert Panel Report: Guidelines for the Diagnosis and Management of Asthma:

Update on Selected Topics. Bethesda, MD, National Heart, Lung, and Blood Institute, 2002.

National Asthma Education and Prevention Program: Expert Panel Report 2: Guidelines for the Diagnosis and Management of Asthma. Bethesda, MD, National Heart, Lung and Blood Institute, 1997.

National Asthma Education and Prevention Program: Full Report of the Expert Panel: Guidelines for the Diagnosis and Management of Asthma (EPR3). Bethesda, MD, National Heart, Lung and Blood Institute, 2007.

Nelson HS, Weiss AT, Bleecker ER, et al: The Salmeterol Multicenter Asthma Research Trial: A comparison of usual pharmacotherapy for asthma or usual pharmacotherapy plus salmeterol. Chest 2006;129:15–26.

O'Byrne PM, Barnes PJ. Rodriguez-Roisin R, et al: Low dose inhaled budesonide and formoterol in mild persistent asthma: The OPTIMA Randomized Trial. Am J Respir Crit Care Med 2001;164:1392–1397.

O'Byrne PM, Bisgaard H, Godard PP: Budesonide/formoterol combination therapy as both maintenance and reliever medication in asthma (STAY). Am J Respir Crit Care Med 2005;171:129–136.

Pauwels RA, Lofdahl CG, Postma DS, et al: Effect of inhaled formoterol and budesonide on exacerbations of asthma. N Engl J Med 1997;337:1405–1412.

Pauwels RA, Pedersen S, Busse WW, et al: Early intervention with budesonide in mild persistent asthma: A randomized, double-blind trial (START). Lancet 2003;361:1071–1076.

Schatz M, Sorkness CA, Li JT, et al: Asthma Control Test: Reliability, validity and responsiveness in patients not previously followed by asthma specialists. J Allergy Clin Immunol 2006;117:549–556.

Vignola AM, Kips J, Bousquet J: Tissue remodeling as a feature of persistent asthma. J Allergy Clin Immunol 2000;105:1041–1053.

Management of Persistent Asthma in Children

Anand C. Patel and Leonard B. Bacharier

CLINICAL PEARLS

- Management of persistent childhood asthma requires assessments of underlying asthma severity and current level of asthma control.

- Controller therapy is indicated for all levels of persistent and uncontrolled asthma.

- Inhaled corticosteroids are the most effective single class of controller medications for childhood asthma.

- A variety of therapeutic options exists for escalation of asthma therapy when inhaled corticosteroids alone do not provide adequate disease control. However, little data currently exist to help guide decision making for step-up care in children.

- Continued reassessment is mandatory in achieving optimal asthma control.

Asthma is the most common chronic disease of childhood, with approximately 9 million children (prevalence of 12.7%) under 18 years of age having a lifetime diagnosis of asthma and 3.8 million having experienced an asthma episode within the preceding year. Childhood asthma exerts a significant burden on society, accounting for nearly 6.5 million outpatient visits in 2004, more than 750,000 emergency department visits, over 198,000 hospitalizations (more than any other condition in children), 186 deaths, total health care costs exceeding $3 billion, and over 14 million missed school days annually.

Over the past decade, the elucidation of the immunologic and inflammatory underpinnings of asthma has transitioned asthma from a condition of abnormal airway smooth muscle function alone to an inflammatory disorder of the airways.[1] The recognition of chronic airway inflammation as the dominant pathophysiologic process underlying asthma has led to a focus on the increased use of anti-inflammatory therapies with consequent improvement in asthma symptom control and quality of life.

WHAT IS PERSISTENT ASTHMA IN CHILDREN?

The term "persistent" has been used to describe at least two different elements of childhood asthma. One use of the term "persistent asthma" denotes the continued presence of asthma-like symptoms over an extended period of time. Alternatively, national and international guidelines have applied the term "persistent" to describe asthma symptoms that occur above a specified frequency, differentiating patients as intermittent or persistent based on recent symptom frequency, rescue medication use, and/or pulmonary function, without indication of long-term prognosis.

The combination of the high prevalence of wheezing in early childhood and several wheezing phenotypes with differing pathophysiologic mechanisms and prognoses suggests that differentiating young children with recurrent wheezing as either at low or high risk for persistence of asthma-like symptoms may help guide asthma diagnosis, treatment, and prognosis. The Tucson Children's Respiratory Study has provided a tool that has proven reliable in categorizing preschool children in terms of subsequent asthma risk. The Asthma Predictive Index (API) (Table 20-1) identifies children with recurrent wheezing with risk factors for active asthma during the school-age years.[2] A positive API at age 3 years indicates a 77% likelihood of having active asthma at some point during the school years, whereas a negative API is associated with not having active asthma during the school years 95% of the time. This clinically applicable approach for assessing the risk of persistence of asthma symptoms following recurrent wheezing in early childhood has recently been incorporated into national guidelines for the determination of children appropriate for initiation of asthma controller therapy.

CLASSIFICATION OF ASTHMA SEVERITY AND LEVEL OF CONTROL

The current approach toward the pharmacotherapy of asthma is based on a combined assessment of the severity and level of control of the patient's disease. The National Asthma Education and Prevention Program (NAEPP) and Global Initiative for Asthma (GINA) Guidelines provide frameworks to categorize asthma severity and control, focusing on symptom frequencies, rescue medication use, need for controller medications, and objective measures of lung function. The most recent NAEPP Guidelines[3] identify two major components of asthma severity and control: current *impairment* and future *risk*. Impairment reflects the frequency and intensity of symptoms and functional limitations the patient is experiencing and includes daytime symptom frequency, nighttime awakenings, interference with exercise/activity, short-acting beta-agonist use, and lung function (for children 5 years of age and older). Risk reflects the likelihood of either asthma exacerbations, progressive decline in lung function or reduced lung growth, or risk of medication-related adverse effects (Tables 20-2 to 20-4). Nighttime symptoms are a particularly important marker of more severe and uncontrolled disease.[4] Awareness of symptom underrecognition and underreporting as common problems in pediatric asthma should reinforce the importance of accurate assessments of asthma symptomatology before determination of asthma severity and control.

Table 20-1
ASTHMA PREDICTIVE INDEX CRITERIA*

Major Criteria	Minor Criteria
Physician-diagnosed parental asthma	Physician-diagnosed allergic rhinitis
Physician-diagnosed eczema	Wheezing apart from colds
	Blood eosinophilia (≥4%)

*For a positive Asthma Predictive Index, the child must have frequent wheezing during the first 3 years of life and one of the two major criteria or two of the minor critieria. Adapted from Castro-Rodriguez JA, Holberg CJ, Wright AL, Martinez FD: A clinical index to define risk of asthma in young children with recurrent wheezing. Am J Respir Crit Care Med 2000;162(4 Pt 1):1403–1406.

Current guidelines include lung function (FEV_1 [forced expiratory volume in 1 second], FEV_1/FVC [FEV_1 to forced vital capacity ratio]) and peak expiratory flow (PEF) criteria to guide severity classification among children 5 years of age and older. Since most children with asthma have FEV_1 percent predicted values in the normal range,[5,6] lung function criteria should be used cautiously for assigning asthma severity in children. Rather, symptom frequency and medication use (both controllers and relievers) may be more sensitive indicators of disease state, and should be the main determinants in classifying a patient's disease severity.

Determination of a level of asthma *severity*, the intrinsic intensity of the disease process, is recommended for patients

Table 20-2
CLASSIFICATION OF ASTHMA SEVERITY (0–4 YEARS OF AGE)

Components of Severity		Intermittent	Persistent — Mild	Persistent — Moderate	Persistent — Severe
Impairment	Symptoms Nighttime awakenings	≤2 days/week 0	>2 days/week but not daily 1–2×/month	Daily 3–4×/month	Throughout the day >1×/week
	Short-acting beta₂-agonist use for symptom control	≤2 days/week	>2 days/week but not daily	Daily	Several times per day
	Interference with normal activity	None	Minor limitation	Some limitation	Extremely limited
Risk	Exacerbations (consider frequency and severity)	0–1/year	≥2 exacerbations in 6 months requiring oral steroids, or ≥ 4 wheezing episodes/1 year lasting > 1 day AND risk factors for persistent asthma		

Frequency and severity may fluctuate over time
Exacerbations of any severity may occur in patients in any severity category

Table 20-3
CLASSIFICATION OF ASTHMA SEVERITY (5–11 YEARS OF AGE)

Components of Severity		Intermittent	Persistent — Mild	Persistent — Moderate	Persistent — Severe
Impairment	Symptoms	≤2 days/week	>2 days/week but not daily	Daily	Throughout the day
	Nighttime awakenings	0	1–2×/month	3–4×/month	>1×/week
	Short-acting beta₂-agonist use for symptom control	≤2 days/week	>2 days/week but not daily	Daily	Several times per day
	Interference with normal activity	None	Minor limitation	Some limitation	Extremely limited
	Lung function	• Normal FEV_1 between exacerbations • FEV_1 > 80% predicted • FEV_1/FVC > 85%	• FEV_1 > 80% predicted • FEV_1/FVC > 80%	• FEV_1 60%-80% predicted • FEV_1/FVC = 75%–80%	• FEV_1 < 60% predicted • FEV_1/FVC < 75%
Risk	Exacerbations (consider frequency and severity)	0–2/year	>2 exacerbations in 1 year		

Frequency and severity may fluctuate over time.
Exacerbations of any severity may occur in patients in any severity category

Table 20-4
CLASSIFICATION OF ASTHMA SEVERITY (≥12 YEARS OF AGE AND ADULTS)

		CLASSIFICATION OF ASTHMA SEVERITY (YOUTHS ≥ 12 YEARS OF AGE AND ADULTS)			
			Persistent		
Components of Severity		**Intermittent**	***Mild***	***Moderate***	***Severe***
	Symptoms	≤2 days/week	>2 days/week but not daily	Daily	Throughout the day
	Nighttime awakenings	≤2×/month	3–4×/month	>1×/week, but not nightly	Often > 7×/week
	Short-acting beta$_2$-agonist use for symptom control	≤2 days/week	>2 days/week but not daily	Daily	Several times per day
Impairment Normal FEV$_1$/FVC	Interference with normal activity	None	Minor limitation	Some limitation	Extremely limited
	Lung function	• Normal FEV$_1$ between exacerbations • FEV$_1$ > 80% predicted • FEV$_1$/FVC normal	• FEV$_1$ < 80% predicted • FEV$_1$/FVC normal	• FEV$_1$ >60% but <80% predicted • FEV$_1$/FVC reduced 5%	• FEV$_1$ < 60% predicted • FEV$_1$/FVC reduced > 5%
Risk	Exacerbations (consider frequency and severity)			0–2/year	>2 exacerbations in 1 year
		Frequency and severity may fluctuate over time. Exacerbations of any severity may occur in patients in any severity category			

not receiving long-term controller therapy, while the level of asthma symptom *control*, an indicator of the degree to which asthma activity is minimized and the goals of therapy achieved, is central in tailoring and optimizing treatment regimens. The goals of asthma therapy (Table 20-5) are to achieve well-controlled status as defined in Tables 20-6 to 20-8. Furthermore, asthma control in children 12 years or older may be assessed using validated control questionnaires. Failure to achieve these targets indicates uncontrolled asthma and suggests a reassessment of diagnosis, medication adherence, environmental controls, and current treatment regimen.

Table 20-5
GOALS OF ASTHMA THERAPY

Reducing Impairment
Prevent chronic and troublesome symptoms (e.g., coughing or breathlessness in the daytime, in the night, or after exertion)
Require infrequent use (≤2 days a week) of short-acting beta$_2$-agonist for quick relief of symptoms (not including prevention of exercise-induced bronchospasm)
Maintain (near) normal pulmonary function
Maintain normal activity levels (inducing exercise and other physical activity and attendance at work or school)
Meet patients' and families' expectations of and satisfaction with care
Reducing Risk
Prevent loss of lung function; for children, prevent reduced lung growth
Prevent recurrent exacerbations of asthma and minimize the need for emergency department visits or hospitalizations
Minimal or no adverse effects of therapy

Adapted from National Asthma Education and Prevention Program: Full Report of the Expert Panel: Guidelines for the diagnosis and management of asthma (EPR-3) (Publication no. TBD). Bethesda, MD, U.S. Department of Health and Human Services, 2007.

APPROACH TO MANAGEMENT

Determination of the appropriate level of asthma severity and control guides the assignment of therapeutic options. While pharmacological interventions are an integral element of management, successful asthma management requires interventions addressing the many factors that contribute to asthma. Environmental control measures may allow for reduction in exposure to allergens and environmental tobacco smoke. Identification and appropriate treatment of the comorbid medical conditions that often complicate asthma are essential, including sinusitis, gastroesophageal reflux, and psychosocial factors. Finally, achieving optimal asthma management demands active understanding and participation of the patient and his or her caregivers, emphasizing the importance of patient and caregiver education and support.

ASTHMA PHARMACOTHERAPY: GOALS OF ASTHMA MANAGEMENT

Excellent asthma control is attainable by the majority of patients with the appropriate combination of therapeutic agents and interventions.[7] However, patients and families often have low expectations in terms of the degree of asthma control that is achievable. Thus, it is incumbent upon health care providers to establish and discuss treatment goals with the family at the outset and continually readdress these goals at follow-up visits. The NAEPP Guidelines provide a set of goals of therapy, focusing on reducing symptoms and, thus quick-reliever medication use (see Table 20-5). If these goals are not being achieved, a reassessment and modification of the treatment approach should be undertaken.

The widespread recognition of asthma as an inflammatory condition has shifted the focus of asthma therapy from the relief of bronchoconstriction to the reduction of airway

Table 20-6
CLASSIFICATION OF ASTHMA CONTROL (0–4 YEARS OF AGE)

Components of Control		CLASSIFICATION OF ASTHMA CONTROL (CHILDREN 0–4 YEARS OF AGE)		
		Well Controlled	Not Well Controlled	Very Poorly Controlled
Impairment	Symptoms	≤2 days/week	>2 days/week	Throughout the day
	Nighttime awakenings	≤1/month	>1×/month	>1×/week
	Interference with normal activity	None	Some limitation	Extremely limited
	Short-acting beta$_2$-agonist use for symptom control	≤2 days/week	>2 days/week	Several times per day
Risk	Exacerbations (consider frequency and severity)	0–1/year	2–3/year	>3/year
	Treatment-related adverse effects	Medication side effects can vary in intensity from none to very troublesome and worrisome. The level of intensity does not correlate to specific levels of control but should be considered in the overall assessment of risk.		

Table 20-7
CLASSIFICATION OF ASTHMA CONTROL (5–11 YEARS OF AGE)

Components of Control		CLASSIFICATION OF ASTHMA CONTROL (CHILDREN 5–11 YEARS OF AGE)		
		Well Controlled	Not Well Controlled	Very Poorly Controlled
Impairment	Symptoms	≤2 days/week but not more than once each day	>2 days/week or multiple times on ≤2 days/week	Throughout the day
	Nighttime awakenings	≤1/month	≥2×/month	≥2×/week
	Interference with normal activity	None	Some limitation	Extremely limited
	Short-acting beta$_2$-agonist use for symptom control	≤2 days/week	>2 days/week	Several times per day
	Lung function			
	● FEV$_1$ or peak flow	>80% predicted/personal best	60%–80% predicted/personal best	<60% predicted/personal best
	● FEV$_1$/FVC	>80%	75%-80%	<75%
Risk	Exacerbations (consider frequency and severity)	0–1/year	≥2 year	≥2 year
	Reduction in lung growth	Evaluation requires long-term follow-up		
	Treatment-related adverse effects	Medication side effects can vary in intensity from none to very troublesome and worrisome. The level of intensity does not correlate to specific levels of control but should be considered in the overall assessment of risk.		

Table 20-8
CLASSIFICATION OF ASTHMA CONTROL (≥12 YEARS OF AGE AND ADULTS)

Components of Control		CLASSIFICATION OF ASTHMA CONTROL (YOUTHS ≥ 12 YEARS OF AGE AND ADULTS)		
		Well Controlled	Not Well Controlled	Very Poorly Controlled
Impairment	Symptoms	≤2 days/week	>2 days/week	Throughout the day
	Nighttime awakenings	≤2/month	1–3/week	≥4×/week
	Interference with normal activity	None	Some limitation	Extremely limited
	Short-acting beta$_2$-agonist use for symptom control	≤2 days/week	>2 days/week	Several times per day
	FEV$_1$ or peak flow	>80% predicted/personal best	60%-80% predicted/personal best	<60% predicted/personal best
	Validated questionnaires			
	● ATAQ	0	1–2	3–4
	● ACQ	≤0.75	≥1.5	N/A
	● ACT	≥20	16–19	≤15
	Exacerbations (consider frequency and severity)	0–1/year	≥2 year	≥2 year
Risk	Progressive loss of lung function	Evaluation requires long-term follow-up		
	Treatment-related adverse effects	Medication side effects can vary in intensity from none to very troublesome and worrisome. The level of intensity does not correlate to specific levels of control but should be considered in the overall assessment of risk.		

inflammation to prevent asthma symptoms and possibly disease progression. This paradigm has driven the current management approach, which includes two general categories of medications: those that provide quick symptom relief and those that confer long-term disease control. Most controller medications target the underlying persistent inflammation, while quick reliever medications treat acute symptoms and exacerbations.

CONTROLLER THERAPY FOR PERSISTENT ASTHMA IN CHILDREN

The current asthma treatment paradigm follows a stepwise approach toward achieving asthma symptom control. The initial assessment of asthma severity determines the initial choice of controller medication regimens (Table 20-9), such that children with mild persistent asthma would begin with step 2 therapy, while those with moderate persistent asthma would begin with step 3 or 4 therapy, and those with severe persistent disease would begin with step 5 or 6 therapy (Tables 20-10 to 20-12). Following initiation of therapy, the level of symptom control determines if modifications to the asthma medication regimen are warranted—a reduction in medications if asthma is well controlled or an augmentation of therapy if control is inadequate. This approach is referred

to as "step down" for a reduction in therapy, and "step up" for increases in therapy. If asthma is well control, current treatment can be continued, or if asthma has been well controlled for at least 3 months, a step down can be undertaken. In contrast, inadequate symptom control should prompt consideration of several factors before a step up in therapy is undertaken. Special attention should focus on adherence to the medication regimen as well as the interaction between the patient and the medication delivery device ([MDI] with or without holding chamber, dry powder inhaler, or nebulizer), as improper inhaler technique reduces medication delivery to the airways, thus reducing efficacy. Consideration of conditions that often complicate or coexist with asthma, including gastroesophageal reflux and rhinosinusitis, should occur before augmentation of asthma therapy. If consideration of these factors yields no other explanation for the lack of symptom control, a step up in therapy may be indicated.

INHALED CORTICOSTEROIDS

Inhaled corticosteroids (ICSs) form the cornerstone of long-term controller therapy. Studies in both children and adults have firmly established that ICS therapy results in significant improvement in asthma control as reflected by reductions in asthma symptoms, exacerbation rates, hospitalizations,

---

Table 20-9
INITIAL STEP THERAPY BY LEVEL OF ASTHMA

	CLASSIFICATION OF ASTHMA SEVERITY			
		Persistent		
	Intermittent	*Mild*	*Moderate*	*Severe*
Lowest level of treatment required to maintain control	Step 1	Step 2	Step 3 or 4	Step 5 or 6

Table 20-10
STEPWISE APPROACH FOR MANAGING ASTHMA IN CHILDREN 0–4 YEARS OF AGE

Intermittent Asthma	Persistent Asthma: Daily Medication					
Consult with asthma specialist if step 3 care or higher is required. Consider consultation at step 2.						
Step 1 Preferred: SABA PRN	Step 2 Preferred: Low-dose ICS Alternative: Montelukast or cromolyn	Step 3 Preferred: Medium-dose ICS	Step 4 Preferred: Medium-dose ICS and either: Montelukast or LABA	Step 5 Preferred: High-dose ICS and either Montelukast or LABA	Step 6 Preferred: High-dose ICS and either: Montelukast or LABA Oral corticosteroids	Step up if needed (first, check adherence and environmental control) Assess control Step down if possible (and asthma is well controlled at least 3 months)
		Patient education and environmental control at each step				

Quick relief medications for all patients
- SABA as needed for symptoms. Intensity of treatment depends on severity of symptoms.
- With viral respiratory infections: SABA every 4–6 hours up to 24 hours (longer with physician consult). Consider short course of systemic corticosteroids if exacerbation is severe or patient has history of severe exacerbations.
- Caution: Frequent use of SABA may indicate need to step up treatment.

LABA, long-acting beta agonist; SABA, short-acting beta agonist.

Table 20-11
STEPWISE APPROACH FOR MANAGING ASTHMA IN CHILDREN 5–11 YEARS OF AGE

Intermittent Asthma	Persistent Asthma: Daily Medication					
Consult with asthma specialist if step 4 care or higher is required. Consider consultation at step 3.						
Step 1 Preferred: SABA PRN	Step 2 Preferred: Low-dose ICS Alternative: LTRA, cromolyn, nedocromil, or theophylline	Step 3 Preferred: Medium-dose ICS OR Low-dose ICS + either LABA, LTRA, or theophylline	Step 4 Preferred: Medium-dose ICS + LABA Alternative: Medium-dose ICS + either LTRA or theophylline	Step 5 Preferred: High-dose ICS + LABA Alternative: High-dose ICS + either LTRA or theophylline	Step 6 Preferred: High-dose ICS + LABA + oral corticosteroid Alternative: High-dose ICS + either LTRA or theophylline + oral corticosteroid	Step up if needed (first, check adherence and environmental control) Assess control Step down if possible (and asthma is well controlled at least 3 months)
			Patient education and environmental control at each step			

Quick relief medications for all patients

- SABA as needed for symptoms. Intensity of treatment depends on severity of symptoms. Up to 3 treatments at 20-minute intervals as needed. Short course of systemic corticosteroids may be needed.
- Caution: Increasing use of beta-agonist, or use > 2 times/week for symptom control (not prevention of EIB) indicates inadequate control and the need to step up treatment.

asthma death, and improved quality of life. In addition, ICSs reduce airway inflammation, as reflected by reductions in airway hyperreactivity[8] and markers of inflammation including exhaled nitric oxide.[9] The Childhood Asthma Management Program (CAMP) trial is the longest prospective randomized trial confirming the efficacy of ICS in childhood asthma. This trial treated 1041 children 5 to 12 years of age with mild to moderate asthma with either placebo, inhaled nedocromil (a nonsteroidal agent), or inhaled budesonide (an ICS, 400 μg/day) daily for 4 to 6 years.[8] As compared with children who received placebo, the children treated with ICSs had significant improvements in airway hyperresponsiveness, fewer asthma symptoms, less albuterol use, longer times until an asthma exacerbation requiring oral corticosteroids, fewer courses of oral corticosteroids, fewer urgent care visits and hospitalizations, and less need for supplemental ICSs because of poor asthma control. The efficacy of ICSs has been established in children as young as 6 months in terms

Table 20-12
STEPWISE APPROACH FOR MANAGING ASTHMA IN YOUTHS ≥ 12 YEARS OF AGE AND ADULTS

Intermittent Asthma	Persistent Asthma: Daily Medication					
Consult with asthma specialist if step 4 care or higher is required. Consider consultation at step 3.						
Step 1 Preferred: SABA PRN	Step 2 Preferred: Low-dose ICS Alternative: Cromolyn, nedocromil, LTRA, or theophylline	Step 3 Preferred: Medium-dose ICS OR Low-dose ICS + LABA Alternative: Low-dose ICS + either LTRA, theophylline, or zileuton	Step 4 Preferred: Medium-dose ICS + LABA Alternative: Medium-dose ICS + either LTRA, theophylline, or zileuton	Step 5 Preferred: High-dose ICS + LABA AND Omalizumab may be considered for patients who have allergies	Step 6 Preferred: High-dose ICS + LABA + oral corticosteroid AND Omalizumab may be considered for patients who have allergies	Step up if needed (first, check adherence and environmental control) Assess control Step down if possible (and asthma is well controlled at least 3 months)
			Patient education and environmental control at each step			

Quick relief medications for all patients

- SABA as needed for symptoms. Intensity of treatment depends on severity of symptoms. Up to 3 treatments at 20-minute intervals as needed. Short course of systemic corticosteroids may be needed.
- Caution: Increasing use of beta-agonist, or use > 2 times/week for symptom control (not prevention of EIB) indicates inadequate control and the need to step up treatment.

of symptom control and rescue bronchodilator use,[10,11] along with improvements in lung function[12] and reductions in an indicator of airway inflammation, exhaled nitric oxide.[13]

The optimal timing for the initiation of ICS therapy remains unclear. An early nonrandomized study by Agertoft and Pedersen suggested that the magnitude of effect of ICSs on lung function (FEV_1) was inversely related to the duration of asthma before initiation of ICSs.[14] However, large trials of continuous ICS therapy[8,15] have failed to demonstrate that early intervention with ICSs alters the natural course of asthma. The Childhood Asthma Management Program (CAMP) trial did not detect a progressive decline in pulmonary function on average,[8] although there were subgroups of children who did experience declines in lung growth.[16] Among patients with mild asthma of less than 2 years' duration, the Inhaled Steroid Treatment as Regular Therapy in Early Asthma (START) trial demonstrated that ICS therapy (budesonide 200 to 400 µg/day) for 3 years resulted in significantly fewer courses of systemic corticosteroids and more symptom-free days compared to treatment with placebo.[17] In an attempt at earlier intervention, the Prevention of Early Asthma in Kids (PEAK) trial examined the effects of continuous ICS therapy among preschool children (2 and 3 years of age) with recurrent wheezing at risk for asthma based on the presence of a positive, modified API consisting of frequent wheezing (at least four episodes in the prior year) and either *one major risk factor* (parental history of asthma, personal history of atopic dermatitis, or aeroallergen sensitization) *or two minor risk factors* (eosinophilia 4% or more, wheezing without colds, or allergic sensitization to food).[15] This trial demonstrated that ICS treatment (fluticasone propionate 176 µg/day) in children with positive asthma predictive indices for 2 years resulted in a significantly greater proportion of episode-free days and lower exacerbation rate compared with placebo, but did not alter the proportion of episode-free days during the year following discontinuation of ICS therapy. Thus, continuous ICS therapy has been convincingly demonstrated to be effective in improving asthma control across a variety of phenotypes of childhood asthma—those with mild persistent disease of recent onset (START),[17] those with mild-moderate persistent asthma with a mean duration of asthma of 5 years (CAMP),[8] children with moderate-severe asthma,[18,19] and among preschool children with recurrent wheezing and risk factors for subsequent asthma (PEAK).[15] However, these beneficial effects occur only while therapy is given, with no substantial evidence indicating long-term disease-modifying effects.

Despite the clear and substantial clinical benefits associated with ICS use, concern over their potential side effects continues to limit their use. In general, ICSs are well tolerated, but potential side effects of ICSs include effects on skeletal growth and bone density, alteration of the hypothalamic-pituitary-adrenal (HPA) axis, and local side effects (i.e., oral candidiasis and hoarseness). Several clinical trials have noted small decreases in growth initially with ICS therapy (approximately 1 cm over 1 year),[8,15,17] although at least one study suggests that final adult height is not affected.[20] Other indicators of ICS safety are evident from the CAMP trial, with no evidence of HPA axis suppression[21] or alterations in bone mineral density[8] with continued use of low-dose ICSs. It should be noted, however, that the excellent safety

data for ICSs has been demonstrated with the use of low-moderate doses. The side-effect profile of higher-dose ICS therapy in children with asthma is less clear, with some evidence for extrapulmonary corticosteroid effects including clinically relevant adrenal insufficiency,[22] reinforcing the importance of continually attempting to reach the lowest ICS dose that provides appropriate asthma control.

Evidence from multiple sources supports the conclusion that the significant benefits of ICS therapy far outweigh the minimal risks associated with their use.[23] When coupled with the substantial morbidity and mortality associated with undertreated asthma this evidence forms the basis for the recommendation of ICSs as first-line controller therapy in all patients with persistent asthma.

LEUKOTRIENE MODIFIERS (LTMs)

The cysteinyl leukotrienes ($LTC_4/LTD_4/LTE_4$) are capable of mediating many of the pathophysiologic processes involved in asthma, including bronchoconstriction, mucus secretion, and increased vascular permeability. LTMs act by either inhibiting leukotriene synthesis by the enzyme 5-lipoxygenase (zileuton) or by antagonizing the binding of leukotrienes to the leukotriene receptor 1 (montelukast, zafirlukast).[24] LTMs are effective in reducing asthma symptoms and, to a lesser extent, in improving lung function,[25,26] bronchial hyperresponsiveness,[27] and air-trapping.[28] Furthermore, montelukast exerts a protective effect in the setting of exercise-induced bronchospasm.[29]

Comparative trials between ICSs and LTMs have demonstrated greater improvements in lung function and/or symptom reduction with ICSs over LTMs in children[30-34] and adults.[35-37] A 1-year comparison between low-dose ICSs and montelukast demonstrated that ICS therapy was associated with significantly greater asthma control and improvements in pulmonary function.[34] A recent crossover trial demonstrated that children experience greater improvements in lung function and other indicators of asthma control with ICS therapy than with LTM if they have lower levels of lung function or high levels of markers of allergic inflammation (exhaled nitric oxide levels or greater airway hyperresponsiveness),[30,31] suggesting that ICSs are preferred over LTM in children with these features. However, age younger than 10 and urinary LTE_4 levels higher than 100 pg/mg were associated with at least a 7.5% improvement in FEV_1 while receiving montelukast over an 8-week period, but were not associated with comparable improvements while receiving ICSs, further emphasizing the significant heterogeneity in response to asthma therapies. Based on their overall efficacy relative to ICSs LTM agents are considered as an alternative to ICSs as monotherapy in mild persistent asthma.

CROMOLYN AND NEDOCROMIL

Cromolyn and nedocromil are nonsteroidal agents that are well tolerated and exert modest anti-inflammatory activity through unknown mechanisms. They are less potent and less effective than ICSs,[8] and may be considered as alternatives to ICSs in children with mild persistent asthma. When given before exercise, both of these agents effectively prevent exercise-induced asthma, and may be used with or without short-acting beta-agonists in this setting.

MANAGEMENT APPROACHES TO PATIENTS WITH ASTHMA INADEQUATELY CONTROLLED WITH INHALED CORTICOSTEROIDS

Patients who do not achieve acceptable asthma control with ICS therapy alone require an escalation of therapy in efforts to achieve good asthma control. Multiple interventions have been examined for patients inadequately controlled with ICSs, including an increase in the dosage of ICSs or the addition of a second controller medication, such as a long-acting beta-agonist, LTM, or theophylline. While these approaches have been well studied in adults, there is a relative paucity of evidence in children to help guide decision making.

Increasing the Dose of Inhaled Corticosteroid

The effects of increasing doses of ICS on the two domains of asthma severity and control, namely impairment and risk, are variable and at least partly dependent on patient age and disease severity. Among children younger than 5, some trials demonstrate a dose-dependent effect of budesonide inhalation suspension on both impairment or risk domains, while others have not.[38] A recent systematic literature review concluded that while there are insufficient data to determine the dose-response of fluticasone in children at doses in excess of 400 μg/day, there was evidence of additional efficacy at higher doses among children with severe asthma,[39] albeit with concomitant adrenal suppression. Thus, while ICS therapy appears to experience a plateauing of effect in terms of reducing impairment with increasing doses, children with greater degrees of asthma impairment may benefit from increasing doses of ICS.

Addition of a Leukotriene Modifier

In addition to their potential use as monotherapy for asthma, the addition of LTM to patients who are uncontrolled on an ICS alone has been shown to produce modest improvement in PEF (but not FEV$_1$), and reduce both rescue albuterol use and percent of exacerbation days.[40] Thus, LTMs may be considered as an adjunct to ICS therapy in patients with more severe or uncontrolled asthma.

Addition of a Long-Acting Beta-Agonist (LABA)

Numerous clinical trials in adult asthma patients whose symptoms remain uncontrolled on low-dose ICS monotherapy have demonstrated that the addition of a LABA to low-dose ICS is superior to doubling the ICS dose[41,42] in terms of lung function and other indicators of asthma control, including exacerbations. The addition of LABA permitted a reduction in ICS dose among adults with asthma.[43] No data are available to judge the efficacy of LABAs in children younger than 4, and little data exist in children older than 4 to determine the efficacy of LABAs when added to ICSs. The addition of salmeterol or formoterol to children with symptomatic asthma despite ICS therapy resulted in significant improvement in morning peak expiratory flow,[44,45] although these interventions were not compared to an increased dose of ICS. The addition of the LABA formoterol to ICS among children with uncontrolled asthma resulted in improvements in lung function, but no advantage in terms of rescue medication use,[46] and in one trial, formoterol use was associated with an increased risk of asthma-related hospitalization.[47] No trial has demonstrated a reduction in asthma exacerbations when a LABA is added to an ICS in children.[48] Only one trial has compared the addition of LABA to an increased dose of ICS among children still symptomatic despite ICS therapy.[49] A total of 177 children (6 to 16 years of age), already treated with ICSs, were randomized in a double-blind parallel study to all receive the ICS beclomethasone dipropionate (BDP) 200 μg twice daily and in addition, either the LABA salmeterol 50 μg twice daily, or an additional 200 μg of BDP twice daily (total BDP dose of 800 μg/day), or placebo (total BDP dose of 400 μg/day). No significant differences between groups were found in FEV$_1$, airway hyperresponsiveness, symptom scores, and exacerbation rates after 1 year. The addition of salmeterol resulted in slightly higher PEF in the first months of treatment. A more recent trial examined the relative efficacies of three treatment approaches in 285 children 6 to 14 years of age with mild-moderate persistent asthma[1]: fluticasone propionate 100 μg twice daily,[2] fluticasone proprionate 100 μg once daily plus salmeterol 50 μg twice daily,[4] and montelukast 5 mg once daily.[34] The proportion of asthma control days over the 1-year trial was comparable between the fluticasone and fluticasone plus salmeterol group, and both groups were superior to the montelukast group. However, the fluticasone group experienced significantly greater improvements in lung function than the group receiving half the dose of fluticasone in addition to salmeterol and the montelukast group. While the addition of LABA to ICSs provides greater clinical improvement than an increased dose of ICS among asthmatic adults inadequately controlled on ICSs alone, children with asthma may or may not respond similarly to adults. Further research is clearly necessary to determine the appropriate use of LABAs in children with uncontrolled asthma.

Addition of Theophylline

Theophylline has been available for the treatment of asthma for more than 50 years. Theophylline use is associated with improvement in pulmonary function and asthma symptoms through unknown mechanisms.[50] Currently, theophylline is suggested for use in combination with other agents (particularly ICSs) in moderate to severe persistent asthma,[51] and is particularly effective in those patients with significant nocturnal symptoms. Theophylline is not recommended in young children because of erratic metabolism induced by intercurrent viral illnesses and fever.

The relative efficacies of these therapeutic strategies among children inadequately controlled on ICSs alone are unknown. However, among adults with asthma under suboptimal control with low-dose ICS therapy alone, the addition of a long-acting beta-agonist to a low-dose ICS has been demonstrated to provide greater improvement in asthma control than the addition of montelukast to ICS therapy.[52]

SPECIFIC IMMUNOTHERAPY

The role of specific immunotherapy in the management of childhood asthma remains unclear. Two meta-analyses have concluded that specific immunotherapy is effective in the management of selected patients with allergic asthma,[53,54] particularly those with sensitization to a single allergen. In contrast, a large placebo-controlled trial evaluating the efficacy of multiallergen immunotherapy for 2 years in asthmatic children did not demonstrate a benefit among children receiving appropriate medical treatment for asthma.[55] A recent trial demonstrated that immunotherapy in monosensitized children with seasonal allergic rhinitis without asthma may prevent the subsequent development of asthma,[56] suggesting that immunotherapy may allow for asthma prevention in children with sensitization to inhalant allergens.

ANTI-IgE THERAPY

Recognition of the high rate of allergic sensitization among patients, particularly children, with asthma led to the development of a humanized monoclonal antibody directed against IgE (anti-IgE or omalizumab), which effectively, rapidly, and significantly reduces circulating levels of IgE. Repeated subcutaneous administration of omalizumab has been demonstrated to be safe[57] and effective in permitting reduction of ICS dosing while preventing asthma exacerbations in placebo-controlled trials in both adults[58,59] and children[60] with moderate-severe persistent allergic asthma receiving ICSs, along with improvement in asthma-related quality of life.[61] Omalizumab is currently approved as an adjunctive therapy for children 12 years and older with moderate-severe persistent allergic asthma whose symptoms are inadequately controlled with ICS therapy.

QUICK-RELIEVER MEDICATIONS

Beta₂-Adrenergic Agonists

Rapid-acting inhaled beta$_2$-adrenergic receptor agonists provide the most effective bronchodilation currently available and serve as the preferred treatment for acute symptoms and exacerbations of asthma as well as the prevention of exercise-induced asthma. Several different beta$_2$-agonists are currently available, and have comparable efficacy and safety properties. The single isomer preparation of albuterol, levalbuterol, has the theoretical advantage of possessing bronchodilatory properties (R-isomer of albuterol) without the presence of the nonbronchodilatory isomer (S-albuterol). Clinical trials with levalbuterol demonstrate minimal clinically relevant differences in bronchodilation or side effects related to beta-adrenergic receptor stimulation, such as tachycardia, tremor, and decreases in serum potassium levels compared to racemic albuterol.[62]

Anticholinergic Agents

The parasympathetic nervous system provides substantial control of airway tone in health and disease. Potential mechanisms by which cholinergic pathways contribute to asthma pathophysiology include bronchoconstriction through increased vagal tone, increased reflex bronchoconstriction due to stimulation of airway sensory receptors, and increased acetylcholine release induced by inflammatory mediators.[63] Patients with asthma experience lesser degrees of bronchodilation with anticholinergic agents (such as atropine and ipratropium bromide) than with beta-agonists. There is presently no indication for anticholinergic agents as a component for long-term asthma control. Evidence supports the use of ipratropium bromide in conjunction with inhaled beta-agonists in the emergency department during acute exacerbations of

asthma in children,[64,65] as the addition of ipratropium has been shown to decrease rates of hospitalization[64] and duration of time in the emergency department.[65] This effect is most evident in patients with very severe exacerbations.

Systemic Corticosteroids

Systemic corticosteroids are considered quick-reliever medications based on their utility in moderate to severe acute exacerbations of asthma. Short courses of systemic corticosteroids may also aid in gaining rapid control of asthma symptoms in patients under poor control. The onset of effect of corticosteroids is more rapid than would be expected by their primary mechanisms of action, including the inhibition of inflammatory cell function and secretion of pro-inflammatory mediators. The rapid up-regulation of beta$_2$-adrenoreceptor number and improved receptor function contributes to the clinical improvements noted within 4 hours of administration.

Systemic corticosteroids accelerate the resolution of acute exacerbations of asthma, and emergency department administration of corticosteroids decreases asthma admission rates[66] and shortens duration of hospitalization. Dosing recommendations for acute asthma range from 1 to 2 mg/kg of body weight per day of prednisone. There is no significant difference in the efficacy of oral or parenteral corticosteroids in acute asthma,[67] unless the child is unable to tolerate oral medications because of vomiting.

Rare patients with severe asthma may require regular corticosteroid therapy (daily or alternate-day dosing) to gain or maintain disease control. Chronic systemic corticosteroid use in severe asthma may be accompanied by hypertension, cushingoid features, decreased morning serum cortisol levels, osteopenia, growth suppression, obesity, hypercholesterolemia, and cataracts.[68] Clinically significant HPA axis suppression does not occur following short bursts of systemic corticosteroids for acute exacerbations of asthma, and tapering of dose is not required with courses of less than 10 to 14 days.

MONITORING AND REASSESSMENT

Continuous monitoring and reassessment are essential in determining the degree of asthma control achieved with a treatment regimen. Several tools aid in monitoring asthma control, including the assessment of symptom frequency and severity using validated questionnaires (Asthma Control Test,[69] Asthma Control Questionnaire[70]) rescue medication use, and home peak flow monitoring.

Serial examinations of pulmonary function are an integral component of asthma monitoring. Effective asthma therapy should lead to an improvement in, and ideally normalization of, FEV$_1$ and FEV$_1$/FVC ratio. Furthermore, in the patient who responds inadequately to asthma therapy, spirometry can detect the presence of other complicating factors such as vocal cord dysfunction. Recent research has suggested that the incorporation of serial measurements of airway inflammation, such as levels of nitric oxide in exhaled air, may allow for titration of ICS dosing as well as improvements in airway hyperresponsiveness[71] and possible identification of patients who would experience a decline in asthma control with a reduction in ICS dosing.[72] Thus, advances in monitoring asthma activity, including measures of symptom frequency, lung function, and noninvasive markers of airway inflammation, will hopefully translate to greater asthma control.

Assessing asthma symptom control, frequency, activity limitation, and school absences are integral components of every asthma visit. Frequency of rescue albuterol use and how long a canister of albuterol lasts (200 actuations = 100 doses) are surrogate indicators of asthma control. Exploring if any changes in the clinical course occur when the patient misses a dose (or several doses) of medications often provides valuable insight into disease activity. These questions, along with a recent (2- to 4-week) history of short-acting beta-agonist use, systemic corticosteroid use, emergency department visits, and hospitalizations provide a complete picture of the patient's current asthma status.

CONCLUSION

Childhood asthma management is highly effective in achieving asthma control, and maximal success occurs in the setting of an active partnership among the clinician, caregiver, and patient in pursuit of the goals of asthma therapy.

REFERENCES

1. Busse WW, Lemanske RF Jr: Asthma. N Engl J Med 2001;344(5):350–362.
2. Castro-Rodriguez JA, Holberg CJ, Wright AL, Martinez FD: A clinical index to define risk of asthma in young children with recurrent wheezing. Am J Respir Crit Care Med 2000; 162(4 Pt 1):1403–1406.
3. National Asthma Education and Prevention Program: Full Report of the Expert Panel: Guidelines for the diagnosis and management of asthma (EPR-3) (Publication No. TBD). Bethesda, MD, U.S. Department of Health and Human Services, 2007.
4. Strunk RC, Sternberg A, Bacharier LB, Szefler S, Group CAMPR: Nocturnal awakening due to asthma in children with mild to moderate asthma in the Childhood Asthma Management Program. J Allergy Clin Immunol 2002;110:395–403.
5. Bacharier LB, Strunk RC, Mauger D, et al: Classifying asthma severity in children: mismatch between symptoms, medication use, and lung function. Am J Respir Crit Care Med 2004;170(4):426–432.
6. Paull K, Covar R, Jain N, et al: Do NHLBI lung function criteria apply to children? A cross-sectional evaluation of childhood asthma at National Jewish Medical and Research Center, 1999–2002. Pediatr Pulmonol 2005;39(4):311–317.
7. Bateman ED, Boushey HA, Bousquet J, et al: Can guideline-defined asthma control be achieved? The Gaining Optimal Asthma Control study. Am J Respir Crit Care Med 2004;170(8):836–844.
8. Childhood Asthma Management Program: Long-term effects of budesonide or nedocromil in children with asthma. N Engl J Med 2000;343(15):1054–1063.
9. Covar RA, Szefler SJ, Martin RJ, et al: Relations between exhaled nitric oxide and measures of disease activity among children with mild-to-moderate asthma. J Pediatr 2003;142(5):469–475.
10. Baker J, Mellon M, Wald J, et al: A multiple-dosing, placebo-controlled study of budesonide inhalation suspension given once or twice daily for treatment of persistent asthma in young children and infants. Pediatrics 1999;103:414–421.
11. Kemp JP, Skoner DP, Szefler SJ, et al: Once-daily budesonide inhalation suspension for the treatment of persistent asthma in infants and young children. Ann Allergy Asthma Immunol 1999;83(3):231–239.
12. Teper AM, Kofman CD, Szulman GA, et al: Fluticasone improves pulmonary function in children under 2 years old with risk factors for asthma. Am J Respir Crit Care Med 2005;171(6):587–590. [Epub 2004 Dec 10.]
13. Moeller A, Franklin P, Hall GL, et al: Inhaled fluticasone dipropionate decreases levels of nitric oxide in recurrently wheezy infants. Pediatr Pulmonol 2004;38(3):250–255.
14. Agertoft L, Pedersen S: Effects of long-term treatment with an inhaled corticosteroid on growth and pulmonary function in asthmatic children. Respir Med 1994;88:373–381.
15. Guilbert TW, Morgan WJ, Zeiger RS, et al: Long-term inhaled corticosteroids in preschool children at high risk for asthma. N Engl J Med 2006;354(19):1985–1997.
16. Covar RA, Spahn JD, Murphy JR, Szefler SJ: Progression of asthma measured by lung function in the Childhood Asthma Management Program. Am J Respir Crit Care Med 2004;170(3):234–241.
17. Pauwels RA, Pedersen S, Busse WW, et al: Early intervention with budesonide in mild persistent asthma: a randomised, double-blind trial. Lancet 2003;361(9363):1071–1076.
18. Ferguson AC, Spier S, Manjra A, et al: Efficacy and safety of high-dose inhaled steroids in children with asthma: a comparison of fluticasone propionate with budesonide. J Pediatr 1999;134(4):422–427.
19. Shapiro G, Bronsky EA, LaForce CF, et al: Dose-related efficacy of budesonide administered via a dry powder inhaler in the treatment of children with moderate to severe persistent asthma. J Pediatr 1998;132(6):976–982.
20. Agertoft L, Pedersen S: Effect of long-term treatment with inhaled budesonide on adult height in children with asthma. N Engl J Med 2000;343(15):1064–1069.
21. Bacharier LB, Raissy HH, Wilson L, et al: Long-term effect of budesonide on hypothalamic-pituitary-adrenal axis function in children with mild to moderate asthma. Pediatrics 2004;113(6):1693–1699.
22. Todd GR, Acerini CL, Ross-Russell R, et al: Survey of adrenal crisis associated with inhaled corticosteroids in the United Kingdom. Arch Dis Child 2002;87(6):457–461.
23. Kelly HW: Potential adverse effects of the inhaled corticosteroids. J Allergy Clin Immunol 2003;112(3):469–478; quiz 479.
24. Drazen JM, Israel E, O'Byrne PM: Treatment of asthma with drugs modifying the leukotriene pathway. N Engl J Med 1999;340(3):197–206.
25. Knorr B, Franchi LM, Bisgaard H, et al: Montelukast, a leukotriene receptor antagonist, for the treatment of persistent asthma in children aged 2 to 5 years. Pediatrics 2001;108(3):E48.
26. Knorr B, Matz J, Bernstein JA, et al: Montelukast for chronic asthma in 6- to 14-year-old children: a randomized, double-blind trial. Pediatric Montelukast Study Group. JAMA 1998;279(15):1181–1186.
27. Hakim F, Vilozni D, Adler A, et al: The effect of montelukast on bronchial hyperreactivity in preschool children. Chest 2007;131(1):180–186.
28. Spahn JD, Covar RA, Jain N, et al: Effect of montelukast on peripheral airflow obstruction in children with asthma. Ann Allergy Asthma Immunol 2006;96(4):541–549.
29. Kemp JP, Dockhorn RJ, Shapiro GG, et al: Montelukast once daily inhibits exercise-induced bronchoconstriction in 6- to 14-year-old children with asthma. J Pediatr 1998;133(3):424–428.
30. Szefler SJ, Phillips BR, Martinez FD, et al: Characterization of within-subject responses to fluticasone and montelukast in childhood asthma. J Allergy Clin Immunol 2005;115(2):233–242.
31. Zeiger RS, Szefler SJ, Phillips BR, et al: Response profiles to fluticasone and montelukast in mild-to-moderate persistent childhood asthma. J Allergy Clin Immunol 2006;117(1):45–52.

32. Garcia Garcia ML, Wahn U, Gilles L, et al: Montelukast, compared with fluticasone, for control of asthma among 6- to 14-year-old patients with mild asthma: the MOSAIC study. Pediatrics 2005;116(2):360–369.

33. Ostrom NK, Decotiis BA, Lincourt WR, et al: Comparative efficacy and safety of low-dose fluticasone propionate and montelukast in children with persistent asthma. J Pediatr 2005;147(2):213–220.

34. Sorkness CA, Lemanske RF Jr, Mauger DT, et al: Long-term comparison of 3 controller regimens for mild-moderate persistent childhood asthma: The Pediatric Asthma Controller Trial. J Allergy Clin Immunol 2007;119(1):64–72.

35. Busse W, Raphael GD, Galant S, et al: Low-dose fluticasone propionate compared with montelukast for first-line treatment of persistent asthma: a randomized clinical trial. J Allergy Clin Immunol 2001;107(3):461–468.

36. Zeiger RS, Bird SR, Kaplan MS, et al: Short-term and long-term asthma control in patients with mild persistent asthma receiving montelukast or fluticasone: a randomized controlled trial. Am J Med 2005;118(6):649–657.

37. Ducharme FM: Inhaled glucocorticoids versus leukotriene receptor antagonists as single agent asthma treatment: systematic review of current evidence. BMJ 2003;326(7390):621.

38. Szefler SJ, Eigen H: Budesonide inhalation suspension: a nebulized corticosteroid for persistent asthma. J Allergy Clin Immunol 2002;109(4):730–742.

39. Masoli M, Weatherall M, Holt S, Beasley R: Systematic review of the dose-response relation of inhaled fluticasone propionate. Arch Dis Child 2004;89(10):902–907.

40. Simons FE, Villa JR, Lee BW, et al: Montelukast added to budesonide in children with persistent asthma: a randomized, double-blind, crossover study. J Pediatr 2001;138(5):694–698.

41. Greening AP, Ind PW, Northfield M, Shaw G: Added salmeterol versus higher-dose corticosteroid in asthma patients with symptoms on existing inhaled corticosteroid. Allen & Hanburys Limited UK Study Group. Lancet 1994;344(8917):219–224.

42. Shrewsbury S, Pyke S, Britton M: Meta-analysis of increased dose of inhaled steroid or addition of salmeterol in symptomatic asthma (MIASMA). BMJ 2000;320(7246):1368–1373.

43. Lemanske RF Jr, Sorkness CA, Mauger EA, et al: Inhaled corticosteroid reduction and elimination in patients with persistent asthma receiving salmeterol: a randomized controlled trial. JAMA 2001;285(20):2594–2603.

44. Russell G, Williams DA, Weller P, Price JF: Salmeterol xinafoate in children on high dose inhaled steroids. Ann Allergy Asthma Immunol 1995;75(5):423–428.

45. Zimmerman B, D'Urzo A, Berube D: Efficacy and safety of formoterol Turbuhaler when added to inhaled corticosteroid treatment in children with asthma. Pediatr Pulmonol 2004;37(2):122–127.

46. Tal A, Simon G, Vermeulen JH, et al: Budesonide/formoterol in a single inhaler versus inhaled corticosteroids alone in the treatment of asthma. Pediatr Pulmonol 2002;34(5):342–350.

47. Bensch G, Berger WE, Blokhin BM, et al: One-year efficacy and safety of inhaled formoterol dry powder in children with persistent asthma. Ann Allergy Asthma Immunol 2002;89(2):180–190.

48. Bisgaard H: Effect of long-acting beta$_2$ agonists on exacerbation rates of asthma in children. Pediatr Pulmonol 2003;36(5):391–398.

49. Verberne A, Frost C, Roorda R, et al: One year treatment with salmeterol compared with beclomethasone in children with asthma. Am J Respir Crit Care Med 1997;156:688–695.

50. Weinberger M, Hendeles L: Theophylline in asthma. N Engl J Med 1996;334(21):1380–1388.

51. Evans DJ, Taylor DA, Zetterstrom O, et al: A comparison of low-dose inhaled budesonide plus theophylline and high-dose inhaled budesonide for moderate asthma. N Engl J Med 1997;337(20):1412–1418.

52. Nelson HS, Busse WW, Kerwin E, et al: Fluticasone propionate/salmeterol combination provides more effective asthma control than low-dose inhaled corticosteroid plus montelukast. J Allergy Clin Immunol 2000;106(6):1088–1095.

53. Abramson MJ, Puy RM, Weiner JM: Allergen immunotherapy for asthma. Cochrane Database Syst Rev 2003;(4):CD001186.

54. Ross RN, Nelson HS, Finegold I: Effectiveness of specific immunotherapy in the treatment of asthma: a meta-analysis of prospective, randomized, double-blind, placebo-controlled studies. Clin Ther 2000;22(3):329–341.

55. Adkinson NF Jr., Eggleston PA, Eney D, et al: A controlled trial of immunotherapy for asthma in allergic children. N Engl J Med 1997;336(5):324–331.

56. Moller C, Dreborg S, Ferdousi HA, et al: Pollen immunotherapy reduces the development of asthma in children with seasonal rhinoconjunctivitis (the PAT-study). J Allergy Clin Immunol 2002;109(2):251–256.

57. Berger W, Gupta N, McAlary M, Fowler-Taylor A: Evaluation of long-term safety of the anti-IgE antibody, omalizumab, in children with allergic asthma. Ann Allergy Asthma Immunol 2003;91(2):182–188.

58. Soler M, Matz J, Townley R, et al: The anti-IgE antibody omalizumab reduces exacerbations and steroid requirement in allergic asthmatics. Eur Respir J 2001;18(2):254–261.

59. Busse W, Corren J, Lanier BQ, et al: Omalizumab, anti-IgE recombinant humanized monoclonal antibody, for the treatment of severe allergic asthma. J Allergy Clin Immunol 2001;108(2):184–190.

60. Milgrom H, Berger W, Nayak A, et al: Treatment of childhood asthma with anti-immunoglobulin E antibody (omalizumab). Pediatrics 2001;108(2):E36.

61. Lemanske RF Jr, Nayak A, McAlary M, et al: Omalizumab improves asthma-related quality of life in children with allergic asthma. Pediatrics 2002;110(5):e55.

62. Gawchik SM, Saccar CL, Noonan M, et al: The safety and efficacy of nebulized levalbuterol compared with racemic albuterol and placebo in the treatment of asthma in pediatric patients. J Allergy Clin Immunol 1999;103(4):615–621.

63. Martinati LC, Boner AL: Anticholinergic antimuscarinic agents in the treatment of airways bronchoconstriction in children. Allergy 1996;51(1):2–7.

64. Qureshi F, Pestian J, Davis P, Zaritsky A: Effect of nebulized ipratropium on the hospitalization rates of children with asthma. N Engl J Med 1998;339(15):1030–1035.

65. Zorc JJ, Pusic MV, Ogborn CJ, et al: Ipratropium bromide added to asthma treatment in the pediatric emergency department. Pediatrics 1999;103(4 Pt 1):748–752.

66. Scarfone RJ, Fuchs SM, Nager AL, Shane SA: Controlled trial of oral prednisone in the emergency department treatment of children with acute asthma. Pediatrics 1993;92(4):513–518.

67. Becker JM, Arora A, Scarfone RJ, et al: Oral versus intravenous corticosteroids in children hospitalized with asthma. J Allergy Clin Immunol 1999;103(4):586–590.

68. Covar RA, Leung DY, McCormick D, et al: Risk factors associated with glucocorticoid-induced adverse effects in children with severe asthma. J Allergy Clin Immunol 2000;106(4):651–659.

69. Nathan RA, Sorkness CA, Kosinski M, et al: Development of the asthma control test: a survey for assessing asthma control. J Allergy Clin Immunol 2004;113(1):59–65.

70. Juniper EF, O'Byrne PM, Guyatt GH, et al: Development and validation of a questionnaire to measure asthma control. Eur Respir J 1999;14(4):902–907.

71. Pijnenburg MW, Bakker EM, Hop WC, De Jongste JC: Titrating steroids on exhaled nitric oxide in asthmatic children: a randomized controlled trial. Am J Respir Crit Care Med 2005:172(7):831–836.

72. Zacharasiewicz A, Wilson N, Lex C, et al: Clinical use of noninvasive measurements of airway inflammation in steroid reduction in children. Am J Respir Crit Care Med 2005;171(10):1077–1082.

Management of Persistent Asthma in Adults

Rodolfo M. Pascual and Stephen P. Peters

CLINICAL PEARLS

- Asthma is characterized by heterogeneity with respect to pathogenesis, severity, symptoms, and response to therapy.

- Patients with risk factors for fatal and near-fatal asthma must be identified and targeted for intensive monitoring and treatment.

- Patients with low lung function or recent asthma exacerbations are at increased risk for future exacerbations and death.

- Inhaled corticosteroids are the most efficacious drugs for persistent asthma and should be the first-line choice in all cases.

- Efficacy translates into effectiveness only when the provider ensures that barriers to the implementation of treatments are removed.

Persistent asthma may be defined as asthma causing symptoms that occur more than twice per week, or asthma that is associated with exacerbations that affect activity, or asthma that is accompanied by nocturnal symptoms occurring more than twice per month; often these characteristics coexist in the same patient. It cannot be overstated that improved asthma management strategies significantly reduce morbidity and reduce mortality. Furthermore, improved asthma control can be achieved in many patients with currently poorly controlled asthma. Somewhat sobering, though, are the observations that most asthmatic patients currently have poor asthma control, and that a significant minority remain poorly controlled, even after rigorous protocols designed to optimize control are used in a controlled trial setting.[1] Certainly, much needs to be done to improve the tools used to treat asthma. Herein we discuss the use of various strategies to identify and modify disease factors with a goal of improving the overall care of the asthma patient.

HETEROGENEITY

There is substantial heterogeneity in asthma with respect to symptoms, underlying pathophysiology, disease natural history, response to therapy, and ability to self-manage that requires flexibility on the part of the provider when designing care. Appreciating the heterogeneity of asthma is crucial when designing a care plan, as it is important to avoid a "one size fits all" approach. For example, with respect to pathophysiology, some asthmatic individuals have complete reversibility of airflow obstruction when treated with beta-adrenergic agonists whereas others do not, indicating interpatient heterogeneity with respect to response to medication. The same patient

who usually demonstrates full reversibility when asymptomatic may not respond as well to medication when experiencing an exacerbation, thus demonstrating intrapatient heterogeneity in response to therapy. In fact, acute resistance to medication therapy is characteristic of exacerbations of asthma. As another example, many asthmatic individuals are atopic, tending to respond to relatively low doses of inhaled steroids or to reductions in antigen exposure while others are nonatopic in whom disease is relatively resistant to corticosteroids.

Some patients with asthma have a good understanding of the inflammatory nature of their disease and command of the proper use of controllers and reliever medications; such patients use self-management plans or written action plans quite effectively. Other patients cannot recall the names of their medications, or how they should be used even with repeated reinforcement; these patients often cannot use written action plans. Finally, the natural history of asthma in many patients waxes and wanes over time so that periods of poor control and greater severity can be interspersed with periods of better control and less severity. To conclude, the heterogeneity of asthma requires a flexible and pragmatic approach that uses frequent reassessment of the current state of the disease and appropriate adjustments of therapy.

EFFECTIVENESS VERSUS EFFICACY

Asthma is a chronic inflammatory disorder causing intermittent symptoms that require some patient self-management. Moreover, most controller and reliever medications are typically inhaled leading to variability in medication effectiveness because of variability in inhaler technique. "Effectiveness concerns the results achieved in the actual practice of healthcare with typical patients and providers, in contrast to efficacy, which is assessed by the benefits achieved under ideal conditions."[2] For providers caring for asthma patients this is an important concept to understand. Efficacy is basically established in the ideal situations created in clinical trials wherein patients are carefully selected and taught how to use their medications and compliance is maximized. Such an ideal cannot be achieved in real practice; however, we will discuss methods that can be instituted in the management of asthma that will enhance the effectiveness of treatment. First, it is important to understand the barriers patients face that prevent them from best using the tools given to them by their physicians. These are listed in Table 21-1.

SEVERITY VERSUS IMPAIRMENT AND RISK

All of the key published asthma management guidelines have emphasized the stratification of asthma based on

Table 21-1
BARRIERS THAT REDUCE THE EFFECTIVENESS OF ASTHMA MANAGEMENT

Barrier	Solution
Poor inhaler technique	Demonstrate proper technique at initial visit, assess and reinforce at each visit, use spacers whenever possible
Inhaler cost	Assist with finding financial resources, use cheaper alternatives
Failure to understand when asthma control worsens based on symptoms	Teach patient to use brief asthma control measurement tools like the Asthma Control Questionnaire or Asthma Control Test, teach use of peak flow meter
Poor environmental control	Reassess environment whenever asthma control worsens, assess for tobacco use or secondhand smoke exposure
General noncompliance	Assess for patient understanding of the role of each treatment, provide written instructions
Frequent use of urgent care or emergency services	Ensure that controllers are available and used appropriately, provide ready access to primary provider via urgent visits when possible, use written action plans when appropriate

severity.[3,4] The newest guidelines recommend defining severity by both the domains of *impairment* (frequency and intensity of daytime or nocturnal symptoms and the extent to which symptoms cause functional limitation) and *risk* (likelihood of exacerbations or progressive loss of lung function).[3] Interestingly, both of these domains correlate with the degree of airflow obstruction (forced expiratory volume in 1 second [FEV_1]). The severity is most easily ascertained in the untreated patient. When medications are already in use, the severity estimate must be adjusted based on the amount of current medication used. For example, a patient with symptoms less than daily and FEV_1 70% predicted while taking medium-dose inhaled corticosteroids (ICSs) is different from one with the same pattern of symptoms and FEV_1 who is dependent on oral steroids. The former has moderate disease while the latter has severe asthma. Generally speaking, a patient with severe asthma suffers from frequent symptoms, excessive use of rescue medications, significant reductions in activity, and severe airflow obstruction. That being said, clinical experience tells us that many asthmatic individuals do not "fit the mold." Some asthmatic individuals with severe airflow obstruction have a relatively stable pattern of symptoms and infrequent rescue medication use that may span years. Still others usually have less severe airflow obstruction but on occasion rapidly develop life-threatening airflow obstruction; this asthma phenotype has been well described but remains poorly understood. Some of the risks associated with asthma that might not necessarily correlate well with current severity include death, severe exacerbations, progressive impairment because of progressive loss of lung function over time, and toxicity from medications. Thus, rather than relying solely on current severity, the provider should also estimate the short- and long-term risk based on each of these factors and adjust therapy accordingly. Once severity has been initially

estimated, the focus shifts during follow-up toward assessing asthma *control*. Poorly controlled asthma requires a step-up in therapy, whereas well-controlled asthma may allow for a step-down in therapy.

SYMPTOM-BASED STRATEGY

Asthma is characterized by heterogeneity in that there is substantial interpatient variability with respect to symptoms. For example, some patients experience intermittent and paroxysmal chest tightness and wheeze, whereas others mainly have a bothersome cough. Moreover, there is only a modest correlation between symptom severity and the degree of baseline airflow obstruction. Importantly, a subgroup of patients seem to poorly sense worsening airflow obstruction; in other words, they do not recognize an exacerbation until it is advanced or even life-threatening. Finally, it is known that some patients have relatively labile disease in that they may have relatively long symptom-free periods interspersed with episodes of severe or even life-threatening airflow obstruction contrasted with those patients who have more continuous symptoms. The pros and cons of managing asthma on a symptom-based strategy are listed in Table 21-2.

For practical purposes, what patients really care about are their symptoms and the effect that these symptoms have on their overall quality of life. Thus, a major advantage to a symptom-based treatment strategy is that it automatically validates the patient's experiences and if symptoms are effectively addressed, patient satisfaction is likely to be high. Types of symptoms present can be elicited with straightforward interview techniques but truly ascertaining the importance of symptoms to the patient can prove to be more challenging. Questionnaires that are thoughtfully constructed can be used to gather valuable information about symptoms that a patient is currently experiencing and also place the current burden of asthma in a historical context. It is important to know how severe current asthma is compared to asthma in the patient's past but also to understand what treatments have been used, how effective they were, and what side effects were experienced. Initial data can be obtained by a questionnaire that can be self-administered or data can be gathered by structured interview; the interviewer can be a trained

Table 21-2
MANAGING PERSISTENT ASTHMA USING A SYMPTOM-BASED STRATEGY

Pros	Cons
Addressing symptoms improves satisfaction	Symptoms correlate poorly with degree of airflow obstruction
Simple	Some asthma patients exhibit a blunted perception of dyspnea
Straightforward data gathering	Measurements lack precision
Improving symptoms improves quality of life	Data are subjective and what is experienced varies substantially patient to patient
Providing clues about concurrent conditions	Symptoms correlate poorly with disease risk
Empowering patient	Symptoms overlap with other diseases
	Requires substantial patient education

"physician-extender." Ultimately, the quality of the data gathered will be limited by the instruments used, the skill of the interviewer, and the motivation and recall of the patient.

If a symptom-based program is used, care must be taken to identify all relevant symptoms and the severity or burden of these symptoms. The caregiver should focus on addressing the symptoms with consideration given to those that are most important to the patient. Moreover, it must be appreciated that some symptoms may be manifestations of other diseases that may or may not be life-threatening. Symptom management is a dynamic process and once the important symptoms are identified they should be addressed in turn. Fortunately, it generally holds that as airway inflammation and bronchial constriction are successfully treated, all symptoms will abate albeit to varying extents. If there appear to be one or more symptoms that are particularly refractory while others improve, alternative mechanisms should be considered. For example, if cough and intermittent chest tightness were initially prominent and the chest tightness has resolved but the cough persists, then other causes of cough like concurrent rhinitis, sinusitis, or gastroesophageal reflux disease (GERD) are considered. Identifying alternative mechanisms has the advantage of allowing for successful treatment of symptoms without overmedicating for asthma per se, improving patient satisfaction and minimizing medication side effects.

Wheezing is a common symptom of asthma especially in the young and is difficult to quantify because the loudness of wheezing does not correlate with the degree of airflow obstruction. It is more helpful to know what triggers wheeze in a given patient and to determine what alleviates it. It is important to differentiate wheeze from stridor; to the patient, a similar sound and sensation but actually a sign of upper airway obstruction often misdiagnosed as asthma and not likely to respond well to bronchodilators. Usually wheezing is absent between attacks of asthma and the patient should be educated that persistent wheezing especially when dyspnea and fatigue are present can be a sign of trouble. Unfortunately, in a small subgroup of more severe asthmatic individuals, exertional wheezing can be continuous even when the patient is relatively well. Besides reliever medications, the patient can be taught to relieve wheezing by resting and slowing down respiratory frequency if possible. Paroxysms of wheezing at night may be signs of GERD or congestive heart failure and these diagnoses should be entertained when wheezing persists when other symptoms improve or if nocturnal wheezing is particularly prominent.

Breathlessness or chest tightness associated with bronchial constriction is usually episodic in nature and if associated with exertion, often is self-limiting not requiring inhaler dosing. In the case of exertional chest tightness, the patient should be encouraged to reduce the level of activity, rest if needed, and remain calm. A reliever medication can be used and the patient should feel relief within several minutes. If a particular activity frequently triggers chest tightness, the patient can be encouraged to use a short-acting relief inhaler as prophylaxis. Typically a short-acting beta-agonist (two puffs) is used 15 to 30 minutes before exposure to a given trigger is expected. Moreover, if the persistent asthma patient is frequently exposed to a given trigger (e.g., daily exercise) a long-acting beta-agonist or a leukotriene antagonist can be employed even if asthma severity otherwise would not require one of these add-on medications. Importantly, chest tightness exacerbated by exertion and relieved with rest, particularly if not associated with cough, might represent angina; this possibility may need to be excluded depending on the overall risk assessment. Although chest tightness associated with asthma often will worsen when exercise is halted, this finding, in and of itself, is not sufficient to exclude angina.

Cough is common in asthma and in some patients it is the dominant symptom. Most patients can tell when cough becomes more frequent because it disrupts sleep and social activities. Whereas cough usually improves when bronchodilation and airway inflammation improve, in some patients it remains a vexing problem. This is because other common comorbidities like rhinitis, sinusitis, and GERD frequently cause cough in their own right. Recognition and specific treatment of these problems early on will lead to speedier improvement and greater patient satisfaction. Careful assessment and judiciously using diagnostic tools with high test specificity and sequential trials of therapy are suggested rather than a shotgun approach or empiric trials because of the cost of medications and increased side effects. It has been our experience that patients on multiple medications will not take them as often as indicated. Because of the cost factor, for many patients it is important to focus on using those therapies that have the most impact. For example, consider that the cost of a proton-pump inhibitor may preclude daily ICS use when both medications cannot be afforded. When we strongly suspect GERD as a cofactor, that is, when there is associated pyrosis or sour brash, we will empirically treat with a proton-pump inhibitor while at the same time recommending a gastroenterology consultation. Additionally, it is important for the patient to know that medication does not stop reflux but only acid irritation. We also discuss strategies to ameliorate reflux including wearing loose-fitting bed clothes, avoiding caffeine and alcohol, and avoiding large meals or those close to bedtime. We suggest that the patient elevate the head of the bed. When allergic rhinitis is a cofactor, topical nasal steroids or leukotriene modifiers are indicated. One or the other should be tried empirically and only continued if they reduce cough. It is our experience that the response to these agents when treating cough is highly variable and sometimes related to the current seasonal allergen pattern. This means that they should only be continued if they have a meaningful effect on cough and should not necessarily be continued when not needed during a "nonallergic" season.

Similar to cough, exertional dyspnea can be a challenging symptom because of common comorbid conditions like congestive heart failure (CHF), obesity, and muscular deconditioning. In the asthmatic individual, unless asthma is severe, exertional dyspnea should be episodic and related to the presence of airflow obstruction and accompanied by other symptoms like wheezing or chest tightness. Consistent exertional dyspnea is a clue that other conditions may be present. The severity of exertional dyspnea during specific tasks can be assessed by using various validated scales like the Modified Borg Scale or Visual Analog Scale. More simply, asking which common tasks (activities of daily living, stair climbing, walking) cause dyspnea provides useful information about the degree of functional impairment. It is also important to determine, on a clinical basis, the impact that each comorbid condition has on dyspnea. Interestingly, obesity is associated with more severe asthma and some studies suggest that weight loss will ameliorate asthma symptoms and dyspnea in obese patients with asthma. At the very least, simple counseling about weight loss should occur at each visit, although multidisciplinary weight-loss programs are more effective and should be used when available. The diagnosis of CHF is usually straightforward, especially when clinical risk factors are present and should be considered when physical exam signs are present. Although very severe asthma can cause cor pulmonale, that situation is probably the exception, as most patients with asthma and cor pulmonale have other concomitant causes of CHF. Muscular deconditioning is invariably present in patients who have sedentary jobs and lifestyles and usually should be treated with a regular exercise program instituted in a graded fashion with frequent assessment for response. A 6-minute walk test done after a bronchodilator is administered can be used to measure exercise capacity. Cardiopulmonary exercise testing can also be useful as a diagnostic tool in selected patients to determine if other conditions are contributing to exertional dyspnea. Exercise testing may be used also to assess the response to therapy especially in athletic patients who are interested in the effect of asthma treatment on the performance of work.

Nocturnal symptoms are very important to many asthmatic individuals and their bed partners. The diurnal variability of asthma is well described and most guidelines and experts use the presence or frequency of nocturnal symptoms as a measure of asthma control. Sleep disruption leads to excessive daytime somnolence, poor performance of daytime activities, and lower quality-of-life scores. Besides intensifying steroid therapy, the use of long-acting beta-agonists or administering theophylline or leukotriene modifiers at bedtime sometimes is helpful when nocturnal symptoms are especially prominent. Assessing and modifying allergen exposure in the atopic asthmatic individual (i.e., reducing dust mites and pet residence in the patient bedroom) may also be helpful. Finally, whether it is because GERD affects asthma or asthma makes GERD worse, the fact that GERD tends to be worse at night means that it should be sought and treated in the patient with nocturnal asthma symptoms.

PULMONARY FUNCTION–BASED STRATEGY

The severity of airflow obstruction (FEV_1) correlates with both impairment and risk in the asthma patient and patients with lower FEV_1 are more likely to suffer severe exacerbations over time.[5] Basing asthma management on changes in pulmonary function offers several potential advantages. First, the measurement of symptoms is imprecise in that there is substantial interpatient variability and also a degree of intrapatient variability. In contrast, spirometry performed on a trained patient by a trained technician is highly precise. A significant change in spirometry is much more likely to signify a real change in the patient's asthma than a change in symptoms. Furthermore, changes in spirometry generally track with changes in airway inflammation, symptoms, quality of life, and exercise capacity. Importantly, until recently, improvement in spirometry was the principal criterion used to determine if an asthma drug was efficacious and hence approved by the Food and Drug Administration. It has been well established that there is heterogeneity of asthma in

Table 21-3 MANAGING PERSISTENT ASTHMA USING A PFT-BASED STRATEGY	
Pros	**Cons**
Spirometry and Peak Flow Meters	
Sensitivity—pulmonary function test changes often occur earlier than symptom changes	May lead to overtreatment
	Additional costs
Measurements easily used in self-management plans	
Spirometry	
Accurate	Requires visit in most cases, although portable home spirometry is becoming available
Precise	
Standardized	
	Requires more training of staff and patient
Peak Flow Meter	
Portable	Multiple measurements required to establish baseline
Simple	
Easier technique	More dependent on effort

response to medications. Spirometry can be used as a tool to determine if a prescribed drug has a measurable effect in a given patient. It can be readily used to determine if a given treatment is improving asthma control. Finally, spirometry provides a rational means to stratify asthma based on severity. The principle of stratification based on severity forms the basis for most current asthma management guidelines. Importantly, daily monitoring for worsening obstruction is especially useful in asthma patients with a blunted "perception of dyspnea," a well-described phenomenon associated with fatal and near-fatal asthma attacks. Hence, we would assert that worsening airflow obstruction is always worrisome even if it occurs without a worsening of symptoms because of the well-described phenomenon; in such patients pulmonary function monitoring can be life saving. Peak flow meters are most commonly used and can be used effectively to assess asthma control. Peak expiratory flow (PEF) variability is minimized and remains close to baseline when asthma is under control. PEF meters can also be used to assess drug efficacy; in fact, several important clinical trials have used improvements in morning peak flow as a primary therapeutic outcome measure.

There are few disadvantages to using pulmonary function to manage asthma and these are mainly related to cost and technical issues (see Table 21-3). However, the widely held assumption that the degree of asthma severity equates with the degree of airflow obstruction is probably not valid. Thus, pulmonary function measurements are not used in isolation but are used in conjunction with a careful assessment of current and future risk based on clinical features including current medication requirements, exacerbation history, the degree of physical impairment, and psychosocial factors that modify risk. While some degree of correlation between airflow obstruction and asthma severity exists in most patients, airflow obstruction usually tracks very well with symptoms and, particularly, impairment.

INFLAMMATORY MARKER–BASED STRATEGY

There are several lines of evidence suggesting that measuring inflammatory markers and using them to make treatment decisions may improve asthma outcomes. First, it is known

Table 21-4
MANAGING PERSISTENT ASTHMA USING NONINVASIVE MARKERS OF INFLAMMATION

Marker	Pros	Cons
Airway hyperresponsiveness	Shown to reduce exacerbations May alter airway remodeling	Lengthy, complex, hence costly test
Exhaled nitric oxide	May allow for steroid reductions	No effect on exacerbation rate
Induced sputum eosinophils count	Reduced exacerbation rates	No effect on quality of life, symptoms, or lung function

that active airway inflammation is present in asthmatic individuals even when no symptoms are present and that this inflammation can be modified using corticosteroids. A number of techniques have been assessed in research settings (Table 21-4) but few have been validated in a prospective manner, thus most remain unavailable for routine clinical use.

Airway hyperresponsiveness is felt to be a marker of airway inflammation and also may be a marker of asthma control. Sont and colleagues in a prospective trial using airway hyperresponsiveness as an adjunctive measure to guide steroid dosing demonstrated reductions in exacerbation rates and reductions in reticular basement thickness when compared to a conventional spirometry approach.[6] Although this is a promising strategy, a simpler, cheaper approach will need to be designed for it to be applied widely in clinical settings.

Exhaled nitric oxide (eNO) levels appear to track well with eosinophilic airway inflammation, are sensitive to steroid therapy, and the technique is reproducible and well tolerated. Unfortunately, studies so far have failed to demonstrate that the use of adjunctive eNO in management strategies reduces exacerbation rates. The technique needs further refinement before it can be recommended for routine use in clinical settings.

Using induced sputum eosinophils counts was shown by Green and colleagues[7] to be a management strategy that can reduce exacerbation rates when compared with a conventional guideline-based strategy. However, in this study there were no differences in lung function, symptoms, or quality of life between the groups. We assert that an exacerbation is a very important outcome making this a promising finding; however, the technical aspects and cost of this test have prevented it from being widely used to date.

OUR RECOMMENDED APPROACH

Guidelines should be integrated into the overall asthma management plan since they have been developed by experts and are evidence based. However, the plan should be tailored to the needs of the individual patient and periodically adjusted because asthma severity will vary over time. Herein we will discuss the following components of asthma management: initial management, continuing management, and the management of acute exacerbations. The suggested pharmacologic regimen is shown in Figure 21-1.

Once the diagnosis has been established, initial management (Table 21-5) includes an assessment of current severity, current symptom control, the prior asthma history,

comorbid conditions, risk factors for asthma exacerbations or fatal asthma (Table 21-6), and an educational process that empowers the patient to comanage his or her asthma whenever possible. Current severity is best determined by combining measurements of lung function with a clinical assessment of control based on symptoms and rescue medication usage. Several useful, validated questionnaires exist that can be used to gauge asthma control including the Asthma Control Questionnaire (ACQ)[8] or the brief Asthma Control Test (ACT) (www.asthmacontrol.com). Recent data from several studies indicate that exacerbations are a very important clinical factor. Data from the TENOR study group shows that recent severe asthma exacerbations or an exacerbation requiring a hospitalization or emergency department visit was a powerful indicator of future severe exacerbations.[9] Furthermore, the use of a recent steroid burst was also a powerful predictor of future severe exacerbations. These data are consistent with several other reports in the literature. Hence, efforts should focus on detecting and arresting exacerbations at an early stage.

Because of the advantages discussed above and the limitation of relying solely on symptoms and medication use, we strongly advocate that baseline spirometry be performed. Monitoring pulmonary function is a more sensitive way to detect exacerbations than symptoms so the patient should be provided with a hand-held spirometer (preferred) or peak flow device and instructed in its use. If peak flow measures are to be used they should be obtained each morning upon awakening and charted for 2 weeks to establish the initial baseline. Because of its inherent precision, once the patient has a spirometer and adequate technique is demonstrated the initial baseline is established. When asthma therapy is felt to be optimized and control maximized in the individual patient, a new "personal best" baseline FEV_1 or PEF should be established and should be used as the benchmark for guiding treatment. Since we all experience loss of lung function normally over time, the goal should be to maintain the FEV_1 percent predicted rather than trying to maintain the absolute volume. Furthermore, maintaining as high an FEV_1 percent predicted as possible as a goal needs to be balanced against the risks imposed by medication toxicity. For example, high-dose prednisone use resulting in obesity in an asthmatic individual will have deleterious effects that might outweigh the generally modest reductions in airflow obstruction.

The best evidence currently available suggests that corticosteroids reduce the risk of death in asthma and should be used in all patients with persistent asthma as shown in Figure 21-1. The corollary in preventing death or serious exacerbation is best accomplished by using adequate doses of steroids. The fact that combination therapy often reduces the dose of steroids needed to reduce the risk of exacerbation does not diminish the central role that steroids play in asthma management. So which is the best steroid to give? Clearly, most patients do not need oral steroids on a daily basis and in most patients properly titrated inhaled steroids provide similar reductions in exacerbations, improvements in lung function, and symptoms. However, some patients cannot afford ICSs and will not take them on a consistent basis. So the best steroid is the one the patient will take on a regular basis, which sometimes means low-dose daily oral steroids. Nevertheless, if an ICS can be used as directed instead of oral prednisone

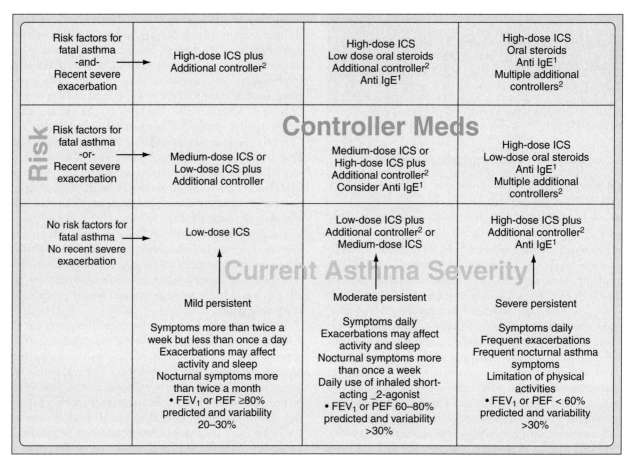

Figure 21-1 Suggested controller medications based on current asthma severity with additional risk modification. To determine recommended therapy first determine current severity then adjust by the appropriate risk modifiers.
[1]Anti-IgE indicated only for atopic asthma; consider cost, should be continued only if it allows for steroid reduction or provides clinically meaningful improvement.
[2]Additional controllers include long-acting beta-agonists, leukotriene modifiers, sustained-release theophylline, cromones, tiotropium.

the ICS is preferred because of its superior side-effect profile. So the principle of maximizing efficacy while minimizing side effects applies, although effectiveness trumps efficacy in clinical practice and steroids are most effective if they are taken consistently. Hence, it is crucial to improve adherence

and this starts with frequent assessment. Another instance where low-dose oral steroids should be considered is when a patient with severe disease suffers frequent exacerbations in spite of taking high-dose ICS or combination therapy; such exacerbations are usually treated with high-dose steroids for 1 or 2 weeks. In this instance, the total steroid use over time and the net effect on the frequency of exacerbations should be taken into account.

Initial education is crucial to improve adherence with asthma monitoring, including self-assessment of symptoms and lung function, and the medication prescription. The patient should understand that daily monitoring can detect exacerbations at an earlier stage when they are more readily treated. Consistency is a key to improving adherence so daily monitoring is recommended. Proper use of inhalers requires personalized attention because of the variety of delivery devices and variable patient ability. Spacers should generally be used with pressurized metered-dose inhalers (MDI). Written asthma action plans should include a brief list of therapeutic goals, instructions for usual medications, and a protocol to intensify management when an exacerbation is detected. Exacerbations are best detected using a method that can detect changes in lung function or symptoms. The plan may use a simple system that stratifies the severity of the exacerbation. The patient should be given clear and explicit instructions about how to deal with each level of severity

Table 21-5
THE INITIAL MANAGEMENT OF PERSISTENT ASTHMA

1. Measure FEV_1 and bronchodilator reversibility
   a. Provide the patient with a device to measure lung function
2. Assess for current severity using a published guideline or Figure 21-1
   a. Adjust severity according to current medication use
   b. Include a risk assessment for exacerbations or potential fatal asthma
   c. Measure impairment
3. Depending on severity, use oral or inhaled glucocorticoids per guidelines
   a. Recent instability: use higher doses
   b. Has risk factor(s) for fatal asthma: use higher doses
4. Provide a rescue inhaler or nebulizer if appropriate
5. Teach proper inhaler technique
6. Provide information and assess understanding of:
   a. Importance of medication adherence in relation to airway inflammation versus symptoms alone
   b. Understanding when asthma is worsening
7. For higher risk, moderate, or severe asthma provide a written action plan; consider written action plans for mild disease
8. Schedule follow-up within a short period of time (2 to 6 weeks) and thereafter follow up frequently until good control is achieved (every 2 to 4 months)

Table 21-6
RISK FACTORS ASSOCIATED WITH FATAL OR NEAR-FATAL ASTHMA

Risk Factor	Comment or Modification
Previous intubation for asthma	Powerful risk factor, consider alternative diagnosis if other findings and lung function inconsistent with moderate-severe asthma
Previous ICU care for asthma	Powerful risk factor
Previous hospitalization for asthma	
Excessive use of asthma medications Beta-agonists Theophylline Glucocorticoids	Carefully assess use of bronchodilators at each visit, intensify anti-inflammatory treatment when appropriate
Severe asthma, low FEV_1	Especially oral steroid-dependent asthma
Frequent emergency department visits for asthma	Not a consistent risk factor Strive to improve adherence Improve outpatient health care access
Labile pulmonary function	High degree of acute reversibility or Large changes in FEV_1 or PEF with exacerbations
Psychosocial factors	Poverty and lack of health care access Psychiatric disease that reduces adherence

Table 21-7
CONTINUING MANAGEMENT OF PERSISTENT ASTHMA NOT IN ACUTE EXACERBATION

1. Measure lung function at each visit, assess patient's technique measuring his or her own lung function
2. Assess asthma control at each visit: symptom frequency, impairment, medication use.
3. Determine if exacerbations have occurred and how they were treated if others are comanaging asthma
4. Determine adherence to the treatment plan at every visit
5. Adjust medications based on current control; step down or step up treatment as appropriate
6. Reinforce correct use of each medication and inhaler technique
7. Review action plans
8. When higher doses of ICS or any oral steroids appear to be needed for control, use combination therapy
   a. Long-acting beta-agonists
   b. Leukotriene modifiers
   c. Theophylline
   d. Omalizumab
9. Control comorbid conditions
   a. Sinusitis or rhinitis
   b. GERD
10. Schedule follow-up interval based on current and prior severity

and should be strongly encouraged to seek medical attention promptly when moderate or severe exacerbations occur.

The continuing management of persistent asthma (Table 21-7) should focus on the detection of exacerbations and a reassessment of asthma control at an interval commensurate with current asthma severity and stability. Unstable severe asthma requires frequent follow-up and reassessment. Regular monthly visits are sometimes needed in difficult to treat cases. Moreover, when severe or unstable asthma is detected, consultation with a specialist is recommended. At each follow-up visit there should be an assessment for current asthma severity and the occurrence of exacerbations. Asthma medication and other medication use should be reviewed and inhaler technique assessed. The patients' understanding of their asthma and the plan of care should be assessed. When there is uncertainty about clinical findings, then the FEV_1 should be measured and the treatment plan modified. If there is improvement and if a step down in therapy is recommended, we recommend that only one medication be reduced or discontinued at a time. Oral or inhaled steroids generally should be tapered gradually. If a step up in treatment is needed, the first consideration is whether an adequate dose of steroid is being used. Combining long-acting beta agonists, leukotriene modifiers, or theophylline with moderate-dose ICS generally is more effective than higher-dose ICS alone and should be considered when moderate doses of ICS alone are insufficient. Again, more complex regimens are more costly and adherence may suffer, so ability to pay should be considered when choosing medications.

When an exacerbation occurs, the first consideration is whether or not hospitalization is required. The management of severe exacerbations is discussed in Chapter 22, Acute

Asthma Management. Less severe exacerbations can usually be successfully treated in the outpatient setting. However a risk assessment should be performed that accounts for current severity, risk factors for fatal asthma, recent exacerbation history, prior response to treatment for exacerbation, and the likelihood of patient nonadherence. All of these factors are predictive of outpatient treatment failure and hospitalization may be considered if these are present even if the current physiological decline would not ordinarily warrant hospital admission. For outpatient treatment of an exacerbation, generally current controller medications are continued, higher dose steroids usually given orally are used, and inhaled bronchodilators are given at higher doses or more frequently for symptom relief. Bronchodilators should never be increased without also intensifying anti-inflammatory steroid therapy. We recommend using 0.25 to 1 mg/kg of oral steroids for a minimum of 4 to 5 days followed by a tapering dose over an additional 7 to 10 days as indicated. The initial dose should be chosen based on the severity of the exacerbation and prior steroid responsiveness. Short acting MDI doses may be doubled and given up to every 3 hours. Spirometry or PEF monitoring should be done every 2 to 4 hours initially and until there is improvement. If improvement does not occur within 12 hours, the patient should be assessed by a health care provider. A follow-up call within 24 hours is advisable. If there is a complete response, the oral steroids may be stopped after 4 to 5 days; for partial responses, tapering steroids are recommended.

Written action plans are a useful adjunct to asthma care and can reduce morbidity and health care use.[10] Plans should be simple, easy to follow, and tailored to the needs of the individual patient. An example of a written action plan is provided in Figure 21-2. Triggers for escalating therapy should be established based on data obtained when the patient is well. For example, the personal best FEV_1 or PEF should be used to

Asthma Action Plan for:_____   Last Revised:_____

Instructions:

1. Using your portable spirometer measure your FEV_1 first thing in the morning
   and late in the afternoon (4 PM), record these numbers
2. Keep track of how many puffs of albuterol you used during each day and if you have
   woken up because of asthma
3. When you check your FEV_1 find your current zone then follow the plan to the right

Green Zone	Action
Your FEV_1 is >_____ L AND You are not waking up at night because of your asthma AND You use your albuterol inhaler less than once daily	Continue to monitor FEV_1 twice daily Continue to take: Budesonide 180 µg, two puffs twice a day Albuterol MDI two puffs every 6 hours as needed
Yellow Zone	**Action**
Your FEV_1 is between _____ L and _____ L for more than 12 hours OR You woke up last night because of asthma OR You are using your albuterol inhaler more than twice a day OR You are more short of breath with exertion or exercise	Increase budesonide to four puffs twice a day AND Monitor your FEV_1, and if it does not improve to greater than _____ within 24 hours *Contact your physician at 555-1234* AND USE Albuterol MDI two puffs every 6 hours as needed
Red Zone	**Action**
Your FEV_1 is less than _____ L at any time OR You are using your albuterol inhaler more than four times a day OR Relief from albuterol lasts less than 4 hours OR You are so short of breath that daily activities are difficult	Immediately go to the emergency room or make an urgent appointment with your physician *555-1234* AND Take prednisone 60 mg once AND USE Albuterol MDI four puffs up to every 20 minutes until you obtain medical attention

Your Asthma Medications

_____ _____

_____ _____

If you have questions contact your physician at:

_____

Figure 21-2   Example of an asthma action plan.

calculate thresholds for increasing treatment. Instructions for modifying both the reliever and controller medications based on current severity should be provided. The patient should be counseled about the warning signs of a severe asthma attack and it is important that the action plan not delay physician assessment. Thus, instructions for contacting the physician or going to an emergency department should be imbedded in the plan and used when signs or symptoms of severe asthma are present, such as large reductions in lung function, resting dyspnea, or lack of relief from short-acting bronchodilators. During follow-up visits, the patient should be asked how often he or she needed to

escalate treatment. Frequent escalations would warrant intensification of the background controller regimen. The plan should be reviewed for effectiveness and the patient's understanding of the plan should be assessed at each follow-up visit.

In conclusion, asthma is a complex, chronic illness that requires an integrated approach to care. Although many studies have demonstrated that several types of medication are efficacious in asthma, actual effectiveness of treatment is reduced by many factors. Recognition of these factors and use of a systematic approach to management and patient education can improve the care of the asthma patient, reducing morbidity and cost.

REFERENCES

1. Bateman ED, Boushey HA, Bousquet J, et al: Can guideline-defined asthma control be achieved? The Gaining Optimal Asthma ControL study. Am J Respir Crit Care Med 2004;170(8):836–844.

2. Aday LA, Lairson DR, Balkrishnan R, Begley CE: Effectiveness: Concepts and Methods. Evaluating the Healthcare System. Chicago, Foundation of the American College of Healthcare Executives, 2004, p 67.

3. National Asthma Education and Prevention Program: Expert Panel Report 3, Guidelines for the Diagnosis and Management of Asthma. Bethesda, MD, National Institutes of Health, National Heart, Lung, and Blood Institute, October 2007.

4. Global Strategy for Asthma Management and Prevention, revised 2006. Available at www.ginasthma.org.

5. Kitch BT, Paltiel D, Kuntz KM, et al: A single measure of FEV1 is associated with risk of asthma attacks in long-term follow-up. Chest 2004;126:1875–1882.

6. Sont JK, Willems LN, Bel EH, et al: Clinical control and histopathologic outcome of asthma when using airway hyperresponsiveness as an additional guide to long-term treatment. The AMPUL Study Group. Am J Respir Crit Care Med 1999;159(4 Pt 1):1043–1051.

7. Green RH, Brightling CE, McKenna S, et al: Asthma exacerbations and sputum eosinophil counts: a randomised controlled trial. Lancet 2002;360(9347):1715–1721.

8. Juniper EF, Svensson K, Mork AC, Stahl E: Measurement properties and interpretation of three shortened versions of the asthma control questionnaire. Respir Med 2005;99(5):553–558.

9. Miller MK, Lee JH, Miller DP, Wenzel SE: Recent asthma exacerbations: a key predictor of future exacerbations. Respir Med 2007; 101(3):481–489.

10. Abramson MJ, Bailey MJ, Couper FJ, et al: Are asthma medications and management related to deaths from asthma? Am J Respir Crit Care Med 2001;163(1):12–18.

Acute Asthma Management

Charles B. Cairns

- Acute asthma exacerbations can result from undertreated disease, recent exposure to triggers, and severe disease unresponsive to conventional therapy.

- Initial acute management strategies include oxygen, beta-agonists, corticosteroids, and anticholinergic agents.

- Additional treatment options include magnesium, xanthines, anesthetics, and ventilatory support.

- While early spirometry will give an objective measure of airflow obstruction, in severe asthma exacerbations, early treatment with oxygen and beta-agonists takes precedence.

- Recognition of the phenotypes of acute asthma patients could enhance management.

Asthma exacerbations remain a common reason why patients seek emergency care, both from general practitioners and emergency departments (ED). Acute asthma presentations account for 2 million ED visits annually in the United States. The etiologies for these presentations range from undertreated or unrecognized disease, exacerbations of stable disease usually due to recent exposure to triggers, and severe disease unresponsive to conventional therapy. Many of these patients exhibit both acute and chronic markers of severe asthma. The recognition of these phenotypes of acute asthma has the potential to enhance the management of these patients in acute and emergency settings. The purpose of this chapter is to describe the characteristics of patients at risk for acute exacerbation, highlight current therapies for acute asthma, and address the management of acute asthma.

CHARACTERISTICS OF PATIENTS WITH ACUTE ASTHMA EXACERBATIONS

Asthma is a chronic disease characterized by recurrent episodes of wheezing, shortness of breath, and cough secondary to reversible airflow obstruction. Bronchial hyperresponsiveness is a hallmark of asthma and a key aspect of asthma is the presence of inflammation. It is well recognized that environmental and other factors cause or provoke the airway inflammation in people with asthma. These factors can result in recurrent acute exacerbations of asthma. In a recent Australian study, 62% of children and 40% of adults re-present for ED care within 1 year.

In the United States, the Multicenter Asthma Research Collaboration (MARC) studied characteristics of adult asthma patients according to frequency of ED visits in the past year. Over 46% of patients had annual ED visits with 21% having six or more visits. Patients with six or more ED visits accounted

for 67% of all prior ED visits in the past year. The number of ED visits was associated with older age, nonwhite race, lower socioeconomic status, and several markers of chronic asthma severity. Better understanding of these characteristics may advance ongoing efforts to decrease health care disparities, including differential access to primary asthma care. A recent review of patients who present to the ED with acute asthma found that the majority of patients had severe asthma with smaller percentages with mild and moderate disease. A summary of the characteristics of patients at risk for acute asthma exacerbations is listed in Table 22-1.

MANAGEMENT OF ACUTE ASTHMA EXACERBATIONS

The management of acute asthma exacerbations includes a review of the clinical history, physiologic assessment, and treatment.

Assessment

AIRWAY FUNCTION

Spirometry is recommended in confirming the diagnosis of asthma and peak flow measurements are recommended in the assessment of patients with acute asthma exacerbations. Spirometry provides more information regarding the pattern of respiratory disease and is more sensitive in measuring airflow obstruction. *While early spirometry will give an objective measure of airflow obstruction, in severe asthma exacerbations, early treatment with oxygen and beta-agonists takes precedence.* Further assessment of severity is accomplished by reviewing speech, vital signs, peak flow measurements, and pulse oximetry as outlined in Table 22-2.

Emergency Treatment

Beta-agonists and systemic corticosteroids remain the cornerstones of initial treatment. Oxygen is recommended for use in all but mild acute exacerbations. Emergency treatment options for acute asthma are summarized in Table 22-3.

BETA-AGONISTS

Intermittent beta-agonist inhalation is the standard method recommended by the National Institutes of Health National Asthma Education and Prevention Program (NIH NAEPP) guidelines for emergency treatment. In the MARC acute asthma studies, patients receive a median of three beta-agonist inhalation treatments in ED, with two of those in the first hour. In the updated NAEPP asthma guidelines, the specific active isomer of albuterol, *levalbuterol*, may be used instead of traditional racemic albuterol in the treatment of asthma exacerbations.

Table 22-1
CHARACTERISTICS OF PATIENTS AT RISK FOR ACUTE ASTHMA EXACERBATIONS

Frequent emergency department visits or hospitalizations for acute asthma within 12 months
Previous life-threatening or intensive care unit admission for asthma
Excessive reliance on inhaled bronchodilator medications
Patient denial of asthma diagnosis or symptoms
Poor adherence to preventive strategies or controller medications
Immediate hypersensitivity to foods, especially nuts
Asthma triggered by aspirin or other nonsteroidal anti-inflammatory medications
Poor access to health services
Older age
Lower socioeconomic status
Chronic severe asthma

Table 22-2
INITIAL CLINICAL ASSESSMENT OF SEVERITY IN ACUTE ASTHMA

Findings	Mild	Moderate	Severe
Speaking in ...	Sentences	Phrases	Words
Heart rate	<100 beats/min	100–120 beats/min	>120 beats/min
Peak Flow/FEV$_1$ (% predicted)	>75%	50%–75%	<50%
Pulse oximetry	>95%	92%–95%	<92%

Table 22-3
THERAPEUTIC OPTIONS IN ACUTE ASTHMA

Acute Asthma Medications	
Oxygen	Initially 100%, titrate to pulse oximetry > 93%
Beta-agonists	Albuterol (inhaled) Adults—0.5 mg every 20 min × 3 Children—0.15 mg/kg every 20 min × 3 (Consider continuous nebulization if severe)
Corticosteroids	Prednisone Adults—60 mg orally Children—1 mg/kg orally (Consider 2 mg/kg methylprednisolone IV if severe)
Anticholinergics	Ipratropium Adults—0.5 mg every 30 min × 3 Children—0.25 mg every 30 min × 3
Additional Therapeutic Options for Severe Exacerbations	
Epinephrine	Adults—0.3 to 0.5 mg SQ every 20 min × 3 Children—0.01 mg/kg SQ every 20 min × 3 (Consider 0.1 mg IV every 30 min in near-arrest states)
Magnesium sulfate	Adults—2 gm IV Children—40 mg/kg IV
Xanthines	Aminophylline Adults—Loading dose 6 mg/kg IV, followed by infusion of 0.9 mg/kg per hour Children—Loading dose of 7.0 mg/kg IV, followed by 0.5–0.8 mg/kg per hour
Heliox	80% helium/20% oxygen, titrate up to 50% helium/50% oxygen to maintain pulse oximetry > 93%.
Anesthetics	Ketamine Adults/children—Loading dose 0.2 mg/kg IV, followed by 0.5 mg/kg per hour × 2 hours

Route of Administration

Delivery of beta-agonists via nebulizer or metered-dose inhaler with spacer device appear to be similarly efficacious. There is no evidence to support the use of intravenous beta-agonists, even in severe, life-threatening asthma.

Continuous versus Intermittent Administration

Intermittent inhalation is the standard method recommended by the NIH NAEPP guidelines for emergency treatment. While it has been proposed that continuous beta-agonist nebulization could provide a more consistent delivery of medication and allow for deeper lung penetration resulting in enhanced bronchodilation, only 5% of EDs use continuous nebulization inhalation for patients with acute asthma exacerbations. Continuous nebulization may reduce hospital admissions in patients with severe asthma.

CORTICOSTEROIDS

Early administration of systemic corticosteroids reduces the need for hospital admission. Double-blind, randomized trials have clearly demonstrated that intravenous (IV) and oral corticosteroids have comparable efficacy. Patients with more severe asthma exacerbations are more likely to receive IV corticosteroids as compared with oral corticosteroids. For moderate or severe exacerbations, intravenous corticosteroids are recommended. Mild to moderate exacerbations can be treated with oral corticosteroids.

IPRATROPIUM BROMIDE

Recent systematic reviews of studies involving children and adults indicate that addition of multiple doses of inhaled ipratropium bromide to early beta-agonist treatments may reduce airway obstruction and reduce hospital admissions, especially for more severe asthma. Thus, ipratropium bromide, in addition to beta-agonists, seems indicated as the standard treatment in children, adolescent, and adult patients with moderate to severe exacerbations of asthma in the emergency setting.

EPINEPHRINE

Epinephrine is recommended for anaphylaxis and respiratory arrest. While subcutaneous or intramuscular administration has been recommended for patients in anaphylaxis, intravenous administration is necessary in arrest and near-arrest states.

DISCHARGE CRITERIA AND INSTRUCTIONS

In the updated NAEPP asthma guidelines, a primary goal of ED therapy is to achieve an FEV$_1$ (forced expiratory volume in 1 second) of more than 70% of the predicted (normal) value.

All patients discharged from the ED should receive necessary medications and education on how to use them, instructions on an asthma action plan, and a referral for follow-up appointment. Treatment for discharged patients should include systemic corticosteroids for 5 to 10 days, for all but the mildest asthma. Inhaled corticosteroids should be also considered for most discharged patients, since evidence suggests that inhaled corticosteroids may reduce relapses and improve quality of life.

Discharge planning should include close follow-up within 1 to 4 weeks and provision of asthma education, including an asthma action plan. Using such evidence-based practices should serve to reduce the burden of acute asthma on patients and the health care system.

PITFALLS AND CONTROVERSIES

Need To Assess Phenotypes of Acute Asthma

Current acute asthma management is dependent upon the applications of assessment and treatment interventions. Yet, the reasons for acute asthma exacerbations can vary and the treatments may not be uniformly successful. Indeed, a recent report found that only 34% of patients presenting with acute exacerbations had potentially preventable causes. Most patients either had acute episodes unresponsive to standard medications or severe asthma at baseline. Thus, patients present for treatment of acute asthma for a variety of reasons, including undertreated or unrecognized disease, exacerbations of stable disease usually due to recent exposure to triggers and severe disease unresponsive to conventional therapy. A summary of an approach to phenotyping acute asthma patients is presented in Table 22-4. Recognition of these phenotypes of acute asthma could enhance the management of these patients.

Airway Function Assessment

Specific criteria for the diagnosis of asthma include reversibility, demonstrated by an increase in the FEV_1 of 12% or 200 mL after a short-acting inhaled bronchodilator. However, this definition has always presented problems and more appropriate ways are needed to define the asthma phenotypes, especially in the acute setting. Most available definitions of asthma provide a qualitative concept of variable airflow obstruction, yet none has yet succeeded in providing quantitative criteria for a "change in severity" in airway narrowing over a "short period" of time. Thus, there is no objective gold standard against which to assess the diagnostic value of objective measures of the disease in the acute setting. In addition, peak flow and other airway measurements have a number of unresolved methodological and analytical issues.

The peak flow meter is an inexpensive and widely used device for assessing lung function in the ED. It is currently recommended that one use the best of three measures made

Table 22-4
APPROACH TO PHENOTYPING ACUTE ASTHMA PATIENTS

Parameter	Assessment
Clinical history	Undertreated asthma
	Acute triggers (infection, allergen)
	Severe disease
Airway function	Peak flow, FEV_1
	Expiratory capnogram
Airway inflammation	Exhaled nitric oxide
	Sputum analysis
Response to medications	Corticosteroids
	Beta-agonists
	Antileukotrienes
Genotypes	Beta$_2$-receptor
	5-Lipoxygenase pathway
	Corticosteroid receptor

at the time of presentation. Available data on the repeatability of estimates of peak flow variability suggest that both short- and long-term repeatability is poor. Furthermore, peak flow variability is increased in the general population in relation to increasing age, female gender, smoking status, and in those with evidence of atopy. In acute asthma exacerbations, this characteristic variability in peak flow values has even been used to predict hospital stay. The ratio between the last and first peak flow values may provide insight into more chronic aspects of the disease and patients with peak flow ratios less than 1 have longer subsequent hospital stays.

However, peak flow does not necessarily correlate with other measures of airway function, or even of airway inflammation in asthma. In adult patients with asthma, peak flow does not correlate with the direct bronchoscopic measurement of the peripheral airway resistance. Reliance on peak flow measurements can markedly underestimate the severity of airway. Because of the above challenges, measures of airway obstruction have been considered relatively insensitive indicators of asthma control and severity during acute exacerbations with questionable practicality and reliability in both acutely dyspneic adults and children.

Airway Inflammation

EXHALED NITRIC OXIDE
Fractional exhaled nitric oxide (FE_{NO}) has been proposed as a marker of bronchial inflammation in asthma. In stable asthma, FE_{NO} levels are elevated above baseline and decrease in response to corticosteroid therapy and demonstrate acceptable reproducibility. FE_{NO} has been proposed as a noninvasive marker of asthma severity and an objective monitor of treatment compliance and effectiveness in acute asthma.

There have been preliminary studies that suggest that FE_{NO} may have utility in acute asthma. In children, the mean peak FE_{NO} level after corticosteroid therapy was significantly less than that measured before treatment in children with acute asthma exacerbations. Concomitant with the decrease in FE_{NO} levels, there was improvement in the spirometry values and physical examination in the asthmatic children. Yet in a larger study of FE_{NO} as a diagnostic tool for assessing severity and response to treatment of acute asthma in the ED, there was poor reproducibility of FE_{NO} measurements, no correlation with clinical severity scores or spirometry, and no meaningful changes in FE_{NO} readings pretreatment and post-treatment. The poor interpatient reproducibility of FE_{NO} measurements appeared to result from the subjects' inability to consistently perform the required forced expiratory maneuver. Thus, it appears that further studies are warranted on the use and impact of FE_{NO} measurements in acute asthma.

SPUTUM ANALYSIS
Direct assessment of airway inflammation using sputum analysis for eosinophils has been associated with improved asthma control and reduced asthma exacerbations and admissions without the need for additional anti-inflammatory treatment. The translation of this strategy to acute asthma may be challenging because the patterns of cellular inflammation can change with asthma exacerbations. In a study of patients with acute severe asthma in the ED, neutrophils made up more than 75% of sputum cells in 10 patients while

eosinophils made up more than 75% of cells in only three patients. The predominance of neutrophils in the acute asthmatic patients suggests that exacerbations may involve the chemoattraction of neutrophils.

Undertreated Asthma

A third of patients with acute exacerbations, predominantly those with chronic mild and moderate asthma, have potentially preventable reasons for their ED presentations. These reasons include poor use of medication, lack of access to specialist care, failure to have a medication review, and poor knowledge of asthma and asthma management. Given these conditions, these patients could be expected to respond to standard asthma medications and control measures in the emergency setting.

Exacerbations of Stable Disease

The link between viral upper respiratory tract infections and asthma exacerbations is well established. In children, viruses are detected in up to 85% of exacerbations. In a recent study, 60% of patients stated that their presentation for emergency asthma care was brought about by a respiratory infection. Most of the time, a visit to their general practitioner had failed to prevent further worsening of their asthma, leading to the need for eventual hospital care. Deterioration in asthma in patients using inhaled controller medications can often be sudden and prolonged. This suggests that inhaled controller therapies may not sufficiently ameliorate airway responses to triggers such as viral infections. Even the use of oral corticosteroids may not prevent acute asthma exacerbations. In a recent Australian study of patients with acute exacerbations, 47% of patients were taking prednisolone to manage their severe asthma.

Variability of Response to Asthma Medications

There is a wide range of individual responses to important asthma medications, including inhaled corticosteroids. Indeed, between 25% and 34% of patients have a minimal FEV_1 response to inhaled corticosteroids. This variability of inhaled corticosteroid response has resulted in the characterization of the response to inhaled corticosteroids to be a "rule of thirds" with a third of the patients having a minimal FEV_1 response, a third with a modest response (5% to 15% improvement in FEV_1) and a third with a marked response (greater than 15% FEV_1 improvement).

Similar variations in response have been reported for montelukast, a leukotriene receptor antagonist when given for chronic asthma management. This variation in response appears to be important in acute asthma as well. A recent study of acute asthma demonstrated significant individual variability in the FEV_1 response in both groups receiving intravenous montelukast as well as in the group receiving standard ED care, including corticosteroids.

Genetic and Pharmacogenetic Aspects of Asthma

The wide variation in responses in therapy can be assessed using the principles of pharmacogenetics, which relates genetic variability to variability in responses to therapy. Potentially, 70% of the variability in therapeutic responses to pharmacotherapy might be due to genetic variability. Recently, specific genetic polymorphisms have been identified that produce biologically plausible effects and could alter clinical responses in asthma.

Beta-Adrenergic Receptor Polymorphisms

Several polymorphisms in the gene coding for the beta-adrenergic receptor have been reported. While several of these polymorphisms produce amino acid changes, changes at 16th and 27th amino acid positions of the beta-adrenergic receptor occur frequently enough to account for some of the clinically observed variability in response to beta-agonists.

Clinical studies demonstrate that patients with polymorphisms in the beta-adrenergic receptor who are homozygous at position 16 (Arg/Arg) do worse when treated regularly with beta-agonists. In contrast, patients treated regularly with beta-agonists who were homozygous for glycine at position 16 (Gly/Gly) did not experience a change in their peak flow throughout the study. Further prospective studies have confirmed that Arg/Arg asthmatic subjects (up to 17% of the population) might experience adverse effects from use of regular beta-agonists rather than benefiting from the treatment.

The impact of the Arg/Arg polymorphism on beta-agonist therapy in acute asthma is currently not known. As the technology for genotyping becomes more clinically accessible, assessment of these polymorphisms (along with the Arg/Gly and Gly/Arg) along with the binding motif of 5-lipoxygenase may be valuable in predicting exacerbation risk and even guiding emergency treatment.

Severe Disease

Severe asthma has heterogeneous pathology and physiology that has been characterized into specific patient phenotypes. The characteristics of these phenotypes include persistent inflammation, corticosteroid unresponsiveness, fixed airflow obstruction, leukotriene prominent disease, and aspirin-intolerant asthma. The persistent inflammation in severe asthma is characterized by a persistence of eosinophils, leukotrienes, and neutrophils, even in the presence of high doses of inhaled and oral corticosteroids. Patients with corticosteroid unresponsiveness exhibit neutrophilic inflammation and an increase in glucocorticoid receptor-β, an endogenous inhibitor of corticosteroid action. The presence of high leukotrienes (LTE_4) in the urine of the patients with severe asthma supports the possibility for this mediator pathway to be operative. Anti-leukotriene treatment has been shown to be of some benefit when added to inhaled corticosteroids in patients with severe asthma. Between 10% and 20% of severe asthmatic patients experience the aspirin-intolerant asthma (AIA) complex of rhinosinusitis, nasal polyposis, and flushing.

Airway Inflammation in Severe Asthma

Studies of the pathologic changes in the airways of chronic, severe asthmatic patients requiring high-dose corticosteroids for control of airway function suggest that inflammation is present in the lungs of these patients despite corticosteroid

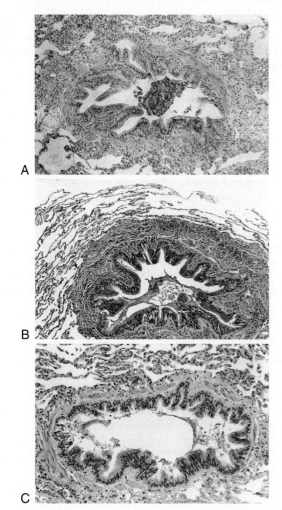

A

B

C

Figure 22-1   Airway thickening and cellular infiltrate in fatal asthma.

treatment. Indeed, inflammation in severe asthma may be distinct from that in mild-to-moderate asthma with marked infiltration of both neutrophils and eosinophils.

Importantly, these patterns of cellular inflammation are dynamic and can change with acute asthma exacerbations. In a study of patients with acute severe asthma in the ED, neutrophils made up more than 75% of sputum cells in 10 patients while eosinophils made up more than 75% of cells in only three patients. The predominance of neutrophils in the acute asthmatic patients suggests that exacerbations may involve the chemoattraction of neutrophils. Furthermore, fatal asthma has been associated with marked neutrophil infiltration of the small airways (Fig. 22-1).

TREATMENT CONTROVERSIES

Magnesium

Magnesium has been shown to have beneficial effects on smooth muscle relaxation and inflammation. Evidence from systematic reviews indicates that intravenous magnesium sulfate may provide benefit in acute asthma, especially in patients with severe asthma exacerbations. Even nebulized

inhaled magnesium sulfate, in addition to beta-agonists in the treatment of an acute asthma exacerbation, appears to have benefit with respect to improved pulmonary function and there is a trend towards benefit in hospital admission.

Leukotriene Antagonists

Intravenous administration of the leukotriene receptor antagonist montelukast to ED patients with acute asthma can result in improved FEV_1 within 20 minutes of administration. In a recent study, patients treated with montelukast tended to receive fewer beta-agonists and have fewer treatment failures than patients receiving placebo. Thus, intravenous montelukast in addition to standard therapy can potentially provide rapid benefit in adults with acute asthma although it is not currently available in the United States. In addition, oral administration of the leukotriene receptor antagonist zafirlukast in acute asthma can also result in a significant improvement in FEV_1 and dyspnea within 60 minutes of administration in the ED. However, the current asthma guidelines state that there is insufficient data regarding the use of leukotriene antagonists in the acute treatment of asthma for it to be recommended.

Intravenous Beta-agonists

In severe patients, airflow can be so limited that many clinicians have proposed that beta-agonists be given intravenously; yet intravenous (IV) beta-agonists have been shown to add little and may increase adverse effects. Systematic reviews have found no significant effect of IV beta-agonists on clinical outcomes in acute asthma, and in two of the larger trials, patients receiving IV beta-agonists actually worsened. The current asthma guidelines do *not* recommend the use of IV beta-agonists in the acute treatment of asthma.

Intravenous Aminophylline

IV aminophylline (theophylline) has been shown to add little bronchodilation and may increase adverse effects. Interestingly in children with a severe asthma exacerbation, the addition of IV aminophylline to beta-agonists and corticosteroids improves lung function within 6 hours of treatment. Yet, there is no apparent reduction in symptoms, number of nebulized treatments, and length of hospital stay in a recent systematic review. Importantly, aminophylline is also associated with a significantly increased risk of vomiting. The current asthma guidelines do *not* recommend the use of aminophylline in the acute treatment of asthma.

Anesthetics

Anesthetics, particularly ketamine, have been proposed as adjuncts for the treatment of severe asthma. A recent study, however, concluded that ketamine provided no incremental benefit to standard therapy in a cohort of children with moderately severe asthma exacerbation.

Heliox (Helium-Oxygen)

In a recent systematic review, the existing evidence does not provide support for the administration of helium-oxygen mixtures to all ED patients with acute asthma. Nonetheless, new evidence suggests certain beneficial effects in patients with more severe obstruction, including patients given albuterol driven via heliox. Starting with 80% helium/20% oxygen, it may be necessary to titrate up the oxygen concentration to 50% helium/50% oxygen to maintain pulse oximetry saturation greater than 93%.

Noninvasive Ventilation

Noninvasive positive pressure ventilation (NPPV) has been shown to be effective in chronic obstructive pulmonary disease patients with acute respiratory failure. NPPV has the advantage that it can be applied intermittently for short periods, which may be sufficient to reverse the breathing problems experienced by patients during severe acute asthma. A recent systematic review concluded that NPPV in acute asthma reduced hospitalizations, increased the number of patients discharged from the ED, and improved respiratory rate and lung function measurements. However, the current asthma guidelines state that there are insufficient data regarding the use of NPPV in the acute treatment of asthma for it to be recommended. One should not delay intubation once it is deemed necessary based on clinical judgment, including impending respiratory failure or severe hypoxia.

Antibiotics

While the updated NAEPP asthma guidelines do not recommend routine antibiotic treatment for asthma exacerbations, infections are thought to be a major cause of acute asthma exacerbations, including viruses in 80% to 85% of exacerbations in children and 57% to 75% in adults. Importantly, 20% of acute exacerbations are due to atypical bacterial infections with mycoplasma and chlamydia.

A recent study of ketolide antibiotic telithromycin in acute asthma exacerbations demonstrated effectiveness in the treatment of acute exacerbations of asthma, although the mechanism or mechanisms of action of telithromycin were not determined. Further studies will be needed to further assess the role of such antibiotic therapies in acute asthma exacerbations.

SUGGESTED READING

Barnard A: Management of an acute asthma attack. Aust Fam Phys 2004;34:7:531–534.

Britton J: Symptoms and objective measures to define the asthma phenotype. Clin Exp Allergy 1998;28(Suppl. 1):2–7.

Cairns CB: Acute asthma exacerbations: phenotypes and management. Clin Chest Med 2006;27(1):99–108.

Gibbs MA, Camargo CA Jr, Rowe BH, Silverman RA: State of the art: therapeutic controversies in severe acute asthma. Acad Emerg Med 2000;7(7):800–815.

Goeman DP, Aroni RA, Sawyer SM, et al: Back for more: a qualitative study of ED reattendance for asthma. Med J Aust 2004;180(3):113–117.

Griswold SK, Nordstrom CR, Clark S, et al: Asthma exacerbations in North American adults: who are the "frequent fliers" in the emergency department? Chest 2005 127(5):1579–1586.

National Asthma Education and Prevention Program: Expert Panel Report 3: Guidelines for the Diagnosis and Management of Asthma. U.S. Department of Health and Human Services, National Institutes of Health, National Heart, Lung, and Blood Institute, Bethesda, MD, NIH Publication No. 07–4051, October 2007.

Rowe BH, Edmonds ML, Spooner CH, Camargo CA: Evidence-based treatments for acute asthma. Respir Care 2001;46(12):1380–1390.

Wakefield M, Campbell D, Staugas R, et al: Risk factors for repeat attendance at hospital emergency departments among adults and children with asthma. Aust N Z J Med 1997;27:277–284.

Management of the Hospitalized and ICU Patient with Asthma

Thomas C. Corbridge and Susan J. Corbridge

CHAPTER

23

CLINICAL PEARLS

- There is a gender and racial gap in adult asthma admissions and asthma death, with women and blacks at greatest risk. Discharged patients are at significant risk for recurrence, stressing the importance of outpatient management.

- Features of severe attacks include upright positioning, diaphoresis, monosyllabic speech, accessory muscle use, widened pulsus paradoxus, and normo- or hypercapnia. Depressed mental status, paradoxical respiration, bradycardia, and a quiet chest warn of impending arrest.

- Inhaled beta-agonists are the preferred drugs to treat the bronchospastic component of acute asthma, but hospitalized patients often demonstrate a lackluster response to albuterol. Addition of ipratropium bromide to albuterol may confer additional benefit.

- Systemic steroids are indicated for hospitalized patients.

- Adjunctive therapies of acute asthma include magnesium sulfate, leukotriene modifiers, and heliox.

- Limited data support the use of noninvasive ventilation in selected patients.

- Prolongation of expiratory time decreases dynamic hyperinflation and auto-positive end-expiratory pressure in intubated patients.

Each year in the United States, acute asthma accounts for approximately 2 million emergency department (ED) visits, 450,000 hospitalizations, and nearly 5,000 deaths.[1] Although the rates have been relatively stable over the past 20 years, analysis of the National Hospital Discharge Survey Database demonstrates that hospitalizations and mortality decreased between 1995 and 2002.[2] This survey further confirmed the gender and racial gap in adult asthma admissions and asthma death, identifying women and blacks at greatest risk. For example, in 2001–2002, the hospitalization rate was 7.46/10,000 for white men compared to 34.42/10,000 for black women; age-adjusted mortality rate in whites was 0.78/100,000 and 2.59/100,000 in blacks.

A minority of patients hospitalized with a primary diagnosis of asthma are admitted to an intensive care unit; even fewer are intubated. Not surprisingly, the risk of in-hospital death is greater for intubated patients and for patients with significant comorbidities. These patients have longer hospital stays and incur additional costs.

PATIENT ADMISSION FROM THE EMERGENCY DEPARTMENT

The magnitude of spirometric improvement in an ED is generally a function of cumulative albuterol dose, but approximately one third of patients demonstrate a blunted response to albuterol, mandating hospitalization or prolonged treatment in an ED holding area.[3] Albuterol unresponsiveness is not necessarily explained by prior albuterol use. Rather, it appears to be a marker of airway wall inflammation, architectural distortion, and the presence of intraluminal mucus. Albuterol nonresponders are identified by inconsequential changes in spirometry after 30 to 60 minutes of bronchodilator therapy, allowing for early decisions regarding admission. Per the Expert Panel 3 Report of the National Institutes of Health (NIH), adequate responders may be discharged home from the ED.[4] But patients with an incomplete response, defined by persistent dyspnea and a PEFR (peak expiratory flow rate) or FEV_1 (forced expiratory volume in 1 second) between 50% and 70% of predicted, should be considered for admission. Severe attacks are characterized by PEFR less than 40% of predicted or personal best, poor response to initial treatment (e.g., less than 10% increase in PEFR), or deterioration despite initial treatment. They include patients with respiratory arrest, progressive hypercapnia, fatigue, depressed mental status, and arrhythmias, and they mandate intensive care unit (ICU) admission.

CLINICAL FEATURES

Dyspnea, cough, and wheeze are the hallmarks of acute asthma. Tachypneic patients speaking in short phrases have at least a moderately severe attack. These patients demonstrate expiratory phase prolongation and audible wheezes. Arterial blood gases typically demonstrate hypoxemia and acute respiratory alkalosis. Sicker patients demonstrate the following features: resting dyspnea, upright positioning, diaphoresis, monosyllabic speech, respiratory rate more than 30/minute, accessory muscle use, pulse greater than 120/minute, pulsus paradoxus more than 25 mmHg, peak expiratory flow rate less than 40% predicted or personal best, hypoxemia, and normo- or hypercapnia. Impending arrest is suggested by depressed mental status, paradoxical respiration, bradycardia, absence of pulsus paradoxus from respiratory muscle fatigue, and a quiet chest. A quiet chest suggests critically low air flow rates, wherein subsequent wheezing marks clinical improvement. Posture, speech pattern, and mental status allow for a quick appraisal of severity, response to therapeutic interventions, and need for intubation.

Supraventricular and ventricular arrhythmias rarely complicate management of acute asthma. Few exacerbations cause clinically apparent right heart strain, myocardial ischemia, and pulmonary edema.

PATHOPHYSIOLOGY OF ACUTE AIRFLOW OBSTRUCTION

Rapid-onset attacks develop in less than 3 to 6 hours. These occur in less than 15% of cases and represent a more pure form of bronchospasm in response to allergens, irritants, stress, inhalation of illicit drugs, and the use of nonsteroidal anti-inflammatory agents or beta-blockers in susceptible patients.[5] Infection is an unlikely trigger.

Most asthma attacks evolve over 24 hours with increasing airway wall inflammation and mucus plugging. These exacerbations may be triggered by viral or mycoplasmal infections and portend a longer time to recovery.

In critical airflow obstruction, the time available for expiration (1 to 5 seconds) is insufficient for full exhalation, resulting in gas trapping and dynamic lung hyperinflation (DHI). This may be self-limiting because DHI increases lung elastic recoil pressure and airway diameter, which augments expiratory flow and allows for enhanced gas emptying at the cost of greater lung volume.

Trapped gas elevates alveolar volume and pressure relative to mouth pressure at end-expiration, a state referred to as auto-PEEP. Auto-PEEP is a pressure that must be overcome during inspiration by more vigorously lowering pleural pressure. It therefore increases inspiratory work of breathing at a time when the diaphragm has been placed in a mechanically disadvantageous position by DHI. Ultimately, this imbalance between load and strength results in respiratory failure.

Hypoxemia is a result of decreased ventilation (V) to perfused (Q) lung units. The severity of hypoxemia roughly tracks the severity of obstruction, but in recovering patients, spirometry may improve faster than PaO_2 and V/Q inequality, indicating that larger airways recover faster than smaller airways.

Large swings in intrathoracic pressure accentuate the normal inspiratory fall in systolic blood pressure, a phenomenon referred to as "pulsus paradoxus." During vigorous inspiration, intrathoracic pressure falls, lowering right atrial and ventricular pressures and augmenting right ventricular (RV) filling. This shifts the intraventricular septum leftward causing a conformational change in the left ventricle (LV), diastolic dysfunction, and incomplete LV filling. Negative pleural pressures further impair LV emptying. During forced expiration, high intrathoracic pressures impede blood return to the RV. The net result is a cyclical change in blood pressure that tracks asthma severity; however, severe acute asthma may not increase the pulsus paradoxus when fatigue diminishes the magnitude of pleural pressure change.

ACID-BASE STATUS

Hypoxemia and respiratory alkalosis are common in acute asthma. Eucapnia and hypercapnia indicate severe obstruction; however, hypercapnia alone is not an indication for intubation, particularly when initial treatment is effective.

Conversely, the absence of hypercapnia does not preclude a life-threatening attack.

In response to acute respiratory alkalosis, patients waste bicarbonate and may develop a post-hypocapneic metabolic acidosis. Lactic acidosis signifies increased work of breathing during a severe attack.

Arterial blood gases are indicated in patients with severe acute asthma. However, serial blood gases are generally not necessary unless the patient is intubated.

CHEST RADIOGRAPHY

In classic cases of acute asthma, the chest x-ray rarely affects management. A chest x-ray should be obtained when there are focal signs on examination, concerns regarding barotrauma or pneumonia, or questions regarding diagnosis. In intubated patients, chest x-rays confirm proper endotracheal tube position.

PHARMACOLOGIC MANAGEMENT

Beta-Agonists

Although beta-agonists are the preferred drugs to treat the bronchospastic component of acute asthma (Table 23-1), hospitalized patients demonstrate a lackluster response (or they would not have been admitted). High-dose beta-agonists, delivered in a repetitive or continuous fashion, are necessary during the initial hospital course. In the sickest patients continuous administration (at the same total dose) appears to be slightly better than repetitive dosing, although these approaches are nearly equal in most cases.

Table 23-1 DRUGS USED IN THE TREATMENT OF ACUTE ASTHMA	
Albuterol	2.5 mg in 2.5 mL normal saline by nebulization every 15–20 minutes × 3 in the first hour or 4–6 puffs by MDI with spacer every 10–20 minutes for 1 hour then as required or 10–15 mg via continuous nebulization over 1 hour for intubated patients, titrate to physiologic effect and side effects.
Levalbuterol	1.25 mg by nebulization every 15–20 minutes × 3 in the first hour, then as required
Epinephrine	0.3 mL of a 1:1000 solution subcutaneously every 20 minutes × 3. Terbutaline is favored in pregnancy when parenteral therapy is indicated. Use with caution in patients over age 40 and in patients with coronary artery disease.
Corticosteroids	Methylprednisolone 40–60 mg IV every 6 hours or prednisone 40 mg PO every 6 hours for the first 48 hours
Anticholinergics	Ipratropium bromide 0.5 mg by nebulization every 20 minutes with albuterol, or 4 puffs by MDI with spacer every 10–20 minutes again combined with albuterol
Aminophylline	5–6 mg/kg IV over 30 minutes loading dose in patients not on theophylline followed by 0.4–0.7 mg/kg/h IV. Check serum level within 6 hours of loading dose. Watch for drug interactions and disease states that alter clearance.
Magnesium sulfate	2 g IV over 20 minutes, repeat once as required (total dose 4 g unless hypomagnesemic)

Albuterol is the most widely used and studied beta-agonist. It can be delivered equally well by metered-dose inhaler (MDI) or hand-held nebulizer. Somewhere between 4 and 10 puffs of albuterol by MDI with a spacer is equivalent to a 2.5 mg nebulizer treatment. MDIs with spacers are cheaper and faster; handheld nebulizers require less supervision and less coordination.

The recommended dose of albuterol is 2.5 mg by nebulization every 20 minutes during the first hour of treatment depending on clinical response and side effects. For more severe exacerbations, 10 to 15 mg of albuterol via continuous nebulization may be used. When treatments are required more often than every 4 hours, ICU admission is desirable for close monitoring and staffing considerations.

Albuterol is a racemate consisting of equal parts of R- and S-albuterol. The R isomer confers bronchodilator effects whereas the S isomer has been viewed as either inert or pro-inflammatory. This provides the rationale for using the R-isomer alone, or levalbuterol. Emerging clinical data suggest that levalbuterol is at least as good as racemic albuterol in children and adults. Results of a large, multicenter, prospective trial of levalbuterol use in the ED treatment of adults with acute asthma have been recently published.[6] Patients with acute asthma and an FEV_1 between 20% and 55% of predicted received prednisone and either 1.25 mg levalbuterol or 2.5 mg of racemic albuterol every 20 minutes for the first hour, then every 40 minutes for three additional doses, and then as needed for up to 24 hours. The primary end point (time to meeting discharge criteria) was not different between groups. Secondary end points included change in FEV_1 and hospitalizations. Levalbuterol improved FEV_1 more than albuterol after the first dose (0.50 L versus 0.43 L, P = .02), particularly for patients not recently on inhaled or oral steroids. Among patients not on steroids, fewer levalbuterol treated patients were admitted (3.8% versus 9.3%, P = .03). Thus, levalbuterol appears to be at least as effective as albuterol, if not more so in steroid-naïve patients. It is unclear whether levalbuterol is cost-effective.

There is no advantage to subcutaneous epinephrine or terbutaline in the initial management of acute asthma, unless the patient is unable to comply with inhaled therapy. In refractory cases, however, it is reasonable to try subcutaneous medication in the absence of contraindications. Fortunately, beta-agonists are generally well tolerated in younger patients; tremor and tachycardia are common, but serious toxicity is rare. Subcutaneous injections are riskier and should be used with extreme caution in older patients at risk for coronary artery disease. Intravenous therapy confers no additional benefit and is even more dangerous.

Long-acting beta-agonists are not recommended in the initial treatment of acute asthma, although formoterol (which has acute onset of action) may prove to be effective and safe in this setting. Long-acting beta-agonists may be added to standard (steroid-containing) therapies in hospitalized patients.

Anticholinergics

The bronchodilating properties of anticholinergic drugs such as ipratropium bromide are modest, precluding their use as sole drugs in acute asthma. However, repetitive doses of ipratropium bromide added to albuterol are effective. Rodrigo and Rodrigo[7] conducted a randomized trial of albuterol and ipratropium bromide (in one container) compared to albuterol alone. After 3 hours of four puffs every 10 minutes, combination therapy resulted in 20.5% and 48.1% greater improvements in PEFR and FEV_1, respectively, compared with albuterol. Hospitalization rates were also less. Subgroup analysis showed that the patients with FEV_1 less than 30% of predicted and symptoms for more than 24 hours were most likely to benefit from combination therapy. Additional studies have demonstrated that combination therapy improves spirometry, but not admission rates, compared with albuterol. Other studies have demonstrated nonstatistical trends or no benefit at all. These studies on the whole used lower doses of ipratropium bromide. Ipratropium should not be continued beyond the first 6 hours of therapy for those patients who require hospitalization.[4]

In children, the data generally demonstrate that combination therapy decreases ED treatment time, albuterol dose requirements, and hospitalization rates.

Corticosteroids

Most acutely ill asthmatic individuals are not taking corticosteroids (either inhaled or oral) before ED arrival. Regardless of prior use, most experts recommend using systemic steroids in the ED, unless the patient has had a marked and immediate response to beta-agonist therapy.

Corticosteroids treat the inflammatory component of asthma by promoting new protein synthesis. Their effects may not be apparent for hours, underlying the importance of early initiation. However, if used within 1 hour of arrival to the ED, corticosteroids may reduce the need for hospitalization.[8] In hospitalized patients, systemic corticosteroids appear to improve the rate of recovery. Oral steroids are as effective as parenteral steroids.

Various dosing regimens have been studied and debate continues regarding the optimal strategy. The Expert Panel 3 Report recommends 120 to 180 mg/day of either prednisone, methylprednisolone, or prednisolone in three or four divided doses for 48 hours, then 60 to 80 mg/day until the PEFR reaches 70% of predicted or the patient's personal best.

There is a limited role for inhaled corticosteroids in acute asthma. Rodrigo and Rodrigo[9] conducted a randomized, double-blinded trial of 400 µg salbutamol with flunisolide 1 mg or placebo every 10 minutes for 3 hours in patients not on systemic steroids. PEFR and FEV_1 were approximately 20% higher in the flunisolide group, beginning at 90 minutes. This quick response may stem from steroid-induced vasoconstriction rather than specific anti-inflammatory effects. Other investigators using different inhaled steroids and protocols have not demonstrated efficacy in this setting.

Inhaled steroids play a pivotal role in achieving outpatient asthma control. Patients discharged from the ED or hospital after successful treatment of an asthma exacerbation should receive an inhaled steroid or an inhaled steroid combined with a long-acting beta-agonist.

Oxygen

Supplemental oxygen should be provided to maintain arterial oxygen saturations greater than 90% (>95% in pregnancy). This increases oxygen delivery to peripheral tissues including the respiratory muscles, reverses hypoxic pulmonary vasoconstriction, and, in and of itself, causes modest bronchodilation. Oxygen further protects against beta-agonist–induced pulmonary vasodilation and increased blood flow to low V/Q units.

Theophylline/Aminophylline

In a recent meta-analysis for the Cochrane Database, Parameswaran and colleagues[10] concluded that use of intravenous (IV) aminophylline does not result in any additional bronchodilation in adults compared to standard care with beta-agonists and that the frequency of adverse effects was higher with aminophylline. This study confirms the findings of numerous others.

Magnesium Sulfate

Prospective trials have yielded conflicting results regarding the efficacy of magnesium sulfate ($MgSO_4$) in acute asthma. Several studies have failed to show a benefit to adding $MgSO_4$ to standard therapies, whereas other studies have demonstrated improved spirometry or rates of admission. Published meta-analyses have also reached different conclusions.

In a recent systematic review by Rowe and colleagues,[11] the data did not support routine use of IV $MgSO_4$ in adult patients with acute asthma. However, $MgSO_4$ was found to be safe and effective in improving spirometry in patients with the most severe exacerbations. The Expert Panel Report 3 recommends consideration of IV magnesium for those patients with life-threatening exacerbations who have failed conventional treatment after the first hour. Further data support the use of inhaled $MgSO_4$ in acute asthma.

Leukotriene Modifiers

Limited data support the use of leukotriene receptor antagonists in acute asthma. The most compelling study is a randomized, double-blinded, parallel group trial by Camargo and colleagues in 201 acute asthmatic individuals.[12] When added to standard therapy, IV montelukast improved FEV_1 over the first 20 minutes (14.8% versus 3.6% with placebo). Effects were seen within 10 minutes and lasted for 2 hours. However, montelukast is not currently available for IV administration in the United States.

Heliox

Heliox consists of 20% oxygen and 80% helium (30%:70% mixtures are also available). It is a less dense gas than air that decreases airway resistance, thereby possibly improving dyspnea and work of breathing when delivered by a tight-fitting facemask. However, several studies have failed to demonstrate a clinical benefit in nonintubated patients, including a recent meta-analysis of six randomized controlled trials involving a total of 369 adults and children.[13] However, methodological differences between studies, small patient numbers, and failure to control for upper airway obstruction (e.g., vocal cord dysfunction) preclude strong conclusions and call for additional data. Heliox may also improve bronchodilator delivery. The Expert Panel Report 3 recommends consideration of heliox for those patients with life-threatening exacerbations who have failed conventional treatment after the first hour.

Antibiotics

The Expert Panel Report 3 states that asthma exacerbation is not an indication for antibiotics unless there is fever with purulent sputum, evidence for pneumonia, or suspected bacterial sinusitis. However, this recommendation is driven more by consensus than data as few well-designed studies are available for review.

NONINVASIVE MECHANICAL VENTILATION (NPPV)

Limited data have demonstrated the use of low levels of nasal continuous positive airway pressure (CPAP) are beneficial, likely by helping to overcome the inspiratory threshold pressure created by auto-PEEP. Soroksky and colleagues[14] reported their experience with BiPAP in 15 patients with acute asthma compared to 15 controls receiving sham bilevel positive airway pressure (BiPAP) for 3 hours. BiPAP improved lung function and reduced the rate of hospitalization.

We consider BiPAP in an alert, cooperative, and hemodynamically stable patient who is not in need of endotracheal intubation to protect the airway or clear secretions. Reasonable initial settings are inspiratory positive airway pressure (IPAP) of 10 cm H_2O and expiratory positive airway pressure (EPAP) of 0 cm H_2O. After the mask is secured and the patient is breathing synchronously, we increase EPAP to 3 to 5 cm H_2O and IPAP as required to lower respiratory rate and improve patient comfort.

Intubation and Mechanical Ventilation

Respiratory arrest and impending respiratory arrest (e.g., extreme exhaustion, a quiet chest, and changes in mental status) are indications for intubation. Oral intubation is preferred because it allows for a large endotracheal tube, which decreases airway resistance and facilitates removal of mucus plugs. Nasal intubation may be attempted in a cooperative patient with a difficult airway, but necessitates a smaller tube and may be complicated by polyps and sinusitis.

Postintubation Hypotension

Postintubation hypotension results from loss of vascular tone with sedation or paralysis, hypovolemia, tension pneumothorax, or mechanical ventilation itself, particularly when insufficient time is allowed for exhalation. When the lung becomes critically inflated, it is difficult to deliver manual breaths during Ambu bag ventilation. Airway pressures increase (discussed later), breath sounds diminish, and blood pressure falls. When critical DHI is suspected, a trial of hypopnea (two to three breaths per minute) or apnea in a pre-oxygenated patient for 30 to 60 seconds is both diagnostic and therapeutic. By allowing for lung deflation, this maneuver helps regain cardiopulmonary stability.

Close inspection of the chest x-ray is mandatory in all hypotensive patients to rule out pneumothorax. When pneumothorax occurs, preferential ventilation to the contralateral lung increases the risk of bilateral pneumothoraces. Management of pneumothorax consists of volume resuscitation and tube thoracostomy (unilateral or bilateral as required).

Initial Ventilator Settings

Expiratory time (Te), tidal volume (Vt), and the severity of airway obstruction all determine the level of DHI during mechanical ventilation.[15] Expiratory time is determined by minute ventilation (respiratory rate [RR] × Vt) and inspiratory flow. To illustrate this point, consider the following hypothetical ventilator settings: RR 15/min, Vt 1000 mL, and an inspiratory flow rate of 60 L/min (or 1 L/sec). In this example, the respiratory cycle time (the total amount of time allowed for one complete breath) is 4 seconds (Fig. 23-1). Inspiratory time (Ti) is 1 second and Te is 3 seconds resulting in an I:E of 1:3. If these settings caused critical DHI, lowering RR to 10/min would prolong respiratory cycle time to 6 seconds and Te to 5 seconds (I:E of 1:5), allowing for greater exhalation of the delivered breath and less DHI. Now consider the effect of increasing inspiratory flow. If inspiratory flow was increased from 60 LPM to 120 LPM, Ti would decrease to 0.5 seconds, and, with an RR of 15/min, Te would increase from 3 seconds to 3.5 seconds. Of course high inspiratory flow rates raise peak airway pressure by elevating airway-resistive pressure, but peak airway pressures per se do not correlate with morbidity or mortality. Consider further that if inspiratory flow is decreased to lower peak airway pressures, Te will fall and DHI will increase. On the other hand, use of high flow rates may have the untoward effect of increasing respiratory rate, thereby decreasing Te.[16]

With these considerations in mind, the initial minute ventilation should be set relatively low in the postintubation period. Limited but compelling data suggest that Ve should be set less than 115 mL/kg/min (or approximately 8 L/m in a 70-kg patient) to avoid dangerous levels of DHI.[17] This can be achieved by setting the RR between 12 and 14/min and Vt between 7 and 8 mL/kg. For inspiratory flow, we recommend 60 LPM using the constant flow regime.

There are no randomized trials of ventilator mode in acute asthma. In paralyzed patients (and other patients not

breathing above the set respiratory rate), synchronized intermittent mandatory ventilation (SIMV) and assist-controlled ventilation (AC) are equivalent. In patients triggering the ventilator, AC may increase Ve more than SIMV, but SIMV may increase work of breathing. Volume-controlled ventilation (VC) is recommended over pressure-controlled ventilation (PC) because of greater staff familiarity with its use. PC offers the advantage of limiting peak airway pressure to a predetermined set value (e.g., 30 cm H_2O) and it has been used successfully in children with severe asthma exacerbation. During PC, Vt is inversely related to auto-PEEP and Ve is not guaranteed. PC also imposes a decelerating inspiratory flow pattern that may shorten Te.

Ventilator-applied PEEP is not recommended in sedated and paralyzed patients because it may increase lung volume if used excessively. In spontaneously breathing patients, however, low levels of machine-set PEEP (e.g., 5 cm H_2O) decrease inspiratory work of breathing by decreasing the pressure gradient required to overcome auto-PEEP, without aggravating lung inflation.

Assessing Lung Inflation

Determining the severity of DHI is central to monitoring the patient and adjusting the ventilator. Numerous methods have been proposed to assess DHI, including the measurement of exhaled gases and the volume at end-inspiration, termed Vei. This volume is determined by collecting expired gas from TLC to FRC during 40 to 60 seconds of apnea. A Vei greater than 20 mL/kg correlates with barotraumas.[17] The utility of this measure is limited by the need for paralysis and staff unfamiliarity with expiratory gas collection. It may also underestimate air trapping if there are slowly emptying lung units.

Alternate measures of DHI include the single-breath plateau pressure (Pplat) and auto-PEEP. Pplat (or lung distension pressure) is an estimate of average end-inspiratory alveolar pressure that is determined by temporarily stopping flow at end-inspiration (Fig. 23-2). Auto-PEEP is the lowest average alveolar pressure achieved during the respiratory cycle. It is obtained by measuring airway-opening pressure during an end-expiratory hold maneuver (Fig. 23-2). Persistence of expiratory gas flow at the beginning of inspiration (which can be detected by auscultation or flow tracings) also suggests auto-PEEP (see Fig. 23-3).

Accurate measurements of Pplat and auto-PEEP require patient-ventilator synchrony and the absence of patient effort. Paralysis is generally not required. Unfortunately neither pressure has been validated as a predictor of complications. Pplat is affected by the entire respiratory system including lung parenchyma, chest wall, and the abdomen. For example, Pplat will be higher in a patient with abdominal distension, for the same degree of DHI. Despite these limitations, experience suggests that outcomes are normally good when Pplat is kept less than 30 cm H_2O. Auto-PEEP can underestimate the severity of DHI if there is poor communication between alveoli and the airway opening. In general, auto-PEEP less than 15 cm H_2O is acceptable.

Ventilator Adjustments

With the above considerations in mind, we offer the following approach to ventilator adjustments. This approach relies

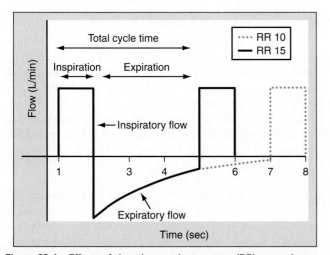

Figure 23-1   Effects of changing respiratory rate (RR) on expiratory time (Te) with a Vt of 1000 mL and a constant inspiratory flow rate of 60 LPM (1 LPS). Note that with a RR of 15/min (*solid line*) the total cycle time (the amount of time allowed for one complete breath) is 4 seconds. Inspiratory time (Ti) is 1 second and Te is 3 seconds resulting in an I:E of 1:3. By lowering RR to 10/min (*dotted line*) the total cycle time increases to 6 seconds and Te is 5 seconds resulting in an I:E of 1:5. Lower RR allows for greater exhalation of the delivered breath and lower Pplat (not shown), although effects are modest because of low end-expiratory flow rates.

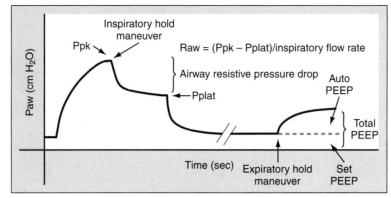

Figure 23-2 Pressure-time tracing during mechanical ventilation demonstrating measurement of the peak inspiratory pressure (Ppk), plateau pressure (Pplat), and auto-PEEP. While delivering a constant inspiratory flow (not shown), airway pressure (Paw) increases to Ppk, the sum of airway resistive pressure and plateau pressure (Pplat). Airway resistive pressure and Pplat are determined by an end-inspiratory hold maneuver during which inspiratory flow is purposely stopped for approximately 0.5 seconds to eliminate airway resistive pressure allowing Paw to fall to Pplat. If inspiratory flow is set at 60 L/min, the resistance pressure drop equals airway resistance (Raw) in units of cm H_2O/L/sec. To measure auto-PEEP, an end-expiratory hold maneuver is performed. During this maneuver, Paw increases by the amount of auto-PEEP present. Note that end-inspiratory and end-expiratory hold maneuvers are performed on different breaths.

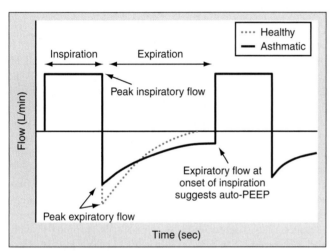

Figure 23-3 Flow-time tracings in a healthy subject and a patient with asthma during mechanical ventilation. Note that peak expiratory flow rates are diminished in asthma because of increased airway resistance and that increased expiratory time is required to exhale the delivered breath. In the asthmatic patient, expiratory flow has not stopped at the time of the next delivered breath (as demonstrated by failure of the exhalation flow tracing to return to baseline), indicating the presence of auto-PEEP.

on Pplat as the measure of lung hyperinflation and arterial pH as an indirect marker of ventilation. If initial ventilator settings result in Pplat more than 30 cm H_2O, RR should be decreased to decrease Pplat below 30 cm H_2O. Although this strategy is sound, the drop in lung volume that follows Te prolongation may be trivial because of low end-expiratory flow.

Decreasing RR may cause hypercapnia. Fortunately, hypercapnia is generally well tolerated in this patient population. Anoxic brain injury and myocardial dysfunction are contraindications to permissive hypercapnia because of the potential for hypercapnia to dilate cerebral vessels, decrease myocardial contractility, and constrict pulmonary vasculature. Lowering RR may not significantly increase $PaCO_2$ if lowering DHI also lowers dead space to improve alveolar ventilation.

If hypercapnia results in a blood pH of less than 7.20 and RR cannot be increased because Pplat is at its limit, we consider an infusion of sodium bicarbonate, although bicarbonate has not been shown to improve outcome. If Pplat is less than 30 cm H_2O and pH is less than 7.20, RR can be safely increased until Pplat nears the 30-cm H_2O limit.

Sedation and Paralysis

Sedation improves comfort, safety, and patient-ventilator synchrony. In patients who may be extubated within hours (such as those with rapid-onset asthma), propofol is a good choice because it can be titrated to a deep level of sedation, but still allow for rapid reversal after discontinuation. Benzodiazepines, such as lorazepam and midazolam, are less expensive alternatives, but time to awakening after stopping these drugs is less predictable.

To provide amnesia, sedation, and analgesia and to suppress respiratory drive, morphine or fentanyl can be added by continuous infusion to propofol or a benzodiazepine. For all patients, daily interruption of sedatives and analgesics avoids uncalled-for accumulation.[18]

Ketamine is an IV anesthetic with sedative, analgesic, and bronchodilating properties. In most cases it is reserved for intubated patients with refractory and critical obstruction. Ketamine must be used with caution because of its sympathomimetic effects and ability to cause delirium.

When safe and effective mechanical ventilation cannot be achieved by sedation alone, consider short-term muscle paralysis. In our ICU we prefer cis-atracurium because it is essentially free of cardiovascular effects, does not release histamine, and does not rely on hepatic and renal function for clearance. Pancuronium is a less expensive alternative, but it lasts longer and may worsen tachycardia. Pancuronium and atracurium both release histamine, but this is of doubtful clinical significance in this setting.

Paralytics may be given intermittently by bolus or continuous IV infusion. Continuous infusions mandate the use of a nerve stimulator (or interruption of drug every 4 to 6 hours) to avoid drug accumulation and prolonged paralysis. Although the use of paralytics likely selects for sicker patients, their use is associated with significant complications including myopathy and ventilator-associated pneumonia. Paralytics should be stopped as soon as possible to minimize risk.

Use of Bronchodilators during Mechanical Ventilation

Additional controlled trials are needed to determine the efficacy of bronchodilators in intubated asthmatic patients and to provide evidence for or against current recommendations. One consistent observation is that intubated patients require higher drug dosages to achieve a clinical effect. This may be because they are refractory to albuterol or that albuterol is inadequately delivered or dosed. When MDIs are used during mechanical ventilation, the use of a spacing device on the inspiratory limb of the ventilator improves drug delivery.[19] When nebulizers are used, they should be placed close to the ventilator, and in-line humidifiers should be stopped during treatments. Inspiratory flow should be reduced to approximately 40 L/min during treatments to minimize turbulence, although this strategy may worsen DHI and should be time-limited. Patient-ventilator synchrony further helps to optimize drug delivery.

Regardless of whether an MDI with spacer or nebulizer is used, higher drug dosages are required and the dosage should be titrated to achieve a fall in the peak-to-pause airway pressure gradient (Figs. 23-4 and 23-5). When no measurable drop in airway resistance occurs, other causes of elevated airway resistance such as a kinked or plugged endotracheal tube should be excluded. Bronchodilator nonresponders should be considered for a drug holiday.

Other Considerations

Rarely, the strategies discussed earlier are unable to stabilize the patient on the ventilator. In these situations, general anesthetic bronchodilators, such has halothane, isoflurane, and enflurane may reduce Ppk and $Paco_2$. These agents are associated with hypotension and arrhythmias, and their

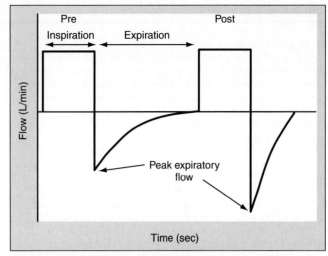

Figure 23-5   Flow-time tracings before and after successful administration of a bronchodilator. Note the increase in expiratory flow and decreased time required for expiratory flow to return to baseline.

benefits are short lived. Heliox delivered through the ventilator circuit may also decrease Ppk and $Paco_2$; however, safe use of heliox requires significant institutional expertise and planning. Gas-density dependent flow meters require recalibration to low density gas and use of a spirometer to measure tidal volume during mechanical ventilation.

Extubation

Weaning and extubation criteria have not been validated for patients with acute asthma. One approach is to perform a spontaneous breathing trial once (1) $Paco_2$ normalizes without significant DHI, (2) airway resistance is less than 20 cm H_2O, (3) the patient follows commands, and (4) neuromuscular weakness has not been identified. Patients with labile asthma may meet these criteria quickly after intubation; more commonly 24 to 48 hours of treatment are required. After extubation, observation in an ICU is recommended for an additional 12 to 24 hours. During this time the focus can switch to safe transfer to the ward and outpatient management.

PROGNOSIS IN PATIENTS REQUIRING ICU ADMISSION

Afessa and colleagues[20] collected data on 132 ICU admissions in 89 patients with acute severe asthma over a 3-year period in the late 1990s. Patients were mainly black (67%), female (79%), and residents of an inner city. Eleven of the 89 patients died; the in-hospital mortality for the 132 admissions was 8.3%. The two most common causes of death were tension pneumothorax and nosocomial infection.

The importance of close follow-up in patients who are successfully discharged after a near-fatal asthma attack cannot be stressed enough. These patients remain at risk for recurrent exacerbations and asthma mortality.

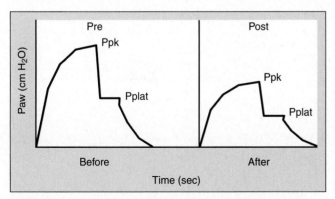

Figure 23-4   Pressure-time tracings before and after successful administration of a bronchodilator. Note the drop in both airway resistive pressure and Pplat reflecting increased airway diameter and decreased lung inflation, respectively.

REFERENCES

1. Mannino DM, Homa DM, Akinbami LJ, et al: Surveillance for asthma—United States, 1980–1999. MMWR Morb Mortal Wkly Rep 2002;51(SS01):1–13.

2. Getahun D, Demissie K, Rhoads GG: Recent trends in asthma hospitalization and mortality in the United States. J Asthma 2005;42:373–378.

3. McFadden ER Jr: Acute severe asthma: state of the art. Am J Respir Crit Care Med 2003;168:740–759.

4. National Asthma Education and Prevention Program: Expert Panel Report 3: Guidelines for the Diagnosis and Management of Asthma. Bethesda, MD, National Institutes of Health, 2007.

5. Barr RG, Woodruff PG, Clark S, Camargo C Jr: Sudden-onset asthma exacerbations: clinical features, response to therapy, and 2-week follow-up. Multicenter Airway Research Collaboration (MARC) investigators. Eur Respir J 2000;15:266–273.

6. Nowak R, Emerman C, Hanrahan JP, et al: A comparison of levalbuterol with racemic albuterol in the treatment of acute severe asthma exacerbations in adults. Am J Emerg Med 2006;24:259–267.

7. Rodrigo GJ, Rodrigo C: First-line therapy for adult patients with acute severe asthma receiving a multiple-dose protocol of ipratropium bromide plus albuterol in the emergency department. Am J Respir Crit Care Med 2000;161:1862–1868.

8. Rowe BH, Spooner C, Ducharme FM, et al: Early emergency department treatment of acute asthma with systemic corticosteroids. Cochrane Database Syst Rev 2006;(1):CD002178.

9. Rodrigo G, Rodrigo C: Inhaled flunisolide for acute severe asthma. Am J Respir Crit Care Med 1998;157:698–703.

10. Parameswaran K, Belda J, Rowe BH: Addition of intravenous aminophylline to beta2-agonists in adults with acute asthma. Cochrane Database Syst Rev 2000;(4):CD002742.

11. Rowe BH, Bretzlaff JA, Bourdon C, et al: Magnesium sulfate for treating exacerbations of acute asthma in the emergency department [systematic review]. Cochrane Airways Group. Cochrane Database Syst Rev 2006;(1):CD001490.

12. Camargo CA Jr, Smithline HA, Malice MP, et al: A randomized controlled trial of intravenous montelukast in acute asthma. Am J Respir Crit Care Med 2003;167:528–533.

13. Rodrigo G, Pollack C, Rodrigo C, Rowe BH: Heliox for nonintubated acute asthma patients. Cochrane Database Syst Rev 2006;(1):CD002884.

14. Soroksky A, Stav D, Shpirer I: A pilot prospective, randomized, placebo-controlled trial of bilevel positive pressure airway pressure in acute asthma attack. Chest 2003;123:1018–1025.

15. Tuxen DV, Lane S: The effects of ventilatory pattern on hyperinflation, airway pressures, and circulation in mechanical ventilation of patients with severe air-flow obstruction. Am Rev Respir Dis 1987;136:872–879.

16. Corne S, Gillespie D, Roberts D, Younes M: Effect of inspiratory flow rate on respiratory rate in intubated patients. Am J Respir Crit Care Med 1997;156:304–308.

17. Williams TJ, Tuxen DV, Scheinkestel CD, et al: Risk factors for morbidity in mechanically ventilated patients with acute severe asthma. Am Rev Respir Dis 1992;146:607–615.

18. Kress JP, Pohlman A, O'Connor MF, Hall JB: Daily interruption of sedative infusions in critically ill patients undergoing mechanical ventilation. N Engl J Med 2000;342:1471–1477.

19. Manthous CA, Hall JB: Update on using therapeutic aerosols in mechanically ventilated patients. J Crit Illness 1996;11:457.

20. Afessa B, Morales I, Cury JD: Clinical course and outcome of patients admitted to an ICU for status asthmaticus. Chest 2001;120:1616–1621.

Environmental Modification: Allergen Avoidance

Elizabeth A. Erwin and Thomas A.E. Platts-Mills

CLINICAL PEARLS

- Identify the sources of exposure that are relevant by a combination of history, knowledge of probable exposure, and definition of specific sensitization.
- Educate patients about the role that exposure plays in the disease and the appropriate measures to control exposure.
- Identify those cases in which the primary or secondary factors are not dependent on the environment.

The word allergen was originally proposed by von Pirquet to encompass all foreign antigens including those that caused "super sensitivity" without immunity.[1] Over the years the word came to be associated only with those antigens that gave rise to immediate or immunoglobulin E (IgE)-mediated hypersensitivity. In keeping with this, the word allergic in common usage implies awareness of a direct relationship between exposure and symptoms. As our understanding of allergic disease has developed, it has become clear that the major role of inhalant allergens in asthma is in maintaining chronic inflammation of the lungs. If the relationship between exposure and symptoms is clear to the patients and their physicians, it is not difficult to make the case for avoidance. An obvious example occurs with occupational asthma, where avoidance is accepted as the first line of treatment. In contrast, for many of the major inhalant allergens associated with asthma, the relevance of exposure to lung symptoms is not apparent to the patients. Such examples include allergens from dust mite, cockroach, and the fungus *Alternaria*. Lack of patient awareness created major problems in the past in establishing the causal relationship between these allergens and asthma and continues to present a challenge in education of both patients and physicians. It is unlikely that any avoidance measures will be successful unless the patient (or parent) is convinced that he or she is allergic.

Establishing a relationship between allergic sensitization and symptoms of asthma is only the first issue; the next question is what measures can be taken to decrease exposure. This is a complex issue for many reasons. Most patients have sensitivities to multiple allergens that may be contributing to their problems. In addition, exposure to some allergens is relatively easier to control than others. Avoidance is not a new treatment. In 1946 the New York City Department of Health initiated "Operation Ragweed," which consisted of spraying ragweed annually in advance of the pollen season with an ultimate goal of eradicating the weed from the city.[2] Over 9 years they estimated a 50% reduction in ragweed acreage.

Pollen measurements throughout the city and even in areas without ragweed that were separated from the city by water did not show any indication of decreases in ragweed indices.[2] We now focus most strategies on decreasing exposure to indoor allergens, but in the mobile society of the 21st century this is complicated by time spent in the homes of relatives and daily exposures at school, daycare, and work.

Avoidance is by no means simple. The goal of this chapter is to provide guidance to individuals caring for people with asthma and to review the existing evidence. The primary concerns in using environmental modification in the treatment of asthma are the following:

1. Identifying the sources of exposure that are relevant by a combination of history, knowledge of probable exposure, and definition of specific sensitization.
2. Educating patients about the role that exposure plays in the disease and the appropriate measures to control exposure.
3. Careful identification of those cases in which the primary or secondary factors are not dependent on the environment.

Each of these issues will be discussed; however, some only in as far as they have direct relationship to understanding allergen avoidance.

THE RELEVANCE OF SENSITIZATION AND THE USE OF SKIN TESTS OR BLOOD TESTS

Although histories are essential, the accounts may be confusing and may only be reliable for the most obvious seasonal exposures. Thus identifying sensitization is essential both to decide what advice to give and to convince the patient that avoidance measures are relevant. Although the time course of inflammatory response to allergen exposure in the lungs is not immediate, the only form of immunity that has been convincingly associated with asthma is immediate or IgE-mediated sensitivity.[3–5] This response can be established either by skin tests or blood tests, and there are good arguments for both approaches. Skin testing either with prick tests or with additional intradermal tests has been the major approach used by allergists because of the advantages in convincing the patients about the role of sensitivity in their disease and decreased sensitivity of older radioallergosorbent testing (RAST) techniques. Although intradermal skin tests are more painful and their role in diagnosing clinically meaningful allergy remains controversial, many practitioners consider them to be essential in identifying or excluding sensitivity to animals and fungi. Blood tests for IgE antibodies were introduced shortly after the discovery of IgE in 1967. The techniques have improved steadily so that today the solid phase used for antigen binding has very high

Table 24-1 PROPERTIES OF INDOOR ALLERGENS			
	Dust mite[50]	Cat[51]	Cockroach[52]
Particle size	>10 μm	<2–15 μm	>10 μm
Exposure	Disturbance	Airborne	Disturbance
Function	Many proteases	Uteroglobin	Many proteases

Table 24-2 EFFECTIVE METHODS FOR DECREASING ALLERGEN EXPOSURE AT HOME
Dust Mite Allergen
Bedding
Allergen-impermeable mattress and pillow encasements
Washing sheets, blankets, and/or duvets in hot water (>130° C)
Removal of stuffed animals (washing or freezing may substitute if removal is refused)
Carpet
Removal
Use of vacuum cleaners with double layer bag or HEPA filter
Cat Allergen
Removal of pet from home
Washing pet for 3 minutes twice weekly
Removal of carpet
Cockroach Allergen
Extermination (professional or gel traps)
Thorough cleaning with solutions containing sodium hypochlorite

capacity and the washing techniques provide consistent low background. In addition, the units for specific IgE are now the same or at least very similar to the units used for total serum IgE. Thus, it is possible to consider the relationship between specific IgE antibodies and total IgE, and even express specific IgE as a percentage of the total IgE. Recent evidence suggests that high-titer IgE response to mite, cockroach, or *Alternaria* may contribute to the strong association between asthma and total IgE. Certainly positive skin tests with a wheal larger than 6×6 mm or IgE antibodies of high titer, that is, greater than 10 IU/mL, are strongly associated with asthma.

The range of allergens used for skin testing is still a subject of debate and varies in different areas of the country.[6,7] Some authorities would restrict testing to approximately 20 antigens, although this requires using tree, weed, and fungal mixes that give less specific information. For the indoor allergens it is essential to test with dust mites, cockroach, cat, and dog (Table 24-1). In any inner-city area mouse and rat allergens should also be tested.[8–10] The range of fungi should at least include *Alternaria*, *Cladosporium*, *Pencillium*, *Aspergillus*, and *Helminthosporum*. There are good arguments for including *Candida* and *Trichophyton* species when testing in adults.[11] However, as mentioned previously only immediate responses have been associated with asthma, and although fungi often give rise to delayed skin responses, those have not been shown to be relevant to asthma.[6]

IDENTIFYING THE SOURCES OF EXPOSURE

This task depends on our understanding of the nature of different allergens and the characteristics of the species from which the allergen is derived. The identification of dust mites as the component of house dust causing reactions in individuals around the world was a major step toward understanding indoor exposures.[12] Isolation of the allergen Der p I from mites made direct measurement of exposure possible, and "bed dust" from blankets and mattresses was found to have the highest levels when compared with other areas of the house.[13] Further understanding of the characteristics of dust mites helps to direct us toward sources of exposure and toward defining strategies for avoidance. Dust mites rely on the relative humidity of the environment to sustain their body water. Levels of humidity from 75% to 80% are optimal and below 60% mites start to desiccate. As a result, mites are not found in areas where high altitude (>1000 m) or cold ambient temperature results in low indoor humidity.[14]

MEASURES TO CONTROL EXPOSURE

Techniques of avoidance have been outlined and updated previously by the contributions of many experts through several workshops and various review papers.[15–18] The overall goal of avoidance is to decrease allergen exposure to a level below which symptoms are thought to occur. For the population as a whole, such levels could be 2 μg/g dust for dust mite allergens as a risk factor for asthma, 8 μg/g dust for Fel d 1, and 2 U/g dust for Bla g 1.[4,5,8] Since individuals vary in sensitivity to allergens, 90% reduction in allergen exposure has been proposed as an alternative goal.[19] Regardless of the target exposure level, effective control of allergen exposure must treat allergen sources or reservoirs by multiple overlapping methods with an approach that can be maintained (Table 24-2).

Dust mite

Dust mite allergen is carried on large particles (20 to 30 μm) that are not detected in the air in the absence of disturbance. Effective avoidance strategies focus on eliminating dust mite reservoirs including bedding. Dust mite encasings have been shown to decrease dust mite measurements in multiple studies.[19–21] Mattress (box spring) and pillow encasings that are permeable to air and water vapor but not mites are used to decrease reaccumulation of dust mites on bedding but should not be used in isolation of other strategies.[16,17] The use of different materials has been evaluated, and tightly woven fabrics with smaller than 10-μm pore size were found to exclude mites below detectable limits.[22] New evidence suggests that the nonwoven fabrics are not impermeable to mites, can accumulate mite allergen, and may not be impermeable to allergen over a long period. Reaccumulation of dust mites and allergen is addressed by modification of laundry habits. In contrast to dry cleaning or washing at cooler temperatures, washing in hot water (above 55° C or 130° F) kills dust mites and removes allergen.[16]

Dust mite eradication from carpeting has not been as successful. Vacuum cleaning can reduce the burden of allergen, but it has no effect on live mites and is not likely to be sufficient to control dust mite exposure. While vacuums vary widely in features and expense, the only specific evidence-based recommendations are that cleaners should have bags with two layers or a HEPA filter on the exhaust.[23,24]

The use of carpet treatments such as acaricides, tannic acid, or a combination of both does not provide much added benefit. Chemical treatments such as benzyl benzoate, pyrethroids, benzyl alcohol, and benzoic acid in the form of powders, foams, and liquids all work in the laboratory to kill mites. Tannic acid decreases allergen levels by its denaturing action on proteins. In homes, a variety of different preparations have shown little effect (less than 50% reduction) and all require reapplication at frequent intervals.[15] It is not known whether the problem of efficacy results from lack of penetration or the effect of dirt in carpets acting as "protection." Furthermore, exposure of carpets to direct sun with concurrent low humidity can kill dust mites but washing or beating is required to remove allergen. Freezing soft toys for 24 hours can be an efficient way of killing mites if the toys cannot be washed.

Cat

Although recent evidence would argue against removal of cats from the home as an effective means of primary prevention of sensitization (this will be discussed in more detail later), no substitute has been found for removal of cats for sensitized children who are symptomatic. In the research setting, bathing can be used to reduce cat allergen levels.[25,26] Avner and colleagues[25] showed that after a bath of longer than 3 minutes, allergen levels were substantially lower 3 hours later. The effect did not persist after 1 week suggesting that cats would have to be washed more frequently than once weekly. In a home it may be necessary to remove carpets and sofas as well as washing the cat.[26] It is possible these measures could provide clinical benefit though, since cat allergen exposure can be reduced to a level that would take 8 hours to induce a bronchial response.[26] It must be noted that even when a cat is removed from the house, although allergen levels gradually decline, it takes about 6 months for levels to be as low as those found in homes without cats.[27] Furthermore, in some homes levels remain persistently elevated. The reduction occurs more rapidly if reservoirs (carpets and furniture) that contain cat allergen are also removed.

Cockroach

In inner-city homes, cockroach exposure is a major burden that can be reduced significantly. Several investigators studied homes that had two extermination visits in which abamectin was applied.[28,29] Allergen levels (Bla g 1) in those homes decreased by 64% and 80% to 90%, respectively. Still, some question the clinical benefits because allergen levels typically remain above the threshold believed to induce symptoms.

EFFICACY OF AVOIDANCE

It has been difficult to design the ideal study to evaluate the success of allergen avoidance, but in examining the results of studies in which a major reduction in exposure was achieved, certain patterns are apparent. First, patients, both adults and children, who are studied while they are staying in the hospital for extended periods of time or while they are undergoing residential treatment at high altitude, consistently show improvements in subjective and objective measures of asthma. An early case report suggested that hospital admission to a dust-free room for a patient with severe asthma could be associated with symptomatic improvement.[30] Platts-Mills and colleagues[31] also found that adult patients with allergic asthma who stayed in a dust-free hospital room experienced fewer symptoms and were able to reduce their medications. Furthermore, morning peak flow measurements improved and most patients showed a highly significant decrease in bronchial hyperreactivity as judged by PC_{30} response to histamine. Similarly, children with allergies and asthma who stayed in the Italian Alps (Misurina, 1756 m) for an extended period of time showed gradual improvement in pulmonary function and a need for fewer medications.[32] A much more difficult issue to interpret is the response to avoidance as a treatment for asthma in the community.

While some studies implementing dust mite avoidance measures have shown benefit, others have failed to show any improvement, leaving room for debate about what conclusions should be drawn (Table 24-3). Most investigations that used mattress and pillow encasings in combination with frequent

Table 24-3
CHARACTERISTICS AND OUTCOMES OF CLINICAL TRIALS INCORPORATING DECREASED DUST MITE EXPOSURE

Investigators	Methods	Less Exposure	Symptom Improvement
Burr et al[53]	Covers	N/A	No
Murray et al[33]	Covers, washing	N/A	Yes
Walshaw et al[34]	Covers, washing, carpet removal	Yes	Yes
Dorward et al[54]	Chemical, vacuuming, washing	N/A	Yes
Ehnert et al[35]	Covers, chemical	N/A	Yes
Marks et al[37]	Covers, chemical	Yes (also placebo)	Yes (also placebo)
Carswell et al[20]	Covers, washing, chemical	Yes	Yes (small effect)
van der Heide et al[36]	Covers, chemical	Yes (covers)	Yes (small effect)
Warner et al[55]	Whole-house ventilation	Yes	No
Carter et al[21]	Covers, washing, cockroach	Yes	Yes
Woodcock et al[39]	Covers	No	No
Terreehorst et al[38]	Covers, washing	Yes	No
Morgan et al[40]	Covers, vacuuming, cockroach	Yes	Yes

N/A, not assessed.

washing of bedding have been associated with decreases in dust mite allergen and improvement in asthma from the standpoint of fewer symptoms or decreased bronchial hyper-reactivity.[20,21,33-36] Sometimes improvements in objective measurements were small, raising doubts about the clinical significance.[20,36] In other cases, patients in both placebo and active treatment groups improved.[37] Overall, the use of acaricides without other measures of avoidance has not produced significant decreases in allergen or symptoms.[20]

Two recent studies that did not support a beneficial effect from mattress encasings used alone were well publicized and have challenged the effectiveness of avoidance.[38,39] Careful evaluation of these studies can highlight some of the difficulties associated with studying allergen avoidance. In one study, coverings were applied without any other advice and the treatment did not produce a significant decrease in exposure at 1 year.[39] In the other study relating to rhinitis, patients were given active or placebo mattress covers; however, all patients were instructed to wash the bedding regularly in hot water.[38] More significantly, it was not clear how the patients were enrolled since the mean total serum IgE was higher than in other studies on allergic rhinitis.[38] In both studies, patients in both placebo and active treatment groups improved with the measures used.[38,39] Another issue raised by these large-scale studies is that in general the same plan for avoidance may not work equally for all patients.

The inner city provides a particular challenge for asthma treatment because of the severe nature of allergic symptoms, primary care that is often fragmented in nature, and high levels of allergen exposure.[8,21,40] Attempts to improve the indoor environment as a whole can be associated with improvements in asthma. Carter and colleagues[21] focused on dust mite avoidance using mattress covers and techniques for washing bedding as well as cockroach avoidance by using bait. Their results were mixed with decreased mite measurements in only one third of homes and decreased acute visits in both the active and placebo groups. However, when children who were sensitized and exposed to dust mite were analyzed separately, the difference in acute visits that was observed was significant.[21] Morgan and associates[40] treated a large group of children with extensive education, implementation of allergen avoidance, and close follow-up. They included allergen impermeable covers, vacuum cleaners with HEPA filters, HEPA filters in bedrooms (for those exposed to tobacco, pets, or fungi), and professional pest control. Although there were no significant effects on lung function, they observed a significant reduction in asthma-related symptoms and fewer unscheduled visits with a physician.

Although most allergists recommend pet removal for children with animal allergies, there are only a few small studies evaluating measures of pet avoidance. In one study, the use of air cleaners was associated with decreased bronchial hyper-reactivity and less variation in peak flows measured in the morning and afternoon.[41] A concurrent change in symptoms was not observed.[41] Another group compared patients who chose to remove pets from their homes with those who did not.[42] They did not find any differences in measures of airway inflammation (induced sputum) between groups.[42] They did observe improvements in PC_{20} with pet removal and some decrease in symptoms as judged by reduction in medications and less need for follow-up.[42]

IMMUNE MECHANISMS

The results of studies on either immune responses or tissue markers of allergic inflammation, in the setting of dust mite allergen avoidance, suggest that inflammation is decreased. Many of the studies were performed on children undergoing the natural means of dust mite avoidance that occurred when they moved to high elevation. Changes have been assessed by measurements of total IgE and specific IgE antibody to dust mite.[14] Although skin test responses did not change, total IgE and specific antibody levels decreased by 40% and 50% respectively over a period of 3 to 9 months of avoidance.[14] These findings were duplicated using markers of eosinophil activity (eosinophil cationic protein [ECP]) and blood eosinophils, as well as serum total and specific IgE antibody responses.[43] Over a period of several months in a sanatorium, significant decreases in ECP, IgE antibody, and total IgE levels were observed. In addition, Piacentini and colleagues[44] reported that antigen-induced histamine release from basophils was decreased after 6 weeks in a dust mite–free environment. Furthermore, re-exposure to dust mite correlated with return of specific IgE and basophil releasability to the levels measured before avoidance.[44] The results were similar for measures of airway inflammation including sputum eosinophils and exhaled nitric oxide levels with decreases observed in both parameters after 3 months of avoidance.[45,46] T-cell studies suggest less activation during avoidance as judged by decreased CD25 expression and an increased ratio of CD45RA to CD45RO cells.[47]

THE CHALLENGE OF DOMESTIC ANIMALS

Although many patients report acute onset of symptoms on entering a house with an animal, the clearest histories of this kind come from patients who do not live in a house with a cat. Indeed, in some studies as many as 80% of the children who are allergic to cats have never lived in a house with a cat. There are at least three parts to this enigma. First, that cat and dog allergens are found both in dust and airborne in places without an animal. Thus, it is not unusual to find more than 2 μg/g Fel d 1/g dust in schools, public buildings, and homes without a cat. These concentrations are sufficient to give rise to both sensitization and symptoms. Second, there are patients who live in a house with a cat and have a positive skin test who report very mild symptoms or are in denial about the role of their own animal. Third, many otherwise allergic individuals who live in a house with a cat are both skin test and serum IgE antibody negative to cat allergens. A wide range of evidence now suggests that the subjects without IgE antibody do develop an immune response to the cat allergen Fel d 1, but this response does not produce symptoms. This response, which can be regarded as a form of immune tolerance, includes antibodies of the IgG4 isotype and T cells that produce interleukin (IL)-10 and interferon gamma (IFN-γ) in vitro. The lack of symptoms in these children argues strongly that it is the IgE antibody element of the immune response that gives rise to the risk of asthma.

Clearly, the fact that some individuals become "tolerant" in the face of high exposure to an allergen poses significant problems for advising avoidance. At a simple level, removing an animal should not be recommended unless the patient is skin test positive. However the more complex question is whether tolerance to animal allergens is reversible. Anecdotally, many college students report that they become allergic to their own home after being away for 2 or more months. The implication is that decreased exposure could lead to an increase in sensitization or allergic symptoms. Similarly it is not known whether exposure can induce this form of tolerance in an allergic individual. The fact that pet removal is only a means of *reducing* exposure must be emphasized. As mentioned, pet exposure occurs to a significant degree in homes without a cat as well as in day-care, school, and other public settings. In our mobile society, even children are exposed to a wide range of environments. Given the complexity of the situation it is not surprising that there have not been any successful controlled trials of allergen avoidance for cat allergens in patients with asthma.

WHEN SENSITIZATION IS IMPORTANT WITHOUT ENVIRONMENTAL EXPOSURE

Especially among adults, the situation may arise where sensitization (i.e., IgE antibodies) is associated with disease but environmental modification is not a solution. This phenomenon is manifested by at least two examples. The first is an association between fungal hypersensitivity and colonization in the lungs. The best-known type is allergic bronchopulmonary aspergillosis (ABPA), but other fungi may also be relevant. It is not clear why some patients develop this complication. Typically these patients have peripheral blood eosinophilia, increased total IgE, specific IgE antibody to the fungus involved, cough, sputum production, and in advanced cases bronchiectasis. Symptoms can be severe and difficult to control with the usual medicines used to treat asthma. Some patients become dependent on steroids. Environmental exposure has not been clearly associated with the risk of developing this complication although some studies suggest that high exposure from chicken or turkey sheds may contribute. Fungal growth in the lungs is the cause of persistent symptoms; and although single sputum cultures may be negative, repeated cultures will usually give a positive result. It is useful to obtain a culture to identify the occasional case caused by other fungi, for example, *Candida* or *Curvularia*. Also, the in vitro sensitivity of the colonizing *Aspergillus* may help predict response to oral antifungal treatment.[48]

Less commonly, *Trichophyton* sensitivity may be identified in association with extensive onychomycosis in men with late-onset and severe asthma.[11] Importantly, these cases respond to antifungal treatment with fluconazole.[49] The syndrome is of mechanistic interest because *Trichophyton* species are strict dermatophytes and cannot grow in the respiratory tract. This implies that antigen absorbed from sites of fungal growth in the skin or nail beds can induce a T-cell–mediated inflammatory response localized to the lungs. Alternatively, almost all these patients have extensive sinus disease, so it seems possible that T cells are primed secondarily in the sinuses and can then localize to the lungs. Whatever the mechanism, as emphasized in this chapter, these patients do not get better when admitted to the hospital

(an early criteria for intrinsic asthma) but may improve with antifungal treatment.[49]

CONCLUSION

Changing a home sufficiently to make a significant decrease in allergen exposure is not easy. Thus, it is important to identify correctly those patients who should decrease exposure and to educate them about the measures necessary to achieve this. As in any proposal about a new treatment, it is important to be aware of the reasons why it might fail. In the case of allergen avoidance, there are several obvious reasons and some less obvious:

1. The patient does not have asthma: e.g., vocal cord dysfunction (VCD) or breathing difficulty secondary to obesity.
2. The patient is not allergic to the allergen.
3. Significant exposure is occurring somewhere other than the patient's home: for example, school or the houses of relatives.
4. Other causes of severity have not been adequately addressed.
5. Measures proposed or carried out will not produce a prolonged decrease in exposure.

Determining sensitization is essential both to decide which allergens are relevant and also to convince patients that the treatment is worth the effort. In patients who have severe disease, it is essential to exclude complications such as sinus disease, VCD, or an infectious component. Equally, other allergens in the environment should be considered, or the possible harmful effects of one of the other treatments.

Having identified a patient who has persistent symptoms and is allergic to one of the indoor allergens that is likely to be present in their environment, it is essential to provide the education and educational materials about the proposed measures. Single measures do not work; thus, vacuum cleaning the carpets, covering the mattress, or removing soft toys are not on their own likely to have any effect. However, taken together, removing carpets; washing the bedding in hot water; covering the mattresses and pillows; and removing excess toys or furniture can produce a more than 90% reduction in mite exposure. Measures of this kind can produce significant improvement in asthma symptoms and particularly in bronchial hyperreactivity among mite-allergic patients. Similarly for cat-allergic patients, it is possible to decrease exposure by a combination of removing carpets, regular cleaning, and air filtration; however, it is simpler to give the cat away.

Education about the role of avoidance should include advice that the improvement that follows successful reduction in exposure will take time, i.e., months, to occur; and that measures ideally should become part of lifestyle and do not need to be carried out at once. Moving from one home to another is a regular part of American life. Measures that may seem impossible or too difficult may be simple if the correct choices are made when moving. Thus, education should recognize the possibility of making choices now or in the future. In all cases, the proposed measures should be designed so that they do not require major effort and can be a part of normal lifestyle in the long term.

REFERENCES

1. von Pirquet CE: Allergy. Chicago, American Medical Association, 1911.
2. Walzer M, Siegel BB: The effectiveness of the ragweed eradication campaigns in New York City. J Allergy 1955;27:113–126.
3. Sears MR, Herbison GP, Holdaway MD, et al: The relative risks of sensitivity to grass pollen, house dust mite and cat dander in the development of childhood asthma. Clin Exp Allergy 1989;19:419–424.
4. Sporik R, Holgate ST, Platts-Mills TAE, Cogswell JJ: Exposure to house-dust mite allergen (Der p I) and the development of asthma in childhood: a prospective study. N Engl J Med 1990;323:502–507.
5. Gelber LE, Seltzer LH, Bouzoukis JK, et al: Sensitization and exposure to indoor allergens as risk factors for asthma among patients presenting to hospital. Am Rev Respir Dis 1993;147:573–578.
6. Bernstein IL, Storms WW, Joint Task Force on Practice Parameters: Summary statements of practice parameters for allergy diagnostic tests. Ann Allergy Asthma Immunol 1995;75:543–625.
7. Esch RE, Bush RK: Aerobiology of outdoor allergens. In Adkinson NF, Yunginger JW, Busse WW, et al (eds): Middleton's Allergy: Principles and Practice. 6th ed. Philadelphia, Mosby, 2003, pp 532–543.
8. Rosenstreich DL, Eggleston P, Kattan M, et al: The role of cockroach allergy and exposure to cockroach allergen in causing morbidity among inner-city children with asthma. N Engl J Med 1997;336:1356–1363.
9. Phipatanakul W, Eggleston PA, Wright EC, Wood RA: Mouse allergen. II. The relationship of mouse allergen exposure to mouse sensitization and asthma morbidity in inner-city children with asthma. J Allergy Clin Immunol 2000;106:1075–1080.
10. Perry T, Matsui E, Merriman B, et al: The prevalence of rat allergen in inner-city homes and its relationship to sensitization and asthma morbidity. J Allergy Clin Immunol 2003;112:346–352.
11. Ward GWJ, Karlsson G, Rose G, Platts-Mills TAE: Trichophyton asthma: sensitization of bronchi and upper airways to dermatophyte antigen. Lancet 1989;1:859–862.
12. Voorhorst R, Spieksma FTM, Varekamp H, et al: The house-dust mite (Dermatophagoides pteronyssinus) and the allergen it produces. Identity with the house-dust allergen. J Allergy 1967;39:325–339.
13. Tovey ER, Chapman MD, Platts-Mills TAE: Mite faeces are a major source of house dust allergens. Nature 1981;289:592–593.
14. Vervloet D, Penaud A, Razzouk H, et al: Altitude and house dust mites. J Allergy Clin Immunol 1982;69:290–296.
15. Platts-Mills TA, Thomas WR, Aalberse RC, et al: Dust mite allergens and asthma: report of a second international workshop. J Allergy Clin Immunol 1992;89:1046–1060.
16. Platts-Mills TAE, Vervloet D, Thomas WR, et al: Indoor allergens and asthma: Report of the Third International Workshop. J Allergy Clin Immunol 1997;100:S1–24.
17. Tovey E, Marks G: Methods and effectiveness of environmental control. J Allergy Clin Immunol 1999;103:179–191.
18. Eggleston PA: Improving indoor environments: reducing allergen exposures. J Allergy Clin Immunol 2005;116:122–126.
19. Owen S, Morganstern M, Hepworth J, Woodcock A: Control of house dust mite antigen in bedding. Lancet 1990;335:396–397.
20. Carswell F, Birmingham K, Oliver J, et al: The respiratory effects of reduction of mite allergen in the bedrooms of asthmatic children—a double-blind controlled trial. Clin Exp Allergy 1996;26:386–396.
21. Carter MC, Perzanowski MS, Raymond A, Platts-Mills TAE: Home intervention in the treatment of asthma among inner-city children. J Allergy Clin Immunol 2001;108:732–737.
22. Vaughan JW, McLaughlin TE, Perzanowski MS, Platts-Mills TAE: Evaluation of materials used for bedding encasements: effect of pore size in blocking cat and dust mite allergen. J Allergy Clin Immunol 1999;103:327–331.
23. De Blay F, Verot A, Ott M, et al: Airborne levels and particle size distribution of cat major allergen (Fel d 1) following use of "anti-allergenic" and standard vacuum cleaners. J Allergy Clin Immunol 1992;89:313–318.
24. Woodfolk JA, Luczynska CM, de Blay F, et al: The effect of vacuum cleaners on the concentration and particle size distribution of airborne cat allergen. J Allergy Clin Immunol 1993;91:829–837.
25. Avner DB, Perzanowski MS, Platts-Mills TAE, Woodfolk JA: Evaluation of different techniques for washing cats: quantitation of allergen removed from the cat and the effect on airborne Fel d 1. J Allergy Clin Immunol 1997;100:307–312.
26. De Blay, Chapman MD, Platts-Mills TAE: Airborne cat allergen (Fel d I). Environmental control with the cat in situ. Am Rev Respir Dis 1991;43:1334–1339.
27. Wood RA, Chapman MD, Adkinson NF, Eggleston PA: The effect of cat removal on allergen content in household dust samples. J Allergy Clin Immunol 1989;83:730–734.
28. Gergen PJ, Mortimer KM, Eggleston PA, et al: Results of the National Cooperative Inner-City Asthma Study (NCICAS) environmental intervention to reduce cockroach allergen exposure in inner-city homes. J Allergy Clin Immunol 1999;103:501–506.
29. Wood RA, Eggleston PA, Rand C, et al: Cockroach allergen abatement with extermination and sodium hypochlorite cleaning in inner-city homes. Ann Allergy Asthma Immunol 2001;87:60–64.
30. Leopold SS, Leopold CS: Bronchial asthma and allied allergic disorders. JAMA 1925;84:731–734.
31. Platts-Mills TAE, Tovey ER, Mitchell EB, et al: Reduction of bronchial hyperreactivity during prolonged allergen avoidance. Lancet 1982;2:675–678.
32. Boner AL, Niero E, Antolini I, et al: Pulmonary function and bronchial hyperreactivity in asthmatic children during prolonged stay in the Italian alps (Misurina, 1756 m). Ann Allergy 1985;54:42–45.
33. Murray AB, Ferguson AC: Dust-free bedrooms in the treatment of asthmatic children with house dust or house dust mite allergy: a controlled trial. Pediatrics 1983;71:418–422.
34. Walshaw MJ, Evans CC: Allergen avoidance in house dust mite sensitive adult asthma. Q J Med 1986;58:199–215.
35. Ehnert B, Lau-Schadendorf S, Weber A, et al: Reducing domestic exposure to dust mite allergen reduces bronchial hyperreactivity in sensitive children with asthma. J Allergy Clin Immunol 1992;90:135–138.
36. van der Heide S, Kauffman HF, Dubois AE, de Monchy JG: Allergen-avoidance measures in homes of house-dust-mite-allergic asthmatic patients: effects of acaricides and mattress encasings. Allergy 1997;52:921–927.
37. Marks GB, Tovey ER, Green W, et al: House dust mite allergen avoidance: a randomized controlled trial of surface chemical treatment and encasement of bedding. Clin Exp Allergy 1994;24:1078–1083.
38. Terreehorst I, Hak E, Oosting AJ, et al: Evaluation of impermeable covers for bedding in patients with allergic rhinitis. N Engl J Med 2003;349:237–246.
39. Woodcock A, Forster L, Matthews E, et al: Control of exposure to mite allergen and allergen-impermeable covers for adults with asthma. N Engl J Med 2003;349:225–236.
40. Morgan WJ, Crain EF, Gruchalla RS, et al: Results of a home-based environmental intervention among urban children with asthma. N Engl J Med 2004;351:1068–1080.
41. van der Heide S, van Aalderen WM, Kauffman HF, et al: Clinical effects of air cleaners in homes of asthmatic children sensitized to pet allergens. J Allergy Clin Immunol 1999;104:447–451.
42. Shirai T, Matsui T, Suzuki K, Chida K: Effect of pet removal on pet allergic asthma. Chest 2005;127:1565–1571.
43. Boner AL, Peroni DG, Piacentini GL, Venge P: Influence of allergen avoidance at high altitude on serum markers of eosinophil activation in children with allergic asthma. Clin Exp Allergy 1993;23:1021–1026.

44. Piacentini GL, Martinati L, Fornari A, et al: Antigen avoidance in a mountain environment: influence on basophil releasability in children with allergic asthma. J Allergy Clin Immunol 1993;92:644–650.

45. Peroni DG, Piacentini GL, Costella S, et al: Mite avoidance can reduce air trapping and airway inflammation in allergic asthmatic children. Clin Exp Allergy 2002;32:850–855.

46. Piacentini GL, Martinati LM, Mingoni S, Boner AL: Influence of allergen avoidance on the eosinophil phase of airway inflammation in children with allergic asthma. J Allergy Clin Immunol 1996;97:1079–1084.

47. Simon H, Grotzer M, Nikolaizik W, et al: High altitude climate therapy reduces peripheral blood T lymphocyte activation, eosinophilia, and bronchial obstruction in children with house-dust mite allergic asthma. Pediatr Pulmonol 1994;17:304–311.

48. Stevens DA, Schwartz HJ, Lee JY, et al: A randomized trial of itraconazole in allergic bronchopulmonary aspergillosis. N Engl J Med 2000;342:756–762.

49. Ward GW, Woodfolk JA, Hayden ML, et al: Treatment of late-onset asthma with fluconazole. J Allergy Clin Immunol 1998;1043:541–546.

50. Tovey ER, Chapman MD, Wells CW, Platts-Mills TAE: The distribution of dust mite allergen in the houses of patients with asthma. Am Rev Respir Dis 1981;124:630–635.

51. Luczynska CM, Li Y, Chapman MD, Platts-Mills TAE: Airborne concentrations and particle size distribution of allergen derived from domestic cats (*Felis domesticus*). Am Rev Respir Dis 1990;141:361–367.

52. deBlay F, Sanchez J, Hedelin G, et al: Dust and airborne exposure to allergens derived from cockroach (*Blattella germanica*) in low-cost public housing in Strasbourg (France). J Allergy Clin Immunol 1997;99:107–112.

53. Burr ML, St Leger AS, Neale E: Anti-mite measurements in mite-sensitive adult asthma. A controlled trial. Lancet 1976;1:333–335.

54. Dorward AJ, Colloff MJ, MacKay NS, et al: Effect of house dust mite avoidance measures on adult atopic asthma. Thorax 1988;43:98–102.

55. Warner JA, Frederick JM, Bryant TN, et al: Mechanical ventilation and high-efficiency vacuum cleaning: a combined strategy of mite and mite allergen reduction in the control of mite-sensitive asthma. J Allergy Clin Immunol 2000;105:75–82.

Teaching Patients to Manage Their Asthma

David Evans

CHAPTER 25

CLINICAL PEARLS

- Assess the patient's knowledge, beliefs, and concerns about asthma by asking open-ended questions like:
  - What do you do to take care of your asthma?
  - What worries you most about your asthma?
  - What concerns do you have about the medicines?
  - What would you like to do that you can't do now because of your asthma?
- Respond to the patient's concerns right away to inform and reassure the patient.
- Teach asthma management skills by:
  - Demonstrating them to the patient
  - Having the patient practice while you give feedback to help the patient learn
  - Asking the patient to demonstrate the skills to you at each visit
- Reach agreement with the patient on short- and long-term goals of asthma management.
- Give verbal praise for things well done.

Successful treatment of asthma requires more than just prescribing appropriate therapy for the patient and giving them a written treatment plan to follow. Meta-analyses of more than 60 controlled trials show that education for the patient and family improves asthma self-management skills, reduces symptoms, and reduces use of emergency care services in both adults and children.[1,2] As a result, asthma self-management education is now accepted as an essential part of treatment for asthma. Teaching the patient and family how to follow the treatment plan is a critical part of successful treatment. This chapter describes the key challenges in assessing and teaching patients and provides simple strategies, based on theories of behavior change, that the clinician can use with patients. Although other health professionals can supplement patient education, the clinician is in the best position to provide the initial assessment and teaching to ensure that a workable treatment plan is developed, agreed upon, and followed by the patient.

Patient education is often thought of as a one-way transfer of information and skills from the doctor to the patient. This model of education, however, is not well suited to patient education in the clinical setting. Most patients bring to the office visit a complex mix of prior experience, information, and beliefs, including worries about asthma and asthma therapy.

These beliefs and concerns influence their ability and willingness to learn from the clinician. Patients typically do not bring up these factors on their own during office visits; to identify them, clinicians need to ask questions. The patient and his or her family may also lack critical skills needed to manage asthma at home, including how to take medicines correctly, or how to recognize changing symptoms and respond appropriately. If these factors are not assessed and addressed, a common result is that patients will not follow the treatment plan, and their asthma control will suffer. To successfully treat asthma, therefore, clinicians need to assess the patient's knowledge, beliefs, and skills, and then build upon that base by correcting inappropriate health beliefs and teaching patients what they need to know to follow the treatment plan willingly and successfully.

In this chapter, we will describe some of the common beliefs and skills that remain unassessed in most office visits. We will also describe two theories of behavior change that provide some relatively simple guidelines and tools for assessing patients and providing them with brief but effective teaching to help them learn to manage their asthma successfully in partnership with their clinician. Finally, we will describe a successful physician education program to provide an example of how theory-based communications and teaching skills can help clinicians educate their patients and achieve better control of asthma.

PATIENT BELIEFS AND SKILLS THAT ARE OFTEN NOT ASSESSED DURING OFFICE VISITS

Korsch and colleagues[3] studied communication between doctors and the parents of sick children during urgent visits to a pediatric walk-in clinic. She tape-recorded 800 visits and conducted an exit interview and a 2-week follow-up interview with parents to assess communication patterns, concerns about the child's health, comprehension of the doctor's advice, and satisfaction with the visit. Only 24% of parents told the doctor about their main worry about the child's health and only 35% told the doctor what they expected from the visit. Simple open-ended questions from the doctor, such as "What worries you most about your child's illness?" helped parents voice their concerns, many of them dramatic and unrealistic fears. Parents who did voice their main worry or expectations were much more satisfied with the visit than parents who did not. It did not matter whether the parent brought up the main worry or the doctor asked about it, but if it was not discussed, parents had poor recall of the doctor's advice at the exit interview, suggesting that unexpressed worries block doctor-patient communication and patient retention of advice. Finally, it is noteworthy that parents' satisfaction was completely unrelated to the length of the visit, which ranged from less than 3 minutes to more than 15 minutes.

The findings from this study provide several key lessons for good communication with patients. These are:

- Identify the patient or family's main worry or concern using open-ended questions;
- Address the patient's concerns immediately using simple everyday language;
- Provide reassurance to the family so they can relax and listen.

Asthma patients and their families have various concerns, many of which are never conveyed to the doctor. These concerns, which may block a patient's ability to listen to the doctor and undermine adherence, include the following beliefs and fears about asthma[4]:

- Every time my child has an asthma attack, I'm afraid he might die.
- Asthma can cause heart attacks (based on observation of rapid heartbeat).
- Having asthma means you can't be physically active.
- Children outgrow asthma as they get older, so it doesn't need regular treatment now.

These concerns also include the following beliefs about asthma treatment[5]:

- Asthma medicines are addictive; if you take them, you won't be able to get off them.
- Asthma medicines are harmful if you take them for a long time.
- If you take the medicines every day, they won't work when you really need them.
- Steroids (of any kind, dose, or route of administration) cause serious side effects.

These beliefs, particularly those about asthma medicines, are likely to lead parents to not use medicines needed to control their child's asthma, or to fail to help the patient live an active life free of limitations.

In addition, critical patient skills and knowledge are often not assessed during the office visit. Patients or families may not know how to use medication devices correctly, and if these are not assessed and corrected, patients cannot improve. Similarly, patients may not know how or when to adjust doses or start additional medicines. Use of a written treatment plan is helpful, but it is essential to review the plan with the patient and have the patient describe how he or she will respond to specific changes in symptoms or peak flow.

Knowledge of what irritants or allergens cause flare-ups of asthma symptoms, and how to control the patient's environment to avoid or reduce them, is also an area that is rarely assessed properly. Developing this knowledge and skill may take time, but the groundwork for these skills must be laid in regular assessment and discussion of these issues.

Finally, patients and their families need to develop the information and skills needed to teach relatives and school or work personnel what they can do to help the patient control his or her asthma. As the patient or family grows more knowledgeable and skilled at controlling asthma, they may do this themselves, but by asking questions about this area, and offering help, such as letters to school officials,

clinicians can stimulate the development of these important self-management skills.

BEHAVIOR CHANGE THEORIES AND STRATEGIES FOR CHANGE

Two theories of behavior change, the health belief model and social cognitive theory, have been widely used to develop strategies to help patients learn to adopt healthy behaviors and to work with their clinicians to improve their health. These theories are summarized below, and specific questions and teaching strategies clinicians can use are presented.

The Health Belief Model (HBM) was developed in the 1950s to explain why people did or did not take part in programs to detect or prevent disease, such as x-ray screenings to detect tuberculosis.[6] The model was later applied to how people responded to illnesses that had been diagnosed, including adherence to medical regimens. Since then, the HBM has been used widely in studies of health behavior. The HBM proposes that preventive or therapeutic recommendations by the clinician are more likely to be followed if the patient feels that:

- I am *susceptible* to this disease.
- I believe that the disease is *serious*.
- I believe that the *benefits* of the recommended treatment will outweigh the *costs* or *barriers* involved in following it.
- I am *confident* that I can carry out the recommended treatment successfully.

In addition, HBM suggests that patients are more likely to follow recommendations if they are exposed to cues to action, such as written or telephone reminders, or public announcements such as posters and public service advertisements on radio.

The HBM provides a useful framework for guiding clinicians' thinking about how to teach their patients and persuade them to follow the treatment plan. A good way to begin, once the initial history or complaint has been discussed, is to ask four basic open-ended questions:

1. What concerns you most about your asthma?
2. What do you know about asthma?
3. What concerns do you have about the medicines?
4. What would you like to do that you can't do now because of your asthma?

These questions invite patients to talk about their feelings, but focus the issue on what matters to them about asthma. The answers will often provide clues the clinician can follow up on to assess specific areas of the HBM. For example, it is often not clear how *susceptible* patients feel about different aspects of asthma or asthma diagnosis. A clinician may not be sure whether the family believes the patient has asthma at all. Other families may readily accept the notion that the patient has asthma, but not believe that it is a chronic problem that exists even when symptoms are not present. Some patients may agree they have asthma, but not believe they are susceptible to having serious asthma exacerbations. These issues can be explored with follow-up questions directed at the issue of susceptibility. For example, "How likely is it that your child will have another asthma attack like this one? or "Do you think you will continue to have asthma symptoms in the next year?" or "How do you feel about the idea that your child has asthma?" Similarly, the patient or family's perception of the *seriousness* of asthma can be explored with questions such as "How serious do you think your asthma is?" or "What do you think will happen if your child's asthma is not treated?" The answers to these questions are likely to bring out the patient's feelings about susceptibility and seriousness, and the clinician can then engage in a discussion with the patient and provide accurate information.

The four basic questions listed above are also likely to provide information about the patient's perception of the potential *benefits* of following the clinician's recommended treatment, as well as perceived *barriers* to doing so. If the recommended treatment is new, the patient is not likely to have given much thought to the potential benefits of following it. The clinician may be able to use the patients' answers to questions about concerns to help patients link the problems they want solved to what the clinician teaches them about the benefits of therapy. For example, "What benefits do you think you might get if you took the inhaled corticosteroid every day?" If the patient is not sure, the clinician can then tie the potential benefits to the patient's expressed concerns: "Earlier you said you were bothered by not being able to sleep through the night. The inhaled corticosteroid that I'd like to prescribe for you will help you to do that. It will also enable you to be physically active without wheezing or coughing. What do you think about that?" A good follow-up question is "Can you think of any other ways this treatment might help your asthma or your ability to do the things you want?" Questions like this will help patients make more connections between the therapy proposed and the benefits they want. With both children and adults, tying the use of the treatment to achieving goals the patients want over a short period of time can help patients perceive the benefits of therapy, motivate them to follow it, and provide them with criteria for recognizing that the treatment is working.

Identifying perceived barriers to following a recommended treatment may be more straightforward, and is one of the goals of the well-known strategy of tailoring the regimen to the patient. Clinicians should discuss specific plans for taking a new medicine at home with the patient, and ask, "What problems do you think you will have in carrying this out the way we have discussed?" A good follow-up question that goes beyond details of administration is "Are there any other problems or concerns you have about following this plan?" Patient beliefs that the medicines may be harmful should be followed with more specific questions, such as "What harm do you think the medicine may cause?" or "What led you to think that this might be a problem?"

Finally, patient or family confidence that the treatment plan can be followed and used to control asthma should be assessed with questions such as "How sure are you that you can give the medicine to your child with the inhaler and spacer?" or "How sure are you that you can control your asthma using the written treatment plan I've given you?" If patients are not sure, then follow up with open-ended probes such as "I can sense you aren't completely sure. What part are you not so sure of?" This approach will enable patients to bring up all the relevant issues before they leave the office.

By using the HBM as a framework for asking questions to assess patients' asthma knowledge, beliefs, and skills, the clinician can identify key issues that need to be addressed to make patients able and willing to follow the treatment plan. The strength of HBM is that it helps identify areas in which discussion and teaching are needed to change patient behavior. Its limitation, however, is that it doesn't tell us much about how behavior change occurs or how the clinician can facilitate change. For that, we turn to cognitive social theory and the self-regulation process.

Social cognitive theory (SCT) describes the process by which people set and achieve goals through a process known as self-regulation.[7,8] Most people self-regulate their behavior to some extent, and can learn, either spontaneously or with coaching, to

- Control problem behaviors, such as smoking;
- Master valued skills, such as playing a musical instrument;
- Achieve goals, such as completing a medical residency.

In self-regulation, the individual attempts to reach desired outcomes by a process that includes controlling three factors: (1) *behaviors*, such as trying out new strategies and self-observation of the results; (2) *personal* thoughts, such as reactions to the success of one's own behavior, or setting new goals; and (3) *environmental* factors. Environmental factors include both physical factors, such as the presence or lack of needed equipment or space, and social factors, such as the presence of a teacher or coach to help acquire knowledge or skills. Self-regulation is the process by which an individual attempts to control the interaction of these three factors to achieve a goal. For example, a student learning to play an instrument may: (1) decide to master a simple piece of music (personal—goal setting); (2) to play the music repeatedly until he or she can do it without mistakes (behavioral—trying a strategy); and (3) finding a place to practice where he or she won't be disturbed by others (environmental).

Coaching by an expert is an important aid in learning to self-regulate behavior. For example, the student might have a teacher who could demonstrate how the music should sound when played correctly, provide feedback about how well the student was playing, and suggest new strategies to help the student play better. Similarly, consider a patient with asthma who has experienced difficulty in controlling flare-ups with a beta-agonist delivered by metered-dose inhaler (MDI). His doctor has suggested that he may not be using the MDI correctly and so is not getting the needed dose of medicine. The patient might (1) decide that he would master MDI technique (personal—goal setting); (2) ask the doctor to demonstrate the correct technique, then practice doing what the doctor did, while reviewing a list to make sure he was following all the steps (behavioral—trying a strategy and self-monitoring the results); and (3) ask the doctor to watch him practice and provide feedback about how he was doing (environmental—use of a coach to assist in self-monitoring and interpreting the results).

Self-regulation is a cyclic process that typically is repeated until a problem is solved or controlled or a skill mastered. The cycle includes (1) deciding to try a specific strategy to reach a goal; (2) initiating the action and self-monitoring to see how it works; (3) making a judgment of success or failure; (4) experiencing an increase or decrease in self-efficacy–self-confidence that the action can be performed successfully and helps achieve the overall goal; and (4) repeating the cycle by modifying the strategy to correct actions that didn't work or to improve on those that did. To amplify the example above, the patient who had just learned proper technique for using a metered dose inhaler from his doctor might (1) decide to try the new technique for the next 2 weeks, while (2) keeping a diary of symptom-free days to see whether his asthma control was improving; (3) review the diary at the end of 2 weeks to decide whether his control had improved; and (4) depending on the result, experience an increase in self-efficacy that he could control his asthma by using the new technique, or perhaps feel a reduction in self-efficacy if the symptom diary didn't show a positive change.

This example highlights the importance of two critical aspects in the self-regulation cycle. The first is that increased self-efficacy is critical to encourage repeated efforts to improve.[7,8] Research shows that as self-efficacy increases, people are more likely to repeat an action, and are more likely to persist in the face of difficulty. For example, as a child makes initial progress in learning a musical instrument and gains confidence that she can play well, she often begins to play the instrument much more frequently, and is willing to tackle more complicated pieces of music. Improvement in self-efficacy is not guaranteed, however, and reduced self-efficacy can bring the cycle to a halt.

The role of coaching is important to help the learner gain confidence and repeat the self-regulation process. Coaches can do this in several ways. First, the coach can help the learner pick goals that can be achieved over a short period of time, to increase the chances of success. Most weight-loss programs, for example, set a goal of losing 1 to 2 pounds per week—a goal that can be readily achieved and builds confidence that the diet is working. Second, the coach can teach the learner how to self-observe, and can provide direct feedback about success. Third, the coach can help learners reach appropriate judgments about success. Many people find it difficult initially to tell if they are doing well, and counseling and problem solving can help their confidence grow as they learn.

There are three ways in which self-efficacy can be increased, and clinicians can make use of all of these with patients learning to control asthma. The first is *verbal persuasion*; that is, telling the patient that he or she is capable of learning the skills needed to control asthma. This is the least effective method, but because these methods are additive in effect, it is a good place to start. The second way is *vicarious experience*, which occurs when the patient talks with or observes another patient who has mastered the same skill. This is more effective because the other patient is a more believable model. For a patient, seeing that another patient has learned to use a metered dose inhaler with a spacer leads to the thought "If she can do it, I can do it too," which is more convincing than the word of the doctor, because the patient is likely to think that "This doctor has had years of training; of course he thinks it is easy." The most effective way in which self-efficacy can be increased, however, is by *direct practice* with feedback that leads to a series of short-term successes as the skill increases. All three approaches should be used when possible. Verbal persuasion can be done to initiate the process. Most clinicians can also allude to the fact that they have other patients who have mastered the skill, which is providing vicarious experience secondhand. In group asthma education

programs, the health educator may be able to have parents who have learned a skill demonstrate it to others to take full advantage of vicarious experience. Finally, by following a model of teaching the skill based on self-regulation theory, most clinicians, alone or with the help of practice staff, can successfully lead the patient to learn the skill with demonstration plus practice with feedback under the guidance of a coach. This model is outlined in Box 25-1.

Repeating the main teaching steps as outlined in step 7 is important for two reasons. First, it takes more time than we usually imagine to fully establish a skill and to work out all the problems in using it. Second, many skills decay over time and need reinforcement. Asking patients to self-monitor for a brief time until they learn key skills is important, because self-monitoring increases the desire to improve performance. By using this teaching process, clinicians can stimulate patients to set goals and start the self-regulation process, thus helping patients improve their control of asthma.

APPLICATIONS OF THE HEALTH BELIEF MODEL AND SOCIAL COGNITIVE THEORY

The HBM and SCT have been used to develop both asthma patient education programs and programs to help clinicians improve quality of care for asthma. To illustrate how these theory-based approaches have been used, the Physician Asthma Care Education (PACE) program will be described.

The PACE program is a 4-hour continuing medical education program for pediatricians and other clinicians treating children with asthma.[9,10] The purpose of the program is to teach clinicians two related sets of skills for managing asthma. The first is how to use the National Heart, Lung, and Blood Institute (NHLBI) guidelines in primary care practice to (1) assess asthma severity; (2) prescribe appropriate therapy; and (3) provide instructions and a written plan to enable the patient to adjust medications when symptoms change. The second set of skills is how to communicate with and teach patients so they will take advantage of treatment recommendations.

Pediatricians are recruited for the PACE program through local networks by an influential pediatrician who serves as the host of the program, which is primarily delivered by an asthma specialist and a specialist in communications or patient education. The program is offered in two evening dinner seminars held a week apart. In seminar 1, the first hour begins with a presentation by the asthma specialist about the three key points listed above: (1) how to assess asthma severity so that children with persistent asthma are identified; (2) how to prescribe appropriate therapy, including daily controller medicines for children with persistent asthma; and (3) how to prepare and teach all patients to use a written treatment plan. The specialist then leads a discussion of these key points.

The second hour of seminar 1 is devoted to communication skills. The educator reviews the link between communications, trust between doctor and patient, and adherence. Physicians are introduced to the HBM as a way to think about patients and to explore patients' beliefs about asthma. A videotape that demonstrates good communication skills (see Box 25-2) is shown, and the educator leads a discussion

BOX 25-1 Asthma Management Using Self-Efficacy

1. Establish overall goals with the patient and family. Explain that you want them to learn how to control asthma and live without restrictions on physical or social activities, and then reach agreement about what that would specifically mean for them. Once the overall goals are agreed upon, you can then introduce the specific skills you want them to learn.

2. Assure them that they can learn to master the skill (verbal persuasion) and that you have other patients who have done so (vicarious experience).

3. Demonstrate the skill yourself and describe the component steps. This should be done in person, but can be supplemented with audiovisual media demonstrations. Encourage the patient to ask questions during the demonstration. If an audiovisual presentation is used, be sure you tell patients you want them to watch it and will talk with them about it after they have watched.

4. Have the patients practice the skill immediately after the demonstration, and provide coaching and feedback to:
   - Correct mistakes and improve technique
   - Teach them how to self-monitor their performance, such as noting posture during inhalation or counting the seconds the breath is held after inhalation

   - Help them recognize that they are successful in improving their skill

5. Establish performance goals to reach by the next visit, including quality of the skill, a schedule for implementing the skill, and criteria for when to use it.

6. Give the patient and family a diary or other self-observation tool to record how they do at home until the next visit. Most patients will not keep diaries for very long, but are often willing to do so for a week or two if you ask them to and schedule a visit to review the results. Another promising strategy is to ask a family member to videotape the patient using the skill at home. Videotapes can capture the quality of performance and also provide rich information about how the patient is managing asthma at home.

7. Review the skill each time the patient returns by:
   - Asking for a repeat demonstration by the patient
   - Correcting mistakes or making suggestions to improve technique
   - Reviewing patient diaries, praising the patient for keeping them, and discussing lessons to be learned
   - Asking about problems encountered and helping the patient devise solutions
   - Praise the patient for progress in learning the skill and sticking to the schedule for using it

---

of which skills the participants already use, and which they might try out. Physicians are asked to try one or more of the skills in their practice during the next week, and to bring a current case they are working with that presents a challenge in managing asthma.

The first hour of seminar 2, held the next week, begins with three short video segments showing how a physician can use the communication skills to teach the patient and family key messages they need to understand and accept to manage asthma successfully. The educator leads a brief discussion after each segment about how the participants teach families about these issues, such as teaching families about the safety and effectiveness of inhaled corticosteroids. The part of the program closes with a review of which communication skills physicians tried during the week, and what the results were.

The second hour of seminar 2 is devoted to discussing clinical cases brought by participating physicians. The discussion is led by an asthma specialist, but includes both therapeutic choices and adherence issues, which are often linked. The specialist adds prepared cases that represent challenging issues in management, and solicits a range of choices about how to handle them. The aim of the discussion is for pediatricians to share ideas and realize that applying the guidelines requires good clinical judgment.

HOW ARE SOCIAL COGNITIVE THEORY AND THE HEALTH BELIEF MODEL USED IN PACE?

Both theories were used in the design of the intervention for pediatricians and in the strategies the physicians were taught to use with their patients. Social cognitive theory was used in all four segments of the two PACE seminars. First,

verbal persuasion was used to help the pediatricians believe they could successfully treat pediatric asthma patients by assessing asthma severity, prescribing appropriate treatment, and using communication skills and patient teaching to help patients understand and follow the treatment plan.

Second, demonstration of new skills coupled with practice and feedback by a coach was used throughout the seminar. In seminar 1, the asthma specialist showed how to use a patient history of recent symptoms to classify asthma severity according to NHLBI guidelines. Then the pediatricians were shown three brief patient accounts of their recent symptoms and, as a group, were asked to practice by classifying severity based on these accounts. In the discussion after each case, the asthma specialist provided coaching and feedback to correct mistakes and increase the participants' confidence that they could accurately classify patients' asthma severity. Similarly, in the second hour of seminar 1, the education specialist used a videotape to demonstrate good communication skills. The specialist also modeled the skills as he or she led the discussion of the videotape. To practice, the pediatricians were asked to use one or more of the skills in their practice during the week. In seminar 2, their experiences were reviewed (coaching and feedback) and successes were identified to increase the self-efficacy of participants directly (for those who tried a skill) and vicariously (for those who did not). A one-page list of the communication skills was provided to enable the physicians to self-monitor their use of the skills during patient visits (see Box 25-2).

Patient teaching skills for the delivery of key educational messages were similarly demonstrated using videotape in the first hour of seminar 2. The discussion following the videotape drew out the physicians' current experiences teaching

BOX 25-2 Teaching and Communications Behaviors

1. Show nonverbal attentiveness
2. Give nonverbal encouragement
3. Give verbal praise for things done well
4. Maintain interactive conversation
5. Find out underlying worries/concerns
6. Give specific reassuring information right away
7. Tailor medication schedule to family's routine
8. Reach agreement on a short-term goal
9. Review the long-term therapeutic plan
10. Help patients use criteria for making decisions about asthma management

Adapted from Figure 1, p. 832, in Clark NM, Gong M, Schork MA, et al: Impact of education for physicians on patient outcomes. Pediatrics 1998;101:831–836.

patients and provided coaching in how they could use the messages presented in the videotape to help their patient teaching. The group discussion also provided vicarious learning by allowing physicians to share successful strategies for teaching key messages, such as the safety of inhaled steroids, or the importance of responding quickly to emerging symptoms. Again, a one-page form listing the key topics and messages was provided to enable the physicians to self-monitor their use, checking off those that have been covered with the patient.

Finally, the discussion of challenging cases in the last hour of seminar 2 allows the physicians to practice applying what they have learned in the first 3 hours to their own patients. The asthma and education specialists provide coaching and feedback to help physicians consider different treatment options to improve therapeutic outcomes and adherence by the family. The specialists stress that there is often not a single solution, and that physicians should have the confidence to apply their clinical judgment.

The HBM was used in PACE to reinforce positive health beliefs about the value of appropriate treatment for asthma and to modify health beliefs that served as barriers to the pediatricians. In the first hour of seminar 1, the asthma specialist emphasizes that undertreatment has *serious* health consequences for children with asthma. The specialist also indicates that such undertreatment is common, and that this *susceptibility* is a major cause of high levels of emergency department (ED) visits and hospitalizations for asthma. The same points are presented in the segments on communication and patient teaching—when the communication and teaching skills are not used, families are less likely to follow the treatment plan. The program also stresses the *benefits* of adopting the recommended treatment practices—better outcomes for patients, more satisfaction for the families and the pediatrician, and for pediatricians, the ability to manage the great majority of their pediatric asthma patients successfully by themselves, referring to specialists only those patients with greater severity or complications.

Finally, the asthma and education specialists address a common belief that serves as a *barrier* to many participating pediatricians. This is the perception that taking a more detailed history of symptoms, using the communication skills, and providing patient teaching will take too much time. Our approach is to indicate that using the communication skills takes no extra time and that the necessary patient teaching can be carried out over several visits scheduled for that purpose. As the findings of the trial indicate, compared with control physicians at 1-year follow-up, physicians who took part in the PACE program estimated that they spent 4 minutes (15%) less time during initial visits for new asthma patients.[9]

The HBM and SCT are also used in the specific communication and teaching strategies that pediatricians are taught to use with patients and families. During the communications segment of seminar 1, the pediatricians are introduced to the HBM as a framework to think about their patients and as a guide for exploring the family's beliefs and concerns about asthma. The HBM is the basis for several of the communication strategies that the pediatrician can use to assess family beliefs about susceptibility to and seriousness of asthma, and the benefits and barriers to following the pediatrician's advice. Referring to Box 25-2, strategy 5 is identifying the family's concerns and worries about asthma or asthma treatment, and is based directly on the HBM. Strategy 4, using interactive conversation, which includes the use of open-ended questions, simple language, and use of analogies to explain medical concepts, is a critical skill for accomplishing strategy 5. Strategy 6, giving reassuring information about these concerns to the family right away, is an important step in helping families change beliefs about almost any aspect of asthma or asthma treatment. This strategy enables the family to set the worry aside and continue to focus on what the pediatrician is teaching. Strategy 7, tailoring the medication schedule to the family's schedule, is familiar to most physicians, and in terms of the HBM, is a way of removing barriers to giving the medicine as prescribed. Eliminating uncertainty about when to give the medicine and developing a practical plan for storing, remembering, and using the medication reduces barriers to adherence.

SCT forms the basis of many of the patient-teaching and communication strategies physicians are taught to use in PACE. First, verbal persuasion that by working with the doctor, the family can learn to control the child's asthma and enable the child to live a normal life is a key message throughout the patient teaching process. Second, the SCT model of demonstration with practice and feedback to master skills needed to control asthma is used repeatedly. For example, in the videotape the pediatrician demonstrates how to use an inhaler and spacer to take medicine, and then gives the child a chance to practice. The doctor makes adjustments in the child's technique if needed and praises her for success, thus increasing her self-efficacy to perform the skill. The doctor also reviews the written plan with the family and at later visits reviews it again so the family has a chance to obtain feedback about how they are using it. Setting short-term goals for asthma control that matter to the patient and family is also derived from SCT: Goals that matter increase motivation to follow the treatment plan, and achievement of goals over the short term increases the patient's confidence that they can control asthma with the treatment plan. The physician also asks the patient to self-monitor by keeping a symptom diary for a short period of time, which focuses the patient's attention on their symptoms and how the treatments are working. This can stimulate patient efforts to improve control and build confidence. Communication strategy 10 (see Box 25-2), helping the family use criteria for making decisions about asthma management at home, such as signs for increasing reliever medicines, increases the family's confidence that they can manage asthma episodes successfully. Finally, praise and nonverbal encouragement for things well done is an essential coaching and feedback strategy that helps the family develop higher self-efficacy for the overall challenge of managing asthma.

PACE was initially evaluated in a controlled trial with 74 pediatricians randomly assigned to intervention or control groups.[9,10] Data were collected from pediatricians and 637 of their patients' families. Patient and family members did not receive any intervention and were blind to their doctor's participation in the program. The pediatricians were surveyed at baseline and 12 months, and patients were surveyed at baseline, 12, and 24 months after intervention. Data were collected from patients' medical records to assess ED visits and hospitalizations.

Two years after intervention, medical record review showed that children seen by physicians who took part in PACE had significantly fewer hospitalizations than controls. Similarly, children with three or more baseline ED visits had significantly fewer ED visits at follow-up than comparable controls. Although these findings for the overall study group were not evident at 1-year follow-up, PACE was able to show that among children who were placed on daily controller therapy for the first time, those treated by physicians who took part in PACE had significantly fewer urgent office visits, ED visits, and hospitalizations than comparable controls. These findings indicate that the PACE program has an overall positive impact on control of asthma and health status, and that among children placed on controller therapy for the first time, the communications and patient teaching components of PACE appear to have helped them adhere to the therapy and thus reduce acute health care visits. A reanalysis of PACE found that low-income families (<$20,000 per year) had significantly greater reductions in hospitalizations and ED visits than families with higher incomes,[11] providing important evidence that low-income families can benefit as much or more than other families from improved asthma care.

Data from the physician surveys at 1-year follow-up showed that treatment physicians were more likely than controls to report that they addressed patients' fears about medicines, reviewed written instructions, provided a sequence of educational messages, wrote down how to adjust the medicines at home when symptoms change, and, as mentioned previously, reported that they spent less time in an initial visit with new asthma patients. At 2-year follow-up, treatment physicians were still more likely than controls to write down how to adjust medicines and provide guidelines for changing therapy, but treatment time with patients, although still less for physicians who took part in PACE, was no longer significantly

shorter than for controls. One interesting finding that emerged at 2-year follow-up was that treatment physicians were more likely than control physicians to use the one-page self-monitoring tool to keep track of what educational messages they had discussed with patients. These findings indicate that physicians who took part in PACE recognized that they were using specific communications strategies and patient education messages with patients.

Data from family interviews show that parents also recognized changes in the physicians' behavior as a consequence of PACE. At 1-year follow-up, parents of intervention physicians were more likely than controls to report that their doctor had been reassuring, described as a goal that the child be fully active, and gave information to relieve specific worries. Parents also were more likely to report that they knew how to make asthma management decisions at home, that their physician had prescribed an inhaled anti-inflammatory medicine, and that the physician had asked them to practice using a metered-dose inhaler in the office to show that they could do it correctly.

At 2-year follow-up, parents scored treatment group physicians higher than control physicians on five positive communication and teaching strategies: paying close attention to the family; praising parents for taking appropriate management steps; using open-ended questions to create an open exchange of information with the family; asking about family concerns about using new medicines; and explaining the treatment plan the family was to follow until the next visit. Again, these changes, reported by parents who were blind to the intervention, provide strong evidence that the communication and teaching strategies based on the HBM and SCT taught in PACE were adopted and used by participating pediatricians.

Finally, the PACE program was replicated in an effectiveness trial to see if the program could be effectively disseminated.[12] Ten small cities in the United States were randomly assigned to treatment or control status, and 101 physicians and 870 of their patients were enrolled in the study. Local faculty teams were trained to deliver the PACE program. At 1-year follow-up, parents reported that treatment group physicians were more likely than control physicians to ask about the parents' concerns about asthma, encourage patients to be physically active, and set goals for successful treatment. Patients of treatment group physicians had greater reductions in days with activity limited by asthma symptoms and ED visits.

SUMMARY

The HBM and SCT provide strategies that can help clinicians identify patient concerns and barriers to adherence, establish open communication, and carry out effective patient teaching to prepare the family to follow the treatment plan. As shown in the PACE program, these strategies have positive impacts on patients' perception of care and on their control of asthma. Use of the strategies does not add to the time spent in office visits by clinicians and is effective in low- as well as middle-income families. Clinicians are encouraged to try these strategies and observe the results in their own practice.

REFERENCES

1. Gibson PG, Powell H, Coughlan J, et al: Self-management education and regular practitioner review for adults with asthma. Cochrane Database Syst Rev 2002;(3):CD001117.
2. Wolf FM, Guevara JP, Grum CM, et al: Educational interventions for asthma in children. Cochrane Database Syst Rev 2002;(4):CD000326.
3. Korsch BM, Gozzi EK, Francis V: Gaps in doctor-patient communication: I. Doctor-patient interaction and patient satisfaction. Pediatrics 1968;42:855–871.
4. Clark NM, Feldman CH, Freudenberg N, et al: Developing education for children with asthma through study of self-management behavior. Health Ed Q 1980;7:278–296.
5. Wasilewski Y, Clark NM, Evans D, et al: Factors associated with emergency department visits by children with asthma and implications for health education. Am J Pub Health 1996;86:1410–1415.
6. Janz NK, Champion VL, Strecher VJ: The Health Belief Model. In Glanz K, Rimer BK, Lewis FM (eds): Health Behavior and Health Education: Theory, Research, and Practice, 3rd ed. San Francisco, Jossey-Bass, 2002, pp 45–66.
7. Clark N, Zimmerman BJ: A social cognitive view of self-regulated learning about health. Health Educ Res 1990;5:371–379.
8. Baranowski T, Perry CL, Parcel GS: How individuals, environments, and health behavior interact: social cognitive theory. In Glanz K, Rimer BK, Lewis FM (eds). Health Behavior and Health Education: Theory, Research, and Practice, 3rd ed. San Francisco, Jossey-Bass, 2002, pp 165–184.
9. Clark NM, Gong M, Schork MA, et al: Impact of education for physicians on patient outcomes. Pediatrics 1998;101:831–836.
10. Clark NM, Gong M, Schork MA, et al: Long-term effects of asthma education for physicians on patient satisfaction and use of health services. Eur Respir J 2000;16:15–21.
11. Brown R, Bratton SL, Cabana MD, et al: Physician asthma education program improves outcomes for children of low-income families. Chest 2004;126(2):369–374.
12. Cabana MD, Slish KK, Evans D, et al: Impact of physician asthma care education on patient outcomes. Pediatrics 2006;117:2149–2157.

Pharmacogenetics: How Will This Change Asthma Management?

John J. Lima

CLINICAL PEARLS

- Several common variants on different genes contribute to the genetic risk of asthma and to variability in response to asthma therapy.

- The relation between variability in response and variants on one or more candidate genes defines pharmacogenetics; the relation between response variability and genomewide variants defines pharmacogenomics.

- The goal of asthma pharmacogenetics/genomics is personalized medicine, or the use of genetic information to manage asthma treatment.

- Genetic polymorphisms in single or multiple genes contribute to variability in response to short- and long-acting bronchodilators, corticosteroids, and leukotriene receptor antagonists, but only explain a small fraction of the variability.

- Genomewide association studies in asthma will lead to personalizing asthma management.

Although there is no cure for asthma, several drug classes and drugs are available to treat symptoms and to control asthma exacerbations; however, depending on the individual drug, 50% or more of the patients receiving treatment do not respond adequately. It has been estimated that as much as 80% of the variability in response to asthma drugs is due to genetic variation.

GENOMIC VARIATION

Begun in 1990, the Human Genome Project (HGP) mapped the locus of each of 30,000 to 35,000 genes on 23 chromosomes, with an estimated 3 billion bases (adenine [A], guanine [G], cytosine [C], and thymine [T]), and identified a number of genetic variants or polymorphisms.[1,2] Recently, phase 1 of the Hap Map project was published.[3] The Hap Map project differs from the HGP in that the HGP is informative about the invariance of the majority of bases across individuals, while the Hap Map project focuses on differences in DNA sequence among individuals. The aim of the Hap Map Consortium was to create a public, genomewide database of common (≥1% frequency) sequence variations. The human genome has about 10 million common polymorphisms. When a mutation arises, it is often strongly associated with particular variants on the same gene or allele as a haplotype, and can be used to "tag" the presence of variants or proxies at another site on the gene.[4] The principal goal of the Hap Map Consortium was to discover haplotypes of single nucleotide polymorphisms (SNPs). SNPs are the most common genetic polymorphisms, and can be either missense or silent coding region SNPs, or they can be found up- or downstream from the coding region or in introns (Table 26-1). Next to SNPs, the most common polymorphisms are addition/deletion polymorphisms, and if located in the coding region, these can lead to frame shift polymorphisms, which can profoundly influence function of the protein(s) a gene encodes.

PERSONALIZED MEDICINE

Since the publication of the HGP and the Hap Map project, numerous lay and professional publications have promoted the potential benefits of these endeavors, which include knowledge of the genetic basis of common complex diseases and their treatment. The contribution of genetic variation to the variability in drug response defines pharmacogenetics and pharmacogenomics, terms that are often used interchangeably. Lay and professional publications have heralded the age of "personalized medicine," that is, using patient-specific information, that is, genetic information, to tailor drug therapy. The relation between pharmacogenetics (or pharmacogenomics) and personalized medicine is illustrated in Figure 26-1.

We have not yet achieved the goal of personalized medicine for asthma or for other common, chronic complex diseases. However, pharmacogenetics/pharmacogenomics has the potential of revolutionizing the management of asthma, and therefore inclusion of this chapter in this book is appropriate.

Asthma is a common, complex disease with important genetic components that contribute to asthma phenotypes, including response to drugs. Unlike diseases involving single gene defects, the genetic contributions to asthma are considered to be susceptibility loci that influence but do not determine the overall disease risk, and thus asthma conforms to the common disease–common variant model.[5] As such, asthma and response to asthma drugs are thought to involve single or multiple variants on multiple genes with each variant contributing modestly to phenotypes. Comparing genetic variation between cases (nonresponders to a drug) and controls (responders to a drug) would enhance our understanding of the genetic contribution of response variability to asthma drugs, and would be expected to lead to the discovery of new drug targets and the development of new drugs. However, genotyping 10 million genomic SNPs in each case and control is not feasible. The Hap Map Consortium however, has now made it possible, depending on ancestry, to capture 80% or more of the common variation in the genome by genotyping 250,000 to 500,000 tagging SNPs (2.5% to 5%).[6] Additionally, technological advances have now made it feasible to genotype

Table 26-1
SINGLE NUCLEOTIDE POLYMORPHISMS (SNP)

SNP Type	Description
Silent	Change in single base that does not result in different amino acid
Missense	Change in single base that results in alternative amino acid
Frame shift	Addition or deletion of one or more bases
Up-, downstream from coding region and introns	Usually thought not to be functional but in linkage disequilibrium with functional polymorphism

5% of the genome in reasonably sized cases and controls. These advances will lead to genomewide association studies of asthma and response to asthma drugs, which will lead to the identification of causal genes and pathways that contribute to asthma phenotypes. Current pharmacogenetic studies in asthma explore associations between response rates and single SNPs or multiple SNPs in single genes or in pathway candidate genes. While these approaches are reasonable and logical, they are also biased by our selection of genes and their variants, and may be responsible, at least in part, for our being able to attribute only a very small fraction of the variability in response to asthma drugs to genetic variants. In genomewide studies, there is little or no selection bias. Associations between responses and "hot spots" in the genome, with subsequent analyses in replicate cohorts, should lead to the

development of genomic algorithms that will allow us to personalize asthma treatment.

PHARMACOGENETIC CONSEQUENCES

The study of associations of single or multiple polymorphisms on one or more genes with response to a drug defines *pharmacogenetics*. The study of genomewide associations with response to a drug defines *pharmacogenomics*. Pharmacogenetics (or pharmacogenomics) has two main domains or consequences: a pharmacokinetic and a pharmacodynamic domain. Genetic variants that influence the activity (affinity; capacity) of phase I drug-metabolizing enzymes (cytochrome p450 enzymes) or phase II enzymes (conjugation reactions; acetylation, sulfation) affect a drug's pharmacokinetics. Polymorphisms that influence a drug's binding to plasma and tissue proteins will also affect a drug's pharmacokinetics. The consequences of a drug's altered pharmacokinetic profile caused by genetic variants can in most cases be mediated by changes in dose rate (i.e., daily dose). Polymorphisms that influence drug targets (receptors, enzymes, transporters) will alter the drug's pharmacodynamics, which usually cannot be mediated by changes in dose rate. Rather, such changes require a different drug to obtain the desired response (see Fig. 26-1). It is possible that genetic variants can alter both a drug's pharmacokinetics and pharmacodynamics.[7]

There are numerous studies of the pharmacodynamic consequences of genetic variation on response to inhaled beta-agonists and inhaled corticosteroids (discussed later). There

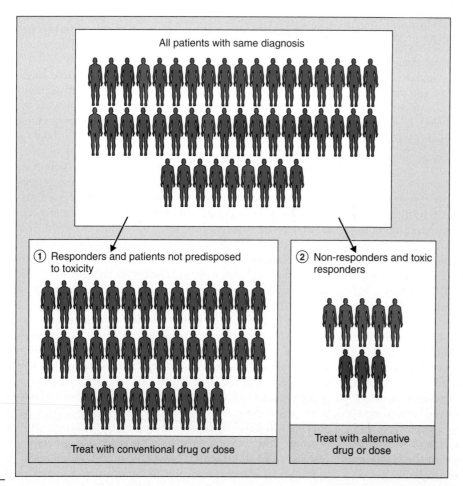

All patients with same diagnosis

① Responders and patients not predisposed to toxicity

Treat with conventional drug or dose

② Non-responders and toxic responders

Treat with alternative drug or dose

Figure 26-1 Role of pharmacogenomics in personalized medicine. A population of patients with a similar diagnosis is prescribed a drug at a conventional dose rate. A group of patients will have a therapeutic response (group 1, *green symbols*); a second group (group 2) will either not respond (*yellow symbols*) or show signs of toxicity (*blue symbols*). It is estimated that 60% to 80% of the variability in response to asthma drugs is related to genetic polymorphisms. Knowledge of the polymorphism(s) that is responsible for a patient being classified as nonresponder would predict that a different drug or dose, depending on the domain affected by the polymorphism (see text), be prescribed for that patient.

are no studies of the pharmacokinetic consequences of genetic variation on these drugs, in part because they are inhaled and evoke their effects locally rather than systemically. Therefore it is expected that the pharmacokinetic consequence of genetic variants would have only a minor influence on the therapeutic benefits of inhaled asthma drugs. Leukotriene receptor antagonists (LTRA) are administered orally or by the intravenous route and thus exert their effects systemically. They are substrate for CYP2C9 and CYP3A4, and possibly drug transporters in the gut, which are polymorphic, and therefore could be subject to pharmacokinetic consequences. To our knowledge, there are no studies of the influence of variants in genes encoding CYP450 that metabolize LTRAs, or transporters that could affect the bioavailability of these drugs.

The clearance of theophylline is influenced in a minor way by a polymorphism in the *CYP1A2* gene.

PHARMACOGENETICS OF ASTHMA DRUGS

The pharmacological treatment of asthma is discussed in Section V, Treatment, Chapters 27–35. The major drug classes used in the treatment of asthma include bronchodilators (short-acting beta-agonists [SABAs], long-acting beta-agonists [LABAs], and anticholinergics), corticosteroids, leukotriene modifiers, and theophylline. While all drugs in each class have proven efficacy and safety, there is substantial interpatient variability in response to treatment. This is shown in Figure 26-2. Depending on the drug, the proportion of individuals responding to SABAs (panel A), ICSs, and/or LTRAs (panel B) can vary between 30% and 70%. It has been estimated that 60% to 80% of the interpatient variability in response to asthma drugs is due to genetic variation.[8] The goals of pharmacogenetics are to identify genetic variants that are responsible for therapeutic

benefits and adverse events, and to use this information to prescribe the drugs that offer the highest probability of therapeutic benefit with minimal side effect, *before* drug therapy is initiated. For example, current guidelines recommend that mild persistent asthma be treated first with inhaled corticosteroids (ICS) monotherapy along with SABA to control acute symptoms. Nearly 50% of patients started on ICS will not respond adequately (see Fig. 26-2), which can result in poor asthma control, increased visits to the emergency room (ER), loss of work or school days, and increased morbidity. Knowledge of the genetic variants that predict non-responsiveness to ICS would dictate use of alternative agents (LTRA, low-dose theophylline) or add-on therapy (LABA, LTRA) thereby minimizing the economic, social, and personal burdens imposed by pharmacological interventions that don't work. Although considerable progress has been made, we are still far away from achieving this goal. In the next section, I review the progress that has been achieved for each of the major drugs used to treat asthma. Additionally, the pharmacogenetics of asthma drugs has been the subject of several excellent reviews; two recent reviews are particularly noteworthy.[9,10]

Bronchodilators

PHARMACOGENETICS OF Beta₂-ADRENERGIC RECEPTOR (β_2AR) AGONISTS

β_2AR agonists include inhaled short-acting agents (SABAs) (albuterol, terbutaline), which are used as rescue bronchodilator medications to treat acute symptoms in asthma, and inhaled long-acting β_2AR agonists (LABAs) (salmeterol, formoterol), which are used as add-on (to ICS) controllers. LABAs are not recommended as long-term monotherapy or as add-on controllers because chronic use can mask and/or

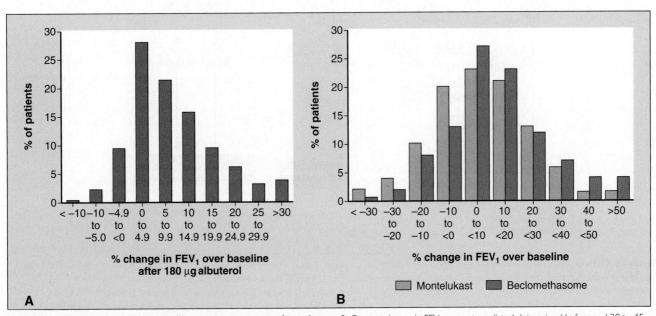

Figure 26-2   Distribution of bronchodilator responses to asthma drugs. A, Percent change in FEV₁ percent predicted determined before and 30 to 45 minutes after two puffs of inhaled albuterol (0.18 mg) in 240 asthmatic individuals. **B,** Response distributions (percentage of patients) at predefined intervals of percent change in FEV₁ in asthmatic individuals treated with 10 mg of montelukast (*tan bars*) and inhaled beclomethasone, 0.2 mg twice daily (*blue bars*). (**A**, *Unpublished data;* **B**, *Data from Malmstrom K, Rodriguez-Gomez G, Guerra J, et al: Oral montelukast, inhaled beclomethasone, and placebo for chronic asthma. A randomized, controlled trial. Montelukast/Beclomethasone Study Group. Ann Int Med 1999;130:487–195.*)

contribute to asthma deterioration. The variability in the bronchodilator response to inhaled albuterol is depicted in Figure 26-2. Only 30% of patients had an increase in FEV_1 (forced expiratory volume in 1 second) of 12% or more after albuterol, which is the minimal increase, typically used to define an acceptable therapeutic bronchodilator response, and thus would be classified as responders. About 50% of the patients had a 0% to 10% increase in FEV_1 and would be classified as nonresponders. A small proportion of patients experienced a decrease in FEV_1 and thus had a negative or adverse response to albuterol. These data suggest that many patients are at risk of inadequate relief of symptoms following a usual dose of albuterol, which could place them at risk for life-threatening consequences.

β_2AR agonists exert their pharmacological effects by binding to and activating the β_2AR as illustrated in Figure 26-3 (and its legend), which depicts the genes known to encode proteins that comprise the β_2AR pathway. Receptor-mediated responsiveness is rapidly desensitized by several mechanisms that lead to receptor uncoupling and a reduction of receptor density, that is, agonist-promoted receptor down-regulation. Common SNPs in the β_2AR gene that are functionally relevant affect receptor density. Thus far no common SNPs are known that influence receptor coupling (discussed later).

The gene encoding the β_2AR is intronless, has one exon, and is located on chromosome 5q31–33. The gene, including the 3' and 5' untranslated regions, is highly polymorphic[11]; at least 56 SNPs and 2 addition/deletion polymorphisms have been identified (Seattle SNPs: http://pga.mbt.washington.edu/). Two common coding region SNPs, Gly16→Arg, Gln27→Glu, and one SNP in the 5' region, Cys-19→Arg, are in tight linkage disequilibrium resulting in common distinct haplotypes (Table 26-2) in both self-described whites and blacks. Functional studies in recombinant cells have revealed that common SNPs at −19, 16, and 27 influence

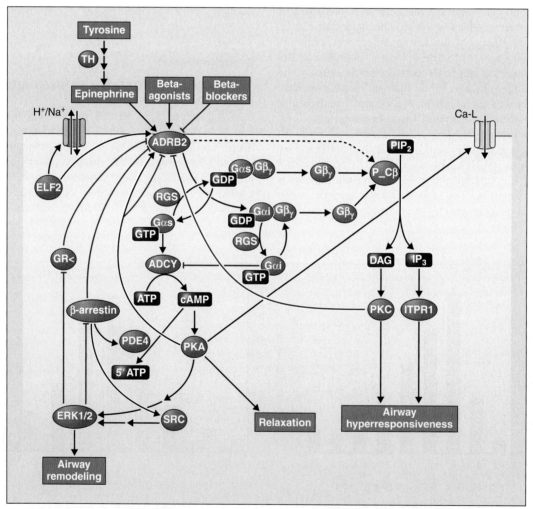

Figure 26-3   Beta$_2$-adrenergic receptor pathway. Agonists bind to a fraction of beta$_2$-adrenergic receptors (β_2AR) coupled to the heterotrimeric G-protein Gs. Gαs dissociates from the complex, GDP is exchanged with GTP, and Gαs activates adenylyl cyclase that catalyzes the conversion of ATP to cAMP, the second messenger. cAMP activates protein kinase A (PKA), which phosphorylates multiple proteins in smooth muscle cells leading to relaxation and bronchodilation. PKA phosphorylates and uncouples the β_2AR resulting in one form of desensitization. The PKA-phosphorylated form of the β_2AR also promotes coupling to inhibitory G-protein Gi. The receptor is also phosphorylated by several members of the G-protein coupled receptor kinase family (GRKs), and serves as a substrate for the binding of b-arrestins. β_2AR-recruited beta-arrestin also initiates activation of C-Src that leads to activation of ERK1 and ERK2 kinases, which participate in airway remodeling. Activated ERK1 and ERK2 phosphorylate both GRK2 and beta-arrestin, decreasing their function and thereby modulating desensitization. Continuous β_2AR activation by agonists also results in receptor ubiquitination, a process that ultimately contributes to receptor degradation, that is, agonist promoted–receptor down-regulation. For more details see http://www.pharmgkb.org/.

Table 26-2
ALLELE FREQUENCIES OF ADRB₂-SINGLE NUCLEOTIDE POLYMORPHISMS AND COMMON (>5%) HAPLOTYPES
IN BLACKS (N = 143) AND WHITES (N = 336)

SNP Position	Alleles or Haplotype	Amino Acid Change	Minor Allele or Haplotype	Frequency, %	
				Blacks	Whites
−1023	G/A	—	A	41	43
−654	G/A	—	A	22	34*
−47	T/C	Cys-19→Arg	C	17	40*
46	G/A	Gly→Arg	A	50	42
79	C/G	Gln→Glu	G	17	40*
523	C/A	—	A	37	19*
Haplotype 1	AGCGGC	—	1	14.3	34.8†
Haplotype 2	GATACC	—	2	19.2	31.6†
Haplotype 3	GGTGCA	—	3	29.7	13.5†
Haplotype 4	AGTACC	—	4	20.6	1.8†

*$P < .05$ blacks vs. whites; Chi Square
†All pairwise comparisons for haplotype by race were significant ($P < .001$) for all combinations except for haplotype 1 versus haplotype 2; chi square.

receptor density by altering receptor translation or by altering the extent of agonist-promoted down-regulation. The Arg16 allele was more resistant to agonist-promoted down-regulation than the Gly16, and the Glu27 was not down-regulated at all.[12]

Pharmacogenetic studies in asthma have focused mainly on the β_2AR. Several early clinical studies explored associations between acute bronchodilator responses to inhaled or systemic SABAs and single β_2AR SNPs and reported that Arg16 alleles were associated with better bronchodilator response to albuterol compared to Gly16 alleles[13,14]; however, the results of subsequent studies of single SNPs were conflicting. This led to the idea that haplotype may be better associated with bronchodilator response than genotype. In one of the early association studies of complex ADBR2 haplotypes and bronchodilator response to albuterol,[11] haplotypes of SNPs designated haplotype 1 in Table 26-2 had a higher bronchodilator response and higher receptor densities compared to haplotypes of SNPs designated haplotype 4. Importantly, no associations between bronchodilator response to albuterol and individual SNPs were found.[11] Later studies, however, using larger patient populations failed to replicate these findings, and more recent ones have focused on genotype (or haplotype) of polymorphisms in additional genes including corticosteroid and adenylyl cyclase genes in different ethnic populations.[9,10] In summary, it is unlikely that a single SNP or multiple SNPs in the β_2AR gene or pathway will account for a significant proportion of variability in the bronchodilator response to SABAs among patients. In order to personalize SABA treatment in asthma, a pharmacogenomic approach is likely to be more informative than a pharmacogenetic approach in characterizing interpatient variability in bronchodilator response.

In contrast to the SABA-evoked bronchodilator phenotype, it is possible that the Gly16→Arg genotype may accurately predict deterioration of lung function following continuous inhaled β_2AR agonist treatment. Since 1990, several large clinical studies reported that regular use of SABA was not beneficial or made asthma worse, thereby concluding that SABAs be used only as rescue medication. Retrospective analysis revealed that during regular use of SABAs, peak expiratory flow rate (PEFR) decreased in Arg16 homozygotes

and increased in Gly16 homozygotes, suggesting that genotype can accurately predict who will benefit and who will be adversely affected by regular use of SABAs. In a prospective trial (the National Institutes of Health [NIH] Asthma Clinical Research Network BARGE trial), regular use of albuterol was associated with an increase in PEFR compared to placebo ($P < .05$) in Gly16 homozygotes (n = 41); whereas PEFR was not different from placebo in Arg16 homozygotes (n = 37) (Fig. 26-4).[15] The authors concluded that Arg16 homozygotes may not benefit from albuterol even when used as rescue medication. The results of these studies are very promising with respect to personalized medicine because they suggest that genotype of the Gly16→Arg SNP predicts which individual will benefit from continuous beta₂-agonist treatment.

However, the results of the BARGE study raise several questions. SABAs are recommended as a rescue medication and not for continuous use, so the clinical relevance of the BARGE trial is not clear. It is also not clear if the results of this study can be extrapolated to LABAs (recent evidence suggests that similar results were obtained during continuous salmeterol treatment). What role does ICS play and how will these results affect the newly established guidelines for LABA use? Also, the SMART (Salmeterol Multi-center Asthma Research Trial) safety trial showed a higher number of primary events and asthma-related events, including deaths in blacks taking salmeterol compared to placebo. Do β_2AR genetic variants predict which patients will experience adverse events while taking LABAs? Finally, although promising, the BARGE trial must be replicated in a larger, more diverse population using ICSs and LABAs not SABAs.

ANTICHOLINERGICS

Anticholinergics (ipratropium, oxitropium, tiotropium) block muscarinic receptors on airway smooth muscles. Five muscarinic receptor subtypes have been identified; however, only three, M1, M2 and M3, subtypes are expressed in human airways. Ipratropium and oxitropium are competitive inhibitors of M2 and M3 receptors, whereas tiotropium selectively blocks M3 receptors. In contrast to SABAs, anticholinergics block or

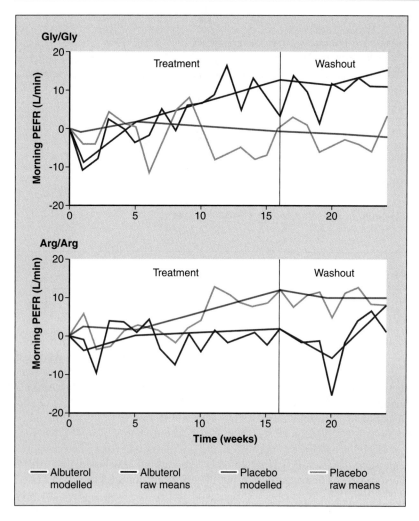

Gly/Gly

Arg/Arg

Time (weeks)

— Albuterol modelled   — Albuterol raw means   — Placebo modelled   — Placebo raw means

Figure 26-4   Change in morning PEFR in Arg16, Gly16 homozygotes. The red and green lines represent the mean PEFR values modeled through the unadjusted mean weekly data (blue and orange lines) in 41 Gly16 homozygotes (Gly/Gly; *top panel*) and 37 Arg16 homozygotes (Arg/Arg; *bottom panel*), at various times during regular use of inhaled albuterol or placebo for 16 weeks. *(Data from Israel E, Chinchilli VM, Ford JG, et al: Use of regularly scheduled albuterol treatment in asthma: genotype-stratified, randomised, placebo-controlled cross-over trial. Lancet 2004;364:1505.)*

antagonize bronchocontriction rather than stimulate broncho-dilation, and the bronchodilation observed with anticholinergics is generally more modest compared to SABAs. M2 and M3 receptors are encoded by *CHM2* (chromosome 7q35–36) and *CHM3* (chromosome 1q41–44) genes respectively. Several databases list polymorphisms in each gene; however, no pharmacogenetic studies involving genetic variants have been reported. The pharmacogenetic importance of anticholinergics may be related to individulas who are poor responders to SABA owing to β_2AR polymorphisms.

Controllers

CORTICOSTERIODS

Corticosteroids are the most potent anti-inflammatory agents used to treat asthma, and ICSs are recognized as the most effective asthma controllers. ICSs reduce airway inflammation and asthma symptoms, improve lung function, and reduce nocturnal symptoms, bronchial responsiveness, asthma exacerbations, and oral steroid dependence. They also improve quality of life and reduce hospital and ED admissions. Corticosteroids exert their effects by binding to cytoplasmic glucocorticoid receptors (GR), which have several major domains including ligand-binding domains, and DNA and transcription factor regulatory domains, followed by hsp90 dissociation allowing nuclear localization (Fig. 26-5). GRs bind to glucocorticoid response elements (GREs), leading to recruitment and activation of transcriptional coactivator molecules (CBP, SRC-1) that have

histone acetyltransferase activity, leading to acetylation of lysine residues on histone proteins, and the unwinding of DNA. This is followed by recruitment of RNA polymerase II and activation of genes encoding anti-inflammatory proteins.[16] Administration of corticosteroids profoundly alters the expression of pro-inflammatory genes triggering the activation of transcription factors including AP-1, NF-κB, NFAT and STAT6, which induce chemoattractants, cytokines, cytokine receptor leukotrienes and cell adhesion molecules that are involved in eosinophil and other leukocyte recruitment.[10]

The interpatient variability in response to ICS is significant (see Fig. 26-2); as much as 50% or more of patients treated with ICS do not respond adequately. However, the study of the genetic contribution to the interpatient variability in response is still in its formative stages. In this regard, one SNP and a haplotype of SNPs in the corticotrophin-releasing hormone receptor 1 (*CRHR1*) gene predicted good FEV_1 responsiveness in adult and pediatric studies; and a functional variant of *TBX21* gene, which encodes for the transcription factor T-bet, was associated with improvement in airway hyperresponsiveness following ICS.[10] The CRHR1 is an important receptor for corticotrophin-releasing factor in the brain, and thereby modulates ACTH and cortisol levels. Given the complexity of the steroid response, a pharmacogenomic approach may be more informative than a candidate gene approach.

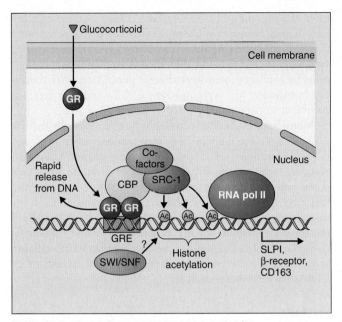

Figure 26-5   Anti-inflammatory gene expression by glucocorticoids. Glucocorticoids bind to glucocorticoid receptors (GR) that translocate to the nucleus, where they bind to glucocorticoid response elements (GRE) leading to recruitment and activation of transcriptional coactivator molecules (CBP, SRC-1) that have intrinsic histone acetyltransferase (HAT) activity leading to acetylation of lysine residues on histone proteins. Chromatin modification leads to local unwinding of the DNA structure, allowing recruitment of large protein complexes, including RNA polymerase II (RNA pol II) resulting in activation of genes encoding anti-inflammatory proteins. *(Adapted from Adcock IM, Ito K, Barnes PJ: Glucocorticoids: effects on gene transcription. Proc Am Thorac Soc 2004;1:247–254.)*

The ICSs in current use undergo hepatic clearance most likely by cytochrome p450 enzymes (mainly CYP3A) and have high hepatic first-pass metabolism and low bioavailability (Table 26-3), properties that decrease the risk of adverse events related to ICS. About 10% to 60% of an inhaled dose of ICS is deposited in the lung, with 40% to 90% of the dose getting swallowed and absorbed. A high first-pass effect minimizes systemic absorption and adverse events including candidiasis, infection, osteoporosis, growth retardations (in children), cataracts, and adrenal suppression. Genetic variation in drug-metabolizing enzymes may contribute to variability in pharmacokinetics, particularly bioavailability, which could increase the risk of adverse events. To our knowledge, there are no studies of the pharmacokinetic consequences of variants in genes encoding these enzymes.

LEUKOTRIENE MODIFIERS

Two classes of drugs are available that modify response mediated through the leukotriene (LT) pathway: leukotriene receptor antagonists (LTRAs: montelukast, pranlukast, zarfirlukast) (see Chapter 29) and inhibitors of 5-lipoxygenase (ALOX5) like zileuton. LTRAs are selective cysteinyl leukotriene (cysLT) 1 receptor inhibitors that antagonize the effects of cysLT (LTC$_4$, LTD$_4$, and LTE$_4$). CysLTs are potent bronchocontrictors and mediators of asthma inflammation and are synthesized from arachidonic acid located in membrane-phospholipids by cyto-solic phospholipase A (cPLA$_2$) in response to stimulation (Fig. 26-6). Arachidonic acid is converted to LTA$_4$ by membrane-bound 5-lipoxygenase (ALOX5) and 5-LO activating protein

Table 26-3
AVERAGE PHARMACOKINETIC PROPERTIES FOR INHALED CORTICOSTEROIDS IN ADULTS*

Corticosteroid	Clearance, L/hr†	Oral Bioavailability, %
Beclomethasone dipropionate	120	26
Budesonide	84	11
Ciclesonide	228	<1
Flunisolide	57	20
Fluticasone	69	11–17
Mometasone furoate	Unknown	11–17
Triamcinolone acetonide	45	11–23

*Adapted in part from Hubner M, Hochhaus G, Derendorf H: Comparative pharmacology, bioavailability, pharmacokinetics, and pharmacodynamics of inhaled glucocorticosteroids. Immunol Allergy Clin North Am 2005;25:469–488.
†L/hr, liters per hour

(FLAP). In human mast cells, basophils, eosinophils, and macrophages, LTA$_4$ is converted to LTB$_4$, a potent chemoattractant, by leukotriene A$_4$ hydrolase (LTA$_4$H), or is conjugated with reduced glutathione by LTC$_4$ synthase to form LTC$_4$. LTC$_4$ is transported to the extracellular space mainly by the multidrug-resistance protein 1 (MRP1) and converted to LTD$_4$ and LTE$_4$ by γ-glutamyltransferase and dipeptidase (see Fig. 26-6).

Numerous clinical trials in adults and children with asthma have established the efficacy and safety of montelukast. However, interpatient variability in response to montelukast in both children and adults with asthma is significant (see Fig. 26-2), which is thought to be due in part to genetic variability. A few studies have reported that the repeat

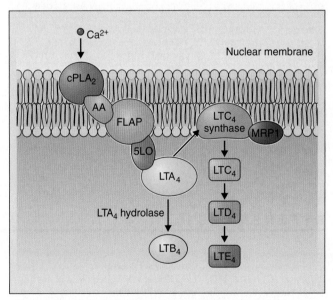

Figure 26-6   The cysteinyl leukotriene pathway. Following stimulation, arachidonic acid (AA) is converted to LTA$_4$ by 5-lipoxygenase (5-LO) and 5-lipoxygenase activating protein (FLAP). LTA$_4$ is converted to LTB$_4$ by LTA$_4$ hydrolase and to LTC$_4$ by LTC$_4$ synthase; LTC$_4$ is actively transported out of the cell by the multidrug-resistance protein 1 (MRP1), and converted to LTD$_4$ and LTE$_4$. The cysteinyl leukotrienes (cysLT: LTC$_4$,LTD$_4$ and LTE$_4$) are potent bronchocontrictors and inflammatory mediators.

(addition/deletion) polymorphism in the *ALOX5* promoter and the *LTC4S* A-444C SNP contributes to the variability in response to montelukast and other LT modifiers.[10] However, the allele frequency of the *ALOX5* repeat polymorphism is too low to contribute much to the variability in response to leukotriene modifiers and the data on the influence of the *LTC4S* A-444C SNP on response to LT receptor antagonists are conflicting.

Recently, the American Lung Association network of Asthma Clinical Research Centers completed a pharmacogenetic study of montelukast in patients with asthma who received montelukast, theophylline, or placebo for 6 months. We typed 28 SNPs in the *ALOX5*, *LTA4H*, *LTC4S*, *MRP1*, and *cysLT1R* genes, and an *ALOX5* repeat polymorphism.[17] Ethnic differences in the allele frequencies of 17 SNPs and the number of *ALOX5* repeats were reported. Because of this and the small number of self-identified black participants, association analyses were restricted to whites. Associations were found between genotypes of SNPs in the *ALOX5* and *MRP1* genes and changes in FEV$_1$ and between two SNPs in *LTC4S* and in *LTA4H* genes for exacerbation rates (Table 26-4). Mutant *ALOX5* repeat polymorphism was associated with decreased exacerbation rates. There was strong linkage disequilibrium between *ALOX5* SNPs. Associations between *ALOX5* haplotypes and risk of exacerbations were found. This study is the first to adopt a candidate gene approach to exploring the contribution of LT-pathway genetic variants to the interpatient variability to montelukast and other LTRAs. The results of this study are encouraging because they support the idea that genetic variation in leukotriene pathway candidate genes contributes to variability in response to LTRA treatment. These associations must be replicated in a large diverse population. Whether or not knowledge of polymorphisms in LT candidate genes is sufficient to personalize LTRA treatment is unclear.

Montelukast is nearly completely cleared mainly by hepatic CYP3A, has a low hepatic clearance (about 50 mL/min), and is well absorbed, yet is only 50% bioavailable. Moreover, plasma concentrations following single or multiple doses vary significantly from patient to patient. Montelukast has properties that suggest it could be a substrate for anionic transporters in the gastrointestinal tract, which demonstrate genetic variation that could contribute to the variation in plasma concentrations. The pharmacokinetic consequences of genetic variation in genes that clear and or transport montelukast and other LTRAs have not been studied.

FUTURE

Despite claims that we can begin to use genotype information to personalize certain asthma treatments, several issues need to be addressed before we can begin to even test whether genotype-driven strategies are superior to conventional modes of asthma management, and some of these have been reviewed.[18] It is clear that although the candidate gene approach yields important clues regarding the contribution of pathway genetic variants to variation in drug response,[17] variants in other unknown genes are likely to contribute to variability in drug response. The solution to this problem is at hand by adopting a *pharmacogenomic* approach. It is now feasible to identify common whole genome variants that contribute to the variability in drug response. To accomplish this we must have relatively large numbers of cases and controls (500 to 1000 or more) with well-characterized phenotypes; and a smaller number of cases from different populations that qualify as replicate cohorts. Once genetic variants are identified and replicated, comparative studies of genotype-driven versus conventional modes of treatment will be performed to evaluate the pharmacoeconomic impact of personalized medicine. Pharmacogenomic studies are currently under way so that it is likely that we will be using genetic information to guide the management of asthma treatment by 2015. Other problems, which 5 to 10 years ago appeared insurmountable—ethical, confidentiality, economic considerations—are now quite manageable.

Table 26-4
INFLUENCE OF VARIANTS IN LEUKOTRIENE PATHWAY CANDIDATE GENES ON THE RISK OF AN ASTHMA EXACERBATION OR CHANGE IN FEV$_1$ IN PATIENTS TAKING MONTELUKAST

LT Genes	Variants	Phenotype/Genotype Association
ALOX5	Repeat variant rs2115819	Risk of exacerbation reduced 73% in mutant variant % predicted FEV$_1$ increased 30% in homozygotes of minor allele
LTA4H	rs2660845	Risk of exacerbation increased four- to fivefold in heterozygotes and homozygotes of minor allele
LTC4S	A-444C SNP	Risk of exacerbation reduced 75% to 85% in heterozygotes and homozygotes of minor allele
MRP1	Rs119774	% predicted FEV$_1$ increased 25% in heterozygotes

REFERENCES

1. Lander ES, Linton LM, Birren B, et al: Initial sequencing and analysis of the human genome. Nature 2001;409:860–921.
2. Venter JC, Adams MD, Myers EW, et al: The sequence of the human genome. Science 2001;291:1304–1351.
3. Altshuler D, Brooks LD, Chakravarti A, et al: A haplotype map of the human genome. Nature 2005;437:1299–1320.
4. Sebastiani P, Lazarus R, Weiss ST, et al: Minimal haplotype tagging. Proc Natl Acad Sci USA 2003;100:9900–9905.
5. Becker KG: The common variants/multiple disease hypothesis of common complex genetic disorders. Med Hypotheses 2004;62:309–317.
6. Hirschhorn JN, Daly MJ: Genome-wide association studies for common diseases and complex traits. Nat Rev Genet 2005;6:95–108.
7. Evans WE, McLeod HL: Pharmacogenomics—drug disposition, drug targets, and side effects. N Engl J Med 2003;348:538–549.
8. Drazen JM, Silverman EK, Lee TH: Heterogeneity of therapeutic responses in asthma. Br Med Bull 2000;56:1054–1070.
9. Hawkins GA, Weiss ST, Blecker ER: Asthma pharmacogenetics. Immunol Allergy Clin North Am 2005;25:723–742.
10. Tantisira KG, Weiss ST: The pharmacogenetics of asthma: an update. Curr Opin Mol Ther 2005;7:209–217.

11. Drysdale CM, McGraw DW, Stack CB, et al: Complex promoter and coding region beta 2-adrenergic receptor haplotypes alter receptor expression and predict in vivo responsiveness. Proc Natl Acad Sci USA 2000;97:10483–10488.

12. Liggett SB: Polymorphisms of the beta2-adrenergic receptor and asthma. Am J Respir Crit Care Med 1997;156:S156–S162.

13. Martinez FD, Graves PE, Baldini M, et al: Association between genetic polymorphisms of the beta2-adrenoceptor and response to albuterol in children with and without a history of wheezing. J Clin Invest 1997;100:3184–3188.

14. Lima JJ, Mohamed M, Eberle LV, et al: Impact of genetic polymorphisms of the beta2-adrenergic receptor on albuterol bronchodilator pharmacodynamics. Clin Pharmacol Ther 1999;65:519–525.

15. Israel E, Chinchilli VM, Ford JG, et al: Use of regularly scheduled albuterol treatment in asthma: genotype-stratified, randomised, placebo-controlled cross-over trial. Lancet 2004;364:1505–1512.

16. Adcock IM, Ito K, Barnes PJ: Glucocorticoids: effects on gene transcription. Proc Am Thorac Soc 2004;1:247–254.

17. Lima JJ, Zhang S, Grant A, et al: Influence of leukotriene pathway polymorphisms on response to montelukast in asthma. Am J Respir Crit Care Med 2006;173:379–385.

18. Weiss ST, Lake SL, Silverman ES, et al: Asthma steroid pharmacogenetics: a study strategy to identify replicated treatment responses. Proc Am Thorac Soc 2004;1:364–367.

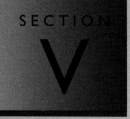

TREATMENT

Bronchodilators: Beta$_2$-Agonists and Anticholinergics

Nicola A. Hanania and Mario Cazzola

CLINICAL PEARLS

- Bronchodilators play a pivotal role in the acute and maintenance management of asthma.

- Beta$_2$-agonists are the most effective bronchodilators in asthma and are well tolerated when given by inhalation.

- Inhaled short-acting beta$_2$-agonists should be limited to rescue and emergency management of asthma symptoms.

- Inhaled long-acting beta$_2$-agonists are currently recommended as add-on therapy to inhaled corticosteroids for maintenance therapy in patients with persistent asthma not controlled with inhaled corticosteroids alone. They should never be used as rescue medication or as monotherapy.

- The use of short-acting anticholinergic bronchodilators is currently limited to management of acute severe asthma when used in conjunction with short-acting beta$_2$-agonists.

- The role of long-acting anticholinergic bronchodilators in the management of asthma requires further evaluation.

- Several novel once-daily inhaled bronchodilators are currently under development.

Bronchial asthma is a chronic inflammatory disease characterized by the presence of airway hyperresponsiveness and airflow obstruction. Airflow obstruction in patients with asthma is usually widespread, but is variable and is often reversible either spontaneously or with treatment. Bronchodilators play a pivotal role in the acute and maintenance management of asthma. The most common groups of bronchodilators currently in clinical use are the beta-agonists and the anticholinergic agents. The inhaled administration of bronchodilators is generally safe and is preferred over their systemic administration. Current national and international asthma guidelines recommend limiting the use of inhaled short-acting beta-agonists (SABAs) for rescue and emergency management and the maintenance daily use of long-acting agents as add-on therapy to inhaled corticosteroids for patients with chronic persistent asthma who are not controlled with inhaled corticosteroids alone (Table 27-1). This chapter focuses on the pharmacology, clinical use, and safety of currently available bronchodilators in the management of acute and chronic asthma.

BETA$_2$-AGONISTS

Historical Perspective

Beta$_2$-agonists play a pivotal role in the acute and chronic management of asthma. Beta-agonists have been used for thousands of years but progress in drug development has

resulted in safer, longer acting and more beta$_2$ receptor-specific agents. In traditional Chinese medicine, the botanical *ma huang* has been used for more than 2000 years for the short-term treatment of respiratory symptoms due to the efficacy of the sympathomimetic agent, ephedrine. Beginning at the turn of the century, the nonselective alpha- and beta-receptor agonist, epinephrine, was introduced and was administered by the subcutaneous route for the treatment of acute asthma. Subsequently, an aerosolized formulation of this drug was introduced and delivered to the lungs using a squeeze-bulb. In the 1940s, isoproterenol was the first beta-agonist to be used in treating airway disease and became the standard of care bronchodilator, although its use was complicated by adverse effects due to activation of the beta$_1$-receptors in nontarget sites. Metaproterenol, a noncatechol resorcinol derivative of isoproterenol was developed in the early 1960s. However, the modern era of selective SABAs did not begin until the simultaneous discovery of albuterol and terbutaline, which remain the SABAs of choice until the present time. The next advance in the development of beta$_2$-agonists was the development of long-acting agents, salmeterol and formoterol, which made their use more appealing for maintenance treatment of asthma. More recently and following suggestion of potential adverse effects associated with one of the two chiral forms of albuterol (S-albuterol), the pure enantiomer, levalbuterol, was developed and is currently in clinical use. At present, several once-a-day ultra–long-acting beta$_2$-agonists are in different stages of clinical development.

Pharmacology of Beta$_2$-Agonists

Beta$_2$-agonists act by binding to the beta$_2$-adrenergic receptor (β_2AR), which is a member of the seven transmembrane domains, G-protein–coupled family of receptors. Although β_2ARs are present in high density in airway smooth muscle

---

Table 27-1
RATIONAL USE OF BETA-AGONISTS IN ASTHMA MANAGEMENT

Short-acting Beta$_2$-Agonists
Drugs of choice for acute bronchospasm
Rapid onset (e.g., albuterol)
Prevention of exercise-induced bronchospasm
Regularly scheduled use *not* recommended
Marker of disease control
Long-acting Beta$_2$-Agonists
Used for maintenance control
Moderate-persistent, severe-persistent asthma
Patients receiving inhaled corticosteroids

Table 27-2
BENEFITS OF INHALED BETA-AGONISTS IN THE MANAGEMENT OF ASTHMA

- Relief of bronchoconstriction due to smooth-muscle relaxation
- Marked protection against all nonspecific constrictor stimuli, such as cold air, methacholine, and exercise
- Reduced vascular permeability and edema
- Increased mucociliary clearance due to increased ciliary beat frequency
- May reduce inflammation due to inhibition of mediator release from inflammatory cells and priming of glucocorticoid receptors

cells, they are also present in submucosal glands, vascular endothelium, ciliated epithelium, mast cells, circulating inflammatory cells such as eosinophils and lymphocytes, Clara cells, type II pneumocytes, and cholinergic ganglia. Upon agonist binding to receptor, adenylyl cyclase is activated via the signal-transducing G_s protein, which results in a rise in cellular cyclic AMP (cAMP) levels and activation of protein kinase A (PKA). The precise PKA phosphorylation targets mediating bronchial smooth muscle relaxation are not fully understood but likely include myosin light-chain kinase and Ca^{2+}-dependent K^+ (K_{ca}) channels. One feature possessed by most G-protein–coupled receptors, including β_2AR, is a mechanism by which the signal is turned off following receptor activation. This process, termed desensitization, is discussed later. Although the major action of beta₂-agonists on airways is relaxation of airway smooth muscles, they also exert several effects mediated through the activation of beta₂-receptors expressed on resident airway cells such as epithelial cells and mast cells and circulating inflammatory cells such as eosinophils and neutrophils (Table 27-2).

Numerous beta₂-agonists of differing pharmacological properties are available for clinical use (Table 27-3). Beta₂-agonists are classified by their onset and duration of action, receptor selectivity, affinity, potency, and efficacy. *Affinity* refers to the attraction between the agonist and its receptor, *potency* refers to the dependency of receptor activation on drug concentration, and *efficacy* refers to the ability of the agonist to activate its receptor without regard to its concentration and is detailed below.

Onset and Duration of Action

The onset of action of inhaled beta₂-agonists is primarily determined by their lipophilicity. Relatively hydrophilic drugs such as albuterol have a very rapid onset of action as they activate the receptor in the aqueous phase, whereas lipophilic drugs such as salmeterol have a slower onset. It is worth mentioning that while formoterol has an intermediate lipophilicity, it is still able to activate the receptor in the aqueous phase and thus also has a rapid onset of action similar to albuterol. The duration of action is similarly determined by lipophilicity, as well as by resistance to metabolism. For instance, salmeterol and formoterol have a longer duration of action than albuterol, and because of their lipophilicity may have a depot effect in the cell membrane. The slow onset and prolonged action of salmeterol both appear to be primarily due to its extreme lipophilicity, with some contribution from quasi-specific interaction of the tail with hydrophobic regions of the beta₂-adrenoceptor (see Table 27-2).

RECEPTOR SELECTIVITY

To minimize side effects, it is essential that a beta-agonist activates its target receptor without activating other receptors. Endogenous catecholamines activate alpha₁-, alpha₂-, beta₁-, beta₂-, and beta₃-adrenoceptors to varying degrees, but synthetic agonists are capable of exquisite specificity. Currently used synthetic beta₂-agonists are moderately to highly selective agonists at the beta₂-receptor. For example, the most widely used beta₂-agonist, albuterol, has a beta₂:beta₁ selectivity −650:1. It is unlikely that greater selectivity is of clinical significance because the heart contains abundant beta₂-adrenoceptors capable of regulating its chronotropic and inotropic properties, so increased selectivity does not avert cardiac stimulation.

STEREOSELECTIVITY

Catecholamines and related beta₂-agonists contain a chiral (asymmetric) center at the hydroxyl carbon of the side chain. As a result, they can exist as either of two stereoisomers, typically designated *R* and *S*. Only the *R* stereoisomer is active at the β_2AR, but most currently available beta₂-agonists are equal (racemic) mixtures of both stereoisomers. Such formulations are based on the assumption that *S* stereoisomers have no activity, but this assumption may be incorrect as there is some evidence that the *S* stereoisomers of albuterol for example may potentiate the response to bronchoconstrictors in vivo and in vitro, possibly by inducing a calcium rise in airway smooth muscle cells. Levalbuterol, the *R*-isomer of albuterol, is the only isomeric beta₂-agonist currently available, beta for clinical use in asthma. Arformoterol, the *RR*-isomer of formoterol was recently approved by the U.S. Food and Drug Administration (FDA) for clinical use in chronic obstructive pulmonary disease (COPD).

POTENCY

This refers to the concentration-dependency of a drug's effect, with a highly potent drug being effective at low concentrations. Drug potency depends both on the affinity of the drug for its receptor and on the efficacy of the drug-receptor interaction. Potency is an important parameter in drug development, but relatively unimportant in clinical practice because regulatory agencies ensure that marketed drugs achieve clinically effective concentrations.

EFFICACY

This refers to the ability of a drug to exert an effect in a target tissue. The measured effect can be clinical (bronchodilation),

Table 27-3
COMMONLY USED BETA₂-AGONISTS IN ASTHMA MANAGEMENT

Onset of Action	Duration of Action	
	Short-acting	Long-acting
Rapid	Fenoterol*	Formoterol
	Pirbuterol	
	Procaterol*	
	Albuterol	
	Terbutaline	
	Levalbuterol	
Slow		Salmeterol

*Not approved for use in the United States.

physiologic (smooth muscle relaxation), or biochemical (rise in cAMP). Agonists of different efficacy can be compared by measuring their maximal effects. However, efficacy is highly dependent on tissue factors such as receptor density and the degree of functional antagonism by a constrictor agonist such as acetylcholine; therefore, the measured efficacy of an agonist in different tissues or in the same tissue under different conditions may vary. *Intrinsic efficacy* refers to the ability of a drug to interact with a receptor such that its signal transduction pathway is activated independent of tissue factors. It serves as a measure of the relative agonism of a drug, that is, a partial agonist is less efficient than a full agonist in causing a downstream cellular response once bound to its receptor. For example, the long-acting beta₂-agonist (LABA) formoterol has a higher intrinsic efficacy than albuterol, which has a higher intrinsic efficacy than salmeterol. Methods are now available to calculate the intrinsic efficacy of a drug. Efficacy is an important parameter of drug action because it plays a key role in the activation of target and nontarget receptors. For example, beta₂-adrenoceptors are present in high density in airway smooth muscle, and a partial beta₂-agonist of low intrinsic efficacy that activates only a small fraction of airway receptors may nonetheless cause full bronchodilation; in contrast, beta₂-adrenoceptors are present in low density in nontarget tissues such as skeletal muscle and the same partial agonist may not cause sufficient activation to lead to tremor. This phenomenon accounts for the attractive side-effect profile of partial agonists such as albuterol. On the other hand, a partial agonist of low intrinsic efficacy may not provide sufficient therapeutic effect in some situations such as severe disease or during an acute exacerbation.

REGULATION OF β₂AR FUNCTION

Receptor desensitization refers to the decreased responsiveness that occurs with repeated or chronic exposure to agonist and is a general feature of most signaling membrane receptors. Mechanistically, desensitization can be divided into receptor *uncoupling* from downstream signal transduction elements by phosphorylation and reversible binding of the protein arrestin; receptor *internalization* by endocytosis; and receptor *down-regulation* (i.e., reduction in total receptor number) by a combination of increased degradation and reduced synthesis. Of importance, desensitization of the beta₂-adrenoceptor in airway smooth muscle is self-limited such that responsiveness is only partially impaired; this differs from the profound desensitization that can occur in other biologic systems. Some aspects of beta₂-adrenoceptor desensitization depend on agonist occupancy ("homologous desensitization"), whereas other aspects do not ("heterologous desensitization"). Homologous desensitization is sensitive to agonist efficacy such that agonists of higher intrinsic efficacy may induce more desensitization.

GENETIC VARIATIONS OF THE β₂AR

Variations of the β₂AR gene (*ADRB2*) may also have important effects on receptor function and regulation. Of the *ADRB2* single nucleotide polymorphisms (SNPs) discovered to date, three result in amino acid substitutions at positions 16, 27, and 164 of the receptor and alter receptor function. An additional SNP results in an amino acid change (cysteine [Cys] to arginine [Arg]) at position 19 of the receptor's 5' upstream peptide (BUP) and affects receptor expression. Cellular studies

of human airway smooth muscle cells and hamster fibroblasts indicate that β₂AR polymorphisms at amino acids 16 (arginine [Arg] to glycine [Gly]) and 27 (glutamine [Gln] to glutamic acid [Glu]) in the amino terminus may affect agonist-induced receptor down-regulation. Gly16 has been shown in vitro to promote increased receptor down-regulation while Glu27 is believed to confer resistance to down-regulation. However, a recent study of human airway smooth muscle cells suggests that Glu27 actually may be associated with increased acute and chronic receptor desensitization. Although β₂AR polymorphisms do not cause asthma per se, they may be disease modifying. For example, Gly16 has been noted to associate with a nocturnal asthma phenotype and to be more prevalent in moderate asthmatic individuals than mild asthmatic individuals. Further, healthy and asthmatic children homozygous for Gly16 are less responsive to a single dose of inhaled albuterol as compared with children homozygous for Arg16. Alternatively, Glu27 homozygotes exhibit marked reductions in airway reactivity to methacholine while Gln27 is associated with increased levels of immunoglobulin E (IgE). The role of β₂AR polymorphisms on the response to regularly administered albuterol in individuals with asthma recently has been evaluated. Surprisingly, in subjects who were Arg/Arg at position 16, an SNP more prevalent in blacks than in whites, the regular use of albuterol induced an approximately 30 L/min loss in morning PEF while no tachyphylaxis was seen in Gly/Gly individuals . A study currently under way will investigate whether similar relationship can be seen with the long-term use of LABAs such as salmeterol.

ROUTE OF ADMINISTRATION

Aerosol delivery of beta₂-agonists maximizes drug concentration in the target tissue (i.e., airway smooth muscle) with minimal systemic delivery to adrenoceptors in nontarget tissues such as the heart or skeletal muscle. For this reason, the inhaled route is preferred for delivery of beta₂-agonists in the treatment of asthma in all circumstances, except when a patient cannot operate the delivery device or possibly in some cases of severe asthma. Progress in aerosol technology has resulted in the availability of a wide variety of nebulizers, spacers, metered-dose inhalers, and dry powder inhalers capable of delivering drugs to the airway with varying efficiency.

Clinical Use of Beta₂-Agonists

BETA₂-AGONISTS IN THE MAINTENANCE MANAGEMENT OF ASTHMA

Medical therapy on a regular schedule is appropriate for all patients with persistent asthma as defined by the National Asthma Education and Prevention Program (NAEPP) Expert Panel (Fig. 27-1) and the international Global Initiative on Asthma (GINA) guidelines (Fig. 27-2). An anti-inflammatory drug, usually an inhaled corticosteroid, should be the first-line maintenance therapy. A long-acting inhaled beta₂-agonist can be added to an inhaled steroid when adequate symptomatic and physiologic control is not achieved with the inhaled steroid alone.

Two long-acting, highly selective inhaled beta₂-agonists are available worldwide: salmeterol and formoterol. Both are also marketed in the United States for their concomitant twice-daily administration in conjunction with an inhaled corticosteroid. Formoterol and salmeterol are often viewed as

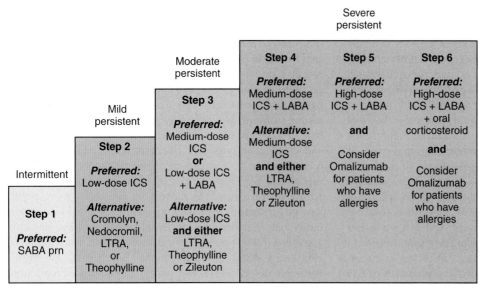

Figure 27-1 **Management approach of asthma severity**. Position of short-acting (SABAs) and long-acting beta₂-agonists (LABAs). *(Adapted from National Asthma Education and Prevention Program: Expert Panel Report 3: Guidelines for the Diagnosis and Management of Asthma [Pub No. 08-5346]. Bethesda, MD, National Institutes of Health, National Heart, Lung, and Blood Institute, October 2007.)*

interchangeable, but as mentioned above, differences in their onset of action, duration of action, and intrinsic efficacy merit consideration. The onset of bronchodilation with formoterol is 2 to 3 minutes, whereas with salmeterol it is approximately 10 minutes and does not peak for hours. The activity of a single 42-μg dose of salmeterol decays only slightly after 12 hours, whereas the activity of a single 12-μg dose of formoterol decays substantially by 12 hours and in some studies does not sustain a 15% increase in FEV₁ (forced expiratory volume in 1 second) for this duration. For this reason, formoterol is sometimes given in higher doses in some countries. Another major difference between formoterol and salmeterol is in their intrinsic efficacies. In vitro, formoterol is almost a full agonist, whereas salmeterol has a very low efficacy for relaxing airway smooth muscle. The intrinsic efficacy of salmeterol is difficult to precisely measure because it partitions into membranes, but its maximal efficacy in relaxing airway smooth muscle has been measured at one third to one half

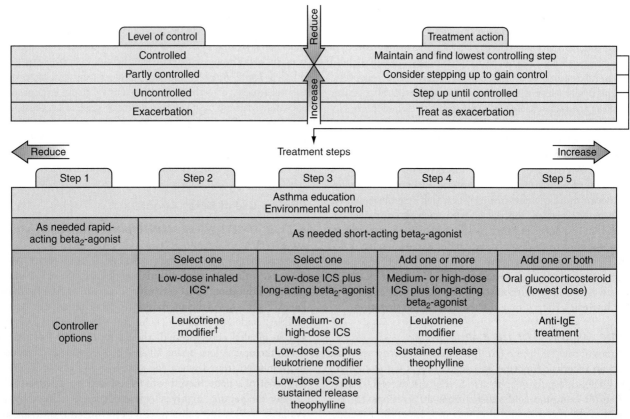

*ICS, inhaled glucocorticosteroids
†, receptor antagonist or synthesis inhibitors

Figure 27-2 **Management of asthma based on control.** Rationale use of short- and long-acting beta-agonists.

that of albuterol, so its intrinsic efficacy must be even less. To put this in perspective, the intrinsic efficacy of albuterol is only 5% that of a full agonist such as epinephrine or isoproterenol. The low efficacy of salmeterol in relaxing airway smooth muscle is mirrored by its low induction of desensitization in vitro. Large controlled, randomized clinical trials with mild to moderate asthmatic individuals show that the maximal bronchodilation achieved with regular administration of salmeterol is comparable to that achieved with albuterol. Side effects from both salmeterol and formoterol are very low at the doses used for maintenance therapy of asthma, and we are not aware of any convincing evidence that side effects from salmeterol are lower than formoterol at equally effective doses. Greater desensitization of bronchodilator effect with formoterol is suggested by the decline in peak expiratory flow that occurred after the first few days of regular treatment with formoterol but not salmeterol, and by the more dramatic shift in beta₂-agonist dose-response curves following regular treatment with formoterol. It is not known whether there is any clinical significance to the subtle bronchodilator subsensitivity caused by LABAs because the improvement they induce in lung function is sustained during long-term trials and is not associated with increases in the frequency or severity of exacerbations. Because of its slow onset of action, low intrinsic efficacy, and risks from accumulation, salmeterol should not be used for rescue therapy. On the other hand, because of its rapid onset of action and high intrinsic efficacy, formoterol has been used effectively as a rescue therapy in some countries. The twice-daily use of either salmeterol or formoterol results in improved lung function, reduced symptoms, fewer exacerbations, and improvement in health status. These agents also protect against exercise-induced asthma for up to 12 hours, and eliminate asthma-related nighttime awakening in most patients.

While the main effect of the existing LABAs is smooth muscle relaxation, the nonbronchodilator activities of beta₂-agonists may enhance their efficacy in the management of asthma (Table 27-4). In preclinical studies, the anti-inflammatory effects of beta₂-agonists are demonstrated through their stabilizing effect on mast cells and their inhibition of mediator release from eosinophils, macrophages, T-lymphocytes, and neutrophils. In addition, beta₂-agonists may inhibit plasma exudation in the airway, the release of neuropeptides from sensory nerves, and mediator release from epithelial cells and may have an effect on mucociliary function. These preclinical observations are not as clearly demonstrated in clinical trials, which may be explained by their induction of rapid desensitization of beta₂-adrenergic receptors on airway inflammatory cells.

Therefore, based on current studies in humans, neither salmeterol nor formoterol is clinically effective in reducing airway inflammation when used as stand-alone medication. However, the beneficial effects of inhaled LABAs have been revealed in multiple studies when regularly used in conjunction with an inhaled corticosteroid; salmeterol and formoterol effectively relieve asthma symptoms and improve physiology without decreasing asthma control or increasing mortality. In this situation, the clinical and functional efficacies of adding a long-acting inhaled beta₂-agonist are greater than doubling the dose of inhaled steroid.

Table 27-4
POTENTIAL NONBRONCHODILATOR ACTIVITIES OF β₂-AGONISTS

Target Site	Effect
Airway smooth muscles	Bronchoprotection—decrease response to nonspecific stimuli (methacholine) and allergens.
Airway mucosa	Increase mucociliary clearance.
Airway inflammatory cells*	Inhibit eosinophil and lymphocyte activation in response to allergen exposure. Reduce serum eosinophilic cationic protein levels. May decrease number of mast cells, eosinophils, lymphocytes, and neutrophils in the bronchial mucosa.* Enhance the effects of inhaled corticosteroids on several inflammatory cells.
Airway vessels	Decrease vascular permeability and airway wall edema, decrease angiogenesis when combined with inhaled corticosteroids.

*Data are controversial.

BETA₂-AGONISTS IN THE RESCUE MANAGEMENT OF ASTHMA

It is generally agreed that the short-acting inhaled beta₂-agonists are by far the most effective drugs for rescue therapy in asthma. Several short-acting inhaled beta₂-agonists are available for use as rescue medication. Albuterol, pirbuterol, terbutaline, and levalbuterol are highly selective beta₂-agonists with onset of action less than 5 minutes and peak action between 60 and 90 minutes. Differences in potency are compensated by differences in dosing such that all available products are essentially equipotent on a "per puff" basis. Older agents, such as isoetharine and metaproterenol, have shorter durations of action and less beta₂-selectivity and will not be further considered here. Along with high receptor selectivity, the excellent side-effect profile of the rescue beta₂-agonists appears to be due in part to their partial agonism. Among these agents, albuterol is the most widely used and the best studied; its intrinsic efficacy has been measured at 5% that of a full agonist such as epinephrine or isoproterenol. As described under pharmacology, a weak partial agonist induces little activation of nontarget tissues due to low density of beta₂-adrenoceptors in these tissues, and clinical studies confirm that the strong agonist fenoterol induces more side effects at comparable target effect than albuterol. The metered-dose inhaler (MDI) is currently the most popular device to deliver these medications, although they can also be delivered using a dry powder device or nebulizer. Although the use of MDI for delivery is more cost-effective in terms of simplicity, targeting medication to the lung, cost, maintenance, personnel time-investment, and risk of contamination when compared to a nebulizer, the use of this device is technique-dependent and its misuse may be associated with inconsistency of the delivered dose of medication. Patients who cannot use an MDI correctly, such as the elderly and young children, may benefit from the use of alternative devices such as breath-actuated devices (e.g., Autohaler), dry powder inhalers, or nebulizers. Historically, MDI technology has used chlorofluorocarbons (CFCs) as propellants, but CFCs will eventually be phased out because of their environmental hazards. Several MDIs for albuterol with hydrofluoroalkane (HFA134a), a nonchlorinated propellant, are currently available.

The frequency of rescue beta$_2$-agonist use is a clinically useful indicator of disease activity, and increasing use has been associated with increased risk of death. This is most likely more a reflection of severe and unstable asthma than a direct toxicity of the drug. In general, the use of more than one canister a month indicates overreliance on rescue drugs and suggests inadequate asthma control. It is recommended that patients who require rescue medication more than two times/week during the day and/or more than two times/month at night take a step-up in therapy such as an increase in the dosage of inhaled corticosteroid or an addition of another medication (e.g., a LABA or a leukotriene modifier).

BETA$_2$-AGONISTS IN THE ACUTE MANAGEMENT OF ASTHMA

Although systemic corticosteroids play an essential role in the therapy of acute severe exacerbations of asthma, these agents act slowly and induce bronchodilation only indirectly. Beta$_2$-agonists, on the other hand, act rapidly and are the most effective bronchodilators available; their use is a cornerstone of the initial management of acute asthma exacerbations. The severity of acute asthma ranges from mild exacerbations that readily respond to initial therapy in the emergency department to severe, life-threatening exacerbations requiring intubation and admission to the intensive care unit. Therefore, a single agent, a standard dose, and a particular route of delivery are not appropriate for all settings. In most cases, an inhaled rescue drug such as albuterol, given more frequently and in higher doses than for simple rescue, will suffice. However, in a patient with impending respiratory failure despite the administration of high doses of a rescue medication, an agonist of higher intrinsic efficacy (full agonist) has theoretical advantages. Beta$_2$-adrenoceptors are functionally antagonized by inflammatory mediators that are present during an acute exacerbation, and they may be desensitized by prior use of beta$_2$-agonists for maintenance and rescue therapy. In this setting, the submaximal efficacy of a partial agonist may become apparent, and a full agonist with a rapid onset of action should be considered. In addition, drug delivery by the inhaled route may be inadequate because of airway obstruction, and parenteral delivery may offer greater benefit. For most patients in the emergency setting, inhaled administration of beta$_2$-agonists is superior and safer than systemic administration. The drug is given at higher doses and more frequently than in the rescue setting to overcome strong constrictive stimulation by inflammatory and neural mediators. In addition, the higher dosing may be necessitated by reduced peripheral airway caliber resulting in poor delivery of beta$_2$-agonists. Most commonly, the drug is delivered by continuous or back-to-back nebulization. Continuous nebulization may be superior to intermittent nebulization and nebulization with a low dose of albuterol (2.5 mg/hour) offers excellent benefit with minimal side effects. In severe asthma, approximately one third of patients have a poor response to a standard dose of nebulized albuterol. In this situation, several options are available. First, a higher inhaled dose of the same medication may be given. Second, a beta$_2$-agonist may be given by the parenteral route in addition to the inhaled route. Third, a beta$_2$-agonist of higher intrinsic efficacy may be given. In a multicenter, randomized, double-blind, parallel-group study, patients receiving inhaled fenoterol had significantly more maximal improvement in airflow than those receiving inhaled albuterol. However, therapy with fenoterol was associated with more systemic adverse effects. Similarly, a recent study demonstrated that isoproterenol administration was associated with superior physiologic and symptomatic response than albuterol in patients with acute severe asthma.

For patients requiring intubation, inhaled bronchodilators have traditionally been administered via nebulization. However, an MDI used with an inline spacer is as efficacious and offers some advantages. In some settings, the nebulizer must be placed in line with the ventilator circuit; in this case, the machine-delivered tidal volume must be reduced to account for the volume added by the nebulizer. Furthermore, contamination of nebulizers can lead to aerosolization of bacteria and thus to respiratory tract infections. Last, the fraction of beta$_2$-agonist aerosol deposited in the lungs of mechanically ventilated patients is higher with an MDI with holding chamber compared with a nebulizer.

Safety of Beta$_2$-Agonists in Asthma

Adverse effects from the highly selective inhaled beta$_2$-agonists are largely due to activation of beta$_2$-adrenoceptors in non-target tissues. These side effects are not usually a problem when the agents are administered by inhalation, but become more frequent with oral and systemic administrations. Most commonly, cardiac stimulation may lead to tachycardia, increased oxygen demand, and occasional arrhythmias, while skeletal muscle stimulation may lead to tremor and hypokalemia. Adverse effects, such as allergic reactions or paradoxical bronchospasm, can also occur but are very rare. Some tolerance has been reported to the bronchoprotective effects of SABAs and LABAs. However, although the reduction in the protective effect of these agents has been demonstrated, this is not progressive and most of the initially observed protective effect is preserved. Modest but nonprogressive tolerance has also been seen in the bronchodilator effects of some beta$_2$-agonists. However, the improvements in lung function induced by LABAs are sustained over long periods and the clinical significance of the tolerance they induce to bronchodilation is unknown.

The regular use of SABAs has been associated with increased asthma mortality. Although, as mentioned earlier, this may be more a reflection of severe and unstable asthma rather than adverse effect from the medication, it is of interest that the two reported asthma mortality epidemics reported in some countries several years ago were observed with the use of the *full* agonists, isoproterenol and fenoterol. More recently, some studies demonstrated that the regular use of short-acting beta-agonists may be associated with poor asthma control in certain individuals with homozygous arginine genotype at position 16 of their *Bin* β_2AR (one sixth of whites and one fifth of blacks in the United States). Whether the above association is present with the use of long-acting agents remains to be determined. However, a recent study suggested an association between the use of LABAs with an increase in asthma-related deaths and life-threatening experiences. The SMART trial (Salmeterol Multicenter Asthma Research Trial) was designed to randomize 60,000 asthma patients to either salmeterol twice daily or placebo. However, following an interim analysis in 26,355 subjects, the study was terminated because of the findings in blacks and difficulties in enrollment. The occurrence of the primary outcome, respiratory-related deaths or life-threatening experiences was low and not significantly different for salmeterol versus placebo (50 versus 36). However, there was a small but significant increase in respiratory-related deaths and asthma-related deaths, and in combined asthma-related deaths or life-threatening experiences in subjects receiving salmeterol. This imbalance occurred largely in the black subpopulation. It is important to note that this subpopulation had more severe asthma at baseline and less than half of subjects were receiving concomitant inhaled corticosteroids. As a consequence of SMART trial results, the FDA issued a public advisory to highlight recommendations about the use of LABAs for asthma. This advisory emphasized the need to use these agents only as add-on therapy in patients who fail to achieve asthma control with the use of moderate doses of inhaled corticosteroids.

ANTICHOLINERGIC (ANTIMUSCARINIC) AGENTS

Historical Perspective

Anticholinergic medications have been used for hundreds of years for the treatment of bronchospasm. A very common treatment for wheezing in ancient India was the inhalation of *Datura stramonium* (Jimson weed), due to the anticholinergic properties of atropine. "Asthma cigarettes" were once a popular method of administering this medication to the lungs. However, because of its systemic effects, atropine was later on replaced by the N-quaternary compounds that do not penetrate the blood-brain barrier. Ipratropium bromide, one of these compounds, has now been used for many years as a bronchodilator of choice in COPD; however, it possesses inferior bronchodilator properties to beta₂-agonists in asthma. Tiotropium bromide, a longer acting anticholinergic, was recently approved for use in COPD but its exact role in asthma remains to be fully explored.

Pharmacology of Anticholinergic Agents

The efferent cholinergic pathway represents a key mechanism in the control of airway smooth muscle tone as well as a number of other physiological and pathophysiological reactions. For many years, the general belief has been that anticholinergics appear to be less effective in asthmatic patients, probably because airway narrowing in asthma is mainly due to the direct effects of inflammatory mediators on airway smooth muscle and not due to increase in cholinergic tone as is the case in COPD. However, although asthma is considered to be an inflammatory disease of the airways, neural mechanisms remain very important. Furthermore, it must be highlighted that an anticholinergic effect on the bronchi in asthma is possible even in the absence of a true bronchodilator effect. In fact, it has been documented that anticholinergic agents can reduce airway hyperresponsiveness.

Interestingly, there is a complex relationship between inflammation and neural control of the airways. Acetylcholine release from parasympathetic nerves activates muscarinic receptors on airway smooth muscle, submucosal glands, and blood vessels to cause bronchoconstriction, mucus production,

and vasodilation. Three muscarinic receptor subtypes are expressed in the lung (Fig. 27-3). M₁ receptors are localized to parasympathetic ganglia in the bronchial plexus that continues into the smaller airways. M₂ receptors are autoreceptors found on the parasympathetic nerve endings and inhibit the release of acetylcholine, while M₃ receptors on airway smooth-muscle cells mediate bronchoconstriction. Since acetylcholine causes not only airway smooth-muscle contraction but also proliferation, it could mediate some aspects of airway remodeling in asthma. In addition, cholinergic receptors are found outside the neuromuscular system, with muscarinic receptors on lymphocytes and neutrophils, and on a variety of other airway cells. Cholinergic neurotransmission may be enhanced by inflammatory mediators; cholinergic nerves are the dominant neural pathway for bronchoconstriction in humans. In particular, it has been suggested that serum IgE may be one of the factors that determine the airway tone, possibly via cholinergic mechanisms, because it has been

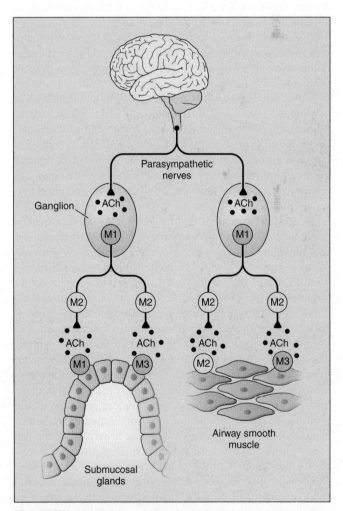

Figure 27-3 Muscarinic receptors in the lung. Vagal parasympathetic nerves from the brain terminate at peripheral ganglia in the lungs. Acetylcholine (ACh) released acts via M₁ muscarinic receptors on postganglionic, nonmyelinated efferent nerves that innervate the submucosal glands and airway smooth muscle. Presynaptic M₂ muscarinic receptors are inhibitory autoreceptors on the postganglionic nerves. ACh released onto the airway smooth muscle causes bronchoconstriction via the M₃ muscarinic receptors and mucus secretion via the M₁ and M₃ muscarinic receptors (*Adapted from Lee AM, Jacoby DB, Fryer AD: Selective muscarinic receptor antagonists for airway diseases. Curr Opin Pharmacol 2001;1:224.*)

observed that higher serum IgE levels were correlated with lower values of FEV$_1$. Furthermore, anticholinergic agents caused more pronounced bronchodilation than beta$_2$-agonists in subjects with high IgE levels. This finding contrasts with the documentation that atopic status appears to have a significant negative effect on the degree of responsiveness to inhaled anticholinergic drugs.

Mucus secretion in airways also plays an important role in asthma, and muscarinic agonists can induce mucus secretion from airway tissue. M$_3$ receptors are involved in mediating cholinergic stimulation of mucus secretion. Ciliary beat frequency is also stimulated by acetylcholine and muscarinic agonists and reduced by muscarinic antagonists.

Clinical Use of Anticholinergic Agents in Asthma

ANTICHOLINERGICS IN THE MAINTENANCE MANAGEMENT OF ASTHMA

As mentioned earlier, the possibility of treating asthma with an anticholinergic agent was suggested many years ago. In 1896, Stewart and Gibson proposed that one of the primary treatments for an asthmatic paroxysm was the use of belladonna alkaloids. However, by 1975, belladonna alkaloids were not considered a significant enough part of asthma treatment to be included in the 14th edition of Cecil's *A Textbook of Medicine*. Nonetheless, the treatment of asthma with ipratropium bromide was introduced in the 1980s, but some studies documented that patients with chronic bronchitis responded better in general to ipratropium bromide, whereas asthmatic subjects responded better to beta$_2$-agonists. Attempts to identify subgroups of asthmatic individuals who respond better to anticholinergic agents have not been very successful. In general, in patients younger than 40, beta$_2$-agonists remain the bronchodilator of choice in asthma. With advancing age, and the apparent decline of beta-adrenergic responsiveness, the initial comparatively small response to ipratropium becomes relatively more important and may predominate. In older patients, the use of anticholinergic agents or continued therapy with both groups of drugs may be preferable.

When given in advance of bronchospastic stimuli, anticholinergic agents provide variable degrees of bronchoprotection. They also have prophylactic effects against the bronchospasm induced in asthmatic patients by beta-blocking agents. Furthermore, a recent genotype-stratified study revealed that patients with certain β_2AR polymorphisms (Arg/Arg genotype at the position 16) might benefit from discontinuation of the use of albuterol as rescue medication and may benefit from the use of as-needed ipratropium bromide instead. Anticholinergic agents may also be useful in patients with chronic asthma who develop fixed airway obstruction. Although "chronic asthma" is a loosely defined disease, it may be equated approximately with nonallergic or "intrinsic" asthma arising in adult life. It has been demonstrated that intrinsic asthmatic individuals and those with longer duration of asthma respond better to anticholinergic agents. However, a Cochrane analysis of randomized controlled trials in which anticholinergic drugs were given for chronic asthma in children older than 2, documented that, although there were some small beneficial findings in favor of anticholinergic therapy, there are insufficient data to support the use of anticholinergic drugs in the maintenance treatment of chronic asthma in children. Another Cochrane analysis, which examined the effectiveness of anticholinergic agents versus placebo and in comparison with beta$_2$-agonists or as adjunctive therapy to beta$_2$-agonists in the management of chronic asthma in adults, concluded that there is no justification for routinely introducing anticholinergics as part of add-on treatment for patients whose asthma is not well controlled on standard therapies. This does not exclude the possibility that there may be a subgroup of patients who derive some benefit and a trial of treatment in individual patients may still be justified.

Nocturnal asthma is considered another likely option for the anticholinergic agents. In fact, it is due, at least in part, to an increase in cholinergic tone during sleep. In one study, vagal blockade with intravenous atropine caused significant bronchodilatation and significantly increased the pulse rate at 4 AM and 4 PM; moreover, nocturnal asthma was almost totally reversed. In another study, morning dipping, assessed by the fall in peak flow overnight, was significantly reduced in the periods when either oxitropium or theophylline was taken, whereas no difference was noticed during the placebo administration. The same finding was demonstrated with the use of ipratropium bromide in 12 patients with morning dipping. Maintenance treatment with ipratropium bromide 40 µg three times daily in 31 children with asthma reduced the provocative dose of histamine, causing a 20% fall in FEV$_1$, despite an 8- to 12-hour gap between the last dose of ipratropium and histamine challenge. It did not, however, diminish the diurnal variation in airway caliber or in bronchodilator responsiveness. These intriguing observations indicate that parasympathetic activity may contribute, but not fully explain, nocturnal airflow obstruction. Therefore, the exact role of anticholinergic agents in nocturnal asthma remains uncertain.

The role of long-term anticholinergics such as tiotropium bromide has yet to be established in patients with asthma and any future trials might draw on the messages derived from this review. It must be highlighted that tiotropium bromide inhibits allergen-induced airway remodeling in a guinea pig model of ongoing asthma. This finding could have important implications for the use of long-acting anticholinergic agents in the treatment of allergic asthma, by protecting against the development of chronic airway hyperresponsiveness and decline of lung function in addition to their acute bronchodilating effects.

ANTICHOLINERGICS IN THE ACUTE MANAGEMENT OF ASTHMA

The rationale for the use of anticholinergic therapy in acute asthma has been the presumption of increased airway vagal tone in these patients. However, the role of anticholinergics has been less well defined than beta$_2$-agonists even in this situation. The overall pooled effect size of trials comparing ipratropium bromide with a beta$_2$-agonist in acute severe asthma shows that a nebulized beta$_2$-agonist produces significantly more bronchodilation than ipratropium. A meta-analysis published in 1993 concluded that anticholinergics should not be used alone to treat acute asthmatic exacerbations. In general, large doses of an anticholinergic agent are required in acute severe asthma, presumably because of increased vagal discharge. In fact, a cumulative dose-response study carried out in patients with acute severe asthma demonstrated that only 0.5 mg ipratropium bromide given by nebulizer produced maximal improvement in peak expiratory flow rates. However, a recent review undertaken to incorporate the more recent evidence available about the effectiveness of treatment with a combination of beta$_2$-agonists and anticholinergics compared with beta$_2$-agonists alone in the treatment of acute asthma suggested that the addition of multiple doses of inhaled ipratropium bromide to beta$_2$-agonists is indicated as the standard treatment in children, adolescents, and adults with *moderate to severe* exacerbations of asthma in the emergency setting. The combined used of these two classes of bronchodilators has been reported to have independent and additive action and reported to attain greater peak and sustained bronchodilatation. This can be accounted for by their different mechanism of action, times of peak effect, and duration of action.

Nonetheless, there is substantial evidence that ipratropium bromide is of limited usefulness in episodes of *mild to moderate* acute asthma. A Cochrane systematic review of acute asthma in children looked at 13 trials of ipratropium bromide. A single dose of ipratropium bromide was of no additional benefit in children with mild to moderate asthma. Multiple doses of ipratropium bromide, while safe, only had sufficient evidence to support its use in school-aged children with acute severe asthma. Another evidence-based review found that whereas multiple doses of ipratropium bromide are indicated in the emergency management of children and adults with severe asthma, there was no apparent benefit of adding single doses of ipratropium bromide to those with mild to moderate asthma. Given that most presentations to the emergency department are mild to moderate in severity, many patients may therefore receive an expensive therapy with little evidence for its efficacy.

Safety of Anticholinergic Agents in Asthma

While atropine produces numerous systemic side effects related to the inhibition of physiological functions of the parasympathetic system, quaternary anticholinergic agents such as ipratropium bromide are poorly absorbed from the mucosa and thus the risk of adverse effects is insignificant. In normal clinical use, the only adverse effects encountered by these agents include dryness of the mouth, which may occur in 5% of patients. However, these agents need to be used with caution in patients with increased intraocular pressure and those with prostatic hypertrophy.

NOVEL BRONCHODILATORS

Novel Beta$_2$-Agonists

After the discovery of formoterol and salmeterol, new candidates for LABAs have emerged. In particular, once-daily beta$_2$-agonists, the so-called ultra-LABAs, are in development for treating asthma in an attempt to simplify its management. Once-daily dosing would allow better compliance and management of patients if desensitization does not occur.

Two compounds, carmoterol and indacaterol, are in advanced phase of clinical development.

CARMOTEROL (CHF-4226, TA-2005)

Carmoterol, a noncatechol beta$_2$-agonist with a *p*-methoxyphenyl group on the amine side chain and a 8-hydroxyl group on the carbostyril aromatic ring, is a pure (R,R)-isomer that has a high potency for the beta$_2$-adrenoceptor and a long duration of action after removal of the drug using both guinea pig tracheal muscle relaxation and bovine trapezium muscle binding experiments. Preliminary clinical trials indicated duration of effect exceeding 24 hours after inhalation of only 3 μg. In a study that evaluated the effects of single doses of carmoterol in mild asthmatic individuals, carmoterol had an exceptional duration of action in man, with significant improvement in FEV$_1$ sustained for 30 hours, twice that of salmeterol or formoterol. Carmoterol restored FEV$_1$ levels to the normal range within 20 minutes of inhalation.

INDACATEROL (QAB-149)

Indacaterol (QAB-149) is another once-daily beta$_2$-agonist that demonstrates a fast onset and long duration of action in vitro and in vivo in the experimental setting. Phase II clinical trials in patients with mild-to-moderate asthma have shown that this ultra-LABA at 200- and 400-μg doses is statistically superior ($P < .05$) to placebo at all time points from 5 minutes to 26 hours post dose, except for 26 hours post dose for the 200-μg dose, but also at a 25-μg dose it has elicited response in mild asthma patients compared to placebo. Improvement in efficacy responses was generally dose dependent and was accompanied by a positive safety profile up to a 2000-μg dose. The efficacy of indacaterol in patients with asthma has further been investigated in longer-term trials in which the 24-hour bronchodilator efficacy of indacaterol observed on the first day was maintained for the duration of the studies, suggesting that regular use of indacaterol is not associated with the development of tolerance, or tachyphylaxis.

OTHER ULTRA-LABAS

The compound GSK-159797 (TD-3327) is an ultra-LABA for the potential once-daily treatment for asthma and COPD, but its structure has not yet been disclosed. It achieved the target increase in FEV$_1$ throughout the 24-hour evaluation period in studies of patients with mild asthma with improvements in efficacy responses that were dose dependent. GSK-159797 was well tolerated, with no increase in heart rate. Also GSK-597901, another ultra-LABA, proved encouraging in early phase II studies, although fewer details have been disclosed. GSK-159802, GSK-642444, and GSK-678007 are three other ultra-LABAs in development.

Novel Long-Acting Anticholinergic Agents (LAMAs)

Several new anticholinergic agents , currently in development mainly for the treatment of COPD, could be considered as potential alternatives or be integrated in the treatment of chronic asthma. NVA237 (AD 237) is a once-daily, long-acting muscarinic antagonist (LAMA) with a fast onset of action. This drug has been identified as glycopyrrolate, a quaternary ammonium anticholinergic compound that has been shown to cause bronchodilatation for at least 12 hours in patients with asthma and has been successfully employed in the treatment of exercise-induced asthma and acute exacerbations of asthma in the past. Recently it has been documented that protection against methacholine-induced bronchospasm after administering glycopyrrolate was maintained to 30 hours, the last time point measured. In addition, glycopyrrolate caused bronchodilation that was fast in onset and sustained at up to 30 hours. Both bronchodilatation and bronchoprotection were significantly longer with glycopyrrolate than after ipratropium bromide, and bronchoprotection was significant at all time points from 2 to 30 hours compared to placebo. LAS-34273 and LAS-35201 are two new LAMAs under development by Almirall, and TD-5742 is a new LAMA under development by Theravance, all with presumably very long duration of effect. Darifenacin is a selective M_3 receptor antagonist but has shown 10-fold and 6-fold less potency in binding to the trachea and salivary gland, respectively, compared with atropine.

Salivary gland responses were inhibited at doses 6 to 10 times higher than those required to inhibit gut and bladder responses. Zamifenacin and darifenacin, which are developed to treat overactive bladder, have the highest affinity for M_3 muscarinic receptors of all the current anti-muscarinic antagonists and these new drugs may be clinically useful for antagonizing M_3 muscarinic receptors on submandibular glands. Increased mucus secretion is seen in exacerbations of asthma and this contributes to airway narrowing; these drugs may decrease mucus secretion in the airways. LAMAs are likely to have additive effects when combined with ultra-LABAs, thus making once-daily combination bronchodilator inhalers a likely development in the future.

SUGGESTED READING

Barnes PJ: Theoretical aspects of anticholinergic treatment. In Gross NJ (ed). Anticholinergic Therapy in Obstructive Airway Disease. London, Franklin Scientific Publications, 1993, pp 88–104.

Cazzola M, Centanni S, Donner CF: Anticholinergic agents. Pulm Pharmacol Ther 1998;11:381–392.

Cazzola M, Matera MG, Lötvall J: Ultra long-acting ß2 agonists in development for asthma and chronic obstructive pulmonary disease. Expert Opin Investig Drugs 2005;14:775–783.

Global Initiative for Asthma (GINA). Global Strategy for Asthma Management and Prevention: NHLBI/WHO Workshop Report (Publication No 02-3659). Bethesda, MD, National Institutes of Health, National Heart, Lung and Blood Institute, 2002 (revised in 2006).

Hanania NA, Moore RH: Anti-inflammatory activities of beta2-agonists. Curr Drug Targets Inflamm Allergy 2004;3:271–77.

Hanania NA, Moore RH, Dickey BF: The rational use of beta2–agonists in the management of asthma: maintenance, rescue and emergency. Sem Respir Crit Care Med 1998;19:613–624.

Hanania NA, Sharafkhaneh A, Barber R, Dickey BF: Beta-agonist intrinsic efficacy: measurement and clinical significance. Am J Respir Crit Care Med 2002;165:1353–1358.

Kanazawa H: Anticholinergic agents in asthma: chronic bronchodilator therapy, relief of acute severe asthma, reduction of chronic viral inflammation and prevention of airway remodeling. Curr Opin Pulm Med 2006;12:60–67.

Kips JC, Pauwels RA: Long-acting inhaled beta2-agonist therapy in asthma. Am J Respir Crit Care Med 2001;164:923–932.

Lee AM, Jacoby DB, Fryer AD: Selective muscarinic receptor antagonists for airway diseases. Curr Opin Pharmacol 2001;1:223–229.

Litonjua AA: The significance of beta2-adrenergic receptor polymorphisms in asthma. Curr Opin Pulm Med 2006;12:12–17.

McDonald NJ, Bara AI: Anticholinergic therapy for chronic asthma in children over two years of age. Cochrane Database Syst Rev 2003;(3):CD003535.

National Asthma Education and Prevention Program. Expert Panel Report 3: Guidelines for the Diagnosis and Management of Asthma (Pub. No. 08-5846). Bethesda, MD, National Institutes of Health, National Heart, Lung, and Blood Institute, October 2007.

Nelson HS: Combination therapy of long-acting beta agonists and inhaled corticosteroids in the management of chronic asthma. Curr Allergy Asthma Rep 2005;5:123–129.

Nelson HS: Long-acting beta-agonists in adult asthma: evidence that these drugs are safe. Prim Care Respir J 2006;15:271–277.

Nelson HS, Weiss ST, Bleecker ER, et al: The Salmeterol Multicenter Asthma Research Trial: a comparison of usual pharmacotherapy for asthma or usual pharmacotherapy plus salmeterol. Chest 2006;129:15–26.

Remington TL, Digiovine B: Long-acting beta-agonists: anti-inflammatory properties and synergy with corticosteroids in asthma. Curr Opin Pulm Med 2005;11:74–78.

Rodrigo GJ, Castro-Rodriguez JA: Anticholinergics in the treatment of children and adults with acute asthma: a systematic review with meta-analysis. Thorax 2005;60:740–746.

Rodrigo GJ, Rodrigo C: The role of anticholinergics in acute asthma treatment: an evidence-based evaluation. Chest 2002;121:1977–1987.

Rodrigo GJ, Rodrigo C, Hall JB: Acute asthma in adults: a review. Chest 2004;125:1081–1102.

Salpeter SR, Buckley NS, Ormiston TM, Salpeter EE: Meta-analysis: effect of long-acting beta-agonists on severe asthma exacerbations and asthma–related deaths. Ann Intern Med 2006;144:904–912.

Sears MR, Lotvall J: Past, present and future—beta2-adrenoceptor agonists in asthma management. Respir Med 2005;99:152–170.

Walters JA, Wood-Baker R, Walters EH: Long-acting beta2-agonists in asthma: an overview of Cochrane systematic reviews. Respir Med 2005;99:384–395.

Westby M, Benson M, Gibson P: Anticholinergic agents for chronic asthma in adults. Cochrane Database Syst Rev 2004;(3):CD003269.

Corticosteroids

Lora Stewart, Stanley J. Szefler, and Ronina A. Covar

CLINICAL PEARLS

- Various structural and pharmacologic features contribute to the efficacy and safety profile of corticosteroids.

- The magnitude of the clinical effects of this class of medication is related to its wide-ranging anti-inflammatory properties which translate into physiologic improvements in airflow limitation, inflammation, and bronchial hyper-responsiveness.

- Corticosteroids are considered preferred therapy in the treatment of severe acute asthma exacerbations and chronic persistent asthma.

- Although most asthmatic patients will respond to corticosteroids, there are distinct features of the disease that can make response to corticosteroids limited or unsustainable.

- The adverse effects related to corticosteroids are dose and duration dependent; at conventional doses, they are preventable and easy to monitor.

From the earliest description of asthma and its "spasms" as a medical condition by Hippocrates (460–370 BC) to the writings by Galen (AD 131–201) that asthma was due to bronchial obstruction for which Romans used owl's blood in wine, chicken soup, and abstinence as remedies, the description and subsequent treatment of asthma have dramatically evolved through the centuries. That asthma was more than just a condition of bronchoconstriction, but perhaps more importantly, one of inflammation, was realized only in the 1960s. This came after significant reports of treatment with corticotropin and cortisone for allergies and asthma were published in the 1950s, shortly after these drugs were first synthesized and demonstrated to be effective in the treatment of another inflammatory condition, rheumatoid arthritis. As asthma is now largely characterized as a chronic disease of airway inflammation, corticosteroids (CSs), and even more specifically glucocorticoids, are considered the most effective class of medications available either for acute and or long-term control. Of all the drugs available for asthma, CSs have had the best record of controlling most clinical, physiologic, and pathologic manifestations of asthma, which then translates into reduction of asthma severity and even mortality.

The application of inhaled CSs for the treatment of asthma has advanced since they first became available over 30 years ago, starting with aerosolized high-dose cortisone suspension to the development of more efficient delivery and spacer devices and newer generation CSs with excellent topical to systemic potency. For most patients, there is little question as to efficacy of CSs but the prevailing challenge is the pursuit of the ideal CS, which provides optimal asthma control with no significant systemic effects. Utilization of CS therapy has been limited by the concern about debilitating adverse effects particularly with long-term use; however, it has also become apparent that CSs do not possess the capacity to induce remission and despite their vast effects on the inflammatory cascade, steroid-independent mechanisms exist and limit the applicability of CSs in cases with refractory disease.

This chapter will provide a broad overview of the structure, pharmacologic properties, mechanisms of action, clinical efficacy, adverse effects, and current issues associated with both systemic and inhaled CS therapy in asthma. In general, CSs refer to the 21 carbon atom molecules synthesized in the adrenal cortex including both the carbohydrate-metabolism regulating glucocorticoids (primarily represented by cortisol) secreted by the inner zonae fasciculata/reticularis and the electrolyte balance–regulating mineralocorticoids (primarily represented by aldosterone) secreted by the outer zona glomerulosa. In this chapter, the term CS is interchangeably used to refer to glucocorticoids, the drug class used for asthma.

PROPERTIES OF CORTICOSTEROIDS

Structure and Chemistry

Alterations made to the basic steroid structure—cortisol molecule—have been created to increase the anti-inflammatory potency and duration of action, and enhance the separation between the glucocorticoid and mineralocorticoid properties (Fig. 28-1A and B). These chemical structure changes improve their pharmacokinetic and pharmacodynamic properties. However, because the anti-inflammatory and metabolic effects of CSs are mediated by the same receptor, the metabolic and hypothalamic-pituitary axis effects of the drug cannot be separated from the anti-inflammatory response. Systemic CSs that have been used for asthma are cortisone, hydrocortisone (cortisol), prednisone, prednisolone, methylprednisolone, and dexamethasone (see Fig. 28-1A). Currently available inhaled CSs are beclomethasone dipropionate (BDP), budesonide (BUD), flunisolide (FLN), fluticasone propionate (FP), mometasone furoate (MF), and triamcinolone acetonide (TAA) (see Fig. 28-1B). Ciclesonide (CIC) has been used in Europe, but is still not currently available in the U.S. market.

While the 4,5 double bond and the 3-keto group on ring A are essential for both glucocorticoid and mineralocorticoid activities, molecular components that increase the glucocorticoid properties over the mineralocorticoid properties include the 11β-hydroxyl group on ring C, the 17α-hydroxyl group on ring D (e.g., prednisone, prednisolone, methylprednisolone,

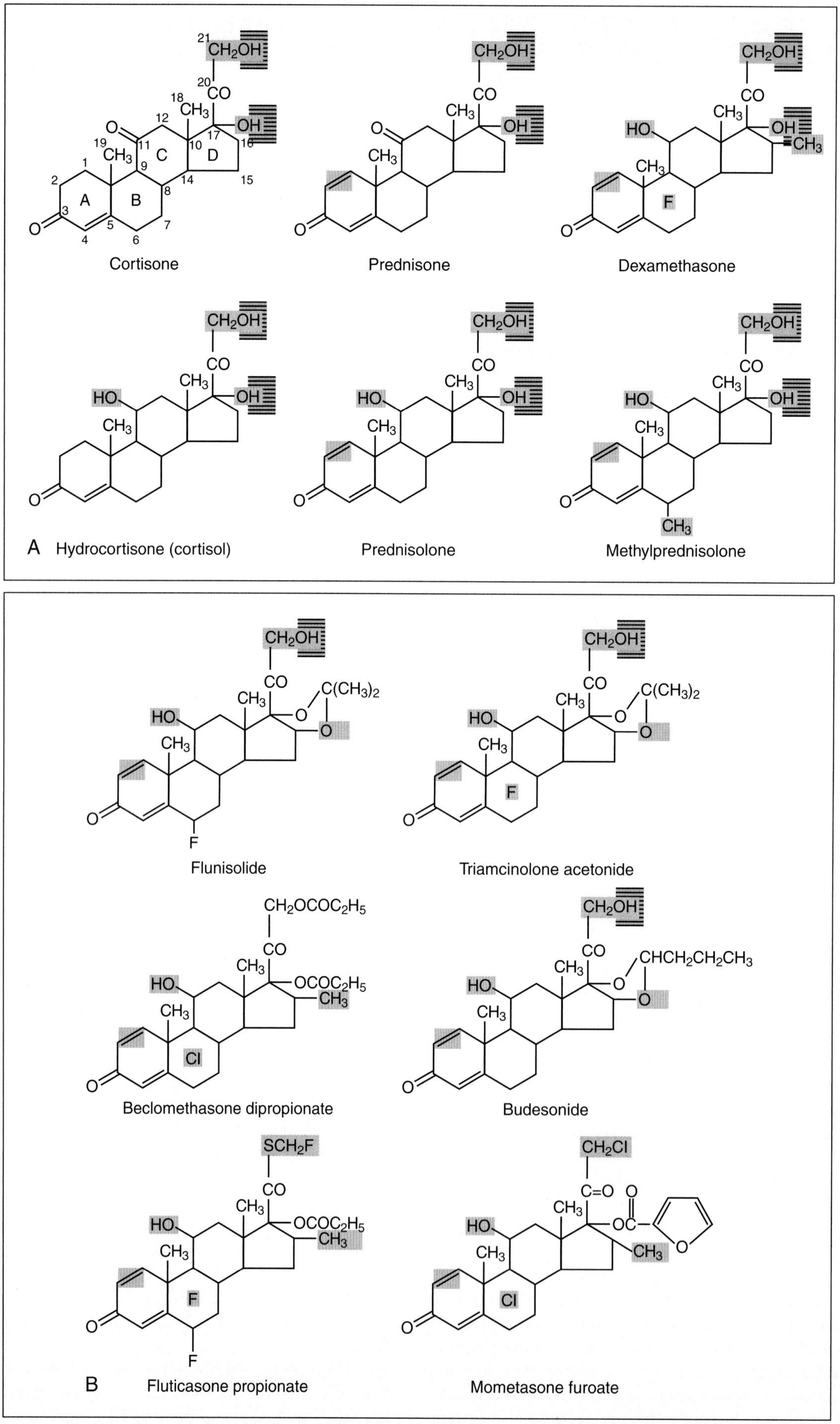

Figure 28-1 **Molecular structures of commonly administered systemic corticosteroids (A) and available inhaled corticosteroids (B) used in the treatment of asthma.** Carbon and ring nomenclature is noted for cortisone. The green-shaded structures confer increased glucocorticoid properties; the blue-shaded structures are esterification sites of the hydroxyl groups at the C-17 and C-21 positions that can improve lipophilicity; and the orange-shaded structures are the free hydroxyl group (or sulfur group in FP) at C-21, which is required for binding to the glucocorticoid receptor.

and dexamethasone), an additional double-bond in the 1,2 position of ring A, and the 9α-fluoro derivatives on ring B combined with other substitutions at C16 on ring D (e.g., dexamethasone, beclomethasone, triamcinolone, and fluticasone) (see Fig. 28-1). The changes in the 9α-position and substitutions at C-16 position result in a 25-fold increase of glucocorticoid with negligible mineralocorticoid activity compared to hydrocortisone. The two systemically administered CSs, cortisone and prednisone, are pro-drugs, that is, they are inactive congeners that require biotransformation of their 11-ketone groups to 11-hydroxy molecules, which results in their active forms, cortisol and prednisolone, respectively. A methyl group at the 6-position of the B-ring of methylprednisolone allows somewhat greater glucocorticoid activity and less mineralocorticoid properties than prednisolone.

Additional modifications increase binding to the receptor and enhance the lipophilicity of the molecules, and subsequently augment topical to systemic potency. The free hydroxyl group (or sulfur group in FP) at C-21 is required for binding to the glucocorticoid receptor. Esterification of the hydroxyl groups at the C-17 and C-21 positions results in increased lipophilicity and improved transport across the cell membrane to reach the CS receptor. Most inhaled CSs are administered in their active forms, with a free hydroxyl group at C-21. BDP and CIC are pro-drugs that are hydrolyzed by pulmonary esterases to form their active moieties, beclomethasone-17-monopropionate (BMP) and desisobutyryl-CIC (des-CIC), respectively.

Pharmacology of Corticosteroids

The pharmacokinetics of a drug, that is, absorption, transport, metabolism, and elimination, determine the extent and duration of its action, thereby influencing dosing strategies to enhance therapeutic benefit and minimize side effects. For systemic CSs, the dosing regimens are not exactly determined by pharmacokinetic properties, as they are largely empirical and the potential for side effects with high dosage and long-term use is unquestionable. Fortunately with the availability of topical preparations, the need for systemic CS has declined considerably; hence a separate discussion on the pharmacology of inhaled CSs is provided.

Hydrocortisone and the synthetic derivatives are highly lipophilic and relatively completely orally absorbed, with peak plasma concentrations evident within 1 to 2 hours for prednisone or prednisolone. Water-soluble esters are administered intravenously to achieve high concentrations rapidly, particularly under circumstances where oral administration is not tolerated. There are no significant factors that affect absorption of systemic CSs but certain medications (antacids by 25% to 40%) and disease states (chronic liver disease by 13% to 35%) can reduce the bioavailability of prednisolone.

Prednisone, the most common systemic CSs used for chronic and acute asthma, is transformed rapidly and almost completely to prednisolone through first-pass metabolism. At least 90% of prednisolone binds to transcortin (also called corticosteroid-binding globulin), albumin, and α1-acid glycoprotein, at low or normal plasma concentrations. It is the unbound fraction that is available for entry into cells, which subsequently binds to the cytosolic glucocorticoid receptor. However, the capacity of protein binding is easily saturated at higher concentrations, such that a much greater fraction of the drug is available in the free state. Protein binding is also reduced with liver disease. Compared to prednisone and prednisolone, methylprednisolone is more slowly absorbed and binds primarily to albumin, which has a large binding capacity. This strong binding capacity may allow for greater penetration and longer retention in the lung tissue but has been demonstrated only in an animal model. Dexamethasone also does not bind as well to transcortin, with protein binding only reported at 68% to 75%, hence increasing its potential for adverse effects.

Certain disease states such as hyperthyroidism and cystic fibrosis can enhance clearance of CSs and minimize therapeutic efficacy. An increased rate of elimination for dexamethasone, prednisolone, and methylprednisolone with concurrently administered anticonvulsants (e.g., phenytoin, phenobarbital, and carbamazepine), and increased clearance for prednisolone and methylprednisolone with rifampin, can also be expected due to similar hepatic cytochrome use, in which case, higher doses may be required. On the other hand, medications that delay CS clearance lead to a higher risk for adverse effects: antifungal (e.g., ketoconazole), reducing both prednisolone and methylprednisolone clearance; oral contraceptives affecting prednisolone clearance; and troleandomycin, erythromycin, and clarithromycin decreasing methylprednisolone elimination.

Pharmacokinetic studies can be obtained for patients with asthma who demonstrate poor response to systemically administered CS, to determine if poor absorption or rapid clearance contributes to poor disease control. A pharmacokinetic abnormality should be considered when there is lack of therapeutic response or adverse effects as expected from chronic systemic CS use. For these patients, a different CS may be offered, or a split-dosing regimen (two thirds in the morning and one third in the afternoon) may be recommended to attain a more normal plasma concentration versus time curve. Comparative pharmacologic features of available systemic CSs for asthma are presented in Tables 28-1 and 28-2.

Pharmacokinetics of Inhaled Corticosteroids

The efficacy and safety of inhaled CSs are influenced by several pharmacokinetic and pharmacodynamic parameters. Factors that promote therapeutic response can be different from those that affect safety. In general, an ideal CS should

Table 28-1
PHARMACOKINETIC AND PHARMACODYNAMIC FEATURES OF SYSTEMIC CORTICOSTEROIDS USED FOR ASTHMA

	Clearance (mL/min/ 1.73 m²)	Volume of Distribution (L/1.73 m²)	Half-life (hr)
Dexamethasone	216	33.4	4.37
Hydrocortisone	425.5	70	1.9
Methylprednisolone	384	91	2.58
Prednisolone	198	53.5	3.25

From Spahn JD: Glucocorticoid pharmacokinetics. In Szefler SJ, Leung DYM (eds): Immunology and Allergy Clinics of North America. Philadelphia, W.B. Saunders, 1999.

Table 28-2
RELATIVE POTENCIES AND PHARMACOLOGIC EFFECTS OF COMMON ORAL CORTICOSTEROIDS

	Anti-Inflammatory Potency	Na⁺-Retaining Potency	Duration of Action	Equivalent Dose (mg)*
Cortisol or hydrocortisone	1	1	S	20
Cortisone	0.8	0.8	S	25
Prednisolone	4	0.8	I	5
Prednisone	4	0.8	I	5
6α-methylprednisolone	5	0.5	I	4
Triamcinolone	5	0	I	4
Dexamethasone	25	0	L	0.75
Betamethasone	25	0	L	0.75

I, intermediate (12–36-hour biologic half-life); L, long (36–72-hour biologic half-life); S, short (8–12-hour biologic half-life).

*Dose comparisons apply to oral and intravenous administration only; GC potencies differ greatly with intramuscular and intra-articular administration.

From Schleimer RP, Spahn JD, Covar R, Szefler SJ: Glucocorticoids: B. Clinical science. In Adkinson NJ, Bochner BS, Busse WW, et al (eds): Middleton's Allergy Principles & Practice, 6th ed. Philadelphia, Mosby, 2003.

have increased lung deposition and pulmonary retention or residence time and high receptor-binding affinity to enhance efficacy but should have poor oral bioavailability, good protein binding, rapid clearance, and have an on-site activation of the prodrug to promote safety (Fig. 28-2). However, a perfect balance between safety and efficacy is yet to be achieved. To understand this in more detail, an overview of the fate of inhaled CSs and a description of relevant pharmacokinetic parameters will be presented.

BIOAVAILABILITY

The amount of an inhaled CS which enters the systemic circulation represents the combination of the orally and pulmonary absorbed fractions. While a large portion of the dose is deposited in the mouth and oropharynx, the swallowed drug is absorbed in the gastrointestinal tract. A highly efficient first-pass metabolism in the liver or gut wall for most CSs allows only minimal yet still highly variable systemic bioavailability through the oral route, that is, the dose that escapes inactivation by first-pass metabolism varies from less than 1% for MF and FP to over 20% for TAA and BMP (Table 28-3).

The remaining portion of the drug is delivered to the respiratory tract, which is the therapeutic target. However, inhaled CSs are not inactivated in the lung, hence pulmonary bioavailability accounts for most of the systemic bioavailability. Inhaled CSs are easily absorbed into the lung tissue and while the deposition in the lungs depends not only on the formulation of the drug itself, the delivery device and method are important components as well, which are covered in a separate chapter. Briefly, particle size less than 2 μm is more likely to reach the small/peripheral airway while particle size between 2 and 5 μm will deliver only up to the bronchi and bronchioles. Delivery of an inhaled CS requires devices such as a pressured metered-dose inhaler (pMDI) with chlorofluorocarbon or hydrofluoralkane propellants, breath-actuated dry powder inhaled devices (DPI), or a compressor nebulizer. The delivery device itself can significantly determine the amount of drug delivered to the lower airway. As an example, the delivery of BUD to the lower airway through the DPI (Turbuhaler, AstraZeneca, Wilmington, DE) is enhanced by twice as much compared to a pMDI. In addition, the use of an ozone-friendly hydrofluoroalkane-propellant pMDI has an additional advantage of improving the delivery of BDP into the lower respiratory tract by as much as 60% compared with the chlorofluorocarbon-propellant pMDI. Furthermore, using the hydrofluoroalkane-propelled pMDI, BDP in a solution allows a smaller particle size and hence better deposition of the drug in the lower airway compared to an FP in a suspension. Last, the delivery of the drug into the lower airways using a pMDI is augmented by 50% to 60% with the use of spacer devices that also decrease the amount of drug deposited in the oropharynx.

PULMONARY RETENTION TIME

The pulmonary retention time of an inhaled drug is an estimate of the duration that the drug exerts its effect. The longer the drug is trapped within the airway, the greater is its ability to interact with the glucocorticoid receptor (GCR). One factor that contributes to this retention time is the rate at which the inhaled particle is released from its vehicle. The other elements that affect pulmonary retention are lipophilicity, lipid conjugation, onsite activation for BDP and CIC,

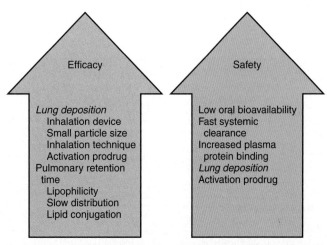

Figure 28-2 Pharmacologic factors that promote efficacy and safety of an inhaled corticosteroid.

Table 28-3
PHARMACOKINETIC AND PHARMACODYNAMIC PROPERTIES OF INHALED CORTICOSTEROIDS

Corticosteroid	Relative Receptor Affinity	Oral Bioavailability, (%)	Unbound Fraction (%)	Clearance (L/hr)	Volume of Distribution at Steady State (L)	Half-Life/ELIM/hr
Mometasone furoate	2300	<1	1–2	54	—	5.8
Fluticasone propionate	1800	<1	10	66-90	318-859	7-8
Beclomethasone dipropionate	53	15–20	13	150	20	0.5
17-Beclomethasone monoprioponate	1345	26	—	120	424	2.7
Beclomethasone	76	—	—	—	—	—
Ciclesonide	12	<1	<1	152	207	0.36
Des-ciclesonide	1200	<1	<1	228	897	3.4
Budesonide	935	11	12	84	183-301	2.8
Triamcinolone acetonide	233	23	29	37	103	2.0
Flunisolide	180	20	20	57	96	1.3

Adapted from Winkler J, Hochhaus G, Derendorf H: How the lungs handle drugs. Proc Am Thorac Soc 2004;1:356–363.

and receptor binding. Receptor binding will be discussed in a subsequent section.

Lipophilicity is an important property of an inhaled CS and one modification to the molecular structure is the addition of lipophilic side chains to the D ring (e.g., FP and BUD in Fig. 28-1B). Lipophilicity affects both drug dissolution (i.e., a drug that is less lipophilic dissolves in the bronchial fluid and is absorbed into the systemic circulation) and the rate at which a drug passes through the cell membranes, both prolonging residence time in the lung. With lipophilicity, however, the distribution of CSs can be affected such that the drug can reside in other tissues of the body for long periods and cause unnecessary side effects.

Intracellular lipid or fatty acid conjugation that involves esterification of the CS is another mechanism by which retention time can be prolonged. This entails an enzymatic reaction between a fatty acid and the hydroxyl group at the C-21 position (see Fig. 28-1B). Although BMP, BUD, flunisolide (FLU), and TAA have this C-21 hydroxyl group, only BUD (and soon to be available CIC) has been shown to undergo this mechanism. Again, the clinical relevance of this property is uncertain but may be a basis for once-daily dosing.

Most CSs are inhaled in their pharmacologically active forms, except BDP and CIC, which are hydrolyzed by intracellular esterases in the lung tissue to their active forms, 17-BMP and des-CIC, respectively. The main advantage of on-site activation is reduction of local effects in the mouth and oropharynx (e.g., oral candidiasis). In addition, since the drugs become active only upon reaching the targeted lung, increased pulmonary retention time can be expected, although the clinical implication of this is still not fully realized.

PROTEIN BINDING

Once the inhaled CS enters the systemic circulation, the molecule reversibly binds to proteins, mainly albumin. The unbound portion of the drug is available for binding to the GCR in various tissues, so that the greater the protein-binding capacity, the better is the safety profile of the drug. Protein binding, in the case of CSs, however, does not influence systemic clearance much since they are "high-extraction drugs,"

that is, they have a high metabolic activity and high hepatic clearance. Again, the different CSs available in the U.S. market have variable protein-binding properties, with MF having well over 90% protein binding.

ELIMINATION

A drug's elimination half-life that measures the rate of change of its plasma concentration is dependent on both the systemic clearance rate and the volume of distribution (Vd). A drug that is removed quickly from the systemic circulation and resides in small amounts within tissues will have a short half-life, translating to lower potential for side effects.

Systemic clearance, expressed as the volume of fluid cleared per unit time (L/h or mL/min), is the sum of the clearance by various organs, primarily the liver where CSs are mostly cleared. The systemic clearance for most CSs such as BUD and FP (84 and 66 to 90 L/hr) approximates the maximum rate, at 90 L/hr determined by the hepatic blood flow, since the liver rapidly metabolizes the drug. However, for 17-BMP and des-CIC, which are converted metabolites, the apparent clearance values are much higher, suggesting extrahepatic metabolism. The faster the systemic clearance, the higher the therapeutic index and lower side-effect potential.

The Vd is a measure of drug distribution within tissues and is related to the lipophilicity of the drug. In light of FP having a large Vd, it also has the long elimination half-life of greater than 3 hours (see Table 28-3). However, for BMP and des-CIC, which also have large Vd, their systemic clearance is much higher as well, that their half-life is not necessarily more prolonged. A large Vd does not necessarily imply greater potential for systemic effects, because CSs circulate primarily in an inactive protein-bound form. The free, unbound form is independent of the Vd; clearance and extent of protein binding are more important determinants.

Pharmacodynamics of Inhaled Corticosteroids

Unlike most drugs, the pharmacodynamic properties of CSs are not tied to their pharmacokinetic characteristics, that is, their efficacy is not dependent on their plasma levels. Upon absorption into the cells, the molecule undergoes a series of steps that leads up to regulation of gene transcription that impacts both the anti-inflammatory and metabolic effects.

All free, unbound CSs are able to diffuse through the cell membrane easily because of their lipophilicity. In the cytoplasm, they bind to the GCR, and each CS possesses different receptor binding affinities. The range of receptor-binding affinities (expressed as relative receptor affinity [RRA] with reference to that of dexamethasone as 100) for the inhaled CSs available is wide: 2300 for MF and 1800 for FP to 53 for BDP and 12 for CIC (see Table 28-3). However, for both BDP and CIC, which are inhaled in their inactive forms, their RRAs upon activation in the body increase to 1345 and 1200, respectively. For reasons still not entirely clear, the CS that binds to the GCR with the greatest affinity has the greatest anti-inflammatory activities. In other words, the higher the binding affinity, the lower the concentration necessary to induce an effect.

The GCR is a large heteromeric complex (90kd) which includes the heat shock proteins (hsp) 90 dimer, a subunit of p23 protein, and any one of immunophilin-related proteins. The hsp associated with GCR maintain the conformation of the GCR for protein binding and inhibit GCR nuclear translocation. Once the CS is bound to the GCR, the GCR dissociates from the complex proteins and the CS-GCR complex undergoes nuclear translocation. GCRs are recycled back to the cytoplasm and reassociation with HSP takes place before binding to another CS (Fig. 28-3).

Within the nucleus, the molecular basis for the anti-inflammatory effects of CS is due to either transactivation or transrepression (see Fig. 28-3). Transactivation refers to a direct GCR-mediated induction of specific target genes (e.g., synthesis of lipocortin 1, type II interleukin [IL]-1 receptor [a decoy molecule for IL-1], secretory leukocyte proteinase inhibitor, and inhibitory κBA [IκBA]) as a result of sequence-specific DNA binding. The CS-GCR complex dimerizes and binds to specific regulatory DNA sites, termed glucocorticoid response elements (GRE). Coactivator proteins, such as chromatin-binding protein (CBP), p300, and steroid receptor coactivator 1 (SRC-1), help the CS-GCR homodimer interact with the basal transcriptional complex, which includes TATA-binding protein, associated transcription factors (TAFs and TFIIs), and RNA polymerase (pol II). These coactivator proteins also have another important property—as histone acetyltransferase activity, which allows unfolding of the chromatin structure for binding to the GCR.

Transrepression is the other process by which CSs exert their anti-inflammatory effects. CS-GCR prompts

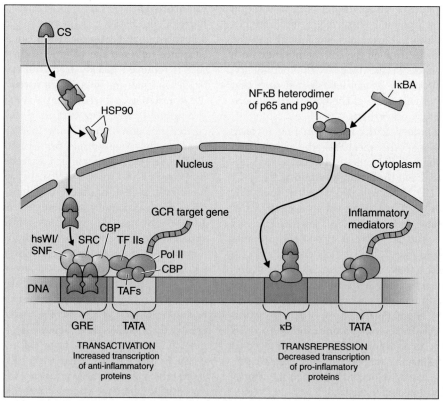

Figure 28-3   A schematic representation of the corticosteroid-receptor pathway. Due to its lipophilicity, the corticosteroid (CS) molecule is able to diffuse through the cytoplasmic membrane. On binding of the CS molecule to the glucocorticoid receptor (GCR), which exists as a large heteromeric complex with other proteins (heat shock proteins 90 dimer, a subunit of p23 protein, and immunophilin-related proteins), the GCR dissociates from the complex proteins. The CS-GCR complex translocates into the nucleus where it affects gene transcription via transactivation or transrepression. In transactivation, the CS-GCR homodimer binds to a specific DNA sequence in the regulatory regions of target genes, called *glucocorticoid response elements* (GRE). Coactivator proteins (chromatin-binding protein [CBP], p300, and steroid receptor coactivator 1 [SRC-1]) allow the GCR homodimer to interact with the basal transcriptional complex (TATA-binding protein, associated transcription factors [TAFs and TFIIs], and RNA polymerase [pol II]). This interaction between GCR and basal transcription complex results in transcription of the GCR target gene. In transrepression, inhibition of gene expression of multiple inflammatory cytokine, adhesion molecules, and enzymes might occur through GCR-mediated interference on the interaction between transcription factors, such as nuclear factor κB, and the basal transcriptional complex. GCRs are recycled back to the cytoplasm and integration to form the heteromeric complex takes place before binding to another CS.

transrepression either by preventing transcription factors (e.g., NFκB) from interacting with the transcription initiation complex or by a DNA-independent interaction with coactivator proteins (e.g., AP-1). Both result in inhibition of gene expression of multiple inflammatory cytokines (e.g., IL-1, IL-2, IL-3, IL-4, IL-5, IL-6, IL-11, IL-13, IL-16, granulocyte-macrophage colony-stimulating factor [GM-CSF], tumor necrosis factor [TNF]-α, matrix metalloproteinase 9, and the chemokines IL-8, RANTES, eotaxin, macrophage inflammatory protein 1a, and the monocyte chemoattractant protein 1); adhesion molecules (e.g., intercellular adhesion molecule 1 and vascular adhesion molecule 1); and various enzymes (IL-4 receptor, high-affinity immunoglobulin E [IgE] receptor, nitric oxide synthase).

Since both the positive and negative effects of CS are produced by this cascade of events, the development of newer CS preparations should incorporate changes that will provide selective stimulation of the transrepression CS-GCR pathway (e.g., blocking the transcription activation of AP-1 and NF-κB) and less on the stimulation of the transactivation pathway that causes the adverse effects.

Cellular and Molecular Effects of Corticosteroids

The superiority of CSs over any other asthma controller therapy is attributed to the multiple effects on the complex cascade of airway inflammatory response features of asthma including mast cell degranulation, eosinophilic infiltration, and increased T-cell activation. CSs suppress circulating eosinophils, basophils, monocytes, mast cells, dendritic cells, and to a smaller degree lymphocytes (particularly T lymphocytes). However, their principal effect comes mainly from their ability to inhibit the synthesis, release, and expression of cytokines, inflammatory peptides, chemokines, growth factors, adhesion molecules, and lipid mediators involved in the inflammatory response. Additional cellular sources of these inflammatory mediators include airway smooth muscle cells, endothelial cells, and fibroblasts. There is increased recognition of the importance of epithelial cells as a major cell target for inhaled CSs as well, as they easily are the first cells to be encountered by outside triggers. Regulation of these proteins is via increased gene transcription and controlled by transcription factors AP-1 and NF-κB, which in turn are inhibited by CSs. The overall effects on the inflammatory response in the airway result in the reduction of cell numbers including inhibition of recruitment or migration, activation, survival, and proliferation of cells. In addition, other important effects of CS therapy that are especially relevant to asthma are the up-regulation of beta-adrenergic receptors on airway smooth muscle cells and inhibition of formation of arachidonic acid metabolites. CSs also are able to induce vasoconstriction, causing decreased capillary permeability and plasma exudation at sites of inflammation, resulting in a reduction in the concentration of inflammatory and chemotactic factors and ultimately in a decrease in the inflammatory response.

ROLE OF CORTICOSTEROIDS IN ACUTE AND CHRONIC ASTHMA

CSs are considered preferred therapy in the treatment of severe acute asthma exacerbation and chronic persistent asthma because of proven efficacy for the treatment of airflow limitation and airway inflammation, as well as bronchial hyperresponsiveness, which are the cardinal features of asthma.

Indications for Corticosteroids

ACUTE ASTHMA

In addition to the risk of mortality, acute asthma accounts for the high morbidity and tremendous cost associated with this condition, in the form of hospitalization, emergency department utilization, and missed work days. Currently, systemic CSs added to bronchodilator therapy are the cornerstones of management of significant asthma exacerbations. Several studies have shown the efficacy of systemic CS therapy in combination with bronchodilator treatments in preventing hospital admissions and reducing relapse rate, and hastening recovery. Systemic CSs also facilitate improvement of asthma symptoms and lung function and reduced need for beta-agonist therapy.

The National Heart, Lung, and Blood Institute (NHLBI) Expert Panel Report 3 (EPR 3) Asthma Guidelines recommend the prompt initiation of oral CS therapy for all moderate to severe asthma exacerbations. The oral route is preferred, unless difficult to tolerate, as it is less invasive compared to parenteral administration, and considered equally efficacious, given the drug's excellent absorption characteristics. The dose and duration of systemic CS treatment necessary for acute asthma have remained largely empiric. For oral therapy, a dose of 1 to 2 mg/kg/day of prednisone for 3 to 10 days is generally used and a taper is not necessary for courses of 10 days or less. Although prednisone is the most frequently used oral preparation, oral dexamethasone and methylprednisolone can be acceptable alternatives for the treatment of acute asthma in an outpatient setting.

In recent years, questions have been raised about the potential benefit of inhaled CSs in the management of acute asthma, for the purpose of minimizing the risk of undesirable adverse effects resulting from frequent systemic CS use. A recent meta-analysis of four studies comparing inhaled CSs to oral CSs in the setting of acute asthma demonstrated no difference between the two interventions in regard to relapse rate, bronchodilator use, or adverse events; however, because of small numbers and inclusion of mild asthma exacerbations, equivalency could not be claimed. In addition, available studies also have demonstrated contradictory results in regard to the superiority of inhaled over oral delivery at the time of an acute exacerbation, by considering various outcomes, that is, symptom resolution, improvement in lung function, or prevention of hospitalization. While initiating or doubling the dose of inhaled CS during acute mild asthma exacerbation has emerged to be a common practice among practitioners in an attempt to prevent the need for systemic CS therapy or development of more severe symptoms, there is no clear consensus of its exact role in the management of exacerbations in general.

In summary, systemic CSs administered orally or parenterally have proven to be efficacious in the treatment of acute asthma. The role of inhaled CSs in the setting of acute asthma is promising, but their efficacy as well as the optimal dose and timing still warrant clarification.

CHRONIC ASTHMA

The clinical goals of asthma controller therapy are to minimize symptoms, decrease bronchodilator rescue use, improve lung function, and prevent exacerbations, using the least amount of medication necessary. These improvements in clinical parameters are attributed to the anti-inflammatory effects of CSs. Before the advent of inhaled CSs, medication options for asthma control included systemic CSs but long-term treatment is associated with unacceptable risk of steroid side effects. Having inhaled CSs with a much-improved topical-to-systemic ratio now available, long-term oral CS therapy, ideally at alternate-day dosing, is now reserved for the maintenance treatment of severe persistent asthma, uncontrolled on high-dose inhaled CSs, and nonsteroidal long-term control therapy.

Numerous studies have shown that inhaled CS treatment results in decreased asthma symptoms, use of rescue bronchodilator, and frequency of acute asthma symptoms, and improved lung function and bronchial hyperresponsiveness. The largest and longest pediatric study, the Childhood Asthma Management Program (CAMP), demonstrated that regular treatment with inhaled CSs was superior to both nedocromil and placebo. The subjects receiving inhaled CSs experienced fewer hospitalizations and emergency care visits, decreased symptoms and use of albuterol rescue therapy, and fewer episodes of acute asthma requiring oral prednisone. Additionally, similar to the adult trials, the inhaled CS group also had a more significant improvement in bronchial hyperresponsiveness.

No asthma controller therapy has been shown to influence asthma mortality and morbidity to a considerable degree other than inhaled CSs. In a nested case-control study from Canada, subjects on inhaled CS therapy were much less likely to die or suffer from a severe exacerbation compared to those who were not on inhaled CSs. For one additional CS canister dispensed, a 21% reduction in the rate of asthma death was found and for six canisters of inhaled CS dispensed per year, the rate of mortality was reduced to half. Donahue and colleagues reported an overall relative risk (RR) of hospitalization of 0.5 (95% confidence interval [CI], 0.4–0.6) among those who received inhaled CSs enrolled in a health maintenance organization compared with those who did not receive inhaled CSs. Last, low-dose inhaled CS was found to impact the number of severe and life-threatening asthma exacerbations in newly diagnosed mild persistent asthmatic individuals.

The key component of asthma management is control of the inflammatory response. With the availability of the flexible bronchoscope in the past 2 to 3 decades, a more detailed evaluation of the mechanisms and pathologic changes associated with treatment response has been evaluated. These studies have employed bronchoscopy with bronchoalveolar lavage (BAL) and/or endobronchial biopsy before and following a course of inhaled CS therapy. However, this is still primarily used at a research level, because of ethical constraints and technical limitations. At a cellular level, inhaled CSs inhibit inflammation by decreasing the number and/or activation of inflammatory cells in the lung including eosinophils, mast cells, and T lymphocytes as seen in studies with biopsy and BAL fluid.

Given the limitation of bronchoscopy in the clinical evaluation of asthma, using noninvasive tools to assess airway inflammation is ideal. Numerous studies have shown reduction in exhaled nitric oxide (NO), sputum eosinophil count and cytokine levels, and even down-regulation of T-lymphocyte activation in peripheral blood associated with inhaled CS therapy.

According to the NHLBI EPR 3 guidelines, inhaled CSs are indicated as first-line therapy, as mono- or combination therapy with adjunctive medications, in asthmatic patients of all ages with persistent disease, regardless of severity. However, a stepwise approach to management with increasing doses of inhaled CS for persistent asthma based on asthma severity (i.e., mild, moderate, and severe) is encouraged, such that low dose is recommended for mild persistent and high dose for severe persistent asthma. The classification of asthma severity is based on the following parameters: (1) frequency of daytime or (2) nighttime symptoms, (3) degree of airflow obstruction by spirometry, and/or (4) peak expiratory flow rate variability defined by frequent symptoms. Patients should be monitored closely for response including improvement in asthma symptoms reported, decreased rescue albuterol use, and improved lung function. Once adequate control is obtained, a "step-down" approach may be appropriate. If control is not achieved, and nonpharmacologic interventions have been pursued, using combination therapy and/or increasing the dose of inhaled CS are currently the options.

When inhaled CSs were introduced, it was assumed that there was a linear relationship between the dose administered and response. Several studies have demonstrated a dose-response effect, but it has been difficult to clearly define. This difficulty is likely because the severity of asthma influences the response to therapy. In addition, different outcomes including symptoms control, improvement in lung function, and improvement in bronchial hyperresponsiveness may be maximized at variable doses. In general, milder patients will achieve maximal control with a lower dose of inhaled CS compared with more severe asthmatic patients likely requiring higher doses of inhaled CS. Finally, once asthma control is achieved as defined by the absence of symptoms and limitations of physical activity with optimal lung function, many patients will tolerate a lower dose of inhaled CS, and reduction of inhaled CS to the lowest required dose is recommended to minimize potential side effects.

It is important to note that the onset of response to an inhaled CS varies with the outcome of interest. For example, improvement in lung function may be apparent within 1 month with improvement in airway inflammatory markers in as early as 2 weeks. However, improvement in bronchial hyperresponsiveness may continue over time. Table 28-4 lists the available preparations and dosing ranges for children and adults.

VARIABILITY AND PREDICTORS OF RESPONSE TO INHALED CORTICOSTEROIDS

Since early introduction of inhaled CSs for persistent asthma has been advocated by most national and international guidelines, the ability to predict response is important. Historically, a CS response was defined as a 15% or more increase in pre-bronchodilator FEV_1 (forced expiratory volume in 1 second) after a 14-day course of oral CSs. Clinically, a response of reported symptom control and lung function is sought after the addition of inhaled CSs to a patient's treatment regimen.

Table 28-4
DOSAGE GUIDELINES

Drug	Low Daily Dose Child 0–4yr	Child 5–11yr	Adult	Medium Daily Dose Child 0–4yr	Child 5–11yr	Adult	High Daily Dose Child 0–4yr	Child 5–11yr	Adult
Beclomethasone HFA, 40 or 80µg/puff	NA	80–160µg	80–240µg	NA	>160–320µg	>240–480µg	NA	>320µg	>480µg
Budesonide DPI 90, 180, or 200µg/inhalation	NA	180–400µg	180–600µg	NA	>400–800µg	>600–1200µg	NA	>800µg	>1200µg
Budesonide inhaled suspension for nebulization, 0.25-, 0.5-, and 1.0-mg dose	0.25–0.5mg	0.5mg	NA	>0.5–1.0mg	1.0mg	NA	>1.0mg	2.0mg	NA
Flunisolide 250µg/puff	NA	500–750µg	500–1000µg	NA	1000–1250µg	>1000–2000µg	NA	>1250µg	>2000µg
Flunisolide HFA 80µg/puff	NA	160µg	320µg	NA	320µg	>320–640µg	NA	≥640µg	>640µg
Fluticasone HFA/MDI: 44, 110, or 220µg/puff	176µg	88–176µg	88–264µg	>176–352µg	>176–352µg	>264–440µg	>352µg	>352µg	>440µg
DPI: 50, 100, or 250µg/inhalation	NA	100–200µg	100–300µg	NA	>200–400µg	>300–500µg	NA	>400µg	>500µg
Mometasone DPI, 220µg/inhalation	NA	NA	220µg	NA	NA	440µg	NA	NA	>440µg
Triamcinolone acetonide, 75µg/puff	NA	300–600µg	300–750µg	NA	>600–900µg	>750–1500µg	NA	>900µg	>1500µg

DPI, dry powder inhaler; HFA, hydrofluoroalkane; NA, not available (not approved, no data available, or safety and efficacy not established for this age group).
Adapted from the National Asthma Education and Prevention Program: Expert Panel Report 3 (EPR 3): Guidelines for the diagnosis and management of asthma. J Allergy Clin Immunol 2007;120:S94–S138, http://www.nhlbi.nih.gov/guidelines/asthma/asthgdin.htm.

Failure to demonstrate a positive response to inhaled CSs should prompt a short course of systemic CSs. Apart from FEV_1, additional long-term outcomes indicating response to CS therapy include prevention of progressive lung function decline, control of asthma symptoms, and decreased rates of acute asthma exacerbations.

Several biomarkers such as bronchial hyperresponsiveness, eosinophilic inflammation, and exhaled nitric oxide have been studied for their ability to predict CS response and guide CS dosing. For example, predictors of a good response based on the change in FEV_1 of more than 15% in patients with moderate to severe asthma may include high exhaled nitric oxide, increased bronchial hyperresponsiveness, and low FEV_1/FVC (FEV_1 to forced vital capacity) ratio at the initiation of therapy. In contrast, predictors of a significantly improved bronchial hyperresponsiveness (>3 doubling doses of PC_{20}) were high sputum eosinophils and older age at onset of asthma. Treatment strategies directed at titrating bronchial hyperresponsiveness, or sputum eosinophilia, or exhaled nitric oxide levels have been shown to result in decreased rate of exacerbations or improved FEV_1, with concomitant control of surrogate markers of disease activity.

LIMITATIONS OR PITFALLS OF CORTICOSTEROID THERAPY
Clinically, most patients with asthma will respond favorably to CSs, and poor response is commonly attributed to poor compliance, poor technique, or suboptimal dose. Although inhaled CS therapy has been shown to suppress inflammation, it does not completely abolish airway inflammation. In a subset of patients, the inflammatory process may not totally be sensitive to CSs, and thus termed refractory, steroid-resistant asthma (SR). Traditionally, SR asthma is usually defined clinically by a failure to improve the morning FEV_1 by at least 15% after a 7- to 14-day course of oral CS therapy. Within the diagnosis of SR there are two classifications: types I and II. Type I is seen in patients who experience the adverse side effects of chronic CS therapy without benefit to their asthma. Type I SR is thought to be an acquired condition specific to the airway inflammatory cells and the local cytokine milieu; and thus the other tissues in the body are still quite sensitive to the unwanted effects of systemic steroids since the anti-inflammatory effects of CSs are mediated through the same receptors. It has been proposed that type I can still be divided into two subtypes: a primary SR involving immune responses that might be associated with genetic polymorphisms, which lead to overproduction of certain cytokines (e.g., IL-4) or various mediators that can themselves generate SR. The other subtype is acquired SR, which might result from an exuberant cell activation secondary to allergen, infection, chronic exposure to medications, such as beta-agonists or even CS.

The clinical, biochemical, and immunohistologic features that have been associated with type I SR are cushingoid features and adrenal suppression on systemic CS therapy; increased T-cell activation; increased IL-2 and IL-4 gene expression in the airway; failure of CSs to inhibit mitogen-induced T-cell proliferation, persistent T-cell activation and inflammatory cytokine production, reduce eosinophils, suppress monocyte-macrophage IL-8 secreetion, and inhibit a delayed type tuberculin skin reaction; decreased glucocorticoid receptor (GR) DNA- and ligand-binding affinity of mononuclear cells; enhanced AP-1 transcriptional activity in peripheral blood mononuclear cells; and increased GR expression in both peripheral blood mononuclear and airway cells.

The molecular mechanisms or etiology of type I SR can conceivably result from an alteration anywhere in the complex pathway from the GCR protein expression (i.e., relative amounts of isoforms α and β), to its activation, nuclear translocation, phosphorylation, and posttranslational modifications. The end result could affect GR-mediated transcriptional activation or repression of target genes. Other mechanisms could involve inflammatory mediators that could produce SR by affecting the levels or function of any of the coactivator or chromatin structure through modification of histone proteins. Some evidence has been shown in regard to increased GRβ formation, MAPK (mitogen-activated protein [MAP] kinase) activation, and reduced GRα nuclear translocation.

The type II SR phenotype is congenital and fortunately rare. It exemplifies a generalized SR syndrome characterized by lack of both steroid beneficial and adverse effects, since it affects all tissues. Type II SR resistance is likely associated with a mutation in the GR gene or in genes that modulate GR function.

Identification of the molecular basis for SR is critical for the development of new treatment approaches for the patients who do not respond to steroid therapy and may provide new insights into the pathogenesis of chronic inflammation.

Although most of the pathophysiologic course of asthma is inflammation based, there may be elements that are not. A critical feature of asthma that has elicited significant interest is airway remodeling, characterized by thickened basement membrane, smooth muscle hyperplasia/hypertrophy, and mucous gland hyperplasia. While a few studies have demonstrated that inhaled CS therapy not only induces amelioration of airway inflammation but also a reduction in the thickness of the bronchial lamina reticularis, it is uncertain if, or to what extent, these specific features impact the control, severity, progression, and morbidity associated with asthma. Complete asthma control is only attainable in less than 50% of patients despite inhaled CS alone or as combination therapy. It might be possible that interventions to modify the structural changes previously noted may also be related to improvement in the clinical course of the disease.

While long-term inhaled CS therapy is effective in improving multiple parameters of asthma control, for most patients, these effects manifest only during treatment. A sustained clinical remission off inhaled CS therapy is possible only for a minority of patients. Thus, there is little evidence to suggest inhaled CSs have any disease-modifying effects, although a minority of subjects with mild asthma may have a sustained remission following discontinuation of long-term therapy.

Last, other aspects of modifying the disease process in asthma such as its natural history may be limited. Early use of continuous or intermittent inhaled CSs in children at high risk for developing asthma does not prevent the development of asthma.

In summary, inhaled CS therapy results in reductions in inflammatory cell infiltration into bronchoalveolar lavage fluid, the epithelium, and within the lamina propria. In addition, there is preliminary data suggesting that inhaled CSs can reduce the thickness of the lamina reticularis. These data support the hypothesis that inhaled CSs act topically by suppressing allergic airway inflammation, albeit not completely. Of importance, inhaled CSs may also attenuate airway remodeling, but there is still no clear evidence that inhaled CSs alter the natural course of asthma.

Safety Profile of Corticosteroids

SYSTEMIC CORTICOSTEROIDS

In general, the development of adverse effects from systemic CS therapy appears to be dose and duration of treatment dependent. Hence, if frequent or long-term oral CS therapy is anticipated, alternative therapy with steroid-sparing properties should be considered. Alternate-day compared to daily dosing of systemic CSs is preferred. The most common adverse effects of systemic CSs are shown in Figure 28-4. Because the GCR is present in almost all cells in the body, the effects of CSs are multisystemic.

Adrenal suppression occurs soon after institution of chronic systemic CSs, as the CS directly impacts the hypothalamic-pituitary axis (HPA) resulting in decreased production of adrenocorticotrophic hormone (ACTH). Without ACTH stimulation, the adrenal glands will not produce cortisone. Manifestations of adrenal insufficiency include cushingoid features of moon facies, buffalo hump, and central obesity. Patients may also develop striae and hirsuitism. Even without these obvious signs, adrenal suppression should be assumed in a patient on chronic CS therapy. These patients should be treated with stress doses of CS in the event of a serious illness, trauma, or surgery.

CS-induced osteoporosis is well established and the mechanism by which CSs affect bone includes inhibition of bone formation and increased bone reabsorption. CSs also alter calcium metabolism by decreasing calcium absorption through the gastrointestinal tract and increased calcium waste through the renal system. Thus, for patients in whom alternative therapies are not available or effective, close monitoring in combination with calcium and vitamin D supplementation is critical. Additionally, treatment with bisphosphonates should be considered.

The formation of posterior subcapsular cataracts is also seen in up to 30% of patients receiving chronic CS therapy. Although there seems to be some variability, the formation of cataracts appears to be dose and duration dependent. Yearly ophthalmologic examination is recommended. Steroid-induced proximal muscle myopathy can also be found in a subset of patients who are treated long-term with systemic CSs. Detection is by isokinetic muscle testing of the hip flexor strength and is most likely in patients receiving daily high-dose CSs.

An additional side effect of chronic CSs, which is specific to the pediatric population, is linear growth suppression. The mechanism of suppression is unclear, but likely results from decreased growth hormone production or direct effects on bone and connective tissue. It is believed that alternate-day dosing of chronic CS therapy decreases the risk of linear growth suppression and doses less than 10 mg every other day of prednisone do not routinely affect growth velocity.

Chronic systemic CS therapy is associated with many potentially deleterious side effects, or debilitating side effects such as hypertension, gastric ulcer disease, and diabetes mellitus. The best approach is to use the lowest necessary dose to minimize the risk. In the instance that chronic therapy is unavoidable, the physician must closely monitor and treat any side effects.

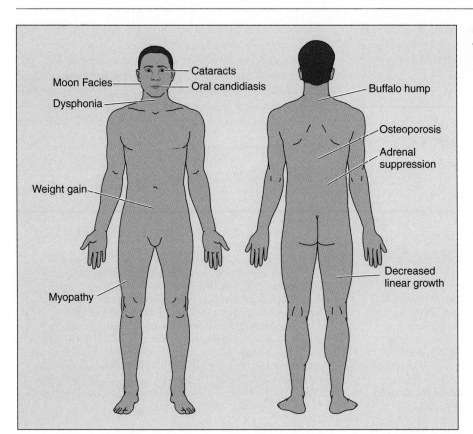

Figure 28-4 Systemic adverse effects of corticosteroids.

Inhaled Corticosteroids

Because of topical delivery, for most patients, local side effects such as hoarseness or dysphonia, cough, and oral candidiasis are the most commonly reported problems associated with inhaled CSs. Although the exact cause for these local effects is unclear, it may be due to local irritation. The stringent use of mouth rinsing can dramatically reduce the likelihood, as does the use of a spacer device. When oral candidiasis occurs, it is typically easily managed with topical antifungal therapy.

As with oral CSs, the systemic adverse effects can be expected from topical CSs particularly at high doses, including adrenal suppression, growth suppression, decreased bone density, myopathy, and weight gain, since CSs reach systemic circulation either through the gastrointestinal tract or absorption through the lung. CS therapy is also thought to be dose and duration dependent, so at low to medium doses, inhaled CSs have a favorable benefit-to-risk profile. In addition to dose, there are other properties of inhaled CSs (e.g., receptor binding and pharmacokinetic parameters), which may make certain drugs of more concern than others, as discussed in an earlier section. For example, because of the high lipophilicity, large Vd, and longer terminal half-life, and high GCR-binding affinity, FP and MF may be expected to have greater potential to cause suppression of the HPA axis as compared to the other formulations. Suppression of the HPA axis by inhaled CSs is rare but has been reported and has been limited to high doses. Currently, HPA axis monitoring is not necessary in children with low- to moderate-dose inhaled CSs unless additional evidence such as growth suppression is present.

Many parents and pediatricians are still concerned about the risk of growth suppression, for fear that this can be a marker of development of other adverse effects. CSs suppress growth by blunting growth hormone release, down-regulating growth hormone expression, inhibiting insulin-like growth factor 1 and osteoblast activity, and altering calcium balance. Even small amounts of exogenous CS have the potential to suppress growth. Thus far, previous studies have shown that there is a detectable but small effect on growth in the first year on moderate doses of inhaled CSs, and much less so with low doses, but the long-term effect on adult height is virtually undetectable. Additionally, the decreased bioavailability of many first-pass inhaled CSs, which are removed on first pass through the hepatic system, decreases the risk of growth suppression. The risk may be increased in patients who are concurrently treated with additional topical steroids for their skin or nasal mucosa.

In summary, the risk of systemic side effects from low to moderate doses of inhaled CSs is low, but the potential from higher doses of inhaled CSs is far greater aggravated by the fact that the patients who require the high doses have also the most exposure to oral CSs. Studies comparing doses between the commercially available inhaled CSs that will produce specific adverse outcomes will be difficult to perform. Despite the low risk, vigilance in following linear growth is still recommended for children on any dose of inhaled CS. Titration to the lowest effective dose of inhaled CS for optimal disease control minimizes the possibility of adverse side effects. What could make this more complicated is finding the ideal parameter of disease control that the clinician could measure against potential risk for side effects. For example, doses that may modulate structural or inflammatory changes and bronchial hyperresponsiveness may be higher than those that would only target lung function or symptoms.

CONCLUSION

Inhaled and systemic CS therapies have provided significant advances for the management of asthma. However, CSs do not prevent the natural history of the disease nor do they control symptoms in all patients. Therefore, further advances in asthma therapeutics must be developed to achieve full control of the evolution of this disease and its management once it is established. Advances are now being made in predicting and monitoring response to CS therapy. Perhaps knowledge from these studies will yield insights for new treatment strategies.

SUGGESTED READING

Barnes PJ, Pedersen S: Efficacy and safety of inhaled corticosteroids in asthma. Am Rev Respir Dis 1993;148:S1–S26.

Leung DY, Bloom JW: Update on glucocorticoid action and resistance. J Allergy Clin Immunol 2003;111:3–22.

National Asthma Education and Prevention Program: Expert Panel Report 3 (EPR 3): Guidelines for the diagnosis and management of asthma. J Allergy Clin Immunol 2007;1220:S94–S138, http://www.nhlbi.nih.gov/guidelines/asthma/asthgdln.htm.

Scarfone RJ, Friedlaender E: Corticosteroids in acute asthma: past, present and future. Pediatr Emerg Care 2003;19:355–362.

Schimmer BP, Parker KL: Adrenocorticotropic hormone; adrenocortical steroids and their synthetic analogs; inhibitors of the synthesis and actions of adrenocortical hormones. In Hardman JD, Limbard LE (eds): Goodman & Gilman's The Pharmacologic Basis of Therapeutics, 10th ed. Mc-Graw-Hill, 2001.

Schleimer RP, Spahn JD, Covar R, Szefler SJ: Glucocorticoids: B. Clinical science. In Adkinson NJ, Bochner BS, Busse WW, et al (eds): Middleton's Allergy Principles & Practice, 6th ed. Philadelphia, Mosby, 2003, pp 870–913.

Spahn JD: Glucocorticoid pharmacokinetics. In Szefler SJ, Leung DYM (eds): Immunology and Allergy Clinics of North America. Philadelphia, W.B. Saunders, 1999, pp 709–723.

Szefler SJ, Martin RJ, King TS, et al, Asthma Clinical Research Network of the National Heart Lung, and Blood Institute: Significant variability in response to inhaled corticosteroids for persistent asthma. J Allergy Clinn Immunol 2002;109:410–418.

Umland SP, Schleimer RP, Johnston SL: Review of the molecular and cellular mechanisms of action of glucocorticoids for use in asthma. Pulm Pharmacol Ther 2002;15:35–50.

Winkler J, Hochhaus G, Derendorf H: How the lung handles drugs. Proc Am Thorac Soc 2004;1:356–363.

CLINICAL PEARLS

- Leukotrienes cause airway constriction, inflammation, and mucous secretion: important features of asthma pathophysiology.

- Leukotriene modifiers (LTMs) may have a particular role in the treatment of allergen induced, aspirin-sensitive, and exercise-induced asthma.

- For clinical presentations such as cough-variant asthma, viral-induced wheeze, and the management of acute asthma exacerbations, there may be an evolving role for LTMs.

- While inhaled corticosteroids are first-line controller agents for the management of persistent asthma, LTMs may offer the ability to avoid escalating dosages of ICS as steroid-sparing agents.

- Significant side effects of LTMs are rare and limited to case reports of Churg-Strauss syndrome that is more likely due to corticosteroid withdrawal than to the LTMs.

Leukotriene modifiers (LTMs) are one of the relatively novel classes of medications introduced for the chronic treatment of asthma. Excitement surrounding this class of medications has arisen for many different reasons. First, unlike corticosteroids, LTMs target a specific pathway of the inflammatory cascade thought to play a significant role in asthma pathogenesis. Second, and possibly due to the specificity with which they act, this class of medications has very few side effects. Third, these medications are relatively easy to administer in comparison to inhaled agents. Based on their systemic absorption, there is limited concern for effective delivery, which may become more important in the pediatric patient. These reasons, among others, have created interest in using the LTMs as controller medications in the treatment of asthma.

In 1997, the National Institutes of Health and the National Heart, Lung, and Blood Institute (NIH/NHLBI) published recommendations for a stepwise approach to asthma management. Included in their discussion was the potential use of the LTMs. Specifically, the NIH/NHLBI stated that for mild persistent asthma, "zafirkulast and zileuton may also be considered for those at least 12 years old, although their position in therapy was not fully established." Based on the availability of clinical data primarily in adult patients with very limited studies in children, in 2002, the NIH/NHLBI's updated recommendations (Table 29-1) suggested that these drugs may be used as the alternative, but not preferred, agents for the treatment of persistent asthma. Additionally, they supported the use of LTMs as potential alternatives to escalating doses of inhaled corticosteroids (ICSs) or the addition of long-acting beta agonists (LABAs).

The most recent NIH/NHLBI guidelines reinforced a role for the LTMs in the management of persistent asthma; however, they did not endorse the use of LTMs as first-line controller medications in persistent asthma. It is clear, however, that asthma is a very heterogeneous entity, thus it is necessary to evaluate the effect of LTMs in the various asthma phenotypes. The intent of this chapter is to identify the rationale for using LTMs, describe what agents are available, and examine what specific situations in the treatment of asthma might warrant the use of these medications.

NATURAL HISTORY OF TREATMENT—EVOLUTION IN CLINICAL PRACTICE

Asthma is a disease of airway hyperresponsiveness, mucous plugging, and inflammation. The importance of inflammation is now accepted as central to the pathogenesis of asthma resulting in a heightened fervor to establish anti-inflammatory therapeutic agents. The pathways that lead to an inflammatory asthmatic response are quite complex and involve intricate interplays of various cells and mediators. Because of the marked heterogeneity of asthma, identifying therapies to target these processes has been difficult. Kellaway initially identified leukotrienes (LTs) in 1938 as "slow-reacting substance of anaphylaxis, SRS-A" based on their ability to cause significant contraction of guinea pig lung smooth muscle in the presence of cobra venom. Brocklehurst subsequently linked these mediators to asthma and allergic reactions in the 1960s. By the 1970s, the LTs were identified to have important effects on airway constriction, mucous hypersecretion, and inflammation. With the subsequent elucidation and characterization of their potent biological properties in relation to the pathogenesis of asthma, the LTs have become targets for novel therapeutic development. Leukotriene modifiers (LTMs) emerged as the first new approach in asthma therapy in 30 years to target a specific component of this inflammatory process.

PATHOGENESIS—RATIONALE FOR THERAPY

Leukotrienes are products of arachidonic acid (AA) and its metabolism. Cell membrane phospholipids activated by phospholipase A2 produce AA, which can then be metabolized by one of two pathways: the cyclo-oxygenase pathway or the 5-lipoxygenase (5-LO) pathway (Fig. 29-1). Metabolism via the 5-LO pathway results in the production of LTs. Once activated, 5-LO moves to the cell membrane where, in conjunction with the 5-lipoxygenase activating

Table 29-1
NATIONAL HEART, LUNG, AND BLOOD INSTITUTE RECOMMENDATIONS FOR THE TREATMENT OF ASTHMA

Asthma Severity	Daily Treatment Recommendations for Children ≤ 5 Years	Daily Treatment Recommendations for Children > 5 Years and Adults
Severe persistent	Preferred: high-dose ICS and LABA If needed: OCS 2mg/kg/day (do not exceed 60mg/day)	Preferred: high-dose ICS and LABA If needed: OCS 2mg/kg/day (do not exceed 60mg/day)
Moderate persistent	Preferred: low-dose ICS and LABA OR medium-dose ICS Alternative: low-dose ICS and either LTRA or theophylline If needed: medium-dose ICS add LABA (preferred) OR medium dose ICS add LTRA or theophylline (alternative)	Preferred: low- to medium-dose ICS and LABA Alternative: Increase ICS within medium-dose range OR add LTM or theophylline If needed: increase ICS within medium-dose range add LABA (preferred) OR increase ICS within medium-dose range add LTM or theophylline (alternative)
Mild persistent	Preferred: low-dose ICS Alternative: cromolyn or LTRA	Preferred: low-dose ICS Alternative: cromolyn, LTM, nedocromil, or theophylline
Mild intermittent	No daily medication needed	No daily medication needed

Updated in 2002. LTMs are recommended as alternatives to preferred therapies.
ICS, inhaled corticosteroid; OCS, oral corticosteroid.

protein (FLAP), it forms leukotriene A4 (LTA$_4$). At this point, LTA$_4$ can either be metabolized to form LTB$_4$ or the cysteinyl LTs: LTC$_4$, LTD$_4$, and LTE$_4$. Neutrophils, monocytes, and macrophages transform LTA$_4$ via LTA$_4$ hydrolase to produce LTB$_4$, a potent neutrophil and eosinophil chemoattractant. The other arm of the 5-LO pathway occurs in alveolar macrophages, eosinophils, and mast cells where LTA$_4$ is conjugated with LTC$_4$ synthase. It is this arm of the LT pathway that produces the cysteinyl LTs that can induce significant atopic reactions, bronchoconstriction, inflammation, and mucous production.

Two types of LT receptors occur in the human body: cysteinyl leukotriene receptor 1 and 2 (CysLTR$_1$ and CysLTR$_2$). Activated mostly by LTD$_4$ and LTE$_4$, the CysLTR$_1$ is found in the spleen, peripheral blood, airway smooth muscle cells, and macrophages. The other receptors, CysLTR$_2$, are activated mostly by LTC$_4$ and are found in airway macrophages and smooth muscle cells, cardiac Purkinje fibers, brain, adrenal medullary cells, and peripheral blood leukocytes. In the presence of LTs, these receptors are responsible for initiating the pathophysiologic effects of asthma, namely airway bronchoconstriction, mucus hypersecretion, and inflammation.

As potent bronchoconstrictors, LTs not only induce airways constriction in asthmatic subjects, but also in nonasthmatic airways. Smooth muscle proliferation and contraction have been shown to occur in vitro when myocytes are exposed to LTs. Leukotrienes are 100 to 1000 times more potent bronchoconstrictors than histamine and 10,000 times more potent bronchoconstrictors than methacholine. Leukotrienes are also potent mucus secretagogues. This has been demonstrated in both animal and human studies. They are more potent than histamine and prostaglandins in producing airway mucus. Along with airway inflammation and smooth muscle

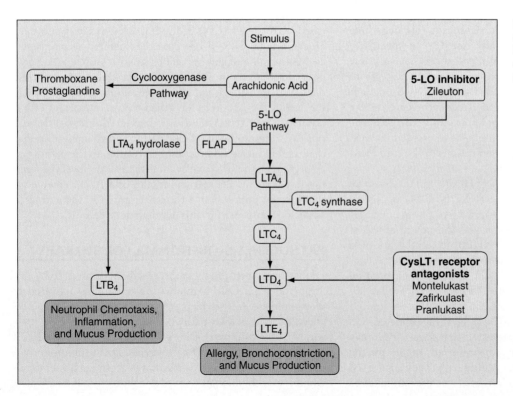

Figure 29-1 Generation of leukotrienes, sequellae of leukotrienes, and site of action of leukotriene modifiers. 5-LO, 5-lipoxygenase.

contraction, mucus hypersecretion can cause significant disruption to airflow and even result in mucus plugging that obstructs conducting airways of the lung potentially leading to atelectasis and ventilation/perfusion inequality seen during exacerbations of asthma.

Finally, LTs also incite a potent inflammatory response in the airways, particularly asthmatic airways. They increase cellular influx of neutrophils and eosinophils by promoting vascular permeability. This effect is not confined to the lower airways, as it is present in the upper airway causing nasal obstruction as well. Importantly, this nasal obstruction persists even after administration of antihistamine medications. It is only after administration of LT modifiers that this nasal obstruction is relieved. Altogether, LTs are responsible for a significant component of the asthmatic reaction that occurs in the lower and upper airways.

THE LEUKOTRIENE MODIFIERS

There are two points in the leukotriene cascade where commercially available medications can block the effects of leukotrienes (see Fig. 29-1). The leukotriene synthesis inhibitor (LTI), zileuton, inhibits 5-LO and FLAP and thus blocks the cascade early in the production of LTs. Leukotriene receptor antagonists (LTRAs), also modify the inflammatory cascade by selectively antagonizing the $CysLT_1$ receptor.

Zileuton (Zylfo, Abbott, Abbott Park, IL) is the only LTI licensed for use in asthma. The recommended oral dosing regimen in asthmatic patients 12 years or older is currently 600 mg four times a day. The adverse effects profile includes headache, dizziness, insomnia, and gastrointestinal upset. This drug is contraindicated in those with hepatic insufficiency and hepatic failure based on its metabolism. Accordingly, it is recommended that serum alanine aminotransferase be measured prior to administration, monthly for the first 3 months, and then every 2 to 3 months for the remainder of the first year. Precautions must be taken when zileuton is administered to patients already taking theophylline, propranolol, and warfarin as it will increase the serum drug levels of these medications. Zileuton is classified as pregnancy category C and it is not known whether it is excreted in breastmilk.

There are three commercially available LTRAs for use in asthma: montelukast (Singulair, Merck & Co., Inc., White House Station, NJ), zafirlukast (Accolate, AstraZeneca, Wilmington, DE), and pranlukast (Onon, Ono Pharmaceuticals Ltd, Ono, Japan). Montelukast and zafirlukast are available in the United States while pranlukast is available in Asia and Central and South America.

Montelukast is usually dosed in adults as 10 mg once a day, while the dosing in children is available in three preparations: a 4-mg granule preparation for those 1 year or older, a 4-mg chewable tablet for those 2 to 5 years of age, and a 5-mg chewable tablet for those 6 to 14 years of age. It is recommended that montelukast be dosed at bedtime. While montelukast is approved by the Food and Drug Administration (FDA) for children down to 1 year, the 4-mg granule dose has been demonstrated to be well tolerated in the 6- to 24-month age group based on a recent 6-week clinical trial. Additionally, this formulation has been FDA approved for the treatment of allergic rhinitis in children 6 months or older. Zafirlukast is administered twice daily at 20 mg for adults and

10 mg for children ages 5 to 12 years. This LTRA must be taken on an empty stomach, either 1 hour before a meal or 2 hours after a meal, as food can decrease its bioavailability by 40%. Zafirkulast, unlike montelukast, does inhibit cytochrome P450, so there is a possibility of drug interactions. Pranlukast, which is unavailable in the United States, is dosed in adults as 337.5 or 450 mg orally twice daily after meals and there are preparations that are available for children as young as 1 year of age that are based on weight in kilograms. Pranlukast should be taken after meals as food increases the absorption.

The LTRAs are generally well tolerated and have a favorable side-effect profile (Table 29-2). While Churg-Strauss syndrome has been previously associated with the use of LTRAs, a causal relationship has never been demonstrated and, in fact, appears to be primarily related to steroid withdrawal rather than the addition of LTRA therapy. Both montelukast and zafirlukast are rated as pregnancy category B. Montelukast has no human data available with regard to breastfeeding, while zafirkulast is deemed unsafe for use while breastfeeding. All of the LTRAs are metabolized through the liver, and therefore monitoring may be necessary in hepatic insufficiency or hepatic failure. It is not necessary, however, in healthy individuals to routinely monitor liver function as in the case of zileuton. In general, dosing adjustments are not necessary for renal insufficiency or even in the elderly except for pranlukast. It is recommended that pranlukast should be decreased to 112.5 mg twice daily in the elderly patient.

Table 29-2
ADVERSE EVENTS ASSOCIATED WITH LTM USE

Drug	Adverse Event*	Antileukotriene Incidence (% of Subjects)	Placebo
Zafirkulast (n = 4058) versus placebo (n = 2032)	Headache	12.9	11.7
	Infection	3.5	3.4
	Nausea	3.1	2.0
	Diarrhea	2.8	2.1
Montelukast (n = 1955) versus placebo (n = 1180)	Headache	18.4	18.1
	Influenza	4.2	3.9
	Abdominal pain	2.9	2.5
	Cough	2.7	2.4
	Dyspepsia	2.1	1.1
Zileuton (n = 475) versus placebo (n = 491)	Headache	24.6	24.0
	Dyspepsia	8.2†	2.9
	Unspecified pain	7.8	5.3
	Nausea	5.5	3.7
	Abdominal pain	4.6	2.4
	Asthenia	3.8	2.4
	Accidental injury	3.4	2.0
	Myalgia	3.2	2.9

*Adverse events listed occurred at an incidence > 2% and at a numerically greater incidence than placebo
†$P < .05$ versus placebo
Reproduced with permission from Spector SL, Antileukotriene Working Group: Safety of antileukotriene agents in asthma management. Ann Allergy Asthma Immunol 2001;86 (6 suppl 1):18–23.

CLINICAL INDICATIONS

The variability in individual response to controller therapies, specifically ICS and LTMs, remains evident. In particular, two studies, one in adults by Malmstrom and colleagues (Fig. 29-2) and one in children by Szefler and colleagues (Fig. 29-3), demonstrated the significant individual variability in response to ICS and LTMs. One reason for such response variability may be the vast heterogeneity of asthma. Despite reinforcing individual variability to these controllers, the pediatric study recommended that children with increased airflow limitation and airway hyperresponsiveness based on methacholine challenge and/or elevated markers of allergic inflammation such as exhaled nitric oxide should be managed with ICS therapy as opposed to LTM. This study in children with mild to moderate persistent asthma suggested that ICS therapy is more effective based on improvement in the forced expiratory volume at 1 second (FEV_1). However, FEV_1 measures particularly in children may not be the best primary outcome measure for such evaluations as has been suggested by several adult and pediatric studies. Specifically, Israel and colleagues have previously challenged the concept that response to LTMs remains limited and underestimated based solely on measures of FEV_1.

The findings of these studies reinforce that one treatment plan cannot be expected to be efficacious for all the different permutations of asthma. In the following section, LTMs will be discussed with regard to their role in several different asthmatic phenotypes based on available clinical evidence. In general, to determine whether LTMs are effective therapy for an individual, one must look at the clinical situation, what is known from the literature, and how that individual responds to the treatment regimen. *Note: In the following sections, the vast majority of data comes from studies involving montelukast and zafirlukast (LTRAs). Therefore, the remainder of this chapter focuses on the use of receptor antagonists (LTRAs) unless zileuton specifically is discussed or the principles of treatment apply to the whole class of LTMs.*

Phenotypes of Asthmatic Disease

ALLERGEN-INDUCED ASTHMA
In the patient with asthma triggered by allergy, two phases typically occur following allergen challenge: the early asthmatic response (EAR) and the late asthmatic response (LAR). In the EAR, acute bronchoconstriction occurs within 15 to 20 minutes of allergen exposure. The LAR takes place in 30% to 70% of atopic asthmatic individuals and typically occurs 3 to 24 hours after initial exposure. The LAR displays not only bronchoconstriction, but also evidence of airways inflammation and increased mucus secretion. Leukotrienes are elevated during the EAR in sputum, bronchoalveolar lavage, and urine. The role of LTs is less clear in the LAR; however several studies have demonstrated heightened LT response in the late phase of allergic asthma.

In general, the LTRAs have demonstrated efficacy in the treatment of atopic asthma compared to placebo. It appears that LTRAs have a more pronounced effect on the EAR by inhibiting bronchoconstriction 50% to 90%, while only 25% to 50% inhibition occurs in the LAR. Furthermore, while it

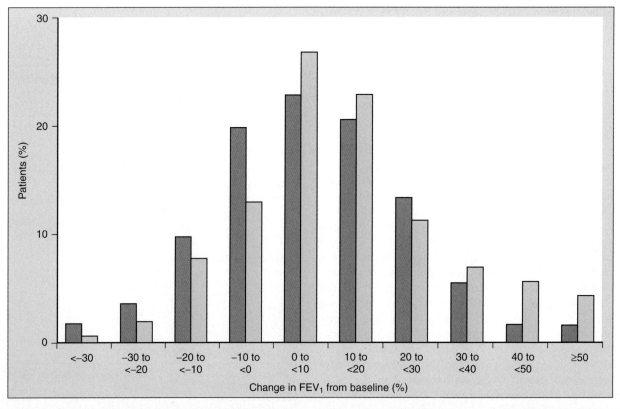

Figure 29-2 **Treatment responses in adults with asthma for FEV₁ with regard to montelukast (green bars) and beclomethasone (yellow bars).** *(Data from Malmstrom K, Rodriguez-Gomez G, Guerra J, et al: Oral montelukast, inhaled beclomethasone, and placebo for chronic asthma. A randomized, controlled trial. Montelukast/beclomethasone study group. Ann Intern Med 1999;130(6):487–495. Used with permission.)*

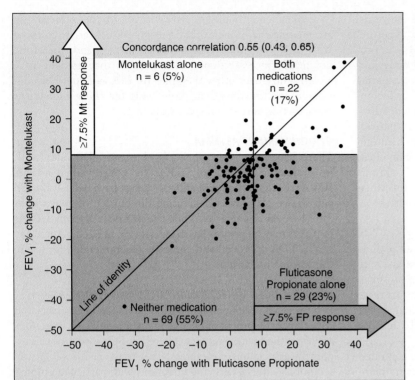

Figure 29-3 Treatment responses in children with asthma for FEV_1 with regard to montelukast (Mt) and fluticasone propionate (FP). Favorable response is defined as change of 7.5% or greater in FEV_1. The line of identity demonstrates favorable response to montelukast above the line and favorable response to fluticasone below the line. *(Data from Szefler SJ, Phillips BR, Martinez FD, et al: Characterization of within-subject responses to fluticasone and montelukast in childhood asthma. J Allergy Clin Immunol 2005;115:233–242)*

is clear that bronchoconstriction is the major factor that is affected by LTRAs in the EAR, it is not clear whether LTRAs have an effect on inhibition of bronchoconstriction, inflammation, or a combination of the two in the LAR. Evidence exists to support the efficacy of LTRAs in attenuating the LAR; however the reason for the attenuation is not clear. While some studies reveal a significant decrease in airway eosinophilia with the use of LTRAs, others do not report such findings. Nevertheless, Leigh and colleagues have shown that montelukast, in comparison to placebo, appears to have a significant effect on reducing airway hyperresponsiveness in both the EAR and the LAR. Furthermore, Rosewich and associates demonstrated that if given during the EAR, montelukast may offer some protection from severe airways obstruction in the LAR by preventing a significant drop in FEV_1. Because of demonstrated effectiveness in the EAR and potential benefit in the LAR, LTRAs have been a useful treatment modality for allergen-induced asthma.

More recently, studies have demonstrated that the LTRAs have the additional advantage of providing relief from other atopic symptoms. In general, the LTRAs can provide symptomatic relief from concomitant symptoms of nasal congestion and sinusitis when compared to placebo. The effect of LTRAs in conjunction with histamine blockers does not appear to be superior to either agent alone and they both appear to be less effective than nasal corticosteroids. However, clinically, there may be a role for LTRAs in the individual with atopic asthma and nasal symptoms in order to consolidate pharmacologic effects and use fewer medications. While the LTRAs appear to be effective in reducing both upper and lower airway symptoms following allergen exposure, this effect is not complete and the allergic asthmatic individual should continue to avoid known allergens even when taking LTRAs. Nevertheless, the advantages of ameliorating symptoms in both the upper and lower airway and the proven efficacy suggest that LTRAs

should be considered as a viable therapeutic option for control of mild persistent atopic asthma or as an adjunct to ICS in the more advanced asthmatic with allergy triggers.

ASPIRIN-SENSITIVE ASTHMA

One phenotype of asthma specifically triggered by the CysLTs is aspirin-sensitive asthma (ASA). Theoretically, when the cyclooxygenase pathway of arachidonic acid (AA) metabolism is blocked by aspirin or nonsteroidal anti-inflammatory drugs (NSAIDs), more AA is metabolized via the 5-LO pathway. This shift to the 5-LO pathway may contribute to more LT formation. The pathophysiology for ASA should, therefore, make LTMs an important therapy. Elevations in LTC_4 can be detected in individuals who are affected by aspirin sensitivity in comparison with healthy subjects and even asthmatic individuals without aspirin sensitivity.

Based on several trials, chronic use of LTRAs, specifically montelukast and pranlukast, has demonstrated that symptoms and lung function improve in individuals with ASA. Additionally, Kuna and colleagues demonstrated in a randomized, double-blind, placebo-controlled trial involving 80 individuals with ASA already on ICS, that 4 weeks of montelukast (10 mg daily) significantly improved FEV_1 by 10.2% ($P < .001$), decreased the need for bronchodilators by 27% ($P < .05$), decreased exacerbations by 54% ($P < .05$), and improved asthma-specific quality of life ($P < .05$). Similar to findings in atopic asthma, LTRAs have some effect in ameliorating upper airway symptoms in patients with ASA as well.

Zileuton, the 5-LO inhibitor, also has beneficial effects on airway hyperresponsiveness in ASA. Zileuton in conjunction with conventional asthma therapy can be a useful adjunct that improves lung function and nasal symptoms and decreases the need for beta$_2$-agonist rescue medications.

While it is clear that LTMs can provide asthma-related symptom relief for those with aspirin sensitivity, it is less clear whether these agents provide protection to the individual when actually challenged with aspirin or NSAID exposure. There are conflicting data regarding whether LTMs can provide bronchoprotection against asthma attacks directly provoked by aspirin or NSAIDs. The majority of trials evaluating this challenge model have demonstrated a lack of or incomplete protection with the use of LTMs in the ASA individual. Therefore, based on the conflicting body of evidence, individuals with ASA should be advised to avoid taking such analgesics even if being treated with LTMs. Nevertheless, individuals with ASA can demonstrate asthma symptoms on a chronic basis in the absence of aspirin challenge and it is for this situation that LTMs appear to be an appropriate consideration.

EXERCISE-INDUCED ASTHMA

Because of the high prevalence of exercise-induced asthma (EIA) in asthmatic individuals (70%), treatments that are effective in preventing EIA are important to most who suffer from chronic asthma. Since LTs have been shown to increase after exercise challenge, LTRAs have been studied and appear to have a beneficial effect in the treatment of EIA in both children and adults.

In children, placebo-controlled trials have demonstrated efficacy of the LTRAs for EIA. Kemp and co-workers demonstrated that children 6 to 14 years old treated with montelukast (5 mg), 20 to 24 hours before exercise challenge had a lower FEV_1 decrease (18% in montelukast group versus 26% in placebo group). In 39 children treated by zafirlukast 4 hours before exercise challenge, Pearlman and associates reported that active therapy limited the FEV_1 drop by 50% compared to placebo. Use of montelukast for a longer period of time has also shown benefit in children with EIA. Melo and colleagues evaluated montelukast versus placebo in 22 asthmatic children aged 7 to 16 years old. In this study, montelukast once daily for 1 week limited FEV_1 decrease by 50%, shortened recovery time, and reduced late-phase response to exercise. Finally, Kim and co-workers demonstrated that children treated with 8 weeks of montelukast demonstrate improved lung function, time to recovery postexercise challenge, and symptom scores. Timing of LTRA dosing may be important in terms of efficacy, as Peroni and associates have shown in 19 children with EIA that administration of a single dose of montelukast 12 hours prior to exercise was more effective than dosing 2 or 24 hours prior to exercise.

In adults, there have been several studies supporting the use of LTRAs in controlling EIA. Similar to the pediatric trials, these studies demonstrate efficacy in reducing bronchoconstriction in comparison to placebo. Leff and co-workers evaluated the effectiveness of montelukast compared to placebo in 110 asthmatic individuals aged 15 to 45 years old. In this double-blind study, treatment with montelukast was associated with a significant reduction in bronchoconstriction ($P = .002$) throughout the 12-week period of testing and also demonstrated less need for bronchodilators during or after exercise challenge.

Compared to other active therapies for EIA, LTRAs fare equally or favorably. Unfortunately, there are no trials that compare LTMs to conventional therapy consisting of beta$_2$-agonist pretreatment. Compared to LABAs, such as salmeterol, LTRAs and zileuton show similar efficacy or even superiority used over a prolonged period of time (4 to 8 weeks).

Leukotriene modifiers have proven to be effective in attenuating the bronchospastic response to exercise in those with EIA. With their ease of administration and, therefore, potentially increased compliance, LTMs may actually have an advantage over other therapies for EIA and could be considered for use on a long-term basis for those individuals participating in seasonal sporting activities.

COUGH-VARIANT ASTHMA

There have only been small placebo-controlled pilot studies evaluating the role of LTRAs for cough-variant asthma (CVA). Both montelukast and zafirlukast have been evaluated and shown efficacy in decreasing the burden of cough after 2 to 4 weeks of therapy. While the prospect of using LTRAs for CVA may be promising, more data are needed before they can be FDA approved and clinically recommended for use in this asthma phenotype.

VIRAL-INDUCED WHEEZE IN INFANTS AND TODDLERS

Recurrent wheeze in infants and toddlers has been associated with the development of persistent asthma and viral infections are often the inciting factors. There is ample evidence to support the association of elevated LTs in upper and lower airway secretions with various viral infections with particular emphasis to date on respiratory syncytial virus (RSV). Leukotrienes also seem to be elevated in children who develop persistent wheeze even when the wheezing episode is not acutely associated with a viral illness.

Because of the association between elevated LTs in acute and persistent viral induced wheeze, Bisgaard and colleagues evaluated the use of montelukast therapy in 130 infants, ages 3 to 35 months, with acute RSV bronchiolitis requiring hospitalization. In this placebo-controlled study, the infants were randomized to montelukast 5 mg or placebo within 7 days of onset of symptoms. The montelukast group displayed significant clinical improvement as measured by symptom-free days, cough, and exacerbations. The same group of investigators also demonstrated that long-term treatment with montelukast for children who intermittently wheeze during viral illness reduced both exacerbations and the need for rescue medication during exacerbations. Unfortunately, the study did not show a decreased hospitalization rate or need for oral corticosteroids in the treatment group. While viral-induced wheeze in children is another clinical area where therapy with a LTRA may prove beneficial, additional studies are warranted.

Acute Asthma

Leukotrienes play an important role in asthma exacerbation. Pathophysiologic evidence is demonstrated by the fact that urinary LT levels rise significantly during an acute exacerbation of asthma. Moreover, these elevated levels of urinary LT correlate with the degree of airflow obstruction.

Because of their relatively rapid onset of action, LTRAs, specifically montelukast, have been evaluated as potential therapies for acute asthma exacerbations. While trials are small, there does appear to be some advantage to adding montelukast to standard treatment such as beta$_2$-agonists and systemic corticosteroids in the acute setting. Cylly and associates demonstrated that oral montelukast added to a standard regimen including intravenous corticosteroids results in a trend toward improved peak flows and a decreased need for bronchodilators. Likewise, Camargo and colleagues demonstrated that montelukast administered intravenously with corticosteroids appears to cause a significant improvement in FEV_1 20 minutes after infusion and a trend toward less bronchodilator use.

In the pediatric setting, montelukast was evaluated for intervention for acute asthma in 201 children 2 to 14 years of age with baseline intermittent asthma. This placebo-controlled trial showed that during a 12-month period with 680 acute episodes, montelukast initiated at the first sign of an upper respiratory tract infection significantly reduced emergency department visits, nighttime awakenings, and absences from school and work. This trial, the Pre-Empt Study, was slightly different from the adult trials of montelukast for acute exacerbations of asthma in that the aim was to prevent acute asthma exacerbations. Nevertheless, data from the Pre-Empt Study support the hypothesis that LTRAs may be useful in the acute setting. Further studies are under way to evaluate the usefulness of LTRAs in the individual with intermittent asthma predisposed to severe exacerbations in response to a viral trigger. At this point, however, the use of LTRAs for acute asthma exacerbations remains limited to clinical research.

Persistent Asthma

The vast majority of asthmatic patients demonstrate persistent symptoms and therefore require daily controller therapy. As previously discussed, the most recent NIH/NHLBI guidelines favor ICS over LTMs as first-line controller medications, but do support the LTMs for use in adults and LTRAs for children as alternative agents for the mild persistent asthmatic and as possible agents for steroid sparing in moderate and severe asthmatics.

LEUKOTRIENE MODIFIERS IN COMPARISON TO PLACEBO
Randomized, placebo-controlled, multicenter trials in adults have shown that LTMs are effective in improving baseline lung function (FEV_1), improving morning peak flow measurements, improving symptom scores, and decreasing the need for rescue medication. These trials were performed in individuals with mild to moderate persistent asthma, but it appears that those with a greater impairment of lung function had greater benefit from these medications compared to placebo. There are limited investigations in the pediatric population that have evaluated LTRAs versus placebo in persistent asthma. The existing data, however, corroborate findings in adults.

LEUKOTRIENE MODIFIERS IN COMPARISON TO ACTIVE THERAPY
There have been many trials in adults comparing LTRAs to other asthma therapies. The previously mentioned Malmstrom and co-workers (see Fig. 29-2) and Szefler and colleagues (see Fig. 29-3) studies demonstrate that individual responses to both LTRAs and ICS vary significantly. Specifically, the study by Szefler and colleagues focused on identifying individual predictors of response to montelukast compared to fluticasone rather than focusing primarily on efficacy. In a direct comparison of montelukast 10 mg daily versus fluticasone propprionate 44 µg twice daily, Busse and colleagues demonstrated that ICS performed better in controlling symptoms and improving lung

function in 533 asthmatic adults (mean FEV_1 66% predicted). Meta-analyses have been performed with the data of several trials comparing LTRAs to ICSs. Based on the available data, ICSs are more effective than LTRAs in preventing asthma exacerbations. Secondarily, ICSs are superior to LTRAs with regard to improvement in FEV_1, symptoms and symptom-free days, reduction of nighttime symptoms, use of rescue inhalers, and quality of life. Trials have also scrutinized asthma-related health care costs of persistent asthmatic adults and children treated with ICSs or LTRAs. In general, ICSs demonstrate better cost-effectiveness due to reduced need for hospitalization or augmentation of asthma treatment with another controller medication.

One of the few pediatric trials to compare LTRAs to other asthma treatments involved 124 patients randomized to either once daily montelukast or beclomethasone 100 µg three times a day. In this trial, Maspero and co-workers demonstrated that compliance was nearly double in the montelukast group in comparison to the beclomethasone group ($P < .05$). While there was a significant increase in patient satisfaction ($P < .001$) in the montelukast group, there was no difference in FEV_1 between the two groups. A "real world" prospective analysis by Bukstein and colleagues has compared montelukast to fluticasone propionate in 104 children aged 6 to 12 years old with mild persistent asthma of greater than 1-year duration. This trial compared adherence of the two drugs over 6 to 12 months and found that while there were no differences in symptoms, spirometry, emergency care visits, hospitalizations, or use of bronchodilator rescue medications, there was a significant increase in compliance in the montelukast group ($P = .0003$).

Whereas the data from randomized, controlled trials clearly support the first-line use of ICSs for persistent asthma, there may be some quality of LTRAs in certain situations that makes them an attractive alternative to ICSs, specifically compliance. It may be that, in situations where compliance becomes a significant factor for asthma management, LTRAs provide a therapeutic treatment strategy for asthma management particularly in the mild persistent patient.

LEUKOTRIENE MODIFIERS AS STEROID-SPARING AGENTS IN PERSISTENT ASTHMA
Based on multiple clinical trials primarily in adults, there may be a role for LTMs as adjuncts to ICSs in moderate to severe persistent asthma. A recent meta-analysis has evaluated the question of whether LTMs are beneficial add-on therapy for patients poorly controlled with baseline ICS therapy. In this review, Ducharme and associates conclude that LTMs have a modest effect of improving peak flow measurements in addition to ICSs. They suggest that LTMs in addition to ICS therapy can provide equal benefit compared to escalating doses of ICSs. They also suggest a benefit of LTM add-on therapy during tapering of ICS doses; however, such claims cannot be quantified or confirmed due to a lack of power of the review.

Two studies in children have investigated the use of LTRAs as adjunct therapy. The first trial by Simons and co-workers evaluated 279 children with persistent asthma (mean FEV_1 78%) receiving ICS controller therapy. This multicenter, double-blind, placebo-controlled trial evaluated the addition of 5 mg of montelukast daily or placebo to budesonide

200 μg twice daily and demonstrated better asthma control and a decrease in exacerbations, despite a minimal additive effect on lung function. The trial implied a steroid-sparing effect given that patients experienced heightened control without the need for increased ICSs. Another pediatric trial by Phipatanakul and colleagues of 36 patients maintained on low-to-medium dose ICSs specifically evaluated the role of montelukast as a steroid-sparing agent. Similar to the previous trial, montelukast demonstrated significant reduction in asthma symptoms and need for rescue inhalers compared to placebo. Additionally, those in the montelukast group were able to decrease their ICS dose by 17% while those in the placebo group needed to increase their ICS dose by 64%. Despite these findings, the actual percentage dose reduction in ICSs was not statistically significant between the two groups ($P = .10$). Admittedly, both the above-mentioned pediatric trials evaluated patients who would be considered mild-to-moderate persistent asthmatic individuals rather than severe persistent asthmatic individuals. Nevertheless, the data do suggest that LTRAs (specifically montelukast) should be considered as an adjunct to baseline therapy in the poorly controlled moderate to severe persistent asthmatic.

Leukotriene modifiers have been compared to other steroid-sparing agents such as LABAs. In general, it appears that LABAs perform more favorably when compared to LTMs in this role. In a systematic review, Ram and associates evaluated 12 randomized controlled trials and determined that LABAs are superior to LTMs when added to ICSs for the adult with uncontrolled persistent asthma. The major outcome evaluated was asthma exacerbations requiring systemic steroids, but LABA also proved to be superior in regard to improving lung function, symptoms, and use of rescue bronchodilators. Not surprisingly, LABAs in addition to ICSs has been shown to be more cost effective than LTMs in addition to ICSs when used for the treatment of persistent asthma.

The addition of leukotriene modifiers for steroid sparing remains an important consideration in the management of the poorly controlled asthmatic patient. Clearly the ability to control the asthmatic patient while limiting ICS dosing is desirable. To date, the NIH/NHLBI suggests that LTRAs in children and LTMs in adults are suitable adjuncts in the treatment of persistent asthma. Furthermore, the addition of LABAs to ICSs for control of moderate to severe asthma may be cautioned in certain patient populations. Specifically, the LABA salmeterol when compared to placebo in a large, randomized trial, published by Nelson and colleagues, has shown a small, but significant increase in asthma-related deaths among adults receiving this medication over 28 weeks. Subgroup analysis suggests that African Americans were the population most at risk. Therefore, LTMs, with their favorable side-effect profile, are an important alternative to escalating doses of ICSs or the addition of LABAs and should be considered when avoiding an ICS dose increase or facilitating an ICS dose reduction.

CONTROVERSIES/CONCLUSION

The NIH/NHLBI guidelines for a stepwise approach to asthma treatment have advanced the understanding of medical providers worldwide and serve as an important tool in the treatment of adults and children with persistent asthma. In the 2002 update, LTMs have established a more defined role as a viable alternative to ICS in the management of persistent asthma. Based on the heterogeneity of the disease, individual responses to asthma control therapies vary. Therefore, while it is important to classify the severity of disease, it is also important to understand the pathophysiology of the different asthma phenotypes. Specifically, the LTMs may be more beneficial for certain types of asthma. In this regard, there have been promising hypotheses put forth and evidence available to support the use of LTMs in certain phenotypes of asthma such as allergen, aspirin and exercise induced asthma.

Because of their ease of administration and relatively benign side-effect profile, LTMs are an attractive pharmacologic therapy for individuals with asthma and prescribing medical practitioners. However, patient adherence does not justify or equal efficacy in the individual patient. Furthermore, the fact that these medications, specifically the LTRAs, have little to no side effects should give one pause. It may be attractive to think that the LTMs target a very specific arm of the asthmatic inflammatory cascade and that is why side effects are limited. It may be, however, that the effectiveness of LTMs is limited by that very reason. With time, research may allow the provider to identify circumstances, individual phenotypes, and even, perhaps, genotypes that respond more favorably to specific therapies. From the data available, it is evident that LTMs have a role in the treatment of allergen-induced asthma, ASA, EIA, and as alternatives or adjuncts to ICS in certain situations when treating chronic asthma. Finally, while there are limited preliminary data to suggest the use of LTMs in CVA, viral-induced wheeze, and acute asthma, these agents are not FDA approved for such therapeutic application at this time. In general, many investigations have been performed to identify a role for the LTMs in asthma and this role continues to evolve.

SUGGESTED READING

Bisgaard H: A randomized trial of montelukast in respiratory syncytial virus postbronchiolitis. Am J Respir Crit Care Med 2003;167:379–383.

Bisgaard H, Gilles L, Menten J, et al: Montelukast reduces asthma exacerbations in 2- to 5-year-old children with intermittent asthma. Am J Respir Crit Care Med 2005;171(4):315–322.

Bukstein DA, Luskin AT, Bernstein A: "Real-world" effectiveness of daily controller medicine in children with mild persistent asthma. Ann Allergy Asthma Immunol 2003;90(5):543–549.

Ducharme FM: Anti-leukotrienes as add-on therapy to inhaled glucocorticoids in patients with asthma: systematic review of current evidence. BMJ 2002;324–1545.

Fish JE, Kemp JP, Lockey RF, et al: Zafirlukast for symptomatic mild-to-moderate asthma: a 13-week multi-center study. The Zafirlukast Trialists Group. Clin Ther 1997;19:675–690.

Israel E, Cohn J, Dube L, et al: Effect of treatment with zileuton, a 5-lipoxygenase inhibitor, in patients with asthma. A randomized controlled trial. Zileuton Clinical Trial Group. JAMA 1996;275:931–936.

Leff JA, Busse WW, Pearlman D, et al: Montelukast, a leukotriene-receptor antagonist, for the treatment of mild asthma and exercise-induced bronchoconstriction. N Engl J Med 1998;339(3):147–152.

Malmstrom K, Rodriguez-Gomez G, Guerra J, et al: Oral montelukast, inhaled beclomethasone, and placebo for chronic asthma. A randomized, controlled trial. Montelukast/beclomethasone study group. Ann Intern Med 1999;130(6):487–495.

Maspero JF, Duenas-Meza E, Volovitz B, et al: Oral montelukast versus beclomethasone in 6-11 year old children with asthma: results of an open-label extension study evaluating long-term safety, satisfaction and adherence with therapy. Curr Med Res Opin 2001;17:96–104.

NIH/NHLBI: Guidelines for the diagnosis and management of asthma. Bethesda, MD, U.S. Department of Health and Human Services, National Institutes of Health, National Heart, Lung, and Blood Institute, 2002.

Phipatanakul W, Greene C, Downes SJ, et al: Montelukast improves asthma control in asthmatic children maintained on inhaled corticosteroids. Ann Allergy Asthma Immunol 2003;91(1):49–54.

Ram FS, Cates CJ Ducharme FM: Long-acting beta2-agonists versus anti-leukotrienes as add-on therapy to inhaled corticosteroids for chronic asthma. Cochrane Database Syst Rev 2005;(1):CD003137.

Reiss TF, Chervinsky P, Dockhorn RJ, et al: Montelukast, a once-daily leukotriene receptor antagonist, in the treatment of chronic asthma: a multicenter, randomized, double-blind trial. Montelukast Clinical Research Study Group. Arch Inter Med 1998;158:1213–1220.

Robertson CF, Henry RL, Mellis C, et al: Short course of montelukast for intermittent asthma in children: the Pre-Empt study. Am J Respir Crit Care Med 2004;169(7):A149.

Simons FE, Villa JR, Lee BW, et al: Montelukast added to budesonide in children with persistent asthma: a randomized, double-blind, crossover study. J Pediatr 2001;138(5):694–698.

Szefler SJ, Phillips BR, Martinez FD, et al: Characterization of within-subject responses to fluticasone and montelukast in childhood asthma. J Allergy Clin Immunol 2005;115:233–242.

Phosphodiesterase-4 Inhibitors and Theophylline

Roy A. Pleasants

CLINICAL PEARLS

- Theophylline is a nonselective inhibitor of PDE3, PDE4, and PDE5. PDE activity is inhibited only ~10% at therapeutic concentrations of theophylline; thus, this mechanism partially explains the clinical benefits of theophylline.

- Bronchodilation by theophylline occurs within hours, whereas anti-inflammatory effects take several days to occur.

- PDE4 is commonly found in inflammatory cells and promotes production of cytokines, chemotaxis, and release of inflammatory mediators. Relevant cells that are affected by PDE4 inhibitors include eosinophils, mast cells, monocytes, and lymphocytes. Dual blockade of PDE3 and PDE4 is needed for maximal effects on macrophages and for relaxation of airway smooth muscle.

- One area of theophylline use not discussed in the GINA or NHLBI asthma guidelines is the patient with clinical features of asthma and COPD. A 1- to 2-month trial is usually adequate to assess response to therapy.

- Roflumilast is the PDE4 inhibitor most studied in asthma and COPD, but is not approved yet. Roflumilast appears to not be PDE subtype selective, as it inhibits PDE4A, PDE4B, PDE4C, and PDE4D.

Theophylline, a methylxanthine, has been used in the treatment of asthma since the 1920s.[1] With clinical use, it became apparent that theophylline had a narrow therapeutic window. Pharmacodynamic studies of theophylline in the 1970s helped establish a therapeutic range for theophylline, subsequently improving the safe and effective use of theophylline. The use of theophylline for asthma peaked in the 1970s and early 1980s with the availability of sustained-release formulations, but its use declined with increased emphasis on the use of inhaled corticosteroids and long-acting beta$_2$-agonists. Despite establishment of a therapeutic range for theophylline to optimize efficacy and minimize toxicity as well as the availability of rapid clinical assays, theophylline toxicity still occurred in some patients. In the United States today, it is considered to be a third-line agent in the acute and chronic management of asthma. Theophylline is still widely used in Asian countries. One recent report in France reported use of theophylline in 15% of asthma patients.

Theophylline has bronchodilatory, anti-inflammatory, and immunomodulator effects among other effects on the respiratory system. The mechanisms of action of theophylline are not well defined, but it appears some of its effects are related to inhibition of phosphodiesterase (PDE) and antagonism of adenosine. Because of the multiple effects that phosphodiesterases

have in the airways of asthmatic patients and the toxicity profile of theophylline, more selective PDE inhibitors are in clinical development. Two selective PDE4 inhibitors, cilomulast and roflumilast, have reached phase III clinical trials in the treatment of asthma and chronic obstructive pulmonary disease (COPD).[2,3] This chapter will review the pharmacology and clinical use of theophylline and PDE4 inhibitors in asthma.

MECHANISM OF ACTION OF THEOPHYLLINE AND PHOSPHODIESTERASE INHIBITORS

Theophylline appears to work through multiple pharmacological mechanisms in the treatment of obstructive lung diseases; it causes weak and nonselective PDE inhibition, antagonizes adenosine, and activates histone deacetylases. Some data indicate that PDE inhibition and adenosine antagonism from theophylline only occur at concentrations greater than 10 µg/mL; thus, clinical benefits of theophylline at lower concentrations are likely through other mechanisms. Anti-inflammatory and immunomodulatory effects occur at lower concentrations (<10 µg/mL). Bronchodilation from theophylline occurs within hours of administration, whereas the anti-inflammatory effects are more delayed.

The breakdown of second messenger molecules, cyclic 3′,5′-adenosine monophosphate (cAMP) and cyclic 3′5′-guanosine monophosphate (cGMP) to monophosphates is catalyzed by the PDE enzymes. cAMP and cGMP are then converted to their inactive 5′-mononucleotides (AMP and GMP). AMP and GMP cannot activate cyclic nucleotide-dependent protein kinase cascades. Preventing the breakdown of cAMP leads to functional antagonism of airway smooth muscle and subsequently results in relaxation of the airway smooth muscle (bronchodilation). PDE4 is the predominant PDE enzyme in inflammatory cells in the airways.

Theophylline is a nonselective inhibitor of PDE3, PDE4, and PDE5. PDE activity is only inhibited approximately 10% at therapeutic concentrations of theophylline; thus, this mechanism partially explains the clinical benefits of theophylline. PDE4 inhibition is probably important regarding certain side effects of theophylline including nausea, vomiting, and headache.

At therapeutic concentrations, theophylline is a potent inhibitor of adenosine receptors, principally A1 and A2 receptors. Inhaled adenosine causes bronchoconstriction; this effect is blocked by theophylline. Seizures and cardiac arrhythmias from theophylline are likely to be related to adenosine antagonism. In addition to these effects, theophylline affects inflammatory gene transcription, apoptosis of eosinophils and neutrophils (Table 30-1). However, the exact mechanism by which theophylline exerts its anti-inflammatory effects is not well understood.

Table 30-1
EFFECT OF KEY DISEASES AND DRUGS ON THEOPHYLLINE CONCENTRATIONS

Drug or Disease State	Impact on Theophylline Blood Levels
Pulmonary edema	Marked increases possible
Congestive heart failure	Marked increases possible
Cor pulmonale	Marked increases possible
Cirrhosis	Marked increases possible
Cystic fibrosis	Moderate decrease with standard doses
Adenosine	Theophylline lessens effects of IV adenosine
Cimetidine	Moderate increases possible
Fluoroquinolones	Moderate increases possible with ciprofloxacin, increases unlikely with levofloxacin or moxifloxacin
Macrolide antibiotics	For erythromycin and clarithromycin, moderate increases possible, azithromycin unlikely to interact
Benzodiazepines	Theophylline lessens antianxiety effects of benzodiazepines
St John's wort	Moderate decreases in theophylline blood levels
Smoking tobacco or marijuana	Moderate decreases in theophylline blood levels—see effects of smoking or marijuana on theophylline decline ~1 wk after stopping smoking
Tacrine	Moderate increases possible
Phenytoin/Phenobarbital	Moderate decreases possible

A relatively recently identified mechanism of theophylline effects involves activation of histone deacetylase.[1,4] Acetylation of histones can result in activation and transcription of inflammatory genes. This process is regulated by histone acetyltransferase activity; there is an increase in histone acetyltransferase activity in asthma. Histone acetylation is reversed by histone deacetylases. Corticosteroids suppress the expression of inflammatory genes through activation of glucocorticoid receptors that recruit histone acetyltransferase, thus reducing histone acetylation and altering gene function activated by inflammation. At therapeutic concentrations, theophylline activates histone deacetylases and subsequently suppresses expression of inflammatory genes (Fig. 30-1). Theophylline appears to augment the effects of corticosteroids on histone acetylation. Cigarette smoking appears to decrease the effect of steroids on histone deacetylases; theophylline helps restore the effects of steroids on histone deacetylases in smokers.

Theophylline can inhibit the development of the late-asthmatic response and also decreases bronchial hyperresponsiveness as measured by methacholine challenge. Theophylline inhibits mast cell degranulation and can reduce the number of mast cells. It does not appear that theophylline modulates allergen-induced bronchial hyperresponsiveness. Theophylline can also decrease the number of activated eosinophils in airways of asthmatic individuals. These effects appear to occur at levels less than $10\,\mu g/mL$. Theophylline appears to accelerate eosinophil apoptosis by inhibiting interleukin (IL)-5. Effects on eosinophils are likely not related to PDE antagonism.

Another clinical effect of theophylline is increased mucociliary clearance, through a direct effect on respiratory ciliary

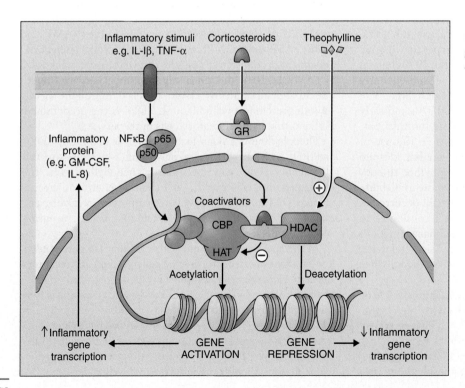

Figure 30-1 **Mechanism of theophylline on HDAC.** *(Adapted from Barnes PJ: Theophylline. New perspectives for an old drug. Am J Respir Critical Care Med 2003;167:813–818.)*

movement and water transport across respiratory epithelium. In addition, theophylline appears to help respiratory muscle function resulting in increased diaphragm contractility and decreased fatigue of the diaphragm and accessory breathing muscles. The clinical significance of these effects in asthma is not known.

PDE4 is commonly found in inflammatory cells and promotes production of cytokines, chemotaxis, and release of inflammatory mediators. Relevant cells that are affected by PDE4 inhibitors include eosinophils, mast cells, monocytes, and lymphocytes. Dual blockade of PDE3 and PDE4 is needed for maximal effects on macrophages and for relaxation of airway smooth muscle

There are more than 10 families of PDE enzymes. Other PDE inhibitors, such as dipyridamole, have been in clinical use for nonpulmonary indications for many years. The PDE5 inhibitor sildenafil is used in the treatment of erectile dysfunction and more recently for the treatment of pulmonary hypertension. PDE5 is a specific inactivator of cGMP. PDE5 is widely distributed in pulmonary vascular smooth muscle of pulmonary arteries and veins, bronchial blood vessels, and airway smooth muscle. Inhibition of PDE5 may also exert anti-inflammatory effects.

There are a number of PDE4 inhibitors in development today; cilomulast and roflumilast are furthest along in clinical development. The development of cilomulast for asthma has been slowed due to a relative lack of efficacy in asthma. Both agents continue to be studied for the treatment of COPD. The anti-inflammatory and immunomodulatory activity of PDE4 inhibitors has been investigated in vitro, in animals and humans. Roflumilast appears to not be PDE subtype selective (inhibits PDE4A, PDE4B, PDE4C, PDE4D), whereas cilomulast has a higher potency for PDE4D compared to PDE4A and PDE4B. One of the important goals for PDE4 inhibitors is to have less gastrointestinal (GI) side effects such as nausea and vomiting, as compared to theophylline. PDE4 receptors are located in the central nervous system (CNS); cilomulast and roflumilast have a lower affinity for the PDE4 receptors in the CNS and thus have less nausea/vomiting associated with them. The PDE4 receptor subtype PDE4B is important in mediating anti-inflammatory effects. PDE4D mediates nausea and vomiting through stimulation of the vomiting center in the brain. Roflumilast has a greater affinity than cilomulast for neutrophils, eosinophils, and CD4-positive T cells. Roflumilast and cilomulast appear to interfere with airway remodeling by decreasing subepithelial collagen, thickening of airway epithelium, and goblet cell hyperplasia.

Pharmacokinetics of Theophylline and PDE4 Inhibitors

PHARMACOKINETICS OF THEOPHYLLINE

The pharmacokinetics of theophylline has been extensively studied. A study by Mitenko and associates[5] in the 1970s demonstrated that in nine acute asthmatic individuals, optimal bronchodilation and minimal adverse effects occurred when blood theophylline levels were maintained between 10 and 20 µg/mL. The relationship between FEV_1 (forced expiratory volume in 1 second) and theophylline blood level was described as log-linear (Fig. 30-2); the majority of the

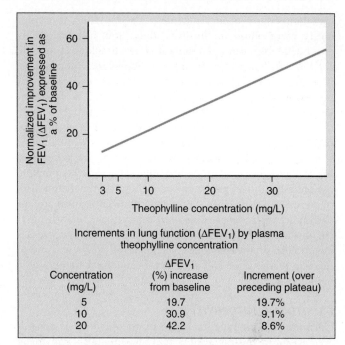

Increments in lung function (ΔFEV_1) by plasma theophylline concentration		
Concentration (mg/L)	ΔFEV_1 (%) increase from baseline	Increment (over preceding plateau)
5	19.7	19.7%
10	30.9	9.1%
20	42.2	8.6%

Figure 30-2 Pharmacodynamic study of theophylline in acute asthma. Dose-response relationship between FEV_1 and log serum theophylline concentration. *(Data from Mitenko PA, Ogilvie RI: Rational intravenous doses of theophylline. N Engl J Med 1973;289:600–605.)*

bronchodilatory effects occurred at blood levels less than 10 µg/mL, with subsequent increases in blood theophylline levels yielding exponentially smaller changes in FEV_1.

Most theophylline preparations are well absorbed. Some sustained-release formulations exhibit bioavailability problems. A proprietary form of ultra-sustained release (given once daily) theophylline used today, Uniphyl (Purdue Pharmaceuticals) has increased absorption when taken with food as compared to taken on an empty stomach. The manufacturer recommends that the patient take the product consistently with or without food. Although there may be less reliable absorption than the previously available brand name formulations, generic sustained-release theophyllines are reasonably well absorbed.

Theophylline is eliminated from the body by hepatic biotransformation into less active metabolites. The normal half-life of theophylline in a healthy adult is typically around 8 hours. There can be marked variation in the half-life as a result of age, drugs, and disease states. In premature infants and newborns, theophylline has a prolonged half-life, but by the age of 4 to 5 years, the half-life is shorter than in an adult (~5 hours). In decompensated congestive heart failure (CHF), cor pulmonale, or liver disease (cirrhosis and hepatitis), the half-life of theophylline may be prolonged to 24 hours. Generally, it is best to avoid theophylline in these types of patients as the degree of cardiac or hepatic impairment tends to wax and wane over time and so does the half-life (and drug clearance) of theophylline, increasing the likelihood of the patient becoming theophylline toxic. However, there is a clinical role for theophylline in patients with apnea associated with heart failure.

There are a number of interacting drugs that can affect theophylline pharmacokinetics. Theophylline is metabolized primarily by the CYT P450 isoenzyme 1A2, but is also metabolized by other isozymes. Theophylline is extensively metabolized in the liver; thus, drug interactions by enzyme inhibition or induction can occur. Smoking of tobacco and/or marijuana can increase theophylline metabolism; it is the inhalation of hydrocarbons that is responsible for this effect. Thus, chewing tobacco or nicotine replacement therapy will not alter theophylline metabolism. However, if nicotine replacement therapy is successful in getting the patient to quit smoking, then metabolism of theophylline is slowed. Generally, 1 week of tobacco abstinence is required for the effects of hydrocarbon inhalation on theophylline metabolism to decline; months are required for metabolism to completely normalize. Some macrolide antibiotics are apt to interact with theophylline (erythromycin and clarithromycin, but not azithromycin). Similarly, ciprofloxacin decreases metabolism of theophylline, but not levofloxacin and moxifloxacin. Cimetidine and allopurinol can inhibit theophylline metabolism.

MONITORING THEOPHYLLINE

Currently the therapeutic range of theophylline is considered to be in the range of 5 to 15 µg/mL (although many clinical laboratories still report the therapeutic range to be 10 to 20 µg/mL). Most patients can be maintained on theophylline for chronic asthma at blood levels between 5 and 10 µg/mL with minimal side effects. Maintaining lower levels decreases the likelihood of levels increasing into the toxic range because of interacting drugs or diseases. Monitoring of blood levels is usually recommended for patients receiving theophylline. Barnes and colleagues suggested that if theophylline is dosed low, side effects and drug interactions are uncommon and drug concentration measurement is not necessary, except to monitor compliance.[1] If a patient has clinical signs or symptoms that could be due to theophylline (nausea, vomiting, and tachycardia are usually first signs that blood levels are excessive), a serum theophylline level should be obtained. For dosage adjustments, serum theophylline concentrations should be measured at steady state. The typical healthy adult patient will have a half-life of 8 hours and steady state is easily achieved within 48 hours of starting theophylline. Patients with liver impairment, CHF, or cor pulmonale will take 3 to 4 days to achieve steady state. Assessing recent compliance is useful before obtaining a theophylline level in the ambulatory setting to ensure the level reflects steady-state dosing. For regular sustained-release formulations (every-12-hour dosing), a level drawn between 6 and 12 hours after a dose is reasonable. For the once-daily formulation, a midpoint level (12 hours postdose) is reasonable. A blood level could also be obtained to assess the impact of a potential drug interaction (e.g., addition of ciprofloxacin), or if the baseline theophylline level is low (5 to 10 µg/mL), monitoring for theophylline toxicity without obtaining a blood level would be acceptable.

Side effects of theophylline are more likely to occur with initiation of therapy or as blood levels increase near or above the upper limits of normal in patients on chronic theophylline. Caffeine-like side effects (nervousness, sleeplessness, tremors) and GI intolerance occur, especially with initiation of therapy. If blood levels remain in the therapeutic range, side effects typically become less within 1 to 2 weeks after initiating theophylline. More serious effects, arrhythmias (premature ventricular contractions, or ventricular tachycardia) and seizures, may occur when blood levels are significantly above the normal therapeutic range. Arrhythmias and seizures are unlikely to occur unless blood levels are substantially above 20 µg/mL (e.g., 40 µg/mL), but are more apt to occur when blood levels rise rapidly (e.g., intentional overdose). Minor side effects do not always occur before the onset of more serious ones.

Dosing of Theophylline

Because theophylline is a drug with a narrow therapeutic window, proper dosing is an important consideration. In children younger than 5, the recommended starting dose of theophylline is 10 mg/kg/day. The maximum recommended dosage (mg/kg/day) in children younger than 1 year = 0.2 (age in weeks) + 5 and is 16 mg/kg/day in children 1 to 5 years old.

In acute asthma, the adult dose of aminophylline is a load of 6 mg/kg, then 0.6 to 0.9 mg/kg by intravenous constant infusion. For acute asthma in children older than 1, a load of 6 mg/kg followed by approximately 1.2 mg/kg/hr is a reasonable starting dose. The constant infusion dose would be lower in a patient with liver impairment, CHF, or cor pulmonale (~0.3 mg/kg/hr). In the treatment of chronic asthma, the average dose in a nonsmoking adult would be 5 to 7 mg/kg/day (e.g., sustained release theophylline 200 mg orally every 12 hours in an 80-kg patient). Low doses used today are typically regular sustained-release theophylline 200 mg orally twice daily or 400 mg ultra-sustained-release theophylline (Uniphyl) orally once daily. If the target dose is 200 mg orally every 12 hours, starting at a lower dose for 1 week (e.g., 200 mg orally every day or 100 mg orally every 12 hours), then increase to 200 mg orally every 12 hours. After reaching the target dose, obtain a level and then adjust the dose as clinically indicated. If increasing the dose, the blood levels typically increase in proportion to the dose increase. However, if making substantial dose increases (e.g., 200 mg twice a day to 400 mg twice a day), nonlinear pharmacokinetics may occur and blood levels may increase disproportionately.

Pharmacokinetics of PDE4 Inhibitors

Roflumilast is moderately well absorbed with an oral bioavailability of about 80%. A clinically insignificant decrease in peak concentrations is seen when given with a high-fat meal. Roflumilast is metabolized by the liver to an active metabolite and exhibits linear pharmacokinetics (increase in dose leads to proportional increases in blood concentrations). The half-life of roflumilast is about 18 hours, allowing for once-daily dosing. Cigarette smoking does not appear to affect the metabolism of roflumilast. There was no interaction with erythromycin by roflumilast. Thus, there are significant pharmacokinetic differences from theophylline.

The pharmacokinetics of cilomulast has been extensively studied. It is well absorbed (rapid and 95% complete), has a half-life of approximately 7 hours, exhibits linear pharmacokinetics, and undergoes extensive metabolism (only 1% excreted unchanged in the urine). Some common drug interactions with theophylline (tobacco smoking) are unlikely with this agent as its metabolism occurs with metabolizing enzymes not typically altered by other agents.

DOSING AND MONITORING OF CILOMULAST AND ROFLUMILAST

Monitoring of blood levels of cilomulast and roflumilast is not recommended. Based on current data in human clinical trials, monitoring of GI side effects is warranted. It is currently unknown what the recommended approach(es) should be if GI side effects are encountered. Because of the long half-life of roflumilast, it was dosed once daily in clinical trials. The most common dose in clinical trials for roflumilast was 500 µg once daily. The dosage of cilomulast in clinical trials was typically 10 or 15 mg orally twice daily. Assuming one or both of these agents reach the market, more information is needed about dosing and monitoring recommendations.

CLINICAL TRIALS OF THEOPHYLLINE—ACUTE ASTHMA

Most clinical studies of IV aminophylline in emergency department (ED) or non–critically ill hospitalized asthmatic patients showed no benefits of the addition of IV aminophylline to inhaled beta$_2$-agonists and steroids. Two studies showed benefits of IV aminophylline in critically-ill patients with impending respiratory failure who have failed first-line therapies (inhaled beta$_2$-agonist and anticholinergic, and corticosteroids).[6,7] One study showed fewer intubations than placebo, another study showed more rapid clinical response. Serum theophylline concentrations of approximately 15 µg/mL were achieved in these patients, at the upper range currently recommended for theophylline. A prospective study in 47 children with status asthmaticus received standard therapy (albuterol and ipratropium via nebulization and IV albuterol, IV methylprednisolone) versus standard therapy plus IV aminophylline.[6] Target theophylline levels ranged from 12 to 17 µg/mL. Subjects receiving theophylline achieved more rapid clinical improvement (18 hours versus 31 hours for target

clinical score). Theophylline had no effect on length of stay in the intensive care unit (ICU). Emesis was common in the theophylline group, whereas tremors were more common in the control patients.

CLINICAL TRIALS OF THEOPHYLLINE—CHRONIC ASTHMA

A number of studies have shown that sustained-release theophylline is effective in controlling the symptoms of asthma and maintaining pulmonary function in persistent asthma. Although suggested as an alternative monotherapy in mild asthma, theophylline likely does not have adequate anti-inflammatory effects for this role. In trials comparing theophylline to inhaled corticosteroids (ICSs) in mild to moderate asthma, both treatments were effective in achieving control of symptoms. ICSs were slightly more effective in reducing symptoms. One clinical use of theophylline is as an add-on to ICS. Studies that have compared increasing the dose of the ICS to maintaining the dose of the ICS and adding theophylline have largely shown adding theophylline is as or more effective than increasing the ICS dose. In a double-blind, placebo-controlled study, 62 asthmatic adults were randomly assigned to receive either low-dose budesonide (400 µg) plus theophylline (250 to 375 mg) or high-dose budesonide (800 µg).[8] The median theophylline level obtained was 8.7 µg/mL. The low-dose budesonide and theophylline group has more significant improvements in spirometry. Similar benefits were seen with both treatments with regard to asthma symptoms, peak flows, and beta$_2$-agonist use (Fig. 30-3). Thus theophylline can serve as a steroid-sparing agent.

Most studies comparing theophylline to salmeterol and formoterol in persistent asthma report greater bronchodilation and better tolerability of the long-acting beta$_2$-agonist (LABA),

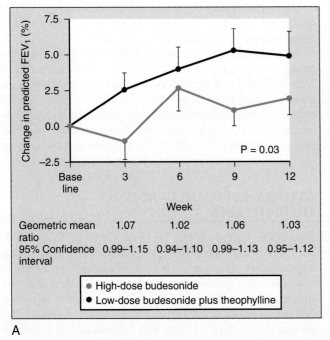

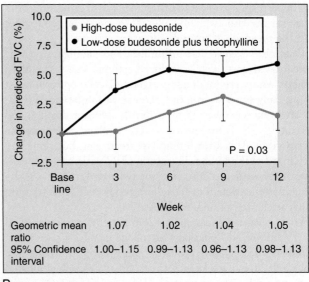

A   B

Figure 30-3   Comparison of high-dose inhaled budesonide (A) versus low-dose inhaled budesonide plus theophylline (B). *(Data from Evans DJ, Taylor DA, Zetterstrom O, et al: A comparison of low-dose theophylline and high-dose inhaled budesonide for moderate asthma. N Engl J Med 1997;337:1412–1418.)*

especially regarding GI side effects. These studies did target higher theophylline levels than typically recommended today. Some studies found combining theophylline with LABA in chronic asthma leads to additive bronchodilation.

Several studies have compared leukotriene modifiers to theophylline in persistent asthma. A recent study compared low-dose theophylline to montelukast in poorly controlled asthmatic individuals. It was a double-blind, randomized, placebo-controlled trial in 489 subjects who were assigned to theophylline 300 mg/day or montelukast 10 mg once daily. Participants were followed for 24 weeks. Neither treatment lowered episodes of poor asthma control, nor improved quality of life. When theophylline was not administered with ICS, significant changes were noted in asthma control symptoms as well as lung function; about three fourths of the subjects were on ICS. Of note, theophylline side effects tended to resolve within a few weeks of starting therapy. Several studies have looked at withdrawal of theophylline in severe asthma. In one study, there were increases in eosinophils and CD4+ cells after withdrawal of theophylline.

CLINICAL TRIALS OF PDE4 INHIBITORS IN ASTHMA

A randomized, double-blind, placebo-controlled study of roflumilast was conducted to assess its effect on the allergen-induced early and late asthmatic responses. Twenty-three patients with mild to moderate asthma received once-daily 250 μg roflumilast, once-daily 500 μg roflumilast, or placebo for 7 to 10 days each. An allergen challenge was done on the last day of each treatment sequence. Both the early and late asthmatic responses were significantly lower with both doses of roflumilast than with placebo. Inhibition of the early asthmatic response amounted to 25% with 250 μg and 28% for 500 μg versus placebo. The percentage inhibition of the late asthmatic response was dose related: 27% with 250 μg and 43% with 500 μg versus placebo. In another study with a single 1000-μg dose of roflumilast given 1 hour before allergen challenge, there was 62% inhibition of the late asthmatic response. Roflumilast also attenuated allergen-induced airway hyperresponsiveness to histamine. These effects of roflumilast on the late asthmatic allergen response are consistent with the presence of anti-inflammatory activity.

Data also suggest that roflumilast and cilomilast provide protection against exercise-induced asthma. In a study of 16 patients who were randomly assigned placebo or roflumilast 500 μg daily for 4 weeks, the percentage inhibition of FEV_1 fall after exercise was 14% on day 1, 24% on day 14, and 41% on day 28. Tumor necrosis factor α blood concentration decreased by 21% after roflumilast treatment, but remained unchanged with placebo. In a study of 27 patients given cilomilast for 1 week at a dose of 10 mg twice daily, there was significant attenuation of exercise-induced bronchoconstriction, which amounted to 34% inhibition.

With regard to cilomilast, 266 patients were enrolled in a randomized, placebo-controlled, parallel-group trial. Cilomilast was given in doses of 5 mg, 10 mg, or 15 mg two times a day for 6 weeks in patients already receiving inhaled corticosteroids. The patients had mean FEV_1 of 66% predicted. At the highest dose of cilomilast, there was a greater improvement in FEV_1 than with placebo, but the difference

was not significant except after 2 weeks when the mean difference between the groups was 0·21 L. In the patients' overall assessment, approximately 70% of patients receiving 15 mg two times daily of cilomilast reported that they were greatly improved compared with 41% of patients on placebo. For the physicians' overall assessment, 59% of patients given cilomilast 15 mg twice daily were improved compared with 29% assigned placebo.

In a 1-year parallel-group study, cilomilast at a dose of 10 mg or 15 mg twice daily was studied in 211 patients; the study was an extension of three double-blind, randomized, phase II studies of 4 to 6 weeks' duration. Fifty-three patients had been assigned placebo and 158 cilomilast. There were only small, nonsignificant improvements in FEV_1 over the 12-month period, and consequently the further development of cilomilast for the indication of asthma was terminated. Another study compared roflumilast 500 μg daily versus beclomethasone dipropionate 200 μg twice a day over 12 weeks. Both drugs resulted in similar improvement in FEV_1 (0.3 L and 0.37 L) along with similar effects on symptoms.

Roflumilast's effects in asthma are more promising, perhaps due to higher in vitro potency than cilomilast. In a randomized, double-blind, parallel-group, dose-ranging study, roflumilast was given for 12 weeks in doses of 100 μg, 250 μg, or 500 μg everyday. At baseline, the mean FEV_1 was 73% of predicted; a total of 690 patients were enrolled. Roflumilast led to significant increases in FEV_1 in all three treatment groups: 11% increase at 100 μg, 13% at 250 μg, and 16% at 500 μg. The response at 500 μg was significantly better than that at 100 μg. Roflumilast also produced significant dose-dependent improvements in morning peak expiratory flow (PEF) in all three treatment groups, respectively (10 L/min, 12 L/min, and 20 L/min). The 500-μg dose was superior to the 100-μg dose for both morning and evening PEF. Clinical effects on PEF were observed within 24 hours after initiation.

The most frequent adverse drug effect (ADR) was headache (13%) in the 500-μg group. Diarrhea (8%), nausea (8%), and abdominal pain (4%) were less frequent. Side effects generally were less frequent over the long term, suggesting adverse drug reactions are more likely to occur early in therapy.

In a subsequent 12-month follow-up from the same study, 456 patients received roflumilast 500 μg once daily. Improvements in lung function in patients who had previously received roflumilast 500 μg for 12 weeks were maintained over the 12-month period. In those patients previously treated with the lower doses of roflumilast, there were further increases in FEV_1, which were greatest in those who had previously received the 100-μg dose for 12 weeks.

ASTHMA GUIDELINES—ROLE OF THEOPHYLLINE

The 2006 Global Initiative on Asthma (GINA) guidelines describe theophylline as a bronchodilator with anti-inflammatory effects at lower concentrations. The guidelines state that theophylline should not be used as first-line therapy for chronic asthma and should be reserved as an add-on therapy in patients not responding to other therapies. The guidelines report side effects may be limiting and that lower concentrations are recommended. When low doses are used, theophylline concentrations are not necessary. GINA further suggests that theophylline is an option in acute asthma and that use for this indication is controversial. There may be no benefit of theophylline above that achieved by adequate doses of short-acting bronchodilators. It is recommended not to use IV aminophylline in patients already receiving long-acting theophylline preparations. The GINA guidelines have more favorable comments regarding the role of theophylline in the management of chronic asthma in those older than 5 years. Theophylline is not listed as an option for the treatment of acute asthma in children.

The 2007 National Heart, Lung, and Blood Institute (NHLBI) guidelines place theophylline as an alternative to low dose ICS or as an add-on in less well-controlled asthma in children 5 to 11 years old. Theophylline is not listed as a recommended therapy in children between 0 and 4 years old.

One area of theophylline use not discussed in the GINA or NHLBI asthma guidelines is the patient with clinical features of asthma and COPD. Up to 25% of COPD patients have concurrent asthma. The author is an advocate for theophyl-line use in severe to very severe COPD patients where other bronchodilators have been optimized and the patient still has significant limitations related to airway obstruction. Use of lower doses improves the safety profile of theophylline in these patients. A 1- to 2-month trial is usually adequate to assess response to therapy.

SUMMARY

Overall, the PDE4 inhibitors appear are potential agents for asthma and COPD. Whether they will ultimately be recommended as monotherapy, or as add-on to other controllers such as inhaled corticosteroids or leukotriene modifiers requires further study. Theophylline has been an option for therapy in asthma and COPD for a very long time, but has fallen to third line given the new products available. However, it has anti-inflammatory and steroid-sparing effects that are beneficial in a subset of patients. Dosing to achieve levels 5 to 15 μg/mL reduces toxicity.

REFERENCES

1. Barnes PJ: Theophylline. New perspectives for an old drug. Am J Respir Critical Care Med 2003;167:813–818.
2. Boswell-Smith V, Cazzola M, Page C: Are phosphodiesterase 4 inhibitors just more theophylline? J Allergy Clin Immunol 2006;117:1237–1243.
3. Lipworth BJ: Phosphodiesterase-4 inhibitors for asthma and chronic obstructive pulmonary disease. Lancet 2005;365:167–175.
4. Ito K, Lim S, Caramori G: A molecular mechanism of theophylline: induction of histone acetylase activity to decrease inflammatory gene expression. Proc Natl Acad Sci U S A 2002;99:8921–8926.
5. Mitenko PA, Ogilvie RI: Rational intravenous doses of theophylline. N Engl J Med 1973;289:600–605.
6. Self TH, Redmond AM, Nguyen WT: Reassessment of theophylline use for severe asthma exacerbation: Is it justified in critically-ill hospitalized patients. J Asthma 2002;39:677–686.
7. Ream RS, Loftis LL, Albers GM: Efficacy of IV theophylline in children with severe status asthmaticus. Chest 2001;119:1480–1488.
8. Evans DJ, Taylor DA, Zetterstrom O, et al: A comparison of low-dose theophylline and high-dose inhaled budesonide for moderate asthma. N Engl J Med 1997;337:1412–1418.

CLINICAL PEARLS

- Immunoglobulin E (IgE) is an important mediator of type I hypersensitivity reactions, including asthma, via binding to mast cells and basophils.

- Many severe-persistent asthmatic subjects may be sensitive to common allergens.

- IgE can modulate allergic responses by up-regulating high-affinity receptors and potentiating mast cell and basophil degranulation.

- Omalizumab (Xolair) is a recombinant monoclonal anti-IgE antibody that attenuates the allergic asthma response by binding the constant region of IgE, thereby preventing its interaction with high-affinity receptors.

- Once bound to IgE, the recombinant antibody forms inert complexes that can be cleared by the reticuloendothelial system; these cannot cross-link to effect mast cells' degranulation and cannot activate complement.

- Omalizumab therapy can reduce free IgE levels, down-regulate high-affinity receptor expression on basophils, attenuate basophil sensitivity to allergen challenge, and diminish inflammatory mediator release.

- Clinically, omalizumab has been shown to reduce the frequency of asthma exacerbations and baseline steroid use.

- Omalizumab dosing is standardized to baseline IgE levels and patient weight. While periodic IgE levels do not need to be obtained, patients must be monitored carefully for rare anaphylactoid reactions after each injection.

- Sodium cromoglycate (SCG) has been shown to increase peak expiratory flow rates (by up to 30%), reduce day and night symptom severity, and improve lung function.

- While steroids are the mainstay of persistent asthma therapy, SCG can be a useful adjunct in the treatment of chronic symptoms, and has efficacy in reducing exercise-induced bronchospasm.

PART I: ANTIBODY THERAPY

Immunoglobulin E (IgE) is intrinsic to the pathogenesis of several allergic disease processes, including rhinoconjunctivitis, food allergies, and asthma. These are grouped under type I hypersensitivity reactions, of which IgE is the prime initiator, via binding to high-affinity receptors (FcεRI) on mast cells and basophils (Fig. 31-1)

The clinical burden of asthma reverberates throughout all levels of health care, accounting for millions of urgent provider visits and billions of dollars in treatment and lost wages.[1] Despite pharmaceutical advances and dissemination of the need for vigilant treatment, the prevalence of asthma continues to rise. In Western Europe, asthma affects 10% to 15% of the adult population; in the United States, asthma cases increased 75% from 1980 to 1994.[2] Indeed, many asthmatic patients have failed to achieve optimum symptom control.

A relatively small subset of patients with refractory asthma symptoms is magnified by its disproportionately large fiscal burden.[3] Clearly, there is a need for the evolution of therapy and of symptom control. While the dominant asthma phenotype in severe-persistent cases is nonallergic, at least half of these patients may manifest skin prick sensitivity to common allergens.[4] On a larger scale, IgE-mediated reactions may be involved (to varying degrees) in all phenotypic expressions of asthma.[4] In children, specific IgE sensitivity with skin testing is linked to almost 90% of cases.[5] While circulating IgE levels have been shown to correlate with asthma's prevalence,[4] local production may be as important to clinical symptoms.[4] Recent autopsy data from fatal asthmatic lung tissue demonstrate an increased proportion of FcεRI+ cells, when compared with similar samples from milder or nonasthmatic individuals.[4]

The Role of IgE in Asthma Pathogenesis

Immunoglobulin E is central to the allergic cascade, effecting mast cell degranulation, inflammatory cell influx, and inflammatory mediator elaboration. The synthesis of IgE is T-cell dependent, the culmination of antigen uptake, processing, and presentation by major histocompatibility complex class II molecules. B cells normally synthesizing IgM or IgG are affected to produce IgE by T cells, through two critical signals: (1) interleukin (IL)-4 or IL-13, which bind to B cells receptors and involve the STAT 6 signal transduction pathway and (2) CD40 on B cells binds to its T-cell ligand (CD40 ligand).[4] Ultimately, B cell DNA is rearranged and spliced, favoring IgE production.[4]

IgE receptors on mast cells and basophils are intrinsic to the elaboration of proinflammatory cascades. Mature mast cells can exist in a primed state when IgE molecules are bound to the FcεRI receptor, awaiting allergen attachment. Activation and subsequent degranulation occur as antigen complexes with IgE are formed through FcεRI.[4] While the cellular events that comprise antigen-complex activation of mast cells are not fully understood, umbilical cord blood data provide some insight. After stimulation of FcεRI on umbilical cord mast cells, many hundred gene expression patterns change, resulting in the elaboration of cytokines, chemokines, adhesion molecules, and proteins that modulate T- and B-cell interactions.[4] IgE-mediated basophil responses include the release of a broad spectrum of inflammatory compounds, but fewer cytokines than mast cells[4] (Fig. 31-2).

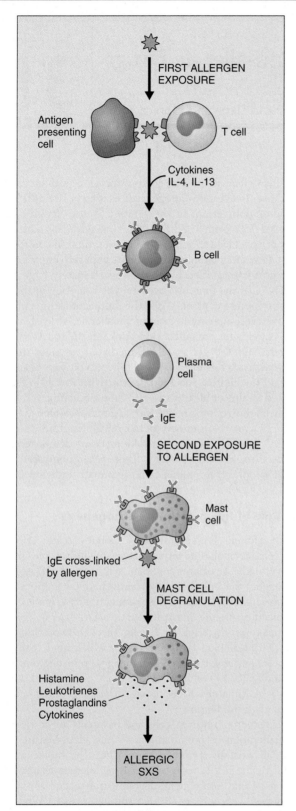

Figure 31-1 The Allergic Cascade. Initial allergen exposure potentiates mast cell degranulation and mediator release. Immunoglobulin E binds to mast cells via its high-affinity receptor and forms cross links with antigens. *(Adapted from Novartis Pharmaceuticals.)*

Labels within figure:
FIRST ALLERGEN EXPOSURE
Antigen presenting cell
T cell
Cytokines IL-4, IL-13
B cell
Plasma cell
IgE
SECOND EXPOSURE TO ALLERGEN
Mast cell
IgE cross-linked by allergen
MAST CELL DEGRANULATION
Histamine Leukotrienes Prostaglandins Cytokines
ALLERGIC SXS

IgE can modulate the expression of its own receptors via mechanisms that upregulate the density of FcεRI, and potentiate mast cell and basophil degranulation.[4] With increased FcεRI expression and high circulating IgE, lower allergen concentrations are needed to stimulate mast cell and basophil responses.[4] IgE may even prolong mast cell survival through the induction of apoptosis resistance, as suggested by murine data.[4] Reduction of circulating IgE levels and IgE receptor levels attenuates the propensity of mast cells and basophils to degranulate. This represents the crux of anti-IgE therapy. The short (less than 2-day) half-life and low circulating levels of IgE are balanced by its high-affinity receptors. This ensures mast cells and basophils exist in a primed state.[4] Once bound to FcεRI receptors, the half-life of IgE increases to 2 weeks.

Omalizumab Structure and Function

In June of 2003, omalizumab (Xolair) (Fig. 31-3), a recombinant monoclonal anti-IgE antibody, received approval by the Food and Drug Administration (FDA) and remains the only specific anti-IgE therapy available for clinical use. It binds the constant region (cε3) of IgE molecules, preventing their interaction with FcεRI and FcεRII receptors on effector cells; residues are 95% human, and 5% murine.[1,4] Murine residues specific to IgE binding are grafted onto a human IgG1 superstructure, with careful extraction of anaphylactogenic units.[1]

However, receptor-bound IgE is unaffected, obviating the potential for cross-linking and omalizumab-mediated mast cell degranulation. Once bound to IgE, the recombinant antibody forms inert complexes (trimers of 2 omalizumab molecules linked to one IgE molecule) that cannot activate complement, but can be cleared by the reticuloendothelial system[1] (Fig. 31-4).

Published data confirm omalizumab's actions at a molecular level, with statistically significant reductions in free IgE levels and down-regulation of FcεRI receptor expression on basophils.[4] Concomitant with receptor down-regulation is a loss of basophil sensitivity to allergen challenge, and diminution of mediator release.[4]

While its primary mechanism of action reduces circulating IgE levels, omalizumab also attenuates FcεRI and CD23 (a low-affinity IgE receptor). Human studies have shown reduced numbers of FcεRI receptors on basophils after treatment: from about 220,000 to about 8300 receptors per cell.[1] Functionally, after ex vivo dust mite challenge, there was a 90% decrease in histamine release by basophils.[1] Similarly, other studies demonstrate a rapid decrease in the expression of dendritic cell FcεRI, which may inhibit antigen processing and presentation to T cells, and an overall reduction in the elaboration of T_H2 cytokines.[4]

Published Efficacy Data

Proof-of-concept studies demonstrated omalizumab's clinical efficacy through inhibition of early and late phase bronchoconstrictor responses after inhaled allergen challenges (Fig. 31-5). When compared with placebo, omalizumab reduced the mean maximal decrease in FEV_1 (forced expiratory volume in 1 second) in early responses by 85%, and in late responses by 65%.[4]

Further data from phase III studies expanded recruitment to include moderate-to-severe asthmatic patients, with a mean age range of 9 to 39 and positive skin prick testing. Standard subcutaneous injections were given every

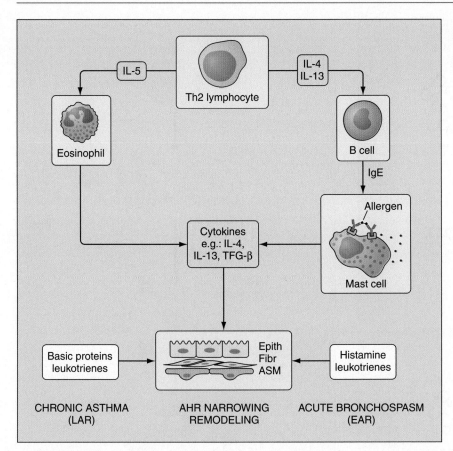

Figure 31-2 Pathways of acute and chronic allergic asthma. Acute airway constriction is precipitated by mast cell degranulation and the elaboration of mediators like histamine and leukotrienes. Late-phase effects include diverse changes in airway structure (airway remodeling), which encompass smooth muscle hyperplasia and hypertrophy, fibroblast proliferation, subepithelial fibrosis, basement membrane thickening, vascular reorganization, and other stigma. *(Adapted from Jonkers RE, van der Zee JS: Anti-IgE and other new immunomodulation-based therapies for allergic asthma. Neth J Med 2005;63:121–128.)*

2 to 4 weeks, at first as an adjunct to inhaled corticosteroid therapy (16 weeks, steroid stable phase), and then continued over a 12-week steroid-reduction phase. Three pivotal phase III (two including adults and adolescents, one including children) studies showed a significant reduction in the frequency of exacerbations in treated patients.[6]

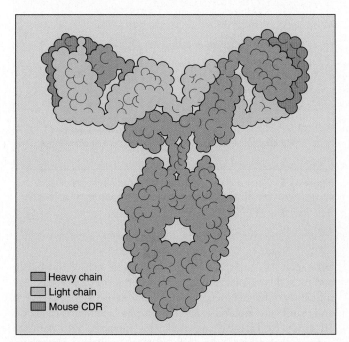

Figure 31-3 The three-dimensional structure of Xolair. *(Adapted from Boushey H: Anti-allergic drugs. J Allergy Clin Immunol 2004;113 [2 Suppl]:279–284.)*

During the steroid-stable phase, pediatric data supporting a reduction in asthma exacerbations did not bear statistical significance, contrasting findings in adolescents and adults. However, during the steroid-withdrawal phase all three trials manifested statistically significant reductions (approximately 50%) per patient. A significantly greater proportion of patients treated with omalizumab reduced their inhaled corticosteroid (ICS) dose; the number of individuals able to achieve complete ICS withdrawal was nearly doubled in the treatment group. Omalizumab demonstrated a similar impact on asthma symptoms. In all three studies, nocturnal symptom scores, daytime symptom scores, and the number of beta-agonist puffs needed per day were reduced in the recipient group. The efficacy of omalizumab persisted during the extension phase of these trials, lasting up to 52 weeks during treatment. The two adult trials showed no exacerbations during the extension phase in 68% and 76% of patients, with nearly one third able to remain steroid free. Pediatric data showed that 91% of patients who achieved ICS withdrawal were able to remain steroid free by the end of the extension phase. Corren and colleagues conducted a pooled data analysis of the three phase III studies, to examine the impact of specific IgE therapy in serious asthma exacerbations, measured as emergency department visits and hospitalizations.[6] Omalizumab-treated patients had fewer unscheduled outpatient visits (21.3 versus 35.5), emergency department visits (1.8 versus 3.8), and hospitalizations (3.42 events versus 0.26) per 100 patient years.[7] Those treated solely with ICS were expected to have more exacerbations per year (1.56 exacerbations per patient-year) than subjects whose therapy included

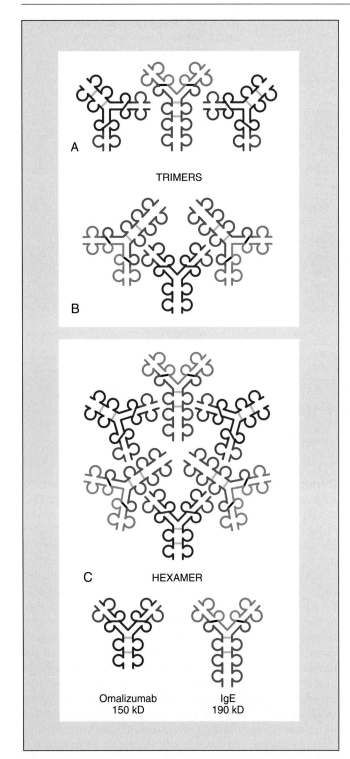

Figure 31-4 Omalizumab binds the constant region of IgE molecules, preventing their attachment to high-affinity receptors on mast cells and basophils. Complexes are usually trimers, but can be more complex. These inert molecules do not cause mast cell degranulation or the activation of complement. *(Adapted from Brownell J, Casale TB: Anti-IgE therapy. Immunol Allergy Clin North Am 2004;24:551–568.)*

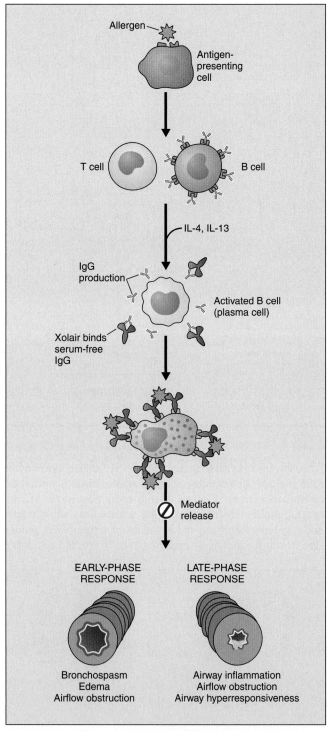

Figure 31-5 Xolair attenuates early- and late-phase allergic responses by binding only to free IgE molecules and preventing their attachment to mast cells and basophils. *(Adapted from Novartis Pharmaceuticals.)*

omalizumab (0.69 exacerbations per patient-year). From these data it is estimated that 44 exacerbations may be prevented per 100 treated patients.

The multicenter INNOVATE trial sought to examine severe asthmatic individuals whose symptoms were inadequately controlled despite high-dose ICS and long-acting beta-agonists—a population at the highest risk of morbidity and mortality. Omalizumab, administered over 28 weeks, significantly reduced emergency department use as well as severe and nonsevere asthma exacerbation rates. Similarly, a phase III study by Holgate and associates included 246 patients with severe asthma, who suffered from persistent symptoms despite high doses of fluticasone.[8] Overall, recipients showed a significantly greater reduction in steroid use: 74% of those on therapy achieved a greater than 50% reduction in baseline steroid use, versus 51% of placebo patients. The frequency of asthma exacerbations was significantly reduced as well (per subject, exacerbation rates were 0.19 and 0.34 for omalizumab and placebo groups, respectively).

Published Data on Markers of Inflammation

Several studies have examined the effect of omalizumab on inflammatory markers, as indicators of changes in airway biology on therapy. A pilot study of 19 patients found that peripheral blood and sputum eosinophil counts were reduced with omalizumab, yet the degree of reduction did not significantly differ from the placebo group.[9] In a similar experiment, Noga and colleagues found a significant attenuation of peripheral blood eosinophil counts at 16 and 52 weeks of therapy (versus placebo).[10] Further evidence suggests that therapy effects a statistically significant decrease in circulating IL-13 levels.[7] A study of mild asthmatic individuals has shown that omalizumab can reduce sputum eosinophil counts, eosinophilic infiltration of epithelial and submucosal compartments on bronchial biopsy specimens, and circulating IgE levels (to less than 21 IU/mL). Additionally, biopsy samples showed a marked reduction (nearly 80%) of $Fc\varepsilon RI^+$ cells, which correlated directly with the reduction of biopsy-expressed IgE.[7] Djukanovic and associates also found a substantial reduction in cell-surface IL-4—a mediator generated by Th2 cells after allergen exposure that stimulates IgE production by B cells.[11] This suggests that omalizumab may exert its clinical effects via an adjunct pathway that modulate Th2 activity, antigen presentation, and IL-4 production.

Administration and Dosing

Omalizumab is FDA approved for patients 12 years of age or older with moderate-to-severe persistent asthma not controlled with the use of inhaled corticosteroids, who have a positive skin test or in vitro reactivity to a perennial aeroallergen. Additionally, subjects should have a total IgE level between 30 IU and 700 IU and not weigh more than 150 kg. An analysis of previous trials by Bousquet and associates found that subjects with an FEV_1 less than 60% who use emergency care and receive high doses of ICS would derive the greatest clinical benefit from therapy.[3] The dosing of omalizumab is standardized and can be calculated by matching an individual's weight with the IgE level obtained before initiating therapy (Fig. 31-6).

As there is no need to adjust dosages during therapy, periodic monitoring of IgE levels is unnecessary. Total free IgE levels should fall to less than 5% of baseline (0.016 mg/kg of omalizumab per IU/mL per 4 weeks), but may increase secondary to the formation of IgE-omalizumab complexes.[3] Currently, omalizumab is supplied only through five specialty pharmacies. Prior authorization must be obtained, either with or without the involvement of a particular pharmacy, and encompasses a statement of medical necessity.

The preparation of each omalizumab dose has also been standardized. A single vial contains 150 mg of recombinant monoclonal IgG antibody. While dosages peak at 375 mg, no single subcutaneous injection can exceed 150 mg; each vial must be injected separately and reconstituted just before use. A single vial costs approximately $470; yearly expenses range from $6110 to $36,600.[3]

Pre-treatment serum IgE (IU/mL)	Q4-Week dosing table Body weight (kg)			
	30–60	>60–70	>70–90	>90–150
≥30–100	150 mg	150 mg	150 mg	300 mg
>100–200	300 mg	300 mg	300 mg	SEE Q2-WEEK DOSING TABLE
>200–300	300 mg	SEE Q2-WEEK DOSING TABLE	SEE Q2-WEEK DOSING TABLE	SEE Q2-WEEK DOSING TABLE
>300–400	SEE Q2-WEEK DOSING TABLE	SEE Q2-WEEK DOSING TABLE	SEE Q2-WEEK DOSING TABLE	SEE Q2-WEEK DOSING TABLE
>400–500	SEE Q2-WEEK DOSING TABLE	SEE Q2-WEEK DOSING TABLE	SEE Q2-WEEK DOSING TABLE	SEE Q2-WEEK DOSING TABLE
>500–600	SEE Q2-WEEK DOSING TABLE	SEE Q2-WEEK DOSING TABLE	SEE Q2-WEEK DOSING TABLE	SEE Q2-WEEK DOSING TABLE

Pre-treatment serum IgE (IU/mL)	Q2-Week dosing table Body weight (kg)			
	30–60	>60–70	>70–90	>90–150
≥30–100	SEE Q4-WEEK DOSING TABLE	SEE Q4-WEEK DOSING TABLE	SEE Q4-WEEK DOSING TABLE	225 mg
>100–200	SEE Q4-WEEK DOSING TABLE	225 mg	225 mg	300 mg
>200–300	225 mg	300 mg	300 mg	DO NOT DOSE
>300–400	300 mg	150 mg	375 mg	DO NOT DOSE
>400–500	300 mg	375 mg	DO NOT DOSE	DO NOT DOSE
>500–600	375 mg	DO NOT DOSE	DO NOT DOSE	DO NOT DOSE

Figure 31-6 Omalizumab dosing is standardized to a pretreatment IgE determination and patient weight. In certain cases, administration is not recommended.

Safety Data

A meta-analysis of 3041 patients involved in eight phase II and III studies revealed similar numbers of adverse events between omalizumab and treatment groups.[1] Most events were either mild or moderate severity, with comparable frequencies of voluntary withdrawals between groups (0.6% of treated patients versus 1.1% of placebo patients). Cases of serum sickness or serumlike sickness syndrome were not reported in groups receiving the drug. While an expert panel did not believe that omalizumab was associated with development of malignant neoplasms, their incidence was doubled in patients on therapy (0.5% in treated groups versus 0.2% in placebo groups).

Anaphylactoid reactions are rare and have been observed in only three patients (0.1%) of the major clinical trials. Patients must be monitored carefully after the total dose is administered and typical medications needed to treat anaphylaxis should be immediately available. Subjects are generally observed for 2 hours after the initial dose, and for 1 hour after subsequent doses. Injection site reactions are not uncommon, but typically occur within an hour of administration, and become less frequent/intense with further dosing.[3]

Some concern arose over the potential for omalizumab-treated patients to be at an increased risk for malignant neoplasms: 20 out of 4127 (0.5%) developed malignant neoplasms, versus 5 of 2236 (0.2%) controls. Several different types of neoplasms were observed, with only one case of non-Hodgkins lymphoma in the treated group. An independent panel reviewed these data and concluded that treatment was not associated with neoplastic potential, and that there was no significant difference in the rates of malignant neoplasms between the treated and untreated groups.[1] However, the manufacturer has partnered with the FDA to monitor 5000 patients receiving Xolair in a 5-year study slated to end in 2011.

PART II: SODIUM CROMOGLYCATE

Sodium cromoglycate (SCG) was introduced as an asthma therapy during the 1960s; numerous clinical trials have scrutinized its efficacy. Our understanding of the anti-inflammatory properties of SCG has evolved considerably and now encompasses several diverse mechanisms. Of prime interest in the treatment of allergic asthma is SCG's ability to inhibit IgE antibody synthesis and to stabilize mast cell membranes, thereby inhibiting degranulation.[12] More recent work has demonstrated that SCG is able to block the release of mediators from several other cell types, including eosinophils, neutrophils, monocytes, alveolar macrophages, and lymphocytes.[12] Overall, SCG appears to affect a diversity of cells involved in the allergic inflammatory cascade by pathways that include the alteration of leukocyte-specific adhesion molecules, modulation of neurogenic responses to tachykinins, and regulation of calcium gating mechanisms.[12]

Studies from the United Kingdom have shown that sodium cromoglycate can be effective in controlling symptoms in nearly 70% of adult and pediatric asthmatic patients.[13] Studies of lung deposition support metered dose actuation as an effective form of delivery: a 5-mg inhaled dose is capable of depositing 0.88 mg of drug into the lung, and up to 1.13 mg if a spacer is used.

Similarly, Cockcroft and colleagues have shown that SCG can prevent increases in airway hyperresponsiveness and can attenuate late asthmatic reactions in response to allergen challenges.[14] Chronic cough induced by angiotensin-converting enzyme inhibitors and capsaicin has also been attenuated with regular use of SCG as two actuations of a 5-mg metered-dose inhaler per day.

Further trials have reaffirmed SCG's place as an adjunct to other current asthma therapies. Evidence has shown that regular SCG use can increase peak expiratory flow rates (by up to 30%), reduce day and night symptom severity, and improve lung function. Long-term studies in children have shown consistent lung function improvements in some patients.

In addition to utility as an asthma-controller medication, a single dose of SCG can attenuate bronchospasm when taken 20 minutes before exercise or cold air exposure. The benefits of inhalation have a mean duration of 2 hours, and are independent of a bronchodilatory response.[12] Those who engage in competitive sports or in exercise of long duration may safely use SCG every 2 hours. However, the combination of SCG with a traditional beta$_2$-agonist bronchodilator is superior to either therapy alone.

Some sources question SCG's place in current asthma control therapy, asserting that it has not uniformly shown benefit. While many pillar studies do not meet inclusion criteria for modern meta-analyses, the burden of evidence indicates that SCG is relevant and efficacious even today. While it is indicated as an alternative to daily inhaled corticosteroids in step two therapy for mild persistent asthma, steroids are the mainstay of treatment. SCG, when used, is often an adjunct to inhaled steroids and other controller medications for chronic symptoms.

REFERENCES

1. Brownell J, Casale TB: Anti-IgE therapy. Immunol Allergy Clin North Am 2004;24:551–568.
2. Jonkers RE, van der Zee JS: Anti-IgE and other new immunomodulation-based therapies for allergic asthma. Neth J Med 2005;63:121–128.
3. Marcus P: Incorporating anti-IgE (omalizumab) therapy into pulmonary medicine practice. Chest 2006;129:466–474.
4. Holgate S, Casale T, Wenzel S, et al: The anti-inflammatory effects of omalizumab confirm the central role of IgE in allergic inflammation. J Allergy Clin Immunol 2005;115:459–465.
5. Milgrom H, Berger W, Nayak A: Treatment of childhood asthma with anti-immunoglobulin E antibody (omalizumab). Pediatrics 2001;108(2): E36.
6. Corren J, Casale T, Deniz Y, Ashby M: Omalizumab, a recombinant humanized anti-IgE antibody, reduces asthma-related emergency room visits and hospitalizations in patients with allergic asthma. J Allergy Clin Immunol 2003;111(1):87–90.
7. Holgate ST, Djukanović R, Casale T, Bousquet J: Anti-immunoglobulin E treatment with omalizumab in allergic diseases: an update on anti-inflammatory activity and clinical efficacy. Clin Exp Allergy 2005;35:408–416.
8. Holgate S, Chuchalin A, Herbert J, et al: Omalizumab, a novel therapy for severe allergic asthma. Eur Respir J 2001;18(Suppl 33): AbstP346.
9. Fahy JV, Fleming HE, Wong HH, et al: The effect of an anti-IgE monoclonal antibody on the early- and late-phase responses to allergen inhalation in asthmatic subjects. Am J Respir Crit Care Med 1997;155(6):1828–1834.
10. Noga O, Hanf G, Kunkel G: Immunological and clinical changes in allergic asthmatics following treatment with omalizumab. Int Arch Allergy Immunol 2003;131(1):46–52.
11. Djukanović R, Wilson SJ, Kraft M, et al: Effects of treatment with anti-immunoglobulin E antibody omalizumab on airway inflammation in allergic asthma. Am J Respir Crit Care Med 2004;170(6):583–593.
12. Storms W, Kaliner MA: Cromolyn sodium: fitting an old friend into current asthma treatment. J Asthma 2005;42:79–89.
13. Holgate ST: Inhaled sodium cromoglycate. Respir Med 1996;90:387–390.
14. Cockcroft DW, Murdock KY: Comparative effects of inhaled salbutamol, sodium cromoglycate, and beclomethasone dipropionate on allergen-induced early asthmatic responses, late asthmatic responses, and increased bronchial responsiveness to histamine. J Allergy Clin Immunol 1987;79(5):734–740.

Immunosuppression and Immunomodulation

CHAPTER
32

C. J. Corrigan

CLINICAL PEARLS

- Most asthmatic individuals are sufficiently well controlled by currently available inhaled and add-on therapies.

- Approximately 10% are not and suffer greatly from persistent symptoms, poor quality of life and the unwanted effects of therapy, particularly those of systemic corticosteroids.

- Immunosuppressive therapy for asthma is of limited clinical application because many patients do not respond, many therapies reduce systemic steroid requirement but do not improve lung function, and there are many contraindications to the use of specific drugs and worries about their longer term benefits and short- and long-term unwanted effects.

- Anticytokine therapies, with notable exceptions, have also so far been generally disappointing and are expensive and cumbersome to administer.

- Failure in this field has highlighted our poor understanding of the relationship between asthmatic inflammation and clinical symptoms and highlights the need for better understanding of this critical relationship.

Asthma affects approximately 12% of children and 6% of adults, with an overall prevalence of 6% (over 3 million patients) in the United Kingdom and many more worldwide. Inhaled corticosteroids form the mainstay of asthma therapy for most patients. Topical corticosteroids are relatively free of unwanted effects and offer a very favorable benefit/risk ratio. Mortality from asthma is relatively low (1200 deaths in the United Kingdom in 2000), but considerable morbidity arises from disease in that a minority of patients have symptoms inadequately controlled by conventional therapy (inhaled corticosteroids, long-acting beta$_2$-agonists, leukotriene receptor antagonists, and theophylline derivatives), even when optimal delivery has been ensured, compliance has been verified, and the effects of other exacerbating factors minimized. In these patients, oral glucocorticoids are often employed, but even then patients may remain symptomatic and also frequently suffer from unwanted effects of therapy. Estimates from studies of prescribing practice in the United Kingdom suggest that approximately 6% of asthmatic individuals are receiving therapy (Fig. 32-1) that would place them at steps 4 or 5 of the British Thoracic Society asthma treatment guidelines (patients taking regular systemic or inhaled corticosteroids at high dosage with other medications). Although in a minority, these patients account for the majority of the costs of asthma care because of their frequent need for physician consultations and emergency and inpatient care. For such patients, new approaches to therapy are urgently required.

ASTHMA PATHOGENESIS AND THE EVOLUTION OF IMMUNOSUPPRESSIVE THERAPY

Asthma is associated with chronic, cell-mediated inflammation of the bronchial mucosa in which cytokines and chemokines play a critical role. Activated T cells are a prominent source of these mediators (Fig. 32-2) but some are produced by granulocytes such as eosinophils and mast cells, as well as structural cells of the bronchial mucosa (epithelial and endothelial cells, fibroblasts and smooth muscle cells). Evidence suggests that corticosteroids ameliorate asthma at least partly through inhibition of T cells and elaboration of their cytokine products. There has been a great deal of research directed at why T cells in some asthmatic individuals are relatively resistant to glucocorticoid inhibition, but it will be some time before this research evolves toward new approaches to therapy. In the meantime, other T-cell immunomodulatory agents have been investigated for their possible therapeutic effects in asthma. Since many of these agents have potentially serious unwanted effects, attention has generally been focused on those asthmatic patients who continue to have severe disease despite maximal topical and additional continuous systemic

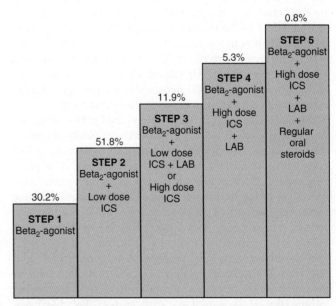

Figure 32-1 Proportions of adult asthmatic patients in the United Kingdom at each step of the UK (British Thoracic Society) asthma therapy guidelines. *(Data from Neville RG, Pearson MG, Richards N, et al: A cost analysis of asthma prescribing in the UK. Eur Respir J 1999;14:605–609.)*

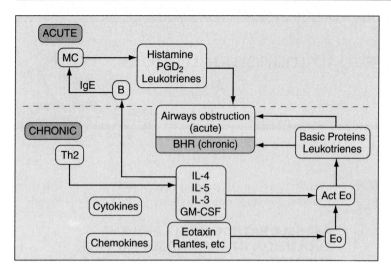

Figure 32-2 Overview of asthma pathogenesis. In all asthmatic individuals, cytokines and chemokines from Th2 T cells and other cells control the influx and activation of effector granulocytes such as eosinophils (Eo, Act Eo) into the bronchial mucosa. Direct effects of these cytokines and certain products of the granulocytes (such as eosinophil basic proteins and leukotrienes) are thought to cause chronic bronchial hyperresponsiveness (BHR), although the precise mechanisms are unclear. In atopic asthmatic individuals, allergen exposure may in addition cause acute release of mediators (histamine, prostanoids, leukotrienes) from IgE-sensitized mast cells (MC) causing acute exacerbation of disease on the background of T-cell–mediated BHR. There is a link between these mechanisms in that the Th2 cytokines IL-4 and IL-13 are responsible for switching of B lymphocytes (B) to IgE synthesis, thus initiating the inappropriate IgE response that characterizes atopy.

corticosteroid therapy (that is, in those patients in whom the benefit/risk ratio of therapy is most likely to be acceptable).

Gold Salts and Methotrexate

Evaluation of these drugs for asthma was originally based on empirical observation of their anti-inflammatory effects in diseases such as rheumatoid arthritis, rather than cogent hypotheses regarding their possible mechanisms of action. It has since become clear, however, that both drugs may exert inhibitory effects on T cells.

Actions of gold salts, which may be relevant to a corticosteroid-sparing effect in asthma, are ill defined, but may include inhibition of T-cell proliferation, interleukin (IL)-5-mediated prolongation of eosinophil survival, immunoglobulin E (IgE)-mediated degranulation of mast cells and basophils, and leukotriene production by granulocytes. Some of these effects may be secondary to inhibition by gold salts of pro-inflammatory transcriptional regulatory proteins, in particular NFκB. Two double-blind, placebo-controlled parallel group studies in which oral gold salts were administered for 6 months showed a modest but significant glucocorticoid-sparing effect of the therapy as compared with placebo (Fig. 32-3). Lung function was not improved, and additional anti-asthma therapy not reduced. Not all of the patients showed a significant response. Unwanted effects of oral gold salt therapy include dermatitis, hepatic dysfunction, proteinuria, interstitial pneumonitis, and, rarely, blood dyscrasias.

Methotrexate is a folic acid analogue used at low dosage for its anti-inflammatory activity in an increasing variety of chronic diseases. It exerts a delayed but sustained therapeutic effect even with intermittent, weekly dosage regimens. This probably reflects its accumulation in cells as polyglutamate complexes, resulting in accumulation of S-adenosyl methionine and adenosine, both of which are inhibitory to T-cell function. Indeed, it has recently been shown that methotrexate therapy increases the sensitivity of blood T cells from oral corticosteroid–dependent asthmatic patients to corticosteroid inhibition (Fig. 32-4). Several blinded, placebo-controlled trials of methotrexate therapy in severe, oral corticosteroid–dependent asthma (Fig. 32-5), as well as a meta-analysis (Fig. 32-6) suggested an oral corticosteroid–sparing effect (overall 20%, but only in about 60% of responding patients) of concomitant methotrexate therapy if used for a minimum of 3 to 6 months,

with no significant improvement in lung function. A more exacting Cochrane analysis of these trials concluded, however, that existing trial data do not justify the premise that methotrexate is corticosteroid sparing. The most serious potential unwanted effect of methotrexate therapy is cumulative hepatic toxicity and hepatic fibrosis, with isolated reports of deaths from opportunistic infections and pneumonitis.

Cyclosporin A

Cyclosporin A (CsA) is a lipophilic, cyclic undecapeptide derived from the fungus *Tolypocladium inflatum*. In a complex with the cytoplasmic binding protein, cyclophilin, it inhibits calcineurin-mediated dephosphorylation and nuclear translocation of the cytoplasmic subunit of the T-cell transcriptional activator NF-AT, thus inhibiting T-cell proliferation and cytokine production relatively specifically (Fig. 32-7). It has been widely used to prevent allograft rejection. Investigation of the effects of cyclosporin A in asthma was probably the first trial of immunosuppressive therapy in

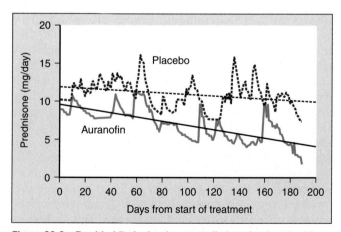

Figure 32-3 Double-blind, placebo-controlled study of oral gold (auranofin) therapy in corticosteroid-dependent asthma. Thirty-two patients were treated with auranofin (3 mg twice daily) and oral prednisone tapered from 12 weeks if disease remained stable. The total prednisone reduction (mean 4 mg/day) achieved in the actively treated group was significantly greater (0.3 mg/day) than that achieved in the placebo-treated group, with fewer exacerbations. *(Data from Nierop G, Gijzel WP, Bel EH, et al: Auranofin in the treatment of steroid dependent asthma: a double blind study. Thorax 1992;47:349–354.)*

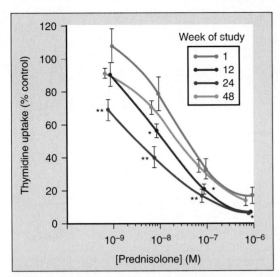

Figure 32-4 **Methotrexate therapy of corticosteroid-dependent asthmatic patients increases susceptibility of their blood T cells to corticosteroid inhibition.** The figure shows concentration-response curves for prednisolone-induced inhibition of lectin-induced T-cell proliferation (measured by tritiated thymidine uptake) at 1, 12, and 28 weeks of therapy with methotrexate 15 mg intramuscularly, and again at 40 weeks, 12 weeks after withdrawal of methotrexate. T cells became progressively more senitive to the inhibitory effects of methotrexate over the 28-week period, with reversal when the methotrexate was withdrawn. *(Data from Corrigan CJ, Shiner R, Shakur BH, Ind PW: Methotrexate therapy in asthma increases T cell susceptibility to corticosteroid inhibition. Clin Exp Allergy 2003;33:1090–1096.)*

asthma based on a rational knowledge of the mechanism of action of the immunosuppressive agent.

Two blinded, placebo-controlled trials in severe, oral corticosteroid–dependent asthmatic patients together showed that concomitant CsA therapy improved lung function while reducing oral prednisolone requirements (Fig. 32-8). As with methotrexate, not all patients showed a significant response.

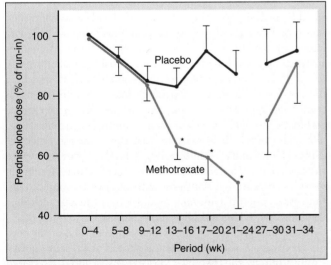

Figure 32-5 **Double-blind, placebo-controlled study of methotrexate in corticosteroid-dependent asthma.** Sixty-nine patients were treated with intramuscular methotrexate 15 mg weekly or placebo and oral corticosteroid tapered every 4 weeks if lung function did not deteriorate. After 34 weeks of treatment, mean starting prednisolone dosages could be reduced by a significantly greater percentage in the active (50%) as compared with the placebo-treated (14%) group, but the reduction was not sustained when the treatment was discontinued. *(Data from Shiner RJ, Nunn AJ, Chung KF, Geddes DM: Randomised, double-blind, placebo-controlled trial of methotrexate in steroid-dependent asthma. Thorax 1990;336:137–140.)*

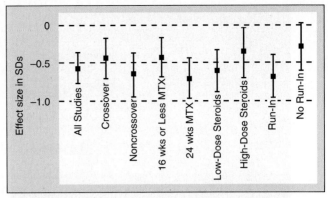

Figure 32-6 **Effect size (in standard deviations, with bars showing 95% confidence intervals) of all double-blind trials (parallel group or crossover) of methotrexate therapy in reducing oral corticosteroid requirement in severe, corticosteroid-dependent asthmatic patients.** *(Data from Marin MG: Low dose methotrexate spares steroid usage in steroid-dependent chronic asthmatic patients: a meta-analysis. Chest 1997;112:29–33.)*

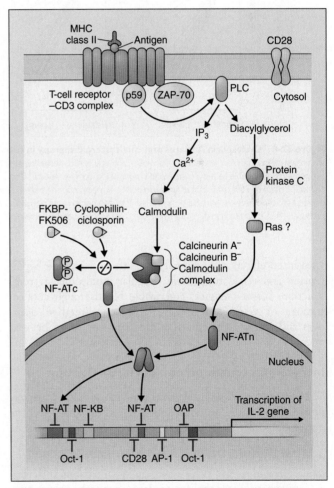

Figure 32-7 **Mechanism of action of cyclosporin A and FK506 (tacrolimus).** These agents bind to specific binding proteins in the cytoplasm of T cells, and in doing so block the formation of the calcineurin/calmodulin complex which is necessary for phosphorylation of the cytoplasmic portion of the transcriptional regulatory factor Nuclear Factor of Activated T cells (NF-ATc), which in turn allows it to migrate into the cell nucleus. There, it binds to its nuclear portion (NF-ATn) and the complex binds to promoter sites on the interleukin-2 (IL-2) gene, thus initiating its transcription. IL-2 is an essential growth factor for T cells, and so these drugs block the initiation of T-cellular proliferation. *(Adapted from Schreiber SL, Crabtree GR: The mechanism of action of cyclosporin A and FK506. Immunol Today 1992;13:136–142.)*

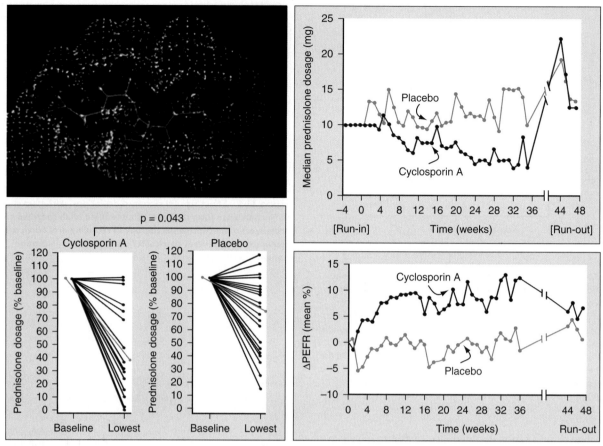

Figure 32-8 Cyclosporin A spares oral corticosteroid therapy in severe, corticosteroid-dependent asthma. Thirty-nine patients were randomized to receive cyclosporin A or placebo for 36 weeks, and oral corticosteroid tapered at 2-week intervals if disease remained stable or improved. Patients receiving cyclosporin A were able to reduce initial oral prednisolone dosages (mean 10 to 3.5 mg/day, 62%) to a significantly greater extent than those receiving placebo (10 to 7.5 mg/day, 25%) (*top right of figure*). In addition, mean morning peak expiratory flow rate (PEFR) improved in the actively treated group (*bottom right*). The effect of cyclosporin A was variable between patients, and not all responded (*bottom left*). *(From Lock SH, Kay AB, Barnes NC: Double-blind, placebo-controlled study of cyclosporin A as a corticosteroid-sparing agent in corticosteroid-dependent asthma. Am J Respir Crit Care Med 1996;153:509–514.)*

Unwanted effects of low-dosage CsA therapy include hypertension and renal impairment. Regular monitoring of renal function, blood pressure, and whole blood trough concentrations of CsA is necessary. Lymphoproliferative disorders and serious opportunistic infections appear to be very uncommon.

Intravenous Immunoglobulin (IVIG) Therapy

Therapy with pooled intravenous immunoglobulin, originally designed to restore immune deficiency, also appears to have immunomodulatory effects in diseases involving immune effector mechanisms. In a blinded, parallel group study of oral corticosteroid–dependent asthmatic patients, patients were randomized to receive IVIG 2 g/kg, 1 g/kg, or albumin (placebo) 2 g intravenously monthly for a total of 6 months (seven infusions). During therapy, oral prednisone requirements were reduced to an almost identical extent (33% to 39%) in all three groups, with no significant differences in changes in symptoms, lung function, and the frequency of disease exacerbations. In a second, similar blinded trial, treatment of patients with both IVIG and placebo allowed significant reduction in oral prednisone dosages, which was significantly greater in the IVIG-treated group when only those asthmatic individuals on relatively high initial dosages of oral prednisone were included

in the analysis. Another double-blind, placebo-controlled study of IVIG therapy in severe childhood asthma failed to show any benefit of IVIG over placebo in terms of changes in symptoms and lung function. The possible mechanisms by which IVIG therapy could exert a beneficial effect in asthma are not clear. Some of the benefits may result from immunoglobulin replacement itself, since a proportion of chronic asthmatic patients have depressed serum IgG concentrations, although there is little evidence that this results in defective humoral immunity. Additionally, IVIG has been shown to increase T-cell susceptibility to glucocorticoid inhibition in vitro, to abrogate IgE synthesis by B cells in vitro, and to contain other potential immunomodulatory products including soluble CD4, CD8, and HLA molecules and cytokines.

In summary, however, the evidence that IVIG is of any benefit in corticosteroid-dependent asthma is at present equivocal. In addition, the therapy is very expensive and is associated with a high incidence of unpleasant urticarial and anaphylactic reactions, as well as fever and aseptic meningitis.

NEW IMMUNOSUPPRESSIVE DRUGS

Tacrolimus (FK506) is a macrolide derived from the soil organism *Streptomyces tsukudaiensis*, which, despite having a different structure from CsA, similarly inhibits NF-AT activation. Its increased potency may be outweighed by similarly increased toxicity.

Sirolimus (rapamycin) is another macrolide derived from *Streptomyces hygroscopius*. It has a fundamentally different inhibitory action on T cells, since it inhibits IL-2 signaling at least partly by inhibiting phosphorylation/activation of the kinase p70 S6 (p70^{S6k}), and by inhibiting the enzymatic activity of the cyclin-dependent kinase cdk2-cyclin E complex.

Other new immunomodulatory drugs, the inhibitory actions of which are relatively specific for T cells, continue to appear, including brequinar sodium and mycophenolate mofetil (inhibitors of de novo synthesis of pyrimidines and purines respectively, particularly in T cells), leflunomide, and the napthopyrans. Whether or not these drugs will offer opportunities for the therapy of severe asthma with a more favorable benefit/risk ratio remains to be seen. One new immunosuppressive agent, suplatast tosilate, appears to inhibit the production of asthma-relevant cytokines relatively selectively, and early studies suggest clinical benefit in asthma.

CYTOKINE-DIRECTED THERAPY IN ASTHMA

T helper 2 (Th2) lymphocytes are thought to play a key role in asthma pathogenesis since they are a principal source of asthma-relevant cytokines (see Fig. 32-2). Therapeutic strategies directed toward inhibition of Th2 cytokines would thus seem to offer an attractive immunomodulatory strategy for asthma (Table 32-1). Alternatively, because a range of Th1 cytokines are inhibitory to the development of Th2 T cells, or antagonize the actions of Th2 cytokines on target pro-inflammatory leukocytes, therapy with key Th1 cytokines may also be effective in asthma (see Table 32-1).

Inhibition of Th2 and Other Cytokines

Of the Th2 cytokines, IL-5 has been regarded as of particular importance because it is the only cytokine that exerts

Table 32-1
CYTOKINE-DIRECTED THERAPEUTIC STRATEGIES IN ASTHMA

Inhibition of Proinflammatory Cytokines	Therapy with Inhibitory Cytokines
IL-5	IL-10
IL-4	IL-12
IL-13	Interferon-α/γ
IL-9	IL-18
IL-25	IL-23
TNF-α	

IL, interleukin; TNF, tumor necrosis factor.

its actions specifically on eosinophils, increasing their expression of adhesion molecules, priming them for elevated mediator release and selectively prolonging their survival in tissues (all of which may result in the accumulation of eosinophils in the bronchial mucosa, which is one of the most constant features of asthma). In IL-5 gene-deleted mice, eosinophilic responses and concomitant increases in airways hyperresponsiveness in response to allergen priming and challenge are markedly suppressed, without any apparent significant alteration of global T-cell function. Humanized monoclonal antibodies against human IL-5 have been manufactured. A single intravenous infusion of one of these antibodies (mepolizumab) markedly reduced circulating blood eosinophils and greatly reduced eosinophil recruitment to the airways following allergen bronchial challenge in patients with mild asthma (Fig. 32-9). Unfortunately, however, this had no effect on the early- or late-phase bronchoconstrictor responses to allergen challenge or on basal bronchial hyperresponsiveness (see Fig. 32-9). More prolonged studies on patients with moderate to severe asthma were similarly disappointing in terms of improvements in asthma symptoms or lung function. A biopsy

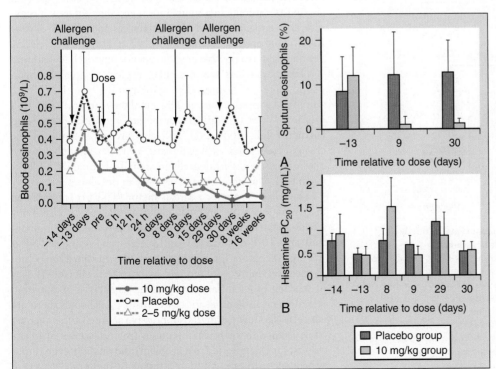

Figure 32-9 Effect of an anti-IL-5 blocking monoclonal antibody (mepolizumab) on the response to allergen bronchial challenge of atopic asthmatics. *Patients were given single infusions of antibody (10 mg/kg or 2.5 mg/kg) or placebo and blood eosinophil counts measured in the ensuing 16 weeks. Treatment with the antibody greatly reduced blood and induced sputum eosinophil counts before and after challenge but did not affect the magnitudes of the early- and late-phase bronchoconstrictor responses to challenge or associated changes in bronchial hyperresponsiveness. (Data from Leckie MJ, ten Brinke A, Khan J, et al: Effects of an interleukin-5 blocking monoclonal antibody on eosinophils, airway hyperresponsiveness and the late asthmatic response. Lancet 2000;356:2144–2148.)*

study suggested that, while anti-IL-5 antibody profoundly reduced circulating eosinophils, it was less effective in removing eosinophils from the bronchial mucosa (Fig. 32-10). There are various possible interpretations of these studies. They may mean that granulocytes such as eosinophils do not play as critical a role in asthma pathogenesis as was thought, but since current strategies have not been effective in removing eosinophils entirely from the bronchial mucosa, this conclusion must be guarded. An alternative view is that, until a strategy is uncovered that completely removes eosinophils from the airways, the case for their noninvolvement in asthma remains

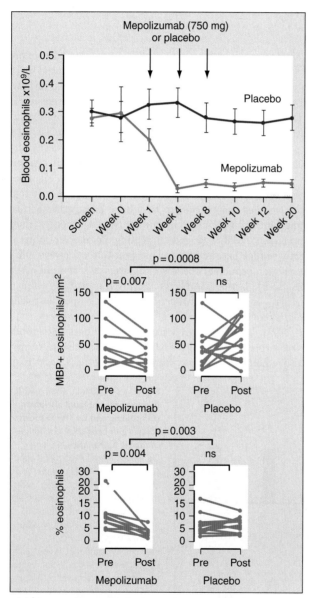

Figure 32-10   Effects of an anti-IL-5 monoclonal antibody (mepolizumab) on airways eosinophils in asthmatic individuals. Mepolizumab (750 mg) or placebo was infused on three occasions separated by 4 weeks into a group of asthmatic individuals, with fiber-optic bronchoscopy beforehand and 4 weeks after the final infusion. Compared with placebo, mepolizumab greatly reduced blood eosinophils (*top*) and significantly reduced, but did not abolish eosinophils in the bronchial mucosa and bronchoalveolar lavage fluid (*bottom*). (*Data from Flood-Page PT, Menzies-Gow AN, Kay AB, Robinson DS: Eosinophil's role remains uncertain as anti-interleukin-5 only partially depletes numbers in asthmatic airway. Am J Respir Crit Care Med 2003;167:199–204.*)

unproven. Whatever the case, these observations have at least temporarily quenched enthusiasm for further evaluation of anti-IL-5 strategies.

IL-4, another Th2 cytokine, is one of only two cytokines (the other being IL-13) that causes switching of B lymphocytes to IgE synthesis and is therefore implicated in the pathogenesis of the inappropriate production of allergen-specific IgE that characterizes atopy. IL-4 is also involved in recruitment of eosinophils to the airways in asthma and acts in an autocrine fashion further to promote the differentiation of Th2 lymphocytes. Soluble, humanized IL-4 receptors (altrakincept), administered by nebulization, have been tested in clinical trials and have been shown to prevent deterioration in lung function induced by withdrawal of corticosteroids in patients with moderately severe asthma, but further, prolonged studies were more disappointing and this strategy is currently also not being pursued.

There is increasing evidence that certain cytokines may cause airway changes in asthma independently of their effects on pro-inflammatory leukocytes such as eosinophils. IL-13 is one such cytokine. In addition to having a range of effects in common with IL-4, since it shares a surface receptor, IL-4Rα, with the latter cytokine, when selectively overexpressed in the airways of mice it causes many of the features associated with airways remodeling, such as mucous hyperplasia and laydown of new extracellular matrix proteins. Deletion of the IL-13 gene in mice prevents development of airways hyperresponsiveness following allergen sensitization and challenge despite the infiltration of eosinophils (another effect of IL-13 is to increase the production of eosinophil-attracting chemokines such as eotaxin by airways epithelial cells). Such observations are providing increasing support for the concept that cytokines may directly cause many changes characteristic of asthmatic airways inflammation without the need for involvement of cells such as eosinophils, which were previously thought to be necessary for such changes. Apart from IL-4Rα, IL-13 has two other specific receptors named IL-13Rα1 and IL-13Rα2. The latter receptor also exists naturally in a soluble form and may act as a "decoy" receptor, scavenging and thus inhibiting the effects of free IL-13. Humanized, soluble IL-13Rα2 is currently in clinical development as a possible new therapeutic approach for asthma.

Other cytokines are of similar interest as possible therapeutic targets in asthma. The cytokines IL-9 and IL-25 both amplify the production of Th2 cytokines. In addition, IL-9 promotes mast cell differentiation and mediator release and augments IgE production, and also promotes some of the changes associated with asthmatic airways remodeling when overexpressed experimentally in animals. Humanized, blocking anti-IL-9 antibodies are currently in development.

The cytokine tumor necrosis factor (TNF)-α is expressed in asthmatic airways and may play a pivotal role in amplifying a wide range of inflammatory responses. A blocking, humanized anti-TNF-α antibody (infliximab) and soluble TNF-α "decoy" receptors (etanercept) have shown remarkable (not to mention unprecedented and unexpected) clinical efficacy in treating other inflammatory diseases such as rheumatoid arthritis and inflammatory bowel disease, although there are concerns about the immunosuppressive actions of this therapy on resistance to microbial infections (recrudescence of tuberculosis, for example, is a real problem) and possibly even tumor surveillance. In one study, treatment of moderate to severe

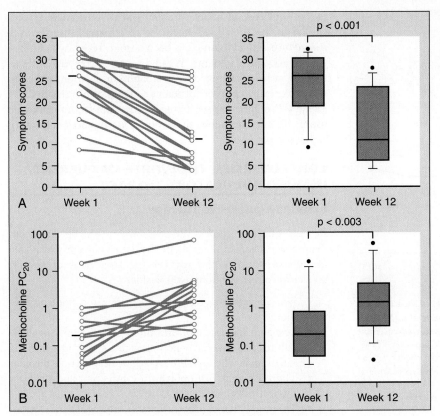

Figure 32-11 Effect of TNF-α blockade in asthma. Seventeen severe asthmatic patients were treated for 12 weeks with the soluble TNF-α receptor/IgG₁Fc fusion protein etanercept in an open-label study. Etanercept treatment was associated with significantly reduced symptoms and bronchial hyperresponsiveness. *(Data from Howarth PH, Babu KS, Arshad HS, et al: Tumour necrosis factor (TNF-alpha) as a novel therapeutic target in symptomatic corticosteroid dependent asthma. Thorax 2006;61:1012–1018.)*

asthmatic individuals with etanercept 25 mg subcutaneously twice weekly for 12 weeks produced impressive improvements in symptoms and reductions in bronchial hyperresponsiveness (Fig. 32-11) to a degree approaching that expected with systemic corticosteroid therapy. Anti-TNF-α therapies thus seem to hold considerable promise, despite their potential unwanted effects. Because these therapies have to be administered by injection, a search is on for small molecule TNF-α inhibitors. TNF-α-converting enzyme (TACE) is a matrix metalloproteinase-related enzyme required for the release of TNF-α from cell surfaces where it is stored in an extracellular matrix "reservoir." Small molecule TACE inhibitors are currently in development.

Therapy with Potential Anti-asthma Cytokines

Some cytokines inhibit the Th2 cytokine responses of T cells that characterize asthma with varying degrees of specificity. While it may not be possible to administer such cytokines to patients in the long term, it may be possible to develop strategies that increase their release or drugs that activate their particular signaling receptors and pathways.

IL-10 has a number of anti-inflammatory properties that may be relevant to asthma therapy. It is one of the few cytokines the expression of which is enhanced, rather than inhibited, by corticosteroids. It inhibits the function of antigen-presenting cells and impairs their ability to prime T cells for Th2 cytokine release. It also reduces Th2 cytokine production by differentiated Th2 T cells and is thought to be one of the principal effector cytokines that mediate the activity of T regulatory cells. In addition, it exerts inhibitory actions on a range of inflammatory leukocytes such as mast cells and eosinophils. Recombinant human IL-10 has proven effective

in controlling other inflammatory diseases such as inflammatory bowel disease and psoriasis, where it is given as a weekly injection. It is reasonably well tolerated, although hematological unwanted effects have been noted. With regard to asthma, peripheral blood T cells from clinically corticosteroid resistant, as compared with sensitive severe asthmatic individuals, showed a marked defect in corticosteroid-induced IL-10 production (Fig. 32-12). There is also evidence that IL-10 production plays a role in the well-known synergistic clinical effects of inhaled corticosteroids and long-acting beta-agonists in asthma (Fig. 32-13). These data strongly support a role for IL-10 in regulating asthma severity. Recent studies suggest that the defect in IL-10 production observed in T cells from corticosteroid-resistant asthmatic patients may be overcome by other agents such as vitamin D3, which are known to increase IL-10 production both in vitro and ex vivo. Manipulation of IL-10 production by such relatively innocuous agents, as distinct from therapy with IL-10 itself, offers great promise for future asthma therapy.

IL-12 is a cytokine produced largely by antigen-presenting cells that is a key regulator of Th1 T-cell development. Th1 cytokines, particularly interferon-γ, strongly inhibit Th2 responses. Recombinant human IL-12 has been administered to humans but has a range of toxic effects that are somewhat minimized by slow escalation of the dosage. In a single study on atopic asthmatic individuals (Fig. 32-14), weekly infusions of IL-12 over 4 weeks at escalating dosage caused a progressive fall in circulating eosinophils and also reduced ingress of eosinophils into induced sputum following allergen bronchial challenge. Unfortunately, as with anti-IL-5, there was no evidence of reduction of the early- or late-phase bronchoconstrictor responses to allergen challenge or alteration of the associated increased bronchial hyperresponsiveness. Most of

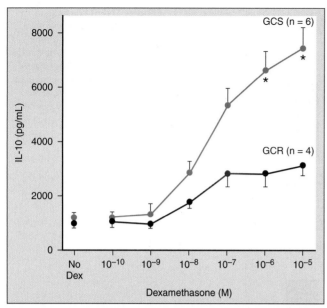

Figure 32-12 Corticosteroid (dexamethasone)-induced IL-10 production is deficient in blood T cells from corticosteroid-resistant (GCS) as compared with resistant (GCR) asthmatic patients. *(Data from Hawrylowicz C, Richards D, Loke TK, et al: A defect in corticosteroid-induced IL-10 production in T lymphocytes from corticosteroid-resistant asthmatic patients. J Allergy Clin Immunol 2002;109:369–370.)*

the patients suffered with malaise and one with cardiac disrhythmia. Consequently, IL-12 is not likely to be used alone as a therapeutic agent for asthma.

Cytokines such as IL-18, which synergizes with IL-12 to enhance the release of Th1 cytokines by T cells, and IL-23, which is related to, and shares some of the effects of IL-12, are also potential therapeutic agents for asthma that are waiting

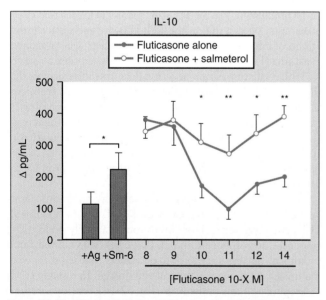

Figure 32-13 Effects of the long-acting beta-agonist salmeterol (SM) and the corticosteroid fluticasone alone and in combination on allergen-stimulated T lymphocytes. Salmeterol alone increased production of the anti-inflammatory cytokine IL-10 and also increased the effect of fluticasone in inducing IL-10 production and regulatory T-cell activity. *(Data from Peek EJ, Richards DF, Faith A, et al: Interleukin-10 secreting "regulatory" T cells induced by glucocorticoids and β2-agonists. Am J Respir Cell Mol Biol 2005;33:105–111.)*

to be explored, although problems with unwanted effects similar to those of IL-12 might be anticipated. Interferon-γ, a signature Th1 cytokine, has been administered by nebulization to asthmatic patients. It did not seem to reduce inflammation, at least as judged by eosinophil infiltration, although it is not certain whether sufficient concentrations reached the airways. Preliminary reports suggest that interferon-α may be useful for the treatment of severe, corticosteroid-refractory asthmatic patients.

CONTROVERSIES: THE WORTH OF CURRENT IMMUNOMODULATORY THERAPY

Immunosuppressive Therapy

In view of these clinical observations, it will be clear that many reservations remain about the use of currently available immunosuppressive therapy for the treatment of severe, corticosteroid-dependent asthma since:

- Not all patients respond, and response cannot be predicted a priori;
- The high incidence of unwanted effects makes it difficult to assess overall benefit/risk ratios even in asthmatic individuals who are able to reduce oral corticosteroids;
- There is a risk of opportunistic infection and (at least theoretically) neoplasia;
- There are many relative or absolute contraindications to therapy, such as pregnancy; and
- There is lack of knowledge about the long-term effects, beneficial or otherwise, of therapy.

Consequently, it is clear that any further investigation of immunosuppressive therapy for asthma should be performed within the confines of a controlled trial. There is an urgent need to produce a global definition of precisely which patients are suitable for such trials, and what constitutes an appropriate trial of therapy. None of the immunosuppressive strategies discussed previously has made a significant impact on the management of severe, oral corticosteroid-dependent asthma, although isolated patients do respond. A large gap in our knowledge is whether or not these drugs do what they are assumed to do in asthma, which is to reduce T-cell activation and cytokine production. Few studies have addressed possible effects of immunosuppressive therapy on the cellular and molecular immunopathology of the disease.

Cytokine-Directed Therapy

The similar general lack of success of cytokine-directed therapy so far in asthma has also been disappointing. The apparent failure of anti-IL-5 (not complete because it has still not been used long enough completely to remove eosinophils from the airways) sent a wave of shock and controversy through the asthma research community, because the eosinophil/IL-5 axis was thought to be fundamental to asthma pathogenesis. These problems have, however, served little more than to highlight the chasm of ignorance about how the cellular, immunological, and structural changes one can observe in asthma are related, if at all, to the clinical manifestations of disease (variable airways obstruction, which may become less reversible, and bronchial hyperresponsiveness). There

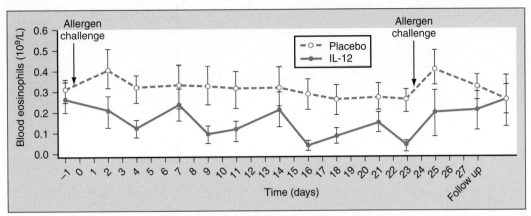

Figure 32-14   Effects of IL-12 on allergen bronchial challenge of mild atopic asthmatic individuals. Mild asthmatic individuals were given increasing weekly injections of 0.1, 0.25, and 0.5 mg/kg or placebo in a double-blind, parallel-group study, with allergen challenge performed beforehand and 24 hours after the final injection. IL-12, compared with placebo, progressively reduced blood, and induced sputum eosinophils after challenge but did not affect the magnitude of the late-phase bronchoconstrictor response or the associated change in bronchial hyperresponsiveness. *(Data from Bryan SA, O'Connor BJ, Matti S, et al: Effects of recombinant interleukin-12 on eosinophils, airway hyperresponsiveness and the late asthmatic response. Lancet 2000;356:2149–2153.)*

is a pressing need to delineate the precise functions of cells and cytokines implicated in asthma pathogenesis, otherwise the success of cytokine-directed strategies (as with TNF-α, perhaps the least "asthma-related" cytokine) will remain serendipitous. It is essential to understand what mechanisms cause irreversible airways obstruction in asthma so that therapy can be directed to these. Specific, cytokine-directed therapies offer perhaps the best chance of "removing particular cytokines from the equation," but owing to the redundancy of cytokine action, and as evidenced by ventures into anticytokine therapy thus far attempted, they may not necessarily offer viable therapeutic solutions.

SUGGESTED READING

Barnes PJ, Chung KF, Page CP: Inflammatory mediators of asthma: an update. Pharmacol Rev 1998;50:515–596.

Corrigan CJ: Asthma refractory to glucocorticoids: the role of newer immunosuppressants. Am J Respir Med 2002;1:47–54.

Cronstein BN: Methotrexate and its mechanism of action. Arthritis Rheum 1996;39:1951–1960.

Davies H, Olson L, Gibson P: Methotrexate as a steroid sparing agent in adult asthma. Cochrane Database Syst Rev 2000(2):CD000391.

Dumont FJ, Su Q: Mechanism of action of the immunosuppressant rapamycin. Life Science 1995;58:373–395.

Eckstein JW, Fung J: A new class of cyclosporin analogues for the treatment of asthma. Expert Opin Investig Drugs 2003;12:647–653.

Hawrylowicz CA, O'Garra A: Potential role of interleukin-10-secreting regulatory T cells in allergy and asthma. Nat Rev Immunol 2005;5:271–283.

Ichinose M, Barnes PJ: Cytokine-directed therapy in asthma. Current Drug Targets Inflamm Allergy 2004;3:263–269.

Ito K, Chung KF, Adcock IM: Update on glucocorticoid action and resistance. J Allergy Clin Immunol 2006;117:522–543.

Woolcock AJ: Steroid resistant asthma: what is the clinical definition? Eur Respir J 1993;6:743–747.

Allergy Immunotherapy

Jeffrey R. Stokes and Thomas B. Casale

- Allergen immunotherapy is the only proven therapy that alters the natural course of allergic disease.

- Allergen immunotherapy is effective for the treatment of allergic rhinitis, allergic asthma, and Hymenoptera allergy.

- Allergen immunotherapy should generally be administered for up to 5 years to attain optimal therapeutic and immunomodulatory effects.

- Allergen immunotherapy should be administered under the direct supervision of health care professionals able to recognize and appropriately treat systemic (anaphylactic) reactions.

Allergic diseases have increased in prevalence over the past 20 years, affecting as many as 40 to 50 million people in the United States. Allergen immunotherapy has been used for over 100 years. Allergen immunotherapy alters the course of allergic diseases through a series of injections of a mixture of extracts composed of clinically relevant allergens. The term *allergen extract* has been replaced by *allergen vaccine* by the World Health Organization. Allergen extract refers to the extract mixture not yet integrated into the vaccine. Once it is incorporated into the vaccine the preferred term is "allergen immunotherapy extract." Other terms used for allergen immunotherapy include hyposensitization, desensitization, allergy shots, or allergy injections.

INDICATIONS

Allergen immunotherapy is used for the treatment of allergic rhinitis, allergic asthma, and stinging insect (Hymenoptera) venom hypersensitivity. The diagnosis of these diseases is made by history and physical exam supported by testing to confirm the presence of allergen-specific immunoglobulin E (IgE) antibodies. Skin testing by prick or intradermal method is the preferred diagnostic method, but in vitro tests such as serological tests for allergen-specific IgE antibody are an alternative, especially when skin testing cannot be performed. In patients with a history consistent with venom allergy but negative skin tests, in vitro testing should be performed to identify the cause. Patients with a history of venom allergy and negative skin tests, but positive serological tests for Hymenoptera allergen–specific IgE antibody, are candidates for immunotherapy. Patients with allergen-specific IgE but no clinical symptoms correlating with the identified allergen are not candidates for allergen immunotherapy.

Candidates for venom or Hymenoptera immunotherapy include all patients who have experienced life-threatening allergic reactions or non–life-threatening systemic reactions to Hymenoptera stings. The risk of anaphylaxis for a venom-allergy patient from an insect sting is greater than the risk of anaphylaxis from immunotherapy. In patients younger than 16 with only urticaria to Hymenoptera stings, immunotherapy is not generally recommended. However, in patients older than 16 with only cutaneous reactions, immunotherapy is a recommended option. Venom immunotherapy is not indicated for patients who have only had local reactions at the stinging site, even large local reactions.

Immunotherapy is also effective for inhalant aeroallergens such as pollen, mold, animal dander, dust mite, and cockroach. Symptomatic patients with allergic rhinitis and asthma despite allergen avoidance and pharmacotherapy are candidates for immunotherapy (Table 33-1). Other candidates include allergic rhinitis or asthma patients having undesirable adverse reactions to medications, or those wishing to reduce or eliminate long-term pharmacotherapy. In addition to reducing symptoms to current allergens, immunotherapy may prevent the development of sensitization to new allergens. In a study of nearly 200 children with allergic rhinitis, treatment with allergen immunotherapy decreased the development of asthma. This was noted both after 3 years of immunotherapy and 7 years after discontinuation of immunotherapy (Fig. 33-1). Food allergy, chronic urticaria/angioedema, and atopic dermatitis are not acceptable indications for allergen immunotherapy. There are limited data to support the use of immunotherapy in patients with atopic dermatitis and aeroallergen sensitivity.

Table 33-1
IMMUNOTHERAPY

Currently indicated	Allergic rhinitis
	Allergic asthma
	Venom allergy
Not indicated	Atopic dermatitis (may be beneficial with concurrent aeroallergen sensitization)*
	Food allergy
	Chronic urticaria
	Chronic angioedema
Relative contraindications	Unstable asthma
	Concurrent use of beta-blockers or ACE inhibitors
	Severe coronary artery disease
	Malignancy
	Unable to communicate clearly (children younger than 5)

Although immunotherapy is not indicated for atopic dermatitis in a specific subset of patients with concurrent aeroallergen sensitization, it may be beneficial.

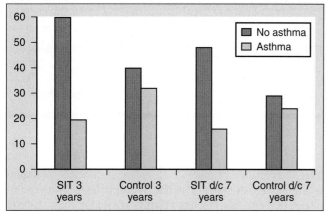

Figure 33-1   Prevention of asthma in children treated for allergic rhinitis with allergen immunotherapy. Children treated for 3 years with immunotherapy had less asthma after the 3 years of therapy (SIT 19/60 patients versus control 32/40) and 7 years later (SIT 16/48 versus control 24/27). *(Data compiled from: Moller C, Dreborg S, Ferdousi HA, et al: Pollen immunotherapy reduces the development of asthma in children with seasonal rhinoconjunctivitis [the PAT-Study]. J Allergy Clin Immunol 2002;109:251–256; and Valovirta E, Jacobsen L, Niggemann B, et al: A 3-year course of subcutaneous specific immunotherapy results in long-term prevention of asthma in children. Ten year follow-up on the PAT-Study. J Allergy Clin Immunol 2006;117:721.)*

MECHANISM

The type I hypersensitivity reaction is the basis of the allergic reaction. The allergen is taken up by antigen-presenting cells, typically dendritic cells. The dendritic cells process and present the antigen to T-lymphocytes. This triggers an "allergic" T-lymphocyte (TH2) response producing interleukin (IL)-4 and IL-5. IL-4 stimulates B lymphocytes to produce IgE while IL-5 stimulates eosinophils. The exact mechanisms of how immunotherapy works are not fully understood, but involve shifting a patient's immune response to an allergen from the predominately "allergic" TH2 to a "nonallergic" T-lymphocyte (TH1) response, producing interferon (IFN)-γ (Fig. 33-2). Allergen immunotherapy has been shown to reduce levels of both IL-4 and IL-5, and increase IFN-γ levels, albeit

inconsistently. What has been consistent is increased production of allergen-specific IL-10, possibly from regulatory T cells. Regulatory T cells can produce transforming growth factor (TGF)-β and IL-10, which cause a shift in allergen-specific IgE to allergen-specific IgG. With allergen immunotherapy, the seasonal increase in allergen-specific IgE is blunted, whereas allergen-specific IgG1 production is increased, initially, but by 2 years of immunotherapy, IgG4 elevation is more pronounced. Efficacy of allergen immunotherapy is not completely dependent on the reduction in specific IgE levels. Periodic skin testing or in vitro IgE antibody measurements are generally not useful in evaluating responses to immunotherapy.

CONTRAINDICATIONS

Relative contraindications for immunotherapy include medical conditions that reduce the patient's ability to survive a serious systemic allergic reaction, such as coronary artery disease or severe asthma (see Table 33-1). Beta-adrenergic blocking agents (including eye drops) may make the treatment of immunotherapy-related systemic reactions more difficult. Despite this, immunotherapy is indicated for patients with life-threatening stinging insect hypersensitivity receiving beta-blockers because the risk of stinging insect allergy is greater than the risk of immunotherapy-related systemic reactions. Allergen immunotherapy should not be initiated in asthmatic patients unless the patient's asthma is relatively stable with pharmacotherapy and their forced expiratory volume in 1 second (FEV_1) is more than 70% of predicted. Patients who are mentally or physically unable to communicate clearly, such as very young children, are not good candidates for immunotherapy, as it may be difficult for them to report early symptoms of a systemic reaction. In addition, patients need to be cooperative and compliant. Pregnancy is not a contraindication for immunotherapy, but by custom immunotherapy is not initiated during pregnancy. If a patient becomes pregnant while already on immunotherapy, the dose is not increased

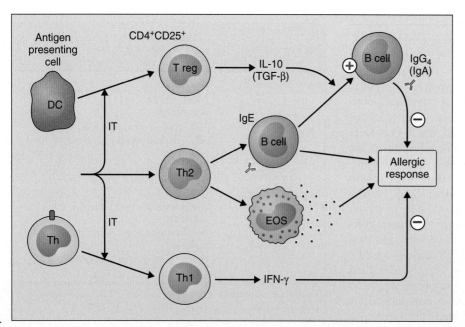

Figure 33-2   Proposed mechanism of immunotherapy. Immunotherapy reduces TH2 responses (IL-4, IL-5) while increasing TH1 responses (IFN-γ). Regulatory T cells seem to play a role via IL-10. *(From Till SJ, Francis JN, Nouri-Aria K, et al: Mechanisms of immunotherapy. J Allergy Clin Immunol 2004;113:1025–1024; permission requested.)*

during the pregnancy but maintained at the current level in an attempt to avoid anaphylactic reactions.

DOSING

Standard allergen immunotherapy is administered as a subcutaneous injection. The allergist/immunologist selects the appropriate allergen extracts based on the patient's clinical history, allergen exposure history, and the results of tests for allergen-specific IgE antibodies to prepare the vaccine. The immunotherapy vaccine should contain only clinically relevant allergens. Standardized extracts should be used, when available, and may be mixed with nonstandardized extracts. Currently the only standardized extracts available are dust mites, grass pollen, cat, and short ragweed. When preparing mixtures of allergen vaccines, the prescribing physician must take into account the cross-reactivity of allergens, the optimal dose of each constituent, and the potential for allergen degradation caused by proteolytic enzymes in the mixture. The highest concentration allergy immunotherapy vial is the "maintenance concentrate" vial. This is used for the "projected effective" dose. The maintenance dose is the dose that best provides therapeutic efficacy without adverse reactions. Thus, the maintenance dose in some cases may not equal the projected effective dose. The maintenance concentrate should be prepared and labeled for each individual patient. The practice of mixing individual antigens in a syringe is not recommended. The efficacy of immunotherapy depends on achieving an optimal therapeutic dose of each allergen extract in the vaccine.

Allergen immunotherapy dosing consists of two treatment phases: the buildup phase and the maintenance phase. The prescribing physician must specify the starting immunotherapy dose, the target maintenance dose, and the immunotherapy buildup schedule. The highest concentration of vaccine that is projected to provide the therapeutically effective dose is called the *maintenance dose* or *concentrate*. In general, the starting immunotherapy dose is 1000- to 10,000-fold less than the maintenance dose. For highly sensitive patients, the starting dose may be even lower. Dilute concentrations are more sensitive to degradation and lose potency more rapidly than the more concentrated preparations. Thus, their expiration dates are much shorter, and must be closely monitored.

The buildup phase involves injections with increasing amounts of allergens. The frequency of the injections can vary depending on the protocol. The most common or "conventional" protocol recommends dosing once to twice a week with at least 2 days between injections (Table 33-2). Patients with greater sensitivity may require a slower buildup phase to prevent systemic reactions. Typically during a patient's "allergic" season the potential for systemic reactions is increased leading to more cautious dosing schedules during that time of year. With a typical buildup schedule, maintenance dosing is usually achieved after 3 to 6 months (Table 33-3). Alternative schedules such as "rush" or "cluster" immunotherapy rapidly achieve maintenance dosing and should only be administered by an allergist/immunologist because of an increased risk for systemic reactions. Immunotherapy dosing schedules should be written by trained allergists/immunologists, and primary care physicians should seek their advice if questions or issues arise during administration.

Table 33-2
CONVENTIONAL IMMUNOTHERAPY

Buildup
- 1000- to 10,000-fold dilution starting dose (depending on sensitivity)
- Very sensitive patients may require a further reduction of the starting dose
- Increase dose once to twice a week with at least 2 days between injections
- Maintenance achieved after 3 to 6 months

Maintenance
- Therapeutic dose administered up to every 4 weeks for inhalant allergens and up to every 8 weeks for venom allergy
- Therapy continued for up to 5 years or more depending upon the circumstances

The maintenance phase begins when the effective therapeutic dose is achieved. This final dose is based on several factors including the specific allergen, the concentration of the extract, and how sensitive a patient is to the extract. Once maintenance is achieved, the intervals for injections range up to 4 weeks for inhalant allergens and up to 8 weeks for venom, but are individualized for each patient. Clinical improvement can be demonstrated shortly after the patient reaches the maintenance dose. If no improvement is noted after 1 year of maintenance therapy, a reassessment should be done. Possible reasons for lack of efficacy need to be evaluated, and if none are found, discontinuation of immunotherapy should

Table 33-3	
TYPICAL BUILDUP SCHEDULE FOR CONVENTIONAL IMMUNOTHERAPY	
1:1000 (V/v)	0.05
	0.10
	0.20
	0.40
1:100 (V/v)	0.05
	0.10
	0.20
	0.30
	0.40
	0.50
1:10 (V/v)	0.05
	0.07
	0.10
	0.15
	0.25
	0.35
	0.40
	0.45
	0.50
Maintenance concentrate	0.05
	0.07
	0.10
	0.15
	0.20
	0.25
	0.30
	0.35
	0.40
	0.45
	0.50

V/v, percent by volume in volume.
Adapted from Li JT, Lockey IL, Bernstein JM, et al: Allergen immunotherapy: A practice parameter. Ann Allergy Asthma Immunol 2003;90:1–40 with permission.

be considered. Patients should be evaluated at least every 6 to 12 months while on immunotherapy by the prescribing allergist/immunologist. Duration of maintenance therapy is up to 5 years. At this point a decision is made about the continuation of immunotherapy based on the severity of disease, benefits from sustained treatment, and the convenience of treatment. Treatment may lead to prolonged clinical remission and persistent alterations in immunologic reactivity, but at this time there are no tests or markers that will distinguish between patients who will stay in remission and those who will relapse.

Many studies, especially from Europe, have shown that high-dose sublingual allergen immunotherapy (SLIT) is effective for certain patients, but generally not as effective as subcutaneous immunotherapy. The greatest advantage of SLIT is safety. Local symptoms such as mouth itching are common but systemic/anaphylactic reactions appear to be less common than with subcutaneous therapy. Many questions still remain unanswered on sublingual immunotherapy including effective dose concentrations, schedule for build-up and maintenance therapy, and timing of dosing, that is, seasonal, preseasonal, or continuous throughout the year. Additionally, sublingual therapy requires much larger doses of allergen to be effective, up to 500 times greater, and at this time no Food and Drug Administration (FDA)-approved extracts are available. Finally, the utility of sublingual immunotherapy for polysensitized patients is not yet determined.

SAFETY

The greatest concern with immunotherapy is safety. Local reactions at the injection site, such as redness, swelling, and warmth, are common. These reactions can be lessened with H1 antagonists before injections. Local reactions can be managed with treatments such as cold compresses or topical corticosteroids. Large, local, delayed reactions (25 mm or larger) do not appear to be predictors of developing severe systemic reactions, and generally do not require adjustment of dosing schedules. However, some patients with a greater frequency of large local reactions (more than 10% of injections) may be at increased risk for future systemic reactions and dosing adjustments may be necessary.

The incidence of systemic reactions, such as urticaria and angioedema, increased respiratory symptoms (nasal, pulmonary, ocular), or hypotension, ranges from 0.05% to 3.2% per injection or 0.84% to 46.7% of patients. Risk factors for systemic reactions include errors in dosing, symptomatic asthma, a high degree of allergen hypersensitivity, concomitant use of beta-blocker medications, injections from new vial, and injections given during periods when allergic symptoms are active, especially during the allergy season. A recent survey of 1700 allergists reported that 58% of responders had an event in which a patient received an injection meant for another patient and 74% reported that patients had received an incorrect amount of vaccine. These errors resulted in a multitude of adverse events including local reactions, systemic reactions, and even one fatality. Thus, it is extremely important to make sure patients are questioned about potential risk factors and the correct vials are used to administer immunotherapy injections.

Premedication with antihistamines may reduce the frequency of systemic reactions in conventional immunotherapy.

In cluster or rush immunotherapy, premedication with antihistamines, and when appropriate, prednisone, can be given before dosing.

The incidence of fatalities due to immunotherapy has not changed much over the past 30 years in the United States. From 1990 to 2001, fatal reactions occurred at a rate of 1 per 2.5 million injections, with an average of 3.4 deaths per year. Most fatal reactions occurred with maintenance doses of immunotherapy. The population at greatest risk was poorly controlled asthmatic patients. In many of the fatalities, there was either a substantial delay in giving epinephrine or epinephrine was not administered at all. The incidence of near-fatal reactions (respiratory compromise, hypotension, or both requiring epinephrine) is 2.5 times more frequent than fatal reactions.

TREATMENT OF ANAPHYLAXIS

Systemic allergic reactions can be life threatening and need to be treated rapidly. Most systemic reactions are limited to the skin, such as urticaria. Respiratory symptoms are seen alone or with skin manifestations in 42% of systemic reactions. Epinephrine is the standard of care for systemic or anaphylactic reactions. Treatment of anaphylactic reactions includes placing a tourniquet above the injection site and immediately injecting epinephrine 1:1000 intramuscularly. For adults, the dose is typically 0.2 to 0.5 mL, and for children, 0.01 mL/kg (max 0.3 mg dose) every 5 to 10 minutes as needed. For convenience, subcutaneous injection at the arm (deltoid) is frequently used, but intramuscular injection into the anterolateral thigh produces higher and more rapid peak levels of epinephrine.

IMMUNOTHERAPY IN GENERAL PRACTICE

Immunotherapy should be administered in a setting that permits the prompt recognition and management of adverse reactions. The preferred setting is the prescribing physician's office, especially for high-risk patients. However, patients may receive immunotherapy injections at another health care facility if the physician and staff at that location are equipped to recognize and manage systemic reactions, in particular, anaphylaxis. Because of the potential for anaphylaxis, immunotherapy should not be administered at home. Informed consent should be obtained before administering immunotherapy. A full, clear, and detailed documentation of the patient's immunotherapy schedule must accompany the patient when receiving injections at another health care facility. Use of a constant, uniform labeling system for dilutions may reduce errors in administration. The maintenance concentration and serial dilutions should be prepared and labeled for each individual patient. The American Academy of Allergy, Asthma, and Immunology's recommended nomenclature and color-coded system is contained in Table 33-4.

A brief review of a patient's current health status is recommended before dosing. It is important to assess any current asthma symptoms, increased allergic symptoms, any new medications, or any delayed reactions to the previous injection. In patients with asthma, peak expiratory flow rate measurements should be obtained before each injection. In general, immunotherapy injections should be withheld if the

Table 33-4
IMMUNOTHERAPY VACCINE LABELING

Dilution From Maintenance	Dilution Designation In Volume Per Volume (V/v)	Color	Number
Maintenance	1:1	Red	1
10-fold	1:10	Yellow	2
100-fold	1:100	Blue	3
1000-fold	1:1000	Green	4
10,000 fold	1:10,000	Silver	5

Adapted from Li JT, Lockey IL, Bernstein JM, et al: Allergen immunotherapy: a practice parameter. Ann Allergy Asthma Immunol 2003;90:1–40 with permission.

patient presents with an acute asthma exacerbation, if peak flow measurements are below 20% of the patient's baseline values, or if the FEV_1 value is less than 70% predicted normal. Immunotherapy may need to be decreased or held if significant allergic symptoms are present before an injection.

Most severe reactions develop within 20 to 30 minutes after the immunotherapy injection, but reactions can occur after this time. Patients need to wait at the physician's office for at least 30 minutes after the immunotherapy injection. In some cases, the wait may need to be longer depending on the patient's history of previous reactions.

It is usual practice to reduce the dose of vaccine when the interval between injections is longer than prescribed (Table 33-5). This reduction in dose should be clearly stated on the patient's immunotherapy schedule. Because of the potential of extract degradation over time, when new vials are started the initial dose is decreased and then built back up to maintenance. When a systemic reaction occurs, the prescribing physician needs to decide if immunotherapy should be continued. If the decision is to continue, the dose of the vaccine needs to be appropriately reduced to decrease the risk of a subsequent systemic reaction.

EFFICACY AND OUTCOMES

Once maintenance dosing is achieved for venom immunotherapy, 80% to 98% of individuals will be protected from systemic symptoms upon sting challenges. Maintenance therapy is generally recommended for 3 to 5 years, with growing evidence that 5 years of treatment provides more lasting benefit. A low risk of systemic reactions to stings (approximately 10%) appears to remain for many years after discontinuing venom immunotherapy. In children who have received venom immunotherapy, the chance of a systemic reaction to a sting after discontinuation of immunotherapy is even lower.

Table 33-5
EXAMPLES OF DOSING ADJUSTMENT

Delay in Dosing	
1–7 days late	Next scheduled dose
8–14 days late	Repeat last dose
15–21 days late	Decrease dose 25%
22–28 days late	Decrease dose 50%
First Injection from New Vial	
Decrease dose 50%	

The efficacy of immunotherapy for allergic rhinitis has been clearly demonstrated in a number of clinical trials. These studies have shown significant improvements in symptoms, quality of life, medication use, and immunologic parameters. Allergen immunotherapy for allergic rhinitis has also been shown to be beneficial for up to 3 to 6 years or more after completion of a 3-year course of treatment.

The efficacy of immunotherapy for asthma has been assessed in many trials, but some studies have been difficult to interpret either because of the use of poor-quality allergen extracts or suboptimal study design. The risk/benefit ratio of immunotherapy for asthma must always be considered. Currently, professional allergy societies recommend that patients with asthma and FEV_1 values less than 70% predicted should not receive immunotherapy. A Cochrane review in 2004 examined the role of allergen immunotherapy for asthma. This review of 75 trials with 3100 asthmatic patients found a significant reduction in asthma symptoms and medication use, and improvement in bronchial hyperreactivity associated with the administration of allergen-specific immunotherapy. It was concluded that immunotherapy was effective in asthma, and noted that one trial found that the size of the benefit was possibly comparable to inhaled corticosteroids. Another meta-analysis of data from 900 asthma patients in 24 studies demonstrated that 71% of trials resulted in beneficial effects, whereas only 17% of the studies showed no efficacy. Overall, immunotherapy improved lung functions, protected against bronchial challenge, and reduced asthma symptoms and need for medications.

Typically, studies evaluating the effectiveness of inhalant allergen immunotherapy are conducted with single allergens. However, most patients in the United States have multiple allergic sensitizations and are treated with extracts containing several allergens.

SUMMARY

Allergen immunotherapy has been a valuable tool in treating allergic rhinitis, asthma, and stinging insect hypersensitivity for decades. Although newer pharmacological agents continue to become available, immunotherapy is still the only available treatment that alters the natural course of allergic diseases. Risks of adverse allergic reactions to the immunotherapy can be minimized when immunotherapy is given in an appropriate environment to carefully selected patients. Recent guidelines have been established to further reduce the risks by establishing a universal system of reporting dilutions and establishing appropriate dosing. Despite a large body of evidence demonstrating the positive therapeutic benefits of immunotherapy, only 3 million patients in the United States are receiving immunotherapy out of a potential 40 to 50 million allergic patients, many of whom could benefit from this therapy. Newer therapies, such as anti-IgE (omalizumab), when used with immunotherapy may improve the efficacy and safety profile of immunotherapy. In addition, newer forms of immunotherapy such as T-cell peptides or immunostimulatory sequences of DNA containing CpG motifs combined with allergens are currently under investigation.

SUGGESTED READING

Aaronson DW, Gandhi TK: Incorrect allergy injections: allergists' experiences and recommendations for prevention. J Allergy Clin Immunol 2004;113:117–121.

Abramson MJ, Puy RM, Weiner JM: Allergen immunotherapy for asthma (Cochrane Review). In: The Cochrane Library. Issue 2. Chichester, UK: John Wiley, 2004.

Bernstein DI, Wanner M, Borrish L, et al: Twelve-year survey of fatal reactions to allergen injections and skin testing: 1990–2001. J Allergy Clin Immunol 2004;113:1129–1136.

Golden DBK, Kagey-Sobotka A, Norman PS, et al: Outcomes of allergy to insect stings in children, with and without venom immunotherapy. N Engl J Med 2004;351:668–674.

Li JT, Lockey IL, Bernstein JM, et al: Allergen immunotherapy: a practice parameter. Ann Allergy Asthma Immunol 2003;90:1–40.

Lieberman P, Kemp SF, Oppenheimer J, et al: The diagnosis and management of anaphylaxis: an updated practice parameter. J Allergy Clin Immunol 2005;115:S483–523.

Moller C, Dreborg S, Ferdousi HA, et al: Pollen immunotherapy reduces the development of asthma in children with seasonal rhinoconjunctivitis (the PAT Study). J Allergy Clin Immunol 2002;109:251–256.

Ross RN, Nelson HS, Finegold I: Effectiveness of specific immunotherapy in the treatment of allergic rhinitis: An analysis of randomized, prospective, single- or double-blind, placebo-controlled studies. Clin Ther 2000;22:342–350.

Ross RN, Nelson HS, Finegold I: Effectiveness of specific immunotherapy in the treatment of asthma: A meta-analysis of prospective, randomized, double-blind, placebo-controlled studies. Clin Ther 2000;22:329–341.

Till SJ, Francis JN, Nouri-Aria K, et al: Mechanisms of immunotherapy. J Allergy Clin Immunol 2004;113:1025–1034.

Treatment Delivery Systems

Bruce K. Rubin and James B. Fink

CHAPTER

34

- The dose of aerosolized medication should be the same at all ages. Although more drug deposits in the airway of adults and older children, because there is a greater airway surface, no age associated dose adjustment is needed independent of the delivery system.

- For the nearly all patients, medications delivered by pressurized metered-dose inhaler (pMDI) or dry powder inhalers (DPI) are equivalent if not superior in efficacy to those administered by currently available jet nebulizers.

- Distress and crying significantly reduce the amount of medications deposited in the infant's airway to almost none. Thus, it is recommended that medications never be administered to a crying child.

- Pulmonary deposition of aerosolized medication falls off precipitously as the facemask or tubing is moved away from the child's face and only a tiny fraction of medication is available to the child when the aerosol is less than 2 cm away. It is never effective to deliver as medication by "blow-by" aerosol

- The most effective aerosol masks are comfortable, make a good seal, and have a minimal amount of dead space.

- Pulmonary deposition of drugs delivered by currently available ultrasonic nebulizers is so poor that these cannot be recommended for the administration of asthma medications.

- Continuous nebulization of high doses of beta-agonist is effective for the emergency treatment of asthma. However, it is recommended that these be administered for no more than 1 hour because of significant and cumulative side effects.

- The change to hydrofluroalkene (HFA) propellant systems provides new opportunities for ultra-fine particle delivery to the lung. However, most of the currently available inhaled corticosteroids and all of the bronchodilator medications have a similar particle size whether in an HFA or a CFC carrier.

- When administering nebulized medications through a mechanical ventilator circuit, it is important that medications be actuated during inspiratory flow and at a velocity sufficiently slow to reduce drug precipitation in the tubing. Go with the flow and go slow.

- In the absence of a dose counter on a pMDI, it is critically important that the patient either counts the number of doses used or calculates when the canister will be depleted. Canisters will continue to puff out propellant long after the medication is gone.

- The most important part of prescribing any aerosol device is education. In the absence of patient education, there is a high risk for medication misuse.

Although "Slick" Willie Sutton (1901–1980) never actually said that he robbed banks because that is where the money is located, the admonition to "go where the money is" appropriately applies to aerosol therapy for the treatment of asthma. Asthma is primarily an airway disease. The airway is the site of inflammation, bronchoconstriction, and mucus secretion. Provoking allergies, irritants, and infectious agents initiate asthma through access to the airway. It makes sense that the most commonly used therapies for asthma would be directed to the airway by aerosols. When aerosol medication is administered to the site of disease, there are topical effects, reduced systemic side effects, and decreased medication costs.

Aerosol delivery can be a challenge under the best of conditions, as the airway limits lung penetration of the many aerosols found in the air around us, ranging from dust and pollen to airborne pathogens. The smaller the airway, the greater the volume of particles filtered, so that delivery of medical aerosols to children may be an order of magnitude less than adults.[1] This challenge is greater when there is airflow limitation, inflammation, excess mucus secretion, and airway remodeling, as with asthma. In this chapter we discuss characteristics of aerosols, techniques for aerosol generation, and best techniques for aerosol delivery in patients with asthma.

AEROSOL GENERATION

An aerosol is a group of particles that remain suspended in air because of a low terminal settling velocity. The settling velocity depends both on the particle size and its density. Aerosol particle size is usually reported as the mass median aerodynamic diameter (MMAD). For a uniformly spherical particle this is defined as the particle diameter multiplied by the square root of the particle density, which, for water, would be 1. Because particles are nonuniform in density and shape, they are usually sized by their settling behavior on a series of baffles in a cascade impactor. This yields information about the MMAD and also the particle size distribution or geometric standard deviation (GSD). The smaller the GSD, the greater the proportion of particles that will cluster around the MMAD. By convention, a GSD of less than 1.22 is described as monodisperse, while aerosols with a GSD greater than or equal to 1.22 are called polydisperse. Until recently, monodisperse aerosols have only been available for investigational use or for radioisotope studies of deposition. However, clinical devices under development produce a near-monodisperse-size distribution of particles. This may allow targeting of particles to specific parts of the airway.

Most therapeutic aerosols are polydisperse; however there is wide variability in the GSD across devices with pressurized metered-dose inhalers (pMDI) and dry powder inhalers

(DPI) generally having a smaller GSD than that produced by jet nebulization (JN). Therefore, although the mean particle size can be similar with these devices, the respirable mass can be quite different. In general, the respirable fraction of a therapeutic aerosol is defined as the volume percent of particles between 0.5 and 5.0 μm MMAD. Up to 80% of the total emitted dose deposits in the oral pharynx leading to swallowing of medication, gastrointestinal (GI) absorption, increased systemic effects, and loss of medication available to the lung. Oral pharyngeal deposition has been associated with thrush or laryngeal dysfunction with inhaled corticosteroids (ICS). Very large particles will deposit in the device itself. Extremely fine particles, less than 0.5 μm are so light that they may not sediment in the airway and can be exhaled. However, nanoparticles, such as those generated in the smoke of cigarettes, have the greatest penetration of and retention in the lungs.

The three major mechanisms of aerosol deposition are inertial impaction, gravitational sedimentation, and diffusion, and each depends on particle size. Inertial impaction is the primary mechanism for deposition of particles larger than 3 μm. Inertial impaction is flow dependent, so that during high inspiratory flow there is a greater tendency for even smaller particles to impact and deposit in the upper airway. In contrast, slow inspiratory flow allows larger particles to pass through the upper airways and into the lungs.

Gravitational sedimentation is the primary mechanism of deposition for particles less than 2 μm, but also affects larger particles when there is low flow. The longer a particle resides in the lung, the greater the likelihood that it will deposit by sedimentation. It is for this reason that breath holding for 5 to 10 seconds is recommended after inhaling. Perhaps of greater importance, breath holding has been shown to improve distribution to the lung parenchyma.

Diffusion primarily affects particles so small that Brownian motion is a greater influence on particle movement than gravity. Random Brownian movement results in both collision and coalescence of particles with both the airway and with other particles. Particles tend to coalesce, or be attracted by the mass of other objects, when they are within a distance of less than 25 times their diameter.

The ability of a device to produce appropriately sized particles is a function of both how the device is designed as well as how the device is used. For example, spontaneous breathing results in 30% greater deposition of aerosol from a jet nebulizer than positive-pressure breaths delivered by intermittent positive-pressure ventilation or mechanical ventilation with that same nebulizer. Problems and challenges of aerosol delivery are both patient and device specific.

DEVICES

The earliest aerosol devices used a bulb atomizer similar to those used for perfume sprays. This was an inefficient means of nebulization, producing only coarse particles. The modern era of aerosol therapy began with the introduction of the Wright pneumatic nebulizer in 1958 and the Medihaler Epi pMDI in 1956. Nebulizers used today include ultrasonic nebulizers (UNs), Venturi-type jet nebulizers (JNs), vibrating mesh (VM), and variations in aerosol generation ranging from continuous, breath-activated, and breath-enhanced nebulizers (Table 34-1).

Aerosol delivery has recently been reviewed by a panel of the American College of Chest Physicians.[2] In this evidence-based review it was determined that for most patients with asthma, nebulizers, DPIs, and pMDIs were equally effective in delivering aerosolized short-acting beta-agonists if the device was used appropriately by the patient. Although equally effective, there are significant differences in the ability of specific patients to use these devices as well as differences in costs, convenience, portability, and particle-generation characteristics (Table 34-2).

Ultrasonic Nebulization

UN uses a vibrating piezoelectric crystal to produce cavitation in a reservoir containing a liquid formulation, producing standing waves that generate aerosols. Particle size varies with frequency and output rate varies with amplitude. One of the

Table 34-1
AVAILABLE DELIVERY DEVICES FOR INHALED ASTHMA MEDICATIONS

Delivery Device	Medication	Recommended Age for Use*	Remarks
Pressurized metered-dose inhaler (pMDI)	Anticholinergics, beta₂-agonists, corticosteroids, cromolyn sodium, nedocromil sodium	>5 years (<5 years with holding chamber and face mask for some children)	The child may have difficulty triggering a puff while inhaling. Helps to use device with a holding chamber.
Breath-actuated MDI	Beta₂-agonists	>5 years	The child may not be able to generate the necessary inspiratory flow; device does not require the use of a holding chamber or spacer.
Dry powder inhaler	Beta₂-agonists, corticosteroids	>6 years (some can be used in some 4-year-olds but delivery is more consistent > 6)	Some devices deliver drug more effectively than an MDI. Some devices may not work in children with low inspiratory volumes.
Nebulizer	Anticholinergics, beta₂-agonists, corticosteroids, cromolyn sodium	Patients of any age who cannot use an MDI with valved holding chamber or with face mask	Useful in infants and very young children, and any child with a moderate to severe asthma episode although MDI with valved holding chamber as may be effective. Delivery method of choice for cromolyn sodium.

*Suggested ages; clinicians should use their own judgment to tailor treatment according to the specific needs and circumstances of the individual child or family.
From Anhoj J, Thorsson L, Bisgaard H: Lung deposition of inhaled drugs increases with age. Am J Resp Crit Care Med 2000;162:1819–1822.

Table 34-2
ADVANTAGES AND DISADVANTAGES OF EACH TYPE OF AEROSOL-GENERATING DEVICE OR SYSTEM CLINICALLY AVAILABLE

Type	Advantages	Disadvantages
Small-volume jet nebulizer	Patient coordination not required Effective with tidal breathing High dose possible Dose modification possible No CFC release Can be used with supplemental oxygen Can deliver combination therapies if compatible	Lack of portability Pressurized gas source required Lengthy treatment time Device cleaning required Contamination possible Not all medication available in solution form Does not aerosolize suspensions well Device preparation required Performance variability Expensive when compressor added in
Ultrasonic nebulizer	Patient coordination not required High dose possible Dose modification possible No CFC release Small dead volume Quiet Newer designs small and portable Faster delivery than jet nebulizer No drug loss during exhalation (breath-actuated devices)	Expensive Need for electrical power source (wall outlet or batteries) Contamination possible Not all medication available in solution form Device preparation required before treatment Does not nebulize suspensions well Possible drug degradation Potential for airway irritation with some drugs
Pressurized MDI	Portable and compact Treatment time is short No drug preparation is required No contamination of contents Dose-dose reproducibility high Some can be used with breath-actuated mouthpiece	Coordination of breathing and actuation needed Device actuation required High pharyngeal deposition Upper limit to unit dose content Remaining doses difficult to determine Potential for abuse Not all medications available Many use CFC propellants in United States
Valved holding chamber, reverse-flow spacer, or spacer	Reduces need for patient coordination Reduces pharyngeal deposition	Inhalation can be more complex for some patients Can reduce dose available if wrong model or not used properly More expensive than MDI alone Less portable than MDI alone Integral actuator devices may alter aerosol properties compared with native actuator
DPI	Breath-actuated Less patient coordination required Propellant not required Small and portable Short treatment time Dose counters in most newer designs	Requires moderate to high inspiratory flow Some units are single dose Can result in high pharyngeal deposition Not all medications available

CFC, chlorofluorocarbon; DPI, dry powder inhaler; MDI, metered-dose inhaler.
From Dolovich MB, Ahrens RC, Hess DR: Device selection and outcomes of aerosol therapy: evidence-based guidelines. Chest 2005;127:335–371.

advantages of UN is that a large volume of solution can be aerosolized in a relatively short period of time; however, the particles in suspension are poorly nebulized and high-volume aerosol can be irritating to the airway.

It can be difficult to detect when the piezoelectric crystal is cracked, caked with dry medication, or otherwise inoperable. These crystals use considerable energy and generate heat through the process of vibrating and denature heat-sensitive medications, especially proteins. UN can also be more expensive than other delivery devices. UN is less efficient at medication delivery than other devices and so we do not recommend their use for delivering therapeutic aerosols.[3]

Small-Volume Nebulizers

Small-volume (SV) pneumatic nebulizers use the Venturi principle to generate aerosol. A jet of compressed gas is directed over a tube, drawing fluid from a reservoir and shearing the fluid into particles that are driven against a baffle or the internal wall of the nebulizer. This causes large particles to impact and return to the reservoir, while smaller particles continue with the gas stream toward the patient. The efficiency of the SVN depends on the gas flow and pressures driving the nebulizer as well as residual drug volume. Higher flows through the nebulizer generally produce smaller particles. Typical home nebulizers use a gas source between 10 and 35 psi, whereas 50 psi is commonly used in hospital.

There is a wide range of efficiency, particle size, and output rate of SVN on the market.[4] The amount of medication remaining in the nebulizer cup at the end of nebulization or at the start of sputtering is referred to as the nebulizer residual volume and this ranges from 0.5 to 1.8 mL, depending on the nebulizer design. Thus the greater the residual volume and the smaller the initial fill volume, the less the amount of medication available for nebulization and inhalation. Most SVNs continuously produce aerosol and medication is lost to atmosphere when the patient is not inhaling. Breath-enhanced nebulizers use vents and valves to collect aerosol between breaths, moderately improving amount of aerosol inhaled.

Breath-Activated Nebulizers

Breath-activated nebulizers are most commonly SVNs that generate aerosol only during inspiration. Negative pressure at the start of inhalation drops a valve into place to allow nebulization to begin and stops when each inhalation is complete. These nebulizers can increase inhaled dose by as much as threefold compared to continuous nebulizers but they take longer to completely nebulize a charge. They have the potential advantage of requiring smaller fill volumes because there is less medication lost.

Large-Volume Nebulizers

Large-volume nebulizers (LVNs) have been used primarily for continuous nebulization of beta-agonist bronchodilators in the emergency department or intensive care unit. LVNs have a greater reservoir volume (20 to 200 mL) to allow aerosol to be generated for extended periods of time, although this may not be therapeutically advantageous.[5]

Vibrating-Mesh Nebulizers

These nebulizers generate aerosols by pushing or drawing fluid through a mesh. This process usually includes the use of a piezoceramic element to vibrate the plate containing the apertures. The vibrating-mesh nebulizer (VM) operates at less than 10% of the frequency and power consumption of the standard UN used in the clinical setting, with less heat transferred to formulation. Particle size is directly related to the exit diameter of the aperture. Less residual drug is left in the nebulizer, making this the most efficient commercially available aerosol-generation technology.

New Nebulizer Technologies

There are various new and promising nebulizer technologies in development. The Respimat (Boehringer Ingelheim) has been released in Europe as a handheld multidose nebulizer used to deliver tiotropium. Aerosol generation through use of electrostatic charge (Ventaira) has been shown to produce small, almost monodisperse particles. Other technology, which incorporates the rapid vaporization of molecules, including proteins, appears to produce highly respirable small particles.

INHALERS

Pressurized Metered-Dose Inhalers

pMDIs were first developed in the early 1950s by the Riker Company, now part of 3M. They use a metering device to nebulize a specific amount of medication from a multiple-dose canister. Each canister has a reservoir that contains a combination of propellants, surfactants/dispersing agents,

and active drug, which is less than 2% of the mixture emitted. The pMDI also includes a boot, which is designed to emit a small aliquot of the canister contents through a mouthpiece when the device is actuated. The traditional asthma "puffers" are the primary means of aerosol medication delivery worldwide and use of the pMDI with the valved holding chamber (VHC) is often considered the standard by which other aerosol delivery devices are judged (Table 34-3).

Few changes were made to the traditional pMDI over the first 40 years until the mandate to seek new, more environmentally friendly propellants. The pMDI is one of the most cost-effective devices for inhaled medication delivery. The pMDI is conveniently lightweight, portable, multidose, and can be stored in any orientation without leakage. They reliably provide consistent dosing during the canister life. The traditional pMDI is a very inexpensive dosage form. In volume, the costs to produce a pMDI are less than US $2.00 each. This is much less expensive than any alternative device with multidose convenience.

Within the stratosphere, 10 to 25 miles above the earth's surface, ozone is highly concentrated protecting the surface from harmful ultraviolet radiation. Once released, chlorofluorocarbons (CFCs) rise to the stratosphere where they are gradually broken down by ultraviolet light to release chlorine that depletes stratospheric ozone. pMDIs have historically used the chlorofluorocarbons trichlorofluoromethane (CFC11) and dichlorodifluoromethane (CFC12) as propellants, both of which are potent and previously common ozone-depleting substances.

With the adoption of the Montreal protocol to reduce emission of fluorocarbons into the atmosphere, there has been a requirement to develop alternative propellants to the traditional CFC11 and CFC12 used for the pMDI since the early 1950s. The Food and Drug Administration (FDA) announced a final rule to amend regulation *21 CFR 2.125* on the use of ozone-depleting substances in medical products. This essential use designation ends December 31, 2008, after which production and sale of single ingredient CFC pMDIs must stop.

Table 34-3
OPTIMAL SELF-ADMINISTRATION TECHNIQUE FOR USING pMDI WITHOUT VHC

1. Warm pMDI canister to hand or room temperature. A cold canister will not deliver the appropriate dose of medication.
2. Shake the canister vigorously.
3. Assemble the apparatus, and uncap the mouthpiece.
4. Ensure that no loose objects are in the device that could be aspirated or could obstruct outflow.
5. Open the mouth wide.
6. Keep the tongue from obstructing the mouthpiece.
7. Hold the pMDI vertically with the outlet aimed at the mouth.
8. Place canister outlet between lips, or position pMDI 4 cm (two fingers) away from the mouth.*
9. Breathe out normally.
10. Begin to breathe in slowly (less than 0.5 L/sec).
11. Squeeze and actuate the pMDI.
12. Continue to inhale to total lung capacity.
13. Hold breath for 4 to 10 seconds.
14. Wait 30 seconds between inhalations (actuations).
15. Disassemble the apparatus, and recap the mouthpiece.

*Open-mouth technique is not recommended with ipratropium bromide.

The hydrofluoroalkane HFA134a (tetrafluoroethane) is a substitute for CFC12 and has been used in a variety of new pMDI devices. HFA134a has a much lower potential for ozone depletion and is considered an acceptable alternative for CFCs under the Montreal protocol. HFA-carrier pMDIs require a different metering valve with a smaller aperture, thus producing a fine particle size for many medications. The particle size is decreased for some lipophilic corticosteroids that dissolve into solution in HFA134a but remain in suspension in CFC carriers.[6] In some cases, the new valves can reduce the particle size from greater than 4 µm MMAD to about 1.2 µm, as is the case with beclomethasone dipropionate (BDP) and flunisolide. These medications are commercially available as QVAR (BDP HFA, Teva Pharmaceuticals) and Aerospan (flunisolide HFA, Forest Pharmaceuticals). Other steroids do not enter solution in the HFA carrier and so the particle size for medications such as budesonide or fluticasone is about the same for these drugs as CFCs. Bronchodilators like albuterol HFA134a do not have a smaller particle size than in CFCs. Most HFA pMDIs are less affected by changes in temperature, and emit aerosol at a lower velocity, tending to reduce pharyngeal deposition. It is probable that a change to HFA devices will require us to reexamine the age-related dose equivalence of CFC pMDIs.

New propellants present a need to change the design of metering valves. One of the difficulties with pMDIs is that it is hard to tell how much medication remains in the canister. Each canister has a listed number of doses. While some pMDIs have an overfill of 10% to 15% of the nominal fill, the amount of drug emitted after the number of doses on the label can vary, alternating between the label dose and no dose at all.[7] Unfortunately, the residual carrier agents and propellants continue to make an audible sound and plume with each actuation, long after medication delivery has been compromised. Although in the past some manufacturers had suggested that the amount of medication remaining in the canister could be ascertained by floating the canister in a bowl of water, it has been shown that this is not only an unreliable method but that water entering the valve stem can alter performance of the pMDI for subsequent doses.[7] The best alternative is to use a dose counter similar to that used in DPIs so that patients will know how many doses remain within the canister. Extra market dose counters can be added to the pMDI boot and advance forward with each activation. Beginning in 2006, all new pMDIs that are developed and introduced to the US market will be required to have a built-in dose counter. In the absence of a dose counter, the best way of determining how much medication remains is to keep a running count of doses used for rescue drugs taken on an as-needed basis. For "preventer" medications that are taken on a consistent basis, patients should be instructed to calculate in advance the number of actuations and the number of puffs per day and to indicate directly on the pMDI exactly when the canister is to be discarded. For example, if an inhaled corticosteroid (ICS) is to be administered as two inhalations twice a day from a pMDI containing 120 actuations, the canister should last for 1 month (30 days × 4 actuations per day) and should be discarded at the end of that time. In reality, most patients do not do this, and are at risk of using their pMDI beyond their ability to provide consistent dosing.

Problems with pMDIs include availability with relatively few formulations, making it difficult for clinicians to prescribe the same type of device for different medications for individual patients. Many pharmaceutical companies do not release newer inhaled drugs as pMDIs. The design of the CFC pMDIs requires initial and frequent priming. Failure to prime the device results in administration of a substantially lower dose than that prescribed. In contrast, frequent priming tends to waste drug to atmosphere. Environmental factors such as temperature contribute to inconsistent doses. As temperature of the canister drops, so does the emitted dose of the CFC pMDI. This is the basis of recommendations to warm the pMDI canister to hand temperature before use. Heating the canister beyond hand temperature can increase the emitted dose.

Breath-Activated pMDIs

Breath activated pMDIs have an inspiratory flow trigger that activates on inhalation only This eliminates many problems with poor hand-breath coordination, such as inhaling before or after the dose is emitted. Because inspiratory flow is needed to activate these devices, the ability of a patient to use the device is age dependent. Maxair (pirbuterol) by 3M (St. Paul, MN) and albuterol HPA (Teva) are available with the Autohaler and in Europe the Easyhaler (Baker Norton Co., Eire) is available as a breath-activated pMDI with a triggering inspiratory flow required of about 30 LPM.

An aftermarket device, the MD Turbo (Respirex, NC) allows most pMDIs with original boot from the manufacturer to be inserted in a device that provides breath actuation and a dose counter.

Dry Powder Inhalers

In the dry powder inhaler (DPI) the medication powder is milled to a respirable size and loosely bound to a much larger (100-µm) carrier such as lactose. The powder can be packed into cakes that act as a bulk reservoir from which a single dose is scraped at the time of administration or the powder is sealed in individual blister packs or capsules that are punctured at time of administration. Once the medication is milled from a reservoir or liberated from a capsule, it needs to be disaggregated and dispersed into an aerosol cloud. This can be done actively or passively, depending on the role of the patient. Most DPIs are passive, meaning that the energy required to disaggregate the powder comes from the patient's inspiratory flow.

An advantage to DPIs is that they are intrinsically breath activated and the medication is not delivered until inhalation is started. The inspiratory flow required for disaggregating can be as little as 30 LPM for devices such as the Diskus or 60 LPM or more for higher resistance devices like the Turbuhaler (Astra) or the Spiriva Handihaler (Pfizer). Older devices such as the Spinhaler required even higher inspiratory flow. There are some DPI devices that can actively disaggregate and disperse the medication as a fine aerosol into a holding chamber, similar to those used for pMDI (as discussed later). The first of these is the Nektar powder-delivery system for the administration of inhaled insulin (Exubera, Pfizer Pharmaceuticals). In this case a controlled blast of compressed air passes through a blister pack containing the milled medication, disaggregating the powder into a holding chamber. This device offers the opportunity for patients to get consistent inhaled dose independent of inspiratory flow. This type of active DPI tends to be more expensive than passive devices, and will not be initially available for asthma medications.

DPIs may provide a single dose (with individual capsules or blister packs) or multidose convenience. Most multidose DPIs have a dose counter incorporated into the device. Disadvantages to DPI include the tight seal needed on the mouthpiece to produce an adequate inspiratory flow, compromise of inspiratory flow during an acute asthma attack, and humidity sensitivity so that condensation on the mouthpiece or in the device can lead to clumping of the drug and severely impaired disaggregation. The risk for humidity affecting these devices is increased when a patient breathes into the cold device (especially when the device is very cold—think of an automobile glove box in a Canadian winter) and saturated exhaled air condenses in the mouthpiece and the device. There can also be problems when the device is used or stored in a warm and moist environment, for example, when a patient with chronic obstructive pulmonary disease (COPD) lines up loaded anticholinergic DPIs on the bathroom counter. Some of these devices are position sensitive and the medication dose can easily be spilled if they are tipped or tilted before inhalation. Each device is different with different requirements for holding the device, inspiratory flow, method of activation, and method of medication loading. For this reason, patients need to be carefully educated in the use of each different device.

ACCESSORY DEVICES

Different accessory devices have been developed to enhance the function of aerosol delivery devices, principally pMDIs. These include spacers, valved holding chambers, actuation enablers, and dose counters. Accessory devices should confer their benefit without reducing the effective dose available to the patient. The pMDI is designed to operate with the actuator/boot provided by the manufacturer. Accessory devices with "universal" actuators that do not allow use of the actuator/boot may have great variability of performance depending on the pMDI, drug, or propellant used.

Spacers

A spacer is a simple tube or chamber that is placed at the end of the actuator boot letting the pMDI aerosol cloud mature, reducing the speed of the plume of aerosol, and allowing larger particles to evaporate or rain out before reaching the patient. Spacers can be as simple as a piece of tubing, a toilet paper roll, or a large plastic drink bottle that has been cleaned with a second hole added. At their best, spacers can reduce pharyngeal deposition up to 90%. They also provide some protection from loss of aerosol when the pMDI is actuated immediately before inspiration. In general, spacers are inexpensive and provide some benefit over using the pMDI alone. However, unlike valved holding chambers described later, spacers do not improve coordination problems such as the patient exhaling during actuation of the pMDI. Some spacers are poorly

designed leading to significant reduction (up to 40%) of medication inhaled. In general, a spacer that has less than 100 mL of internal volume will reduce the available inhaled mass of drug from the pMDI.

Valved Holding Chambers

The valved holding chamber (VHC) is a great improvement over the spacer. VHCs have a one-way valve that prevents medication loss if the patient exhales into the device (Table 34-4). VHCs also allow a patient to dissociate the coordination of medication inhalation with actuation. Several seconds of delay between actuation and inhalation (or even exhalation during actuation) of the medication will not appreciably reduce the amount of medication available to the lung. The placement of the valve between the chamber and the patient's airway also serves to further reduce pharyngeal deposition by two orders of magnitude compared to the pMDI alone (0.9% versus 90%) and one order of magnitude over simple spacers (0.9% versus 9%) thus reducing side effects. VHCs can also increase the available drug for inhalation by up to fivefold compared to the pMDI alone. The most effective VHCs are either metal coated or made of electrostatic resistant plastics that carry little charge.

Desirable characteristics of a VHC include a size large enough to allow the aerosol cloud to develop and remain as an aerosol until inhalation, an easy to open inhalation valve that is not prone to sticking, the ability to accept a variety of pMDI boots into the device, a clear and straight aerosol flow path that decreases precipitation of aerosol within the device, construction using materials that are electrostatically reduced, and of critical importance, a comfortable interface between the device and the patient whether this interface is a mouthpiece or a mask.[8]

Masks

A variety of masks have been used for VHCs; some of these have been masks designed to be used for anesthesia or resuscitation, some have been masks adapted from adult use for children, while others have been specifically designed for inhalation using a VHC (Fig. 34-1). The best masks have a low dead space, fit comfortably on the child's face, and make a complete seal with a minimal amount of pressure.

Table 34-4
OPTIMAL TECHNIQUE FOR USING A pMDI WITH A VHC
1. Warm pMDI to hand or room temperature. A cold canister will not deliver the appropriate dose of medication.
2. Shake the canister vigorously, holding it vertically.
3. Assemble the apparatus.
4. Ensure that no loose objects are in device that could be aspirated or could obstruct outflow.
5. Place holding chamber in the mouth (or place mask completely over the nose and mouth), encouraging patient to breathe through the mouth.
6. Have patient breathe normally, and actuate at the beginning of inspiration.
7. For small children and infants, have them continue to breathe through the device for five or six breaths.
8. For patients who can cooperate and clear the chamber with one breath, encourage larger breaths with breath holding.
9. Allow 30 seconds between actuations.

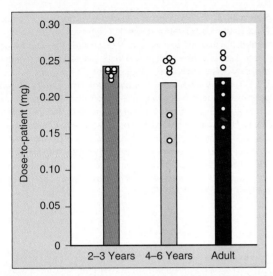

Figure 34-1   Dose to patient: mean and individual values in the three age groups. The 2- to 3-year-old children used the facemask provided with the Nebuchamber and the older patients inhaled through the mouthpiece with a noseclip applied. Budesonide was administered as two separate doses of 200 μg with an interval of 45 seconds. The patients were instructed to inhale each dose from the spacer using slow tidal breathing for 30 seconds. The dose to patient was calculated as the delivered dose of the batch measured in vitro from the pMDI with adapter, after subtraction of the drug recovered from the equipment, facial tissues, and mouth rinses. *(Data from Anhoj J, Thorsson L, Bisgaard H: Lung deposition of inhaled drugs increases with age. Am J Resp Crit Care Med 2000;162:1819–1822.)*

The mask should carry minimal electrostatic charge. For the child's comfort some masks incorporate an exhalation valve. Of all of these characteristics the ability to make a complete and comfortable seal is most important. You can ensure that the mask is completely on the child's face if you can directly observe the valve opening and closing with breathing.

Activation Enablers

Accessory devices have been designed to fit around the boot that holds the pMDI canister, making it easier to press the pMDI and actuate it. These can be useful for the elderly patient with arthritis or with poor grip strength who can find it difficult to actuate the canister.

SPECIAL USES

Neonatal and Pediatric Aerosol Therapy

The smaller diameter of upper and lower airways in infants and children results in a greater percentage of particles impacting in the structures of the upper airway. In addition, preferential nose-breathing filters aerosol from inspired gas reducing the mass of drug available for pulmonary deposition.[9]

There are few indications for administering asthma medication to neonates because asthma is not a neonatal disease. Asthma is also extremely uncommon in infants in the first year of life, and during this period asthma may respond less well to inhaled medications.

Children younger than 3 years are usually not able to make a good seal on a mouthpiece and inhale on command. For these toddlers, it is best that medications be delivered using a device that can be combined with a comfortable, closely

fitting mask (see Fig. 34-1). Today, that would mean using a nebulizer or pMDI and VHC with a mask. If properly used, these two methods of administration are equally effective for the treatment of young children with asthma.[2]

The crying and struggling child or infant has a very short and high flow inhalation and a long exhalation, especially when screaming (Fig. 34-2). This dramatically decreases the amount of medication in the lower respiratory tract and so it is highly recommended that aerosol medication not be given to a child who is upset, fighting the delivery device, or crying.[10] Given this, an absurd scenario is using blow-by aerosols for infants who are distressed. This almost guarantees an angry child who obtains no benefit from the aerosol.

The facemask or mouthpiece appears to be equally effective when using a nebulizer or valved holding chamber with pMDI (Fig. 34-3). Medication should *never* be given by blow-by; that is using a mouthpiece that is not in the child's mouth or a mask that is held some distance in front of the face. Almost no blow-by medication makes it into the lungs.[11]

Older children are usually able to place the device mouthpiece directly in their mouth. When aerosols are given using a mouthpiece, it is important that the patient breathes in slowly and deeply and that the tubing should not increase turbulence as may happen with corrugated tubing. If a child can use a mouthpiece effectively, there should be no reason for them routinely taking asthma medication by nebulizer as all available asthma medications can easily be administered by pMDI with VHC or by DPI.

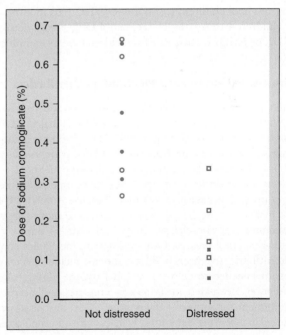

Figure 34-2 Fifteen infants, eight with resolving chronic lung disease of prematurity (mean age, 13 months), and seven with normal birth histories (mean age, 11 months) were studied. Each was given a dose of 20 mg nebulized sodium cromoglycate (SCG) using a Sidestream nebulizer and distress was graded. Urine was collected for 8 hours and analyzed for excreted drug. Estimated absorption of SCG is plotted against the degree of infant distress. Healthy infants are shown with open circles and squares; infants with chronic lung disease of prematurity with solid circles and squares. Distressed infants absorbed significantly less drug than settled infants (P < .001). *(Data from Iles R, Lister P, Edmunds AT: Crying significantly reduces absorption of aerosolised drug in infants. Arch Dis Child 1999;81:163–165.)*

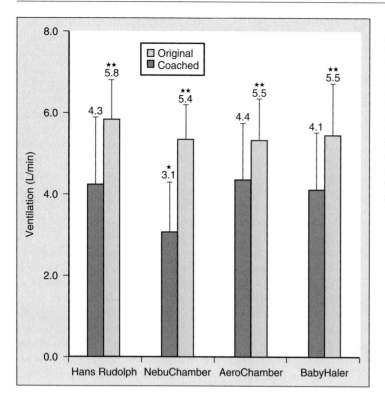

Figure 34-3 Facemask leak was studied in vivo for NebuChamber, AeroChamber, BabyHaler, and Hans Rudolph masks by measuring ventilation with an in-line pneumotachograph while the facemask was held in place by experienced parents who were asked to demonstrate how they deliver medication to their children (N = 30; age: 3.2 ± 1.4 years) without any additional instruction. The first 10 patients performed the tests once again within 1 month while the parents were coached and encouraged to hold the mask tightly against the child's face. The NebuChamber provided the poorest seal, with 45% less ventilation than the Aerochamber and Hans Rudolph masks. All ventilatory volumes during the coached session were significantly greater than during the uncoached session. *(Data from Amirav I, Newhouse MT: Aerosol therapy with valved holding chambers in young children: importance of the face mask seal. Pediatrics 2001;108:389–394.)*

Guidelines from the Global Initiative for Asthma (GINA), a collaboration of the National Heart, Lung, and Blood Institute (United States) and the World Health Organization, recommend a pMDI with VHC plus face mask for infants and preschool children; a pMDI with VHC plus mouthpiece for children 4 to 6 years of age; and a DPI, breath-actuated pMDI, or pMDI with spacer for children 6 years and older.

Administration during Mechanical Ventilation

When the severity of asthma requires intubation and mechanical ventilation, it becomes even more critical that inhaled medications be delivered to the lungs (Table 34-5). Proper techniques of aerosol delivery in mechanically ventilated patients can produce similar deposition to that in ambulatory patients.

It is more difficult to determine the response to aerosols during mechanical ventilation because forced expiratory maneuvers are poorly reproducible. It is more common to monitor pressure changes (peak and plateau) during ventilator-generated breaths. Other changes in mechanics consistent with effective bronchodilator therapy include decreasing pressures needed to deliver a set tidal volume during volume ventilation, decreased mean airway pressure, and decreased requirement for supplemental oxygen. Chest auscultation for changes in wheezing is notoriously inaccurate and should *never* be used as the sole criterion for evaluating the effect of inhaled bronchodilators.

Selection of an effective aerosol delivery system during mechanical ventilation can impact drug delivery. Jet nebulizers have been widely used during mechanical ventilation. While inexpensive and readily available in most clinical settings, they are relatively inefficient, associated with 1% to 3% deposition when used in this setting, compared to 8% to 10% under ambulatory conditions. This suggests that more medication may be required during mechanical ventilation. In

addition, jet nebulizers may add gas to the system, necessitating adjustment of settings and alarms before and after aerosol administration. Nebulizer reservoirs when situated below the ventilator circuit tend to collect condensate and secretions when in the circuit.

Aerosol deposition is affected by inspiratory flow, flow patterns and inspiratory to expiratory ratio. The lower the inspiratory flow and the longer the inspiratory time, the better the aerosol deposition. Efforts should be made to reduce inspiratory flow to 60 LPM or less during aerosol administration, as tolerated by the patient. In other words *go with the flow and go slow.*[12]

Table 34-5
TECHNIQUE FOR USING NEBULIZERS IN MECHANICALLY VENTILATED PATIENTS

1. Place drug solution in nebulizer to optimal fill volume (2 to 6 mL).*
2. Place nebulizer in inspiratory line about 30 cm from patient wye piece.
3. Ensure sufficient airflow (8–10 LPM) to operate the nebulizer.†
4. Ensure adequate tidal volume (about 500 mL in adults). Attempt to use duty cycle greater than 0.3, if possible.
5. Adjust minute volume, sensitivity trigger, and alarms to compensate for additional airflow through the nebulizer, if required.
6. Turn off flow-by or continuous-flow mode on ventilator and remove heat moisture exchanger (if present) from between nebulizer and patient.
7. Observe nebulizer for adequate aerosol generation throughout use.
8. Disconnect nebulizer when no more aerosol is being produced.
9. Rinse with sterile water or air-dry between uses. Store nebulizer under aseptic conditions.
10. Reconnect ventilator circuit, and return to original ventilator and alarm settings. Confirm proper operation with no leaks in circuit.

*The volume of solution associated with maximal efficiency varies with different nebulizers and should be determined before using any nebulizer.
†The nebulizer may be operated continuously or only during inspiration; the latter method is more efficient for aerosol delivery. Some ventilators provide inspiratory gas flow to the nebulizer. Continuous gas flow from an external source can also be used to power the nebulizer.

Humidification of inspired air is essential during mechanical ventilation to prevent airway drying and exacerbation of inflammation. There are no clinical data that support turning off humidification during aerosol administration. It is probably better to give a larger medication dose than to subject patients to the effects of dry air delivered through the ventilator. Heat and moisture exchangers (HME) should never be placed between the nebulizer and the patient airway.

Placing a jet nebulizer 30 cm from the endotracheal tube (ETT) is more efficient than placement between the patient wye connector and the ETT because the inspiratory ventilator tubing acts as a spacer for the aerosol to accumulate between inspirations. Operating the nebulizer only during inspiration is marginally more efficient for aerosol delivery compared with continuous aerosol generation.

The pMDI cannot be used with the actuator/boot designed by the manufacturer, and use of a third-party actuator is required for use with a mechanical ventilator. The size, shape, and design of these actuators greatly affect respirable drug available to the patient and may vary with different pMDI formulations. Use of an effective chamber adapter can deliver as efficiently as during ambulatory conditions (11% to 15%).

Several types of commercial adapters are available to connect the pMDI canister to the ventilator circuit. In vitro and in vivo studies have shown that the combination of a pMDI and an accessory device with a chamber results in a four- to sixfold greater delivery of aerosol than pMDI actuation into a connector attached directly to the ETT or into an in-line device that lacks a chamber. The pMDI with chamber adapter should be placed proximal to the patient, either between the airway and the ventilator circuit, or in the inspiratory limb, proximal to the wye. Actuate the pMDI at the beginning of inspiration. Allow 15 to 20 seconds between actuations. Shake thoroughly before first actuation, then do not remove from actuator or shake between doses.

Emergency Department Aerosol Delivery for Acute Asthma

The goal of asthma therapy in the emergency department (ED) is to quickly reverse underlying bronchospasm, improve airflow, and initiate anti-inflammatory therapy. Fairly high-dose aerosol beta-agonists are often administered with or without anticholinergic bronchodilators. Although there have been small studies that suggest that high doses of ICSs can be nearly as effective as systemic corticosteroids for patients with acute asthma, there is little to recommend ICSs as a substitute for systemic corticosteroids given the high doses of the ICS needed. On the other hand, although subcutaneous or intravenous beta-agonists are effective in treating acute asthma, they are no more effective than these same medications given by aerosol and there is an unacceptably high risk of side affects when beta-agonists are administered systemically.

It has been clearly shown that bronchodilators given by pMDI and VHC are at least as effective as medication administered by JN in the ED[13] (Table 34-6). Although patients with mild asthma may obtain benefit using a DPI, this is not recommended for patients with decreased inspiratory flow and severe acute asthma. Some ED physicians persist in administering asthma medication by JN. Perhaps it is more convenient to charge a nebulizer cup, give it to the patient, and return

after 15 minutes, but this will increase cost and side effects, and an opportunity for teaching is lost. In patients with stable asthma, four inhalations of albuterol (360-μg emitted dose in the United States; 400-μg emitted dose in the rest of the world) is therapeutically equivalent to 2.5 mg by nebulization. However, during acute asthma it may be necessary to initially increase the number of inhalations or the nebulized dose to achieve adequate bronchodilatation. With a higher initial dose of inhaled medications, it is likely that bronchodilators can be administered less frequently. The optimal dose and frequency of aerosol medication administration during acute moderate to severe asthma has not been established and this is likely to be different for patients at different ages, with different duration of symptoms, and other mediations taken.

Beta-agonist bronchodilators can also be delivered by continuous nebulization by placing 10 to 20 mg of albuterol per hour in an LVN and administering this for extended periods of time (8 to 24 hours). Some studies suggest that this may be an effective way to treat patients with severe acute asthma who do not respond with greater than 10% to 15% improvement in flow after initial exposure with high-dose beta-agonists. Randomized controlled trials comparing continuous nebulization with intermittent lower-dose nebulization or frequent inhalation of a pMDI with a VHC have not been reported. If continuous nebulization is used, this should be given with a comfortable and closely fitting mask because holding a mouthpiece in place for extended periods can be tiring. The mask must be vented in order to prevent rebreathing and carbon dioxide retention. The benefits of continuous nebulization probably decrease substantially as the systemic anti-inflammatory drugs take effect. We recommend that if continuous nebulization is used in acute asthma, patients should be closely monitored for tremor and tachycardia, and patients should be evaluated frequently with the goal of returning patients to intermittent pMDI and VHC as soon as the patient demonstrates adverse or therapeutic response to the beta-agonist. Data do not support the use of continuous

Table 34-6
TECHNIQUE FOR USING pMDI IN MECHANICALLY VENTILATED PATIENTS

1. Minimize inspiratory flow during administration.
2. Aim for an inspiratory time duty cycle (excluding the inspiratory pause) greater than 0.3 of total breath duration.
3. Ensure that the ventilator breath is synchronized with the patient's inspiration.
4. Shake the pMDI vigorously.
5. Place the canister in the actuator of a cylindrical spacer situated in the inspiratory limb of the ventilator circuit.*
6. Actuate the pMDI to synchronize with onset of inspiration by the ventilator.†
7. Allow passive exhalation.
8. Repeat actuations after 20 to 30 seconds until total dose is delivered.‡

* With pMDIs, it is preferable to use a spacer that remains in the ventilator circuit so that disconnection of the ventilator circuit can be avoided for each bronchodilator treatment. Although bypassing the humidifier can increase aerosol delivery, it prolongs the time for each treatment and requires disconnecting the ventilator circuit.
† In mechanically ventilated patients in whom a pMDI and spacer combination is used, actuation should be synchronized with onset of inspiration.
‡The manufacturer recommends repeating the dose after 1 minute. However, pMDI actuation within 20 to 30 seconds after the prior dose does not compromise drug delivery

nebulized bronchodilator therapy for patients with mild to moderate acute asthma.

CARE OF DEVICES

Jet Nebulizer Maintenance

JNs should be rinsed and air dried between treatments and routinely washed. Nebulizers should not be stored between treatments still containing medication, as this can be a reservoir for bacteria or fungus. The nebulizer should be routinely checked for leaks and cracks. Nebulizer performance tends to degrade over time; however the newer ones seem to perform more consistently.

Medication should be placed in the nebulizer cup either in unit doses or kept in the refrigerator and discarded once the expiration date is reached. Nebulizers should be inhaled generally from an upright position as tilting the nebulizer cups can cause spillage, loss of medication, and ineffective nebulization. Nebulization should stop once the cup begins to sputter. The fill volume of the cup is particularly important for nebulizers that have a large residual volume.

VHC Maintenance

VHCs also need to be checked to be sure that there are no objects that have entered the chamber during transport. Patients have inhaled safety pins and other small objects that have found their way into the chamber. Clear chambers make it easier to detect if there are foreign objects. The valve should be periodically examined to make sure it is not torn or stuck. This is particularly important for VHCs where the valves are pegged (e.g., Optichamber) rather than using pliant flaps (e.g., Aerochamber). The mask should also be checked to make sure it is not torn and that it sits correctly on the end of the holding chamber.

DPI and pMDI Maintenance

DPIs need to be kept dry when they are not being used. The dose counter needs to be checked periodically to be sure

medication remains in the DPI. The mouth orifice needs to remain clean at all times. Once activated, DPIs should not be flipped as this can cause dumping of medication.

pMDIs need to sit completely in the boot. If they are not properly placed in the boot or if the canister does not go with the boot, this can seriously compromise medication delivery. The boot also should be kept clean and free from foreign objects at all times.

Patients sometimes use a pMDI long after the medication is depleted because they can still hear a sound when the canister is actuated. This happens because the carrier agent can continue to "puff," although after depletion of the nominal medication dose, the amount of medication in each actuation rapidly falls off. Because pMDIs do not usually have a dose counter, it is important that the patient keep track of the amount of medication remaining.

PATIENT EDUCATION

One of the most important factors in the effectiveness of asthma medications, particularly ICS, is adherence to scheduled use. Nonadherence to prescribed ICS is a risk factor for acute severe and fatal asthma. Even during monitored clinical trials, full adherence to prescribed asthma therapy is estimated to be no more than 50%.

One of the most common reasons for nonadherence is the patient being unaware of the correct use of the device or the medication.[14] The best way to ensure adherence is to teach the patient the correct use of medication and device operation, making it easy for them by minimizing the number of drugs and frequency of administration and emphasizing the use of the most important drug, reducing medication costs, and by suggesting administration during times in the day when they are performing other activities, such as tooth brushing, that will remind them to take the medication. The use of medication and devices should be reviewed at every office visit and if there are questions about this, the device use should be directly observed. The keys to good adherence are patient and caregiver education, making medication use important, making it easy, and making it a routine part of the patient's lifestyle.

REFERENCES

1. Rubin BK, Fink JB: Aerosol therapy for children. Resp Care Clinics N Am 2001;7:175–213.
2. Dolovich MB, Ahrens RC, Hess DR, et al: Device selection and outcomes of aerosol therapy: Evidence-based guidelines. Chest 2005;127:335–371.
3. Nakanishi AN, Lamb BM, Foster CF, Rubin BK: Ultrasonic nebulization of albuterol is no more effective than jet nebulization for the treatment of acute asthma in children. Chest 1997;111:1505–1508.
4. Hess D, Fisher D, Williams P, et al: Medication nebulizer performance. Effects of diluent volume, nebulizer flow, and nebulizer brand. Chest 1996;110:498–505.
5. Rodrigo GJ: Inhaled therapy for acute adult asthma. Curr Opin Allergy Clin Immunol 2003;3:169–175.
6. Leach C: Enhanced drug delivery through reformulating MDIs with HFA propellants—drug deposition and its effect on preclinical and clinical programs. Respiratory Drug Delivery V 1996;5:133–143.
7. Rubin BK, Durotoye L: How do patients determine that their metered-dose inhaler is empty? Chest 2004;126:1134–1137.
8. Rubin BK, Fink JB: Optimizing aerosol delivery by pressurized metered-dose inhalers. Respir Care 2005;50:1191–1200.
9. Rubin BK, Fink JB: The delivery of inhaled medication to the young child. Pediatr Clin N Am 2003;50:1–15.
10. Iles R, Lister P, Edmunds AT: Crying significantly reduces absorption of aerosolised drug in infants. Arch Dis Child 1999;81:163–165.
11. Everard ML: Inhalation therapy for infants. Adv Drug Del Rev 2003;55:869–878.
12. Dhand R: Maximizing aerosol delivery during mechanical ventilation: go with the flow and go slow. Intensive Care Med 2003;29:1041–1042.
13. Cates CJ, Crilly JA, Rowe BH: Holding chambers (spacers) versus nebulisers for beta-agonist treatment of acute asthma. Cochrane Database Syst Rev 2006;(2):CD000052.
14. Rubin BK: What does it mean when a patient says, "My asthma medication isn't working?" Chest 2004;126:972–981.

Monitoring for Side Effects from Treatment

Christine A. Sorkness and Valerie A. Schend

CHAPTER

35

- Optimal asthma therapy involves balancing efficacy of a medication with its side-effect profile.

- Patients most at risk for adverse events with the use of inhaled corticosteroids are children, the elderly, diabetic patients, immunocompromised patients, and individuals with a high daily cumulative dose or prolonged multiple-year therapy due to persistent disease severity.

- Prolonged administration of high doses of inhaled corticosteroids has been associated with increased risks of posterior subcapsular cataracts, ocular hypertension, or open-angle glaucoma. Annual eye exams are warranted for patients at risk, especially those requiring intermittent oral corticosteroids and those with concurrent medical risks.

- Side effects of short-acting beta$_2$-agonists are generally transient in nature but can be prolonged with long-acting beta$_2$-agonists. Tachycardia and tremor are the most common side effects. Active investigation is ongoing regarding safety of long-acting beta-agonists. At present, they should be used only in combination with inhaled corticosteroids.

- The most common adverse event noted with leukotriene modifiers is headache and it is not considered a therapy-ending occurrence. The reported incidence of headache is between 12% and 20%, similar to the frequency reported with placebo. With zileuton, liver function monitoring is required at baseline and every 2 to 3 months for a 1-year period, and every 6 months thereafter.

Health care practitioners have the responsibility to balance the anticipated therapeutic benefits versus the potential risks of asthma treatments prescribed. The goal is to achieve the lowest doses of medication needed to achieve and maintain disease control with the fewest adverse effects possible (ideally none) due to the medications. Adverse effects can be deleterious to the patient by causing unwanted physiologic events or misuse or underuse of asthma medications as a means to minimize unwanted side effects. This chapter discusses monitoring approaches for side effects from asthma treatments, with a goal of maximizing therapeutic benefit from these agents.

INHALED CORTICOSTEROIDS

Inhaled corticosteroids (ICSs) are the most effective agents available for the treatment of persistent asthma in both children and adults. Available agents are not equipotent although algorithms exist to estimate microgram dose equivalencies. There is abundant literature describing ICS efficacy in improving all aspects of asthma control including decreased asthma

symptoms and rescue medication use, improved lung function measurements, improved exercise tolerance, decreased rates of exacerbations, and improved quality of life. Due to the robustness of such literature, ICSs are being used more frequently for persistent asthma, in younger and older patients, and for longer durations of treatment. ICSs are generally well tolerated at recommended doses. However, the fear of adverse effects or "steroid-phobia" may result in underuse of these agents. Discussing the differences between glucocorticoids and anabolic steroids may allay some of the patient/family fears of unwanted side effects. The inhaled delivery system allows for the expression of adverse effects both locally (oropharyngeal cavity) and systemically due to absorption of the ICS into the circulation. Systemic absorption occurs through the gut (the portion of the dose deposited on the oropharynx and swallowed) and the lungs (systemic absorption via the lung surface). Patients and physicians voice more concern regarding systemic side effects of ICS even though localized adverse effects are implicated more often in actual physical findings and may lead to underuse or misuse of prescribed therapy. Patients most at risk for adverse events with the use of inhaled corticosteroids are children, the elderly, diabetic patients, immunocompromised patients, and individuals with a high daily cumulative dose or prolonged multiple-year therapy due to persistent disease severity. Monitoring measures to minimize adverse effects of ICS are outlined in Tables 35-1 and 35-2, and are discussed briefly in the following sections.

Table 35-1
MONITORING MEASURES TO MINIMIZE ADVERSE EFFECTS OF ICS

- Use appropriate dosage regimens, with the lowest dose of ICS required to achieve and maintain disease control
- Consider combination pharmacotherapy, e.g., decrease dose of ICS and add long-acting beta-agonists or leukotriene receptor agonists
- Use a spacer device with MDI when appropriate
- Reinforce good administration technique (slow inhalation for metered-dose inhaler, good oral hygiene measures)
- Assess for concurrent risk factors
  - Age/pubertal status
  - Gender
  - Concurrent medical conditions (e.g., diabetes, immunocompromised status)
  - Smoking status
  - Concurrent medications
- Monitor with regular objective measures
  - Oropharyngeal exams
  - Stadiometric height measurements and Tanner staging
  - Ophthalmic examinations of lens and intraocular pressure measurements
  - Bone mineral densitometry
- Initiate specific prevention or treatment strategies

ICS, inhaled corticosteroids.

Table 35-2
SPECIFIC MONITORING PARAMETERS AND PREVENTION STRATEGIES TO MINIMIZE SIDE EFFECTS FROM ASTHMA TREATMENT

Drug	Adverse Effect	Monitoring Parameters	Prevention Strategies
ICS	Growth	Stadiometric measurements starting at 4 months from initiation and then every 6 months	• Decrease ICS dose or frequency; add-on therapy (LABA or LTRA)
	Osteopenia	Bone densitometry (see text for specifics)	• Add calcium and vitamin D to diet, bisphosphonates as indicated
			• Add a program including weight-bearing exercise
	Cataracts and elevated intraocular pressure	Ophthalmic evaluation annually	• Reduce concurrent risks if possible
	HPA axis effects	AM serum cortisol levels	• Decrease ICS dose or frequency, add-on therapy (LABA or LTRA)
		ACTH stimulation test	
		24-hour urinary-free cortisol excretion	• Referral to endocrinologist for specialty testing
	Oral candidiasis	Routine oropharyngeal exam	• Use a spacer with MDI
			• Rinse and spit
			• Decrease frequency of ICS administration
	Dysphonia	Routine query	• Decrease frequency of ICS administration
			• Decrease vocal stress
			• Add a spacer with MDI
			• Rinse mouth and gargle
			• ICS holiday
	Cough	Routine query	• Trial of dry powder inhaler
			• Slower inspiration rate
			• Pre-treat with beta$_2$-agonist
	Skin effects	Routine inspection	• Protective clothing
Anticholinergics	Dry mouth/unpleasant taste		• Rinse mouth and gargle
	Blurred vision		• Close eyes during MDI administration
			• Tight seal around mouthpiece or face mask with nebulizer
Zileuton	Hepatotoxicity	CBC baseline and annually	• Monitor as recommended
		AST or ALT baseline, 30 days after starting therapy, monthly × 3, every other month × 3–4, and then semi-annually	
Theophylline	Multiple	Monitor blood levels if toxicity is suspected or asthma control wanes	• Use low dose therapy (serum concentration < 10 µg/mL)
			• Monitor for drug-drug, drug-disease interactions

ACTH, adrenocorticotropic hormone; HPA, hypothalamus-pituitary-adrenal; ICS, inhaled corticosteroid; LABA, long-acting beta-agonist; LTRA, leukotriene receptor agonist; MDI, metered-dose inhaler.

Growth

Growth effects of ICS continue to be of concern to both clinicians and parents, since current clinical management guidelines recommend early intervention with ICS in appropriate patients, and the prospect of lifelong ICS therapy has clinical implications. The National Asthma Education and Prevention Program (NAEPP) Expert Panel Report 3 (EPR3) recommendations for treating children with mild or moderate persistent asthma were revised in 2007. Based on observational studies, it was the opinion of this Expert Panel that the initiation of long-term control therapy should be considered in infants and young children who have had more than four episodes of wheezing in the preceding year that lasted more than 1 day and affected sleep and who have risk factors for the development of asthma (parental history of asthma or physician-diagnosed allergic rhinitis, wheezing apart from colds, peripheral blood eosinophilia). This recommendation was in addition to previous guidelines for starting long-term control therapy, that is, in infants and young children requiring symptomatic treatment more than two times per week or experiencing severe exacerbations less than 6 weeks apart. The NAEPP has long recommended ICS as preferred therapy for all children who can be classified as having persistent disease.

Childhood growth occurs in three phases. Initially, during the first 2 years, there is a period of rapid but decelerating growth, primarily determined by nutrition. The second phase is a period of relatively steady growth regulated by growth hormone, occurring until the onset of puberty. Finally, the pubertal growth spurt occurs, controlled by both growth hormones and sex steroids. Growth occurs in discontinuous bursts interrupted by long, growth-free periods. These growth patterns likely contribute to the lack of correlation between short- and long-term growth measurements.

Glucocorticoids are potent inhibitors of virtually every component of the growth axis including growth hormone secretion and action, insulin-like growth factor-1 bioactivity, collagen synthesis, and adrenal androgen production. The most important effect responsible for growth failure is still uncertain. The complexity of interactions between glucocorticoids and growth makes it unlikely that a compounding of effects will determine the extent of growth impairment in an individual.

Chronic diseases in children such as asthma may have growth-suppressing actions that are independent of treatment. It has been shown that uncontrolled asthma itself, of at least moderate severity, can have a deleterious effect on growth. Asthma may also delay puberty, and the resulting growth spurts. Bursts of oral corticosteroids to treat asthma exacerbations may also contribute to growth suppression, especially if used frequently.

Use of a quality, accurately calibrated stadiometer is essential for monitoring linear growth of children with asthma. The stadiometer should be installed as directed and carefully calibrated per the manufacturer's instructions. After installation, the stadiometer should be calibrated daily using the metal calibration bar provided by the manufacturer, recording the exact length of the metal bar on the stadiometer. To measure an accurate height, the child should stand erect, with both heels touching the bottom plate of the stadiometer and ankles and feet touching each other. Shoes, thick socks, and headgear all must be removed, and "high" hair dealt with if feasible. Knees should be straight and locked; heels, buttocks, and shoulders should be positioned against the stadiometer. Arms should be hanging freely with the palms facing the thighs and the child should be looking straight ahead without raising his or her chin. While looking eye level at the top of the child's head, the platform is slowly lowered to the child's head; height is then recorded. This procedure is then repeated two more times resulting in three height measurements with a maximum difference of 3 mm or less between any two measurements.

Children prescribed inhaled corticosteroids should be serially evaluated for asthma control and careful height measurements should be performed. This follow-up should begin 4 months after starting ICS and repeated at approximately 6-month increments thereafter. Height measurements should be accurately plotted on growth charts and this information can be used to reassure physician, parent, and child. If a slowing of significant growth rate does occur, a pediatric endocrinologist can be consulted to see if there are other predisposing factors contributing to the growth delay. The health care practitioner should continue to provide reassurance to parents/children of the overall safety of ICS at prescribed doses, the plan to monitor and reevaluate therapy over time and step-down ICS dosages if warranted, and the lack of ICS treatment alone on causing any detectable effect on the final adult height of people who grew up with asthma.

Bone Mineral Density (BMD) and Bone Metabolism

Corticosteroids influence both bone formation and bone resorption. The enhanced resorption is likely explained by both the development of secondary hyperparathyroidism and a direct effect on bone. When given initially, corticosteroids increase secretion of parathyroid hormone, probably because of reduced intestinal absorption and increased renal loss of calcium. There is also evidence that corticosteroids potentiate the activity of parathyroid hormone on osteoblasts. In addition, corticosteroids inhibit calcium absorption.

Corticosteroids affect the secretion of sex hormones, in turn increasing bone resorption. There is a direct effect on gonadal function by inhibition of pituitary gonadotropin secretion and a direct effect on the testes and ovaries. Corticosteroids inhibit secretion of various hormones including estrogen and testosterone, contributing to further bone loss.

The main bone effects of corticosteroids are a diminished amount of new bone formed. This reduced bone formation is attributed to a direct effect on osteoblast function and has been well documented by both biochemical and histomorphometric studies.

Bone mineral density and integrity are difficult to ascertain in children. Bones in children are rapidly changing with rapid increases in both bone mineral content and density, particularly during adolescence. DEXA (dual-energy X-ray absorptiometric) scans of bones in children can give exaggerated results. Larger bones in larger children can appear to have increased bone mineral density while smaller bones in smaller children may seem to have lower bone mineral density. These tests can be properly interpreted by an expert also adjusting the DEXA scan for the child's size, pubertal status, and developmental stage.

Bone density measurements should be performed in any patient requiring oral daily glucocorticoids for longer than 6 months at doses more than 7.5 mg per day, postmenopausal women on oral glucocorticoid therapy at doses of 5 mg/day or greater for 3 months or longer, or any asthmatic patient with a history of fractures that may be related to osteoporosis. BMD screening should also be offered for postmenopausal women requiring more than 2 mg per day of inhaled budesonide or its equivalent or any patient requiring frequent bursts of oral corticosteroids. Follow-up scanning should be repeated annually for patients being treated for osteoporosis, and every 2 years, or as often as every 6 months, for at-risk patients. Osteoporosis is present if the bone density in lumbar spine or femoral neck shows (1) T-score below -2.5 (2.5 standard deviations below the mean value of young normal subjects of the same sex in patients 19 to 69 years] and (2) Z-score below -1 (1 standard deviation below the predicted value for age and sex).

All at-risk patients should also be encouraged to adopt further strategies to improve their overall bone health. Such strategies include smoking cessation, decreasing alcohol consumption if excessive, limiting caffeine and carbonated beverage intake, and starting an exercise routine that includes weight-bearing activities, as well as sufficient calcium (1500 mg/day) and vitamin D (800 IU/day) intake. Special attention should be paid to adolescents with eating disorders, because of menstrual abnormalities. At-risk patients should also be screened for other predisposing factors for fracture such as a history of falls, other fractures, confounding medications that might increase fracture risk (e.g., some antiepileptics) and smoking history.

Eye Effects

The use of systemic corticosteroids is an established risk factor for the development of cataracts, particularly posterior subcapsular cataracts (PSCs). Cataracts are classified according to anatomic location; the most common types are cortical, nuclear, and posterior subcapsular. The most visually disabling type of cataract is the PSC, which accounts for most surgical lens extractions. Cortical and nuclear cataracts become a more frequent cause of vision loss with advancing patient age.

It is also well established that topical ophthalmic glucocorticoids can produce ocular hypertension and secondary open-angle glaucoma in susceptible individuals; most corticosteroid-induced cases of these eye disorders have resulted from topical ophthalmic administration. Case reports of adverse effects with other routes of corticosteroid administration (e.g., oral, periocular injections, eyelid creams or ointments, nasal, inhaled) have surfaced, raising concern in the asthma community.

Prolonged administration of high doses of ICS has been associated with increased risks of PSCs, ocular hypertension, or open-angle glaucoma. Annual eye exams are warranted for patients at risk, especially those requiring intermittent oral corticosteroids and those with concurrent medical risks.

Hypothalamic-Pituitary-Adrenal Axis Effects

Many factors influence the incidence of adrenal suppression with ICS. These factors include dose and frequency of ICS administration, timing of ICS dose, duration of treatment, previous long-term systemic corticosteroid use, patient age, as well as significant interindividual variability. Patients most at risk are those requiring high-dose inhaled corticosteroid treatment as well as supplemental oral glucocorticoids.

The occurrence and magnitude of adrenal suppression are the most extensively evaluated systemic effects of ICS therapy and have been thoroughly reviewed in the literature. Most studies have concluded that with use of low and medium dosage levels of marketed ICS products, the hypothalamus-pituitary-adrenal (HPA) axis is minimally and partially suppressed and there is little risk of adrenal insufficiency in these patients. However, patients requiring high-dose inhaled corticosteroids and additional doses of oral corticosteroids to treat exacerbations (or other disease states requiring the use of glucocorticoids) require monitoring of their fasting morning plasma cortisol levels annually. Patients with below-normal results should be referred to a specialist to determine if clinically significant adrenal sufficiency exists and whether further testing using a low-dose adrenocorticotropic hormone (ACTH) stimulation test would be advised.

Local Side Effects

Local side effects reported with ICS include oral and oropharyngeal candidiasis, pharyngeal inflammation, laryngeal disorders, cough during inhalation, and a sensation of thirst. These problems are probably multifactorial and dependent on the following factors: (1) the corticosteroid itself (preparation, carrier substance, dose, regime); (2) the manner in which it is propelled into the airways (delivery device); (3) intrinsic inflammation of the upper airway in patients with asthma; (4) mechanical irritation due to cough; (5) intercurrent inflammatory disease (rhinitis, gastroesophageal reflux disease [GERD]); (6) intercurrent inflammatory stimuli (smoking,

noxious agents in the environment). The most important clinical problems are discussed below.

ORAL CANDIDIASIS

The development of oral candidiasis in patients using ICS is often associated with administration technique or inadequate oral hygiene. *Candida* is a normal component of the oral microbial flora in 50% of the population. Proliferation of *Candida* may occur with a disruption of the oral environment by the introduction of ICSs resulting in immunosuppression of the normal oral microbial flora. Reported incidence of candidiasis has ranged from none to 77%, with increased incidence at higher ICS doses. However, most manufacturers of ICSs report an incidence of up to 10% (Table 35-3). For pressurized metered-dose inhalers (MDIs), oral candidiasis can be reduced by using certain spacer devices and regular mouth washing (rinsing with water, gargling, and spitting out after inhalation). The use of prodrugs that are activated in the lungs but not in the pharynx (e.g., ciclesonide) and new formulations and devices that reduce oropharyngeal deposition may minimize such effects without the need for a spacer or mouth washing.

Esophageal candidiasis has also been reported. Patients afflicted with esophageal candidiasis should be instructed to use their ICS before eating to further swipe the esophagus and to remain upright after the evening dose instead of going immediately to bed. Patients at increased risk include diabetic patients, immunocompromised individuals, patients on concomitant antibiotic therapy or oral glucocorticoid therapy, and those with poor inhaler technique.

DYSPHONIA/HOARSENESS/COUGH

Dysphonia and hoarseness are terms that can be used interchangeably to describe a change or impairment of vocal quality and have been reported to affect 5% to 50% of patients using ICSs. This wide range of occurrence is likely due to methodologic factors such as use of patient questionnaires or lack of verification by clinical examination. Other patient complaints may include mouth or throat pain, soreness, or irritation. Dysphonia seems to be directly attributable to the effects of ICSs either as a direct effect on the larynx or steroid myopathy affecting the vocal cord muscles. The propellants and lubricants used in traditional MDI preparations have also been shown to have a localized proinflammatory effect. Vocal stress, increasing doses of ICS, and failure to use a spacer with the MDI are all associated with dysphonia. Cough may

Table 35-3
INCIDENCE OF ADVERSE EVENTS REPORTED WITH ICS*

	Beclomethasone HFA MDI	Budesonide DPI	Flunisolide MDI	Fluticasone HFA MDI	Mometasone DPI	Triamcinolone MDI	Fluticasone/Salmeterol HFA and DDI
Dysphonia	<1–6	1–6	3–9	2–6	1–3	1–3	2–5
Cough		5	3–9	4–6			3–6
Candidiasis		2–4	3–9	2–5	4–6	2–4	4–10
URI	3–17	19–24	25	16–18	8–15		10–27
GI	<1–5	1–4	10–25	1–3	1–5	2–5	1–7
Headache	8–17	13–14	25	5–11	17–22	7–21	12–20

*% based on FDA-approved language in package inserts.
DPI, dry powder inhaler; GI, gastrointestinal; MDI, metered-dose inhaler; URI, upper respiratory infection.

also be due to a local irritant effect of the ICS, the propellant, or the excipient (e.g., lactose in DPI) and may be reduced with the use of a spacer. Many factors may be responsible for the local adverse effect of ICS on the throat such as the steroid (dose, regimen, excipients), the inhaler device, and intrinsic inflammation of the upper airway (due to asthma, rhinitis, or irritants such as tobacco smoke). Regardless of the cause, dysphonia can impair quality of life and interfere with work performance. These problems should be addressed at each clinical encounter and strategies implemented.

DENTAL CARIES

Tooth decay and dental erosion of both deciduous and permanent teeth are reported to occur more frequently in children with asthma. Postulated mechanisms for this dental damage include GERD, which is more prevalent in asthma, and the lower pH of asthma medications. MDIs have a pH of 7.0 to 9.3. Dental enamel can begin to dissolve at lower pHs, and powdered formulations of asthma medications may have a pH below 5.5. The dry powdered medication also reduces the production of saliva, affecting the mouth's natural way of maintaining its chemical balance. To offset these side effects, some dentists recommend rinsing with a fluoride mouthwash and chewing sugarless gum to stimulate saliva after inhaling medicine. Some recommend against brushing immediately after inhaling the medication because the action of brushing large particle powder against young teeth may weaken already damaged tooth enamel. Health practitioners should encourage yearly dental exams for these children, to best monitor dental disease and provide ongoing advice.

Skin Effects

Perioral dermatitis can be found as a local irritant effect of ICS around the mouth region in those using spacers with masks, a nebulizer with a face mask, or nebulizing without a mouthpiece. Severe cases may need treatment with topical antibiotics; however, instructions on thorough cleansing of the areas around the mouth in contact with ICS after administration might be sufficient in preventing occurrence. The face should be examined by health care practitioners at each clinical encounter.

Skin thinning and bruising that occur with ICS can be related to increased capillary fragility, increased collagen turnover, or reduced collagen synthesis. This risk increases in older patients and with increased dose of ICS and increased duration of treatment. Cutaneous skin thickness has been shown to decrease 15% to 19% with administration of high-dose ICS and markers of collagen synthesis show a marked decrease in patients treated with moderate-dose ICS. Skin bruising due to ICS usually occurs on the face, neck, or limbs and also on other body areas after slight injury. Almost one half of patients requiring ICS will have some form of skin thinning or bruising and those with lower, although not insufficient, adrenal function seem to be at increased risk. Patients can be advised to wear some protective clothing when performing activities that may cause injury.

ORAL CORTICOSTEROIDS

Most of the aforementioned systemic adverse effects listed for inhaled corticosteroids can occur with oral use of these agents. Multiple body systems can be adversely affected with the use of oral corticosteroids. Obesity, skin thinning with cutaneous striae and bruising, and muscle weakness may also occur as a result of long-term oral corticosteroid therapy.

Hypertension and edema may occur as a result of sodium retention. Hyperglycemia is due to peripheral insulin resistance and pancreatic release of glucagon that causes glycogenolysis. This can lead to the onset of glucose intolerance. Patients should be observed for signs of excessive thirst, frequent urination, fatigue, or unexplained weight loss. Cushing syndrome (either iatrogenic or endogenous) presents as central obesity, moon facies, and buffalo hump and possible psychosis, edema, and delayed wound healing. Gastrointestinal issues beyond nausea and vomiting can include ulceration and/or perforation. Less common, but also of concern, are aseptic necrosis of bone, steroid psychosis, and the possibility of superinfection.

Patients requiring frequent oral corticosteroid bursts or those who are corticosteroid dependent require specialized monitoring. Beyond annual ophthalmic visits and measurement of bone mineral density, these patients should have blood pressures, complete blood counts, glucose levels (hemoglobin AI-C), and cholesterol (lipid panel) measured routinely.

BRONCHODILATORS

Beta$_2$-agonists are an important part of therapy, as rescue medication and as controller medication. Inhaled therapy with these agents causes fewer adverse effects than oral therapy, including cardiac manifestations, muscle tremor, and agitation. Regular use of beta$_2$-agonists can lead to relative refractoriness to these agents.

Short-acting Bronchodilators

Most of the side effects occurring with the short-acting bronchodilators are transient in nature. Adverse effects are heightened when orally administered doses of the medications are used as opposed to inhaled therapy. Some of the adverse events that may occur include tachycardia and palpitations possibly due to beta stimulation and reflex cardiac stimulation. Patient complaints can involve muscle tremor, restlessness, irritability, nervousness, agitation, trouble sleeping, and dizziness. Younger children, especially those receiving oral dosage forms of albuterol, may experience excitability.

Long-acting Bronchodilators

Adverse effects occurring with the long-acting inhaled beta$_2$-agonists are more common in the oral products compared to the inhaled. Cardiovascular overstimulation (such as tachycardia), anxiety, and muscle tremor occur most frequently. There might be an increased risk of asthma-related deaths in a small population of asthmatic patients using salmeterol. The U.S. Food and Drug Administration has issued an advisory, and the NAEPP and Global Initiative for Asthma (GINA) guidelines recommend that these agents should not be used as monotherapy and must always be given as combination therapy with other asthma-controller medications such as ICSs. Evaluation of the long-term effects of long acting beta₂-agonists is currently being actively investigated.

ANTICHOLINERGICS

Ipratropium bromide has bronchial smooth muscle relaxant properties due to its action on muscarinic receptors. The onset of action of ipratropium is slower than that of the beta₂-agonists; however, its duration of action may be somewhat lengthened compared to those agents. Ipratropium is primarily used for acute asthma exacerbations in combination with a beta₂-agonist or as monotherapy in patients unable to tolerate beta₂-agonist agents. These agents are generally well tolerated. Adverse effects are mostly bothersome and include dry mouth and unpleasant taste. Occasionally, blurred vision may occur if the ipratropium gets directly into the eye and causes dilation of the pupil. This can be avoided by closing the eyes while using the MDI or, if nebulized, making sure there is a tight seal around the mouthpiece or face mask.

LEUKOTRIENE RECEPTOR MODIFIERS

Leukotriene receptor antagonists (LRTAs; montelukast and zafirlukast) inhibit the cysteinyl leukotriene CysLT₁ receptor resulting in both anti-inflammatory and bronchodilator effects. Zileuton is an active inhibitor of 5-lipoxygenase, the first step in the enzymatic conversion of arachidonic acid to leukotrienes. These agents are generally well tolerated.

The most common adverse event noted with these agents is headache, which is not considered a therapy-ending occurrence. The reported incidence of headache is between 12% and 20%, similar to the frequency reported with placebo. Gastrointestinal (GI) complaints including nausea, GI pain, and diarrhea may also occur. Patients can be instructed to take this medication with food to ameliorate these effects; however, zafirlukast should be taken on an empty stomach. The bioavailability of zafirlukast can be decreased by 40% if taken with food. Patients may also experience generalized flu-like symptoms, sleep disturbances (including dream abnormalities and insomnia), hallucinations, and drowsiness.

The leukotriene modifiers are almost exclusively metabolized through the liver. Screening for hepatoxicity is necessary for patients using zileuton. A baseline CBC and ALT or AST should be checked, and then liver function tests should be repeated 30 days after starting therapy, monthly thereafter for 3 months, and then every 2 to 3 months for a suggested 10 visits during the first year of therapy. Thereafter, screening should be performed at 6-month intervals.

ANTI-ALLERGY AGENTS

Cromones such as cromolyn and nedocromil have anti-inflammatory activity and are used on occasion to treat allergy-related asthma. Omalizumab is a monoclonal antibody used to treat severe allergic asthma and is discussed in depth elsewhere.

Both cromolyn and nedocromil have good safety profiles and side effects are uncommon. Cough and sore throat may occur, and some patients may object to the taste of nedocromil. Complaints of unpleasant or bitter taste occur in up to 13% of individuals using nedocromil. Use of a spacer might be beneficial in abating the adverse effects.

THEOPHYLLINE

Theophylline is a potent bronchodilator. It is available in a variety of formulations, including once- or twice-daily dosage forms. Theophylline is recommended as adjunctive therapy for patients not receiving sufficient control of their asthma from ICS.

Adverse effects due to theophylline can be significant and limit its role in the treatment of asthma. Routine monitoring of serum concentrations is essential for the safe and effective use of theophylline and cannot be replaced by side-effect monitoring alone. Adverse effects are more common with higher doses; practitioners should aim for theophylline serum concentrations of 10 to 12 μg/mL and no higher than 15 μg/mL. Monitoring is advised when a high dose is started, if the patient develops an adverse side effect on the usual dose, when expected therapeutic aims are not achieved, and when conditions known to alter theophylline metabolism exist. Nausea and vomiting are the most common side effects, and tolerance to these effects can develop. Other adverse effects include GI pain, diarrhea, tremors, cardiac arrhythmias, and seizures. Febrile illnesses, pregnancy, liver disease, and congestive heart failure can alter theophylline metabolism leading to toxicity or lack of therapeutic effectiveness. There are multiple medications that can have an effect on theophylline metabolism either leading to increased metabolism and lower therapeutic levels or decreasing metabolism leading to toxicities, including medications that can be purchased without a prescription (Table 35-4).

CONCLUSION

Many factors influence patient adherence to prescribed therapies. Medication selection should be based on severity of disease as well as patients' perceptions of their disease and their concerns related to potential side effects from the prescribed treatment. Patients should be made aware of potential side effects that might occur as a result of their medication; however, assurance that the patient is being monitored for efficacy and disease control with appropriate step-down therapy, as well as potential side effects can be instrumental in attaining proper adherence. Reassurance that the patient need not fear drug dependency will be beneficial in promoting adherence. Other asthma medication–sparing strategies should be implemented as warranted, such as tobacco cessation, decreased allergen exposure, annual influenza vaccination, and treatment of comorbid diseases (e.g., GERD, sinusitis, allergies).

Table 35-4
THEOPHYLLINE DRUG-DRUG INTERACTIONS

Drug	Mechanism	Result
Allopurinol (high dose)	Decrease theophylline clearance	Elevated serum theophylline concentrations/toxicity
Amiodarone		
Cimetidine		
Ciprofloxacin		
Clarithromycin		
Disulfiram		
Erythromycin		
Fluvoxamine		
Interferon, human recombinant alpha-A		
Methotrexate		
Mexilitene		
Oral contraceptives		
Peginterferon alfa-2a		
Pentoxyphylline		
Propranolol		
Thiabendazole		
Ticlopidine		
Troleandomycin		
Verapamil		
Zileuton		
Alcohol	Large dose can decrease theophylline clearance for up to 24 hours	Increased serum theophylline concentrations
Barbiturates	Induction of hepatic enzymes by barbiturates	Decreased serum theophylline concentrations
Benzodiazepines	Theophylline blocks adenosine receptors, benzodiazepines increase concentrations of adenosine	Larger doses of benzodiazepines may be required to achieve effectiveness
Bupropion	Lowers seizure threshold	Increased serum theophylline concentrations
Carbamazepine Rifampin	Increased theophylline clearance	Decreased serum theophylline concentrations
Lithium	Increased excretion of lithium	Decreased effect of lithium
Phenytoin	Increased hepatic metabolism of theophylline and phenytoin	Decreased effect of both medications
Tacrolimus	Theophylline inhibits the metabolism of tacrolimus	Increased serum tacrolimus concentrations
Tobacco smoke	Decreased half-life of theophylline	Decreased serum theophylline concentrations
Zafirlukast		Decreased zafirlukast efficacy and/or increased serum theophylline concentrations

SUGGESTED READING

Allen DB: Benefits and risks for inhaled corticosteroids in children: an expert interview. Available at http://www.medscape.com/viewarticle/548361?src=mp.

Allen DB: Systemic effects of inhaled corticosteroids in children. Curr Opin Pediatr 2004;16:440–444.

American College of Rheumatology Task Force on Osteoporosis Guidelines: Recommendations for the prevention and treatment of glucocorticoid-induced osteoporosis. Arthritis Rheumatism 2005;39(11):1791–1801.

Global Strategy for Asthma Management and Prevention, Revised 2006. Available at www.ginasthma.org.

Guillot B: Skin reactions to inhaled corticosteroids—clinical aspects, incidence, avoidance and management. Am J Clin Dermatol 2000;1(2):107–111.

Irwin RS, Richardson ND: Side effects with inhaled corticosteroids: the physician's perception. Chest 2006;130:45–53.

National Asthma Education and Prevention Program: Expert Panel Report 3: Guidelines for the diagnosis and management of asthma. National Institutes of Health, National Heart, Lung, and Blood Institute, 2007, available at http://www.nhlbi.nih.gov/guidelines/asthma/index.htm.

Randell TL, Donaghue KC, Ambler GR, et al: Safety of the newer inhaled corticosteroids in childhood asthma. Pediatr Drugs 2003;5(7):481–504.

Roland NJ, Bhalla RK, Earis J: The local side-effects of inhaled corticosteroids: current understanding and review of the literature. Chest 2004;126:213–219.

Sorkness CA: Comparison of systemic effect and safety among different inhaled corticosteroids. J Allergy Clin Immunol 1998;102:S52–S64.

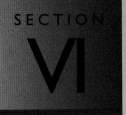

SECTION VI

SPECIAL SITUATIONS IN THE MANAGEMENT OF ASTHMA

The Difficult-to-Treat Asthma Patient

Ilonka H. van Veen and Elisabeth H. Bel

CLINICAL PEARLS

- Not all patients with "difficult-to-control" asthma have "severe asthma." Many of them have an incorrect diagnosis or mild-moderate asthma with unrecognized aggravating factors or are noncompliant with prescribed therapy.

- For a diagnosis of severe asthma, it is necessary to confirm the diagnosis of asthma, to evaluate and treat endogenous and exogenous aggravating factors, and to closely follow the patient for 6 months or longer.

- Severe asthma is a heterogeneous condition with different phenotypes. Defining clinical phenotypes is necessary to improve understanding of underlying mechanisms, to help guide current treatment, and to provide clues for novel therapeutic interventions.

- Despite intensive multidrug treatment with high-dose inhaled and oral corticosteroids, many patients with severe asthma remain uncontrolled. There is an urgent need for new, more effective treatments.

The term *difficult-to-treat asthma* is widely used to describe patients with asthma in whom symptoms are uncontrolled by standard pharmacological and environmental approaches. Although currently available anti-inflammatory and bronchodilator drugs are very effective, and good asthma control can be achieved for most patients, there remains a small but significant number of patients (around 5% of the total asthma population) who continue to experience inadequately controlled symptoms, frequent exacerbations, and objective pulmonary function abnormalities despite maximum standard therapy. These patients represent a heavy burden on health service resources, account for the majority of health care costs related to asthma, and, most importantly, are at greatest risk of death due to asthma. Many terms, including *refractory asthma*, *chronic persistent asthma*, *life-threatening asthma*, *brittle asthma*, and *steroid-resistant asthma*, are being used in different ways by different people to describe difficult-to-treat asthma. In 1999, a European Respiratory Society taskforce defined difficult/therapy-resistant asthma as "asthma, which is poorly controlled in terms of chronic symptoms, episodic exacerbations, persistent and variable airway obstruction and a continued requirement for short acting beta-agonists despite delivery of a reasonable dose of inhaled corticosteroids."[1] One year later, in 2000, an American Thoracic Society workshop on refractory asthma used a similar definition, in which major and minor characteristics were distinguished. For a patient to be diagnosed with "refractory asthma" at least one major and two minor criteria are to be fulfilled[2] (Table 36-1).

Both the European and American definitions are rather inclusive, and there is now consensus among experts that the definition of difficult-to-treat asthma is broader and more inclusive than severe asthma. The term *severe asthma* applies to patients who have refractory asthma who remain difficult to treat despite an extensive reevaluation of diagnosis and management, and following an observational period of at least 6 months by an asthma specialist.[3]

Since patients with difficult-to-treat asthma vary widely in clinical and physiological characteristics, and exhibit different types and degrees of airway inflammation, it is of major importance to subdivide these patients into different subtypes to elucidate the underlying pathophysiological mechanisms and to eventually find new therapies.[4] This chapter describes several clinical and inflammatory phenotypes of difficult-to-treat asthma, provides a guideline for the clinical assessment of this heterogeneous group of patients, and discusses the potential of novel therapeutic agents.

NOT ALL PATIENTS WITH DIFFICULT-TO-TREAT ASTHMA HAVE SEVERE ASTHMA!

When confronted by a patient with inadequately controlled asthma symptoms, frequent exacerbations, or persistent airflow limitation despite maximum standard therapy, one should always ask the following questions:

First, does the patient really have asthma? Second, are there any environmental or comorbid factors worsening

Table 36-1
CRITERIA FOR A DIAGNOSIS OF "REFRACTORY ASTHMA"*

Major Criteria
- Use of oral corticosteroids ≥ 50% of the time
- Continuous use of high doses of inhaled corticosteroids (≥1200 µg/day beclomethasone or equivalent)

Minor Criteria
- Requirement for daily treatment with long-acting beta-agonists, theophylline, or leukotriene antagonists
- Daily asthma symptoms requiring rescue medication
- Persistent airway obstruction ($FEV_1 < 80\%$ predicted); diurnal PEF variability > 20%
- 1 or more urgent care visits for asthma in the last year
- 3 or more courses of oral steroid bursts in the last year
- Prompt deterioration with ≤ 25% reduction in oral or inhaled corticosteroid dose
- Near-fatal asthma event in the past

*At least one major and two or more minor criteria are required for the diagnosis of refractory asthma.

Adapted from Proceedings of the ATS workshop on refractory asthma: current understanding, recommendations, and unanswered questions. American Thoracic Society. Am J Respir Crit Care Med 2000;162(6):2341–2351.

Table 36-2
ALTERNATIVE DIAGNOSES IN DIFFICULT-TO-CONTROL ASTHMA IN ADULTS

Chronic obstructive pulmonary disease
Bronchiectasis
Congestive heart failure
Central airway obstruction by:
    Foreign body
    Tumor (benign/malignant)
    Sarcoidosis
    Tracheobronchomalacia
Cystic fibrosis
Recurrent pulmonary embolism
Obstructive bronchiolitis
Recurrent aspiration
Vocal cord dysfunction
Allergic bronchopulmonary aspergillosis
Churg-Strauss syndrome

asthma symptomatology? Third, is the patient compliant with prescribed therapy and does he or she use it correctly?

Does the Patient Really Have Asthma?

The diagnosis of "difficult-to-treat asthma" is based on a secure diagnosis of asthma. Although this seems a redundant statement, it has been demonstrated that, after thorough evaluation of a group of patients with difficult-to-treat asthma referred for second opinion to a tertiary respiratory unit, 12% left the clinic with an alternative diagnosis (mainly chronic obstructive pulmonary disease [COPD]) and a further 7% with an additional diagnosis.[5] This implies that the diagnosis of asthma needs to be confirmed by the presence of typical symptoms together with objective evidence of variable airflow limitation or bronchial hyperresponsiveness. In addition, alternative diagnoses need to be considered and excluded (Table 36-2). Careful history taking and additional investigations such as high-resolution computed tomography (CT) scanning and bronchoscopy might be needed to exclude these diagnoses. The onset of symptoms, in particular in relation to smoking history, should be carefully reviewed to distinguish asthma from COPD. However, late-onset asthma that has become unresponsive to corticosteroid therapy because of long-standing smoking resembles COPD in many respects, which can make the distinction between both diseases very complicated.

Are There Any Environmental or Comorbid Factors Worsening Asthma Symptoms?

Even after the diagnosis of asthma is confirmed, numerous factors can contribute to continuing respiratory symptoms. Ongoing allergen exposure at home or in the workplace can induce an airway inflammatory process that may increase the severity of asthma. The contribution of chemical or toxic substances at work should also be considered and avoidance measures should be proposed to prevent a worsening of the asthma condition. Smoking is an important factor that may contribute to the development and severity of asthma; smokers

have a reduced response to corticosteroids and a more rapid decline in pulmonary function. Therefore, strategies to encourage smoking cessation are an essential aspect of management of patients with difficult-to-treat asthma.

Several studies have shown that a large proportion of patients with difficult-to-treat asthma have a high incidence of previously unrecognized comorbidities contributing to the continuation and severity of respiratory symptoms. Asthma of any severity may coexist with such comorbidity, resulting in frequent exacerbations, high health care usage, and even risk of serious adverse events. Managing these issues may improve asthma control, and therefore any patient with difficult-to-treat asthma should be systematically assessed to identify and diagnose additional factors influencing the severity of asthma symptoms. Additional diagnoses that can coexist with asthma and may contribute to respiratory symptomatology are hyperventilation, vocal cord dysfunction (VCD), and psychiatric disturbances. The incidence of VCD (upper airway obstruction due to adduction of the anterior two thirds of the vocal cords) is still unclear. In a large series of patients with VCD, predominantly young women, 56% also had asthma. The diagnosis can only be confirmed in a symptomatic patient during laryngoscopy, which is not a very appealing procedure in an already dyspneic patient. Therapeutic options are minimal and although essential, it is often difficult to withdraw (corticosteroid) therapy in these patients.

Compliance with Prescribed Therapy and Correct Inhalation Technique

Other issues that should be addressed in patients with difficult-to-treat asthma are adherence to prescribed treatment and inhalation technique. Adherence is often suboptimal in asthma. In a large study in patients with refractory asthma 32% of the patients who were using high doses of prednisone (more than 15 mg per day) were nonadherent. Checking cortisol levels in these patients may therefore be worthwhile. How to best assess compliance with inhaled therapy in clinical practice is more complicated and remains a significant challenge. Inhalation technique is often far from adequate, and regular checking of correct technique can be rewarding. Proper instruction is essential to improve inhalation technique, while the use of uniform inhaler devices might improve the accuracy of the inhalation technique.

CLINICAL SUBTYPES OF DIFFICULT-TO-TREAT ASTHMA

It has been well established that patients with asthma may vary considerably with respect to clinical characteristics, triggering factors, and type of airway inflammation.[4] Since the beginning of this century, clinicians have recognized various subtypes of asthma, in particular atopic asthma as opposed to intrinsic asthma. Subsequently, many other subtypes of asthma, including aspirin-induced asthma, brittle asthma, and noneosinophilic asthma, have been distinguished. Over the years, clinical researchers have tried to subdivide patients with asthma into distinct phenotypes, but they have failed to reach a definitive classification. One of the reasons for this lack of clear discrimination among various phenotypes is that they were defined by either clinical or physiological characteristics, by environmental triggers, or by underlying pathobiology.

Although there is substantial overlap among the asthma phenotypes, hardly any studies have linked clinical, immunological, and pathological characteristics. For the clinician dealing with patients with difficult-to-treat asthma, identification of the clinical phenotype is important for proper management of the disease. Therefore, the following focuses on three clinical phenotypes of difficult-to-treat asthma that are commonly encountered in the outpatient pulmonary clinic: patients with frequent asthma exacerbations, patients with chronic persistent airflow limitation, and patients who depend on oral corticosteroids to keep their asthma under control.

Asthmatic Patients with Frequent Severe Exacerbations

Despite the clinical and economic importance of asthma exacerbations, only a few studies have examined factors that may contribute to their recurrence. Emergency department visits and hospitalization for asthma seem to be related to several psychosocial factors, such as lower socioeconomic status, inaccessibility of medical care, and coexisting psychiatric diseases. In addition, patient characteristics that are associated with severe life-threatening asthma attacks include female gender, older age, smoking, and noncompliance with recommended therapy. Apart from these patient characteristics and psychosocial circumstances, several endogenous and exogenous aggravating factors have been implicated to contribute to difficult-to-treat asthma. However, factors that contribute to the recurrence of exacerbations among these patients with poorly controlled disease are only beginning to be defined.

PHYSIOLOGIC FACTORS
One of the reasons that some patients exacerbate more easily and frequently than others might be that they detect worsening of their disease only in a late phase. It has been demonstrated that patients with recurrent asthma exacerbations have a poorer dyspnea perception than those with stable severe asthma. This suggests that reduced perception of airway obstruction might be a risk factor of frequent exacerbations. Management of such patients should therefore be focused on self-assessment guided by objective measures of airflow limitation such as home monitoring of peak expiratory flow or spirometry.

Second, patients with frequent exacerbations might suffer from excessive airway narrowing and subsequent airway closure during an asthma attack. It has been shown that patients with frequent exacerbations have more airway closure under stable circumstances than equally severe asthmatic patients without a history of exacerbations. This implies that there are more pathological changes in the smaller airways (airways with a diameter less than 2 mm) of these patients than in patients without exacerbations. During an exacerbation, when further airway obstruction develops due to various triggers, these patients are at risk of dramatic airway narrowing resulting in respiratory insufficiency.

COMORBID FACTORS
Recently, ten Brinke and colleagues investigated clinical and environmental factors potentially associated with recurrent exacerbations in 136 patients with difficult-to-treat asthma, and compared patients with three or more severe exacerbations

in the previous year with those with only one exacerbation per year.[6] A systematic diagnostic protocol was used to assess 13 potential risk factors (Table 36-3). The results of the study showed that frequent exacerbations in difficult-to-treat asthma were invariably associated with one or more contributing factors other than asthma itself. Apart from younger age and shorter asthma duration, frequent exacerbations in these patients was strongly associated with psychological dysfunctioning (odds ratio [OR]: 10.8), recurrent respiratory tract infections (OR: 6.9), gastroesophageal reflux (OR: 4.9), severe nasal sinus disease (OR: 3.7), and obstructive sleep apnea (OR: 3.4). All patients with frequent exacerbations exhibited at least one of these five factors while 52% showed three or even more factors. Furthermore, atopic patients, in particular those with specific immunoglobulin E (IgE) to house-dust mite or cockroach, had more than 10-fold increased odds for frequent exacerbations as compared to nonatopic patients. Psychological dysfunction and severe chronic sinus disease were the only independent contributing factors associated with frequent exacerbations, with adjusted odds ratios of 11.7 and 5.5, respectively. These findings emphasize the high prevalence of mostly unidentified contributing factors in difficult-to-treat asthmatic patients with frequent exacerbations, and suggest that treatment of these specific factors might possibly result in better control of the disease.

Two studies, not specifically focusing on asthma exacerbations, showed that clinical improvement can be anticipated if patients with poorly controlled or difficult-to-treat asthma are submitted to a systematic evaluation protocol, although one study failed to show an improvement in quality of life despite targeted treatment. Psychological disturbances that are recognized and treated in patients with poor asthma control might significantly reduce the morbidity and exacerbation frequency. There is some debate as to whether treatment for gastroesophageal reflux results in overall improvement in asthma, but most authors agree that subgroups of patients may gain benefit. Proper medical and surgical management of sinusitis in asthmatic patients has been shown to result in both

Table 36-3
FREQUENCY OF FACTORS THAT MADE ASTHMA WORSE IN 136 PATIENTS WITH "DIFFICULT ASTHMA"

Factors	%
Endogenous Factors	
Recurrent respiratory infections	58.1
Gastroesophageal reflux	49.3
Severe chronic sinus disease	45.5
Relative immunodeficiency	31.5
Hormonal influences	30.0
Psychological dysfunctioning	20.4
Obstructive sleep apnea syndrome	12.5
Thyroid disease	1.5
Specific Trigger Factors	
Ongoing allergen exposure	38.5
Occupational sensitizers	27.9
Drugs (e.g., beta-blockers, NSAIDs)	9.6
Food allergens	9.4

Adapted from ten Brinke A, Sterk PJ, Masclee AA, et al: Risk factors of frequent exacerbations in difficult-to-treat asthma. Eur Respir J 2005;26(5):812–818.

improved sinonasal and asthmatic symptoms with fewer physician visits and decreased need for medication. Furthermore, nasal continuous positive airway pressure therapy has been demonstrated to improve asthma control in some unstable asthmatic patients.

Asthmatic Patients with Persistent Airflow Limitation

A considerable percentage (around 50%) of nonsmoking adult patients with difficult-to-treat asthma have persistent or "fixed" airflow limitation despite appropriate therapy. Persistent airflow limitation, defined as an FEV_1 (forced expiratory volume in 1 second) less than 75% of the predicted value after maximal bronchodilatation, has been associated with more severe asthma and with increased overall mortality. There is little overlap between patients with recurrent severe exacerbations and those who are well controlled but have fixed airflow limitation, suggesting that either they represent two distinct asthma phenotypes, or that one phenotype develops into the other phenotype. Several factors have been proposed to contribute to loss of lung function and fixed airflow limitation in asthma.

GENETIC AND ENVIRONMENTAL FACTORS

Persistent airflow limitation is believed to be a consequence of structural and functional changes in the airways, possibly related to abnormal injury and repair responses of the bronchial epithelium, either inherited or acquired.[7] Airway inflammation resulting from the interaction between genetic and environmental factors is clearly an important factor contributing to progressive loss of lung function. Studies in severe asthma have indeed shown associations between persistent airway obstruction and eosinophilia in blood, sputum, and bronchial biopsies.

Interestingly, two studies, one cross-sectional and one longitudinal, showed that patients with adult-onset, nonatopic asthma with evidence of previous infection with *Chlamydia pneumoniae* have an increased decline in lung function as compared with other patients with asthma. This suggests that pathogens such as *Chlamydia pneumoniae* might promote the development of persistent airflow limitation in some patients with asthma. Antibiotic treatment with macrolides in patients with asthma of varying severity has indeed shown a small improvement in lung function only in those patients who were polymerase chain reaction (PCR)-positive for *Chlamydia pneumoniae* or *Mycoplasma pneumoniae*. Other studies with macrolides in patients with aspirin-intolerant asthma and corticosteroid-dependent asthma have shown similar results, including an improvement in asthma symptoms.

STRUCTURAL CHANGES OF THE LARGE AIRWAYS AND DISTAL LUNG

How exactly airway inflammation leads to persistent airflow limitation is still unclear. Several pathological changes of the airways, referred to as airway remodeling, have been defined, such as subepithelial fibrosis, increased vascularity of the mucosa, and smooth muscle hyperplasia and hypertrophy. A recent study showed an increase in large airway smooth muscle area in bronchial biopsies from patients with severe asthma as compared to those with moderate asthma, whereas there was no significant difference in subepithelial fibrosis between the two groups. In addition, the amount of smooth muscle mass correlated with the degree of airflow limitation. These data suggest that increased smooth muscle mass might be the key structural change that determines the degree of (persistent) airflow limitation and distinguishes moderate from severe asthma.

A second proposed mechanism of persistent airflow limitation relates to the site of airflow limitation in the bronchial tree. There is now increasing pathologic and physiologic evidence that airway inflammation in asthma not only occurs in the central airways but also extends to the distal lung and the lung parenchyma. Similar structural changes that occur in the large airways have been described for the peripheral airways (airways smaller than 2 mm in diameter) as well. The clinical significance of distal airway inflammation and dysfunction has not yet been clearly determined, but it has been shown that patients with severe asthma, in particular those with persistent airflow limitation, have more peripheral airways dysfunction as compared to those with mild disease. It is therefore conceivable that poorly controlled inflammation in the peripheral airways contributes to the accelerated decline in lung function and airway remodeling. Since peripheral airways are not reached by conventional inhaled steroids, small molecular inhaled steroids (hydrofluoralkane [HFA] steroids), which have a higher lung deposition than conventional steroids, might be an interesting therapeutic option for patients with persistent airflow limitation. One study has shown that a 6-week course of HFA-inhaled steroids suppressed eosinophilic inflammation of the large and small airways and decreased the expression of alpha-smooth muscle actin in peripheral airways; however the effect of these steroids has not yet been compared with that of conventional steroids.

A third explanation of persistent airflow limitation might be the occlusion of the airway lumen by mucus. Abnormalities of the epithelium with increased goblet cell formation and hyperplasia of submucosal glands result in increased mucus production and subsequent plugging of the (smaller) airways.

Finally, changes at the parenchymal level might be responsible for persistent airflow limitation in asthma. Postmortem studies have shown that patients who died from an asthma attack had an increased proportion of abnormal alveolar attachments and a decreased elastic fiber content in the small airway adventitial layer and in the peribronchial alveoli. This suggests that structural alterations at the peribronchiolar level might contribute to the pathogenesis of persistent airflow limitation observed in patients with severe asthma.

Thus, although the pathogenesis of persistent airflow limitation is far from clear, an increase in airway smooth muscle mass, a reduced ability of the airways to dilate, peripheral airway dysfunction, plugging of the airway lumen by mucus, and loss of alveolar attachments resulting in airway collapse are possible mechanisms that can result in persistent airflow limitation in patients with difficult-to-treat asthma.

Patients Who Depend on Oral Corticosteroids to Keep Their Asthma under Control

Patients with difficult-to-treat asthma are per definition characterized by an insufficient response to treatment with inhaled steroids. After exclusion of misdiagnosis, nonadherence with treatment, inadequate inhalation technique, the influence of environmental or comorbid factors that aggravate the disease, and the presence of irreversible airflow limitation, the clinician is left with the true steroid-dependent asthmatic patient. In these patients, there might be several reasons why treatment with inhaled steroids fails to control the disease.

First, the inflammation of the airways might be too severe to respond to "normal doses" of asthma medication. These patients will respond to increasing the dose of inhaled corticosteroids above the recommended dose.

Second, the inhaled corticosteroids do not reach specific sites of inflammation in the lung, for example, the small airways or the upper airways. Asthma is now increasingly recognized as a systemic disease, not only affecting the lower airways, but also the nose and paranasal sinuses. Because of the cross-talk between the upper and lower airways via the bone marrow and systemic circulation, a systemic therapeutic approach can sometimes be more effective than a local approach. This can be observed in clinical practice when patients fail to keep their asthma under control with high doses of inhaled corticosteroids, but are perfectly well controlled by the combination of moderate doses of inhaled corticosteroids and low doses of oral corticosteroids.

A third option is that patients with steroid-dependent asthma have a different profile of inflammatory cells in the airways as compared to steroid-sensitive asthmatic patients. It has been shown that patients with severe steroid-dependent asthma have more neutrophilic airway inflammation that is less likely to respond to steroid treatment than patients with mild asthma.

A fourth explanation might be that the intrinsic effect of the corticosteroid on the inflammatory process in the airways is reduced. The anti-inflammatory effect of corticosteroids can be disturbed due to various mechanisms, such as reduced corticosteroid affinity of the glucocorticoid receptor (GR) or diminished GR translocation into the nucleus.

Other possible mechanisms include interaction with pro-inflammatory transcription factors or impaired activation of anti-inflammatory genes via reduced histone deacetylase [HDAC] function. Smoking and ex-smoking have also been associated with reduced steroid sensitivity. In patients with asthma who smoked, a reduced effect of inhaled and oral steroid treatment has been demonstrated as compared with nonsmoking asthmatic patients. The mechanisms of corticosteroid resistance in smokers are unexplained, but might be due to a more neutrophilic type of inflammation, changes in the glucocorticoid receptor expression, and increased activation of pro-inflammatory transcription factors or reduced HDAC activity.

Finally, persistent viral infection might induce steroid resistance by activation of pro-inflammatory transcription factors that interfere with corticosteroid action. Persistent infection with *Chlamydia pneumoniae* and *Mycoplasma pneumoniae* has been associated with progression of the disease in asthma. Furthermore, it has been demonstrated that latent adenoviral infection in guinea pigs inhibits the anti-inflammatory effects of glucocorticoids. Thus, a combination of extrinsic and intrinsic factors can result in reduced sensitivity to inhaled corticosteroids and dependence on oral corticosteroids, resulting in a difficult-to-treat asthmatic patient.

WHICH PATIENTS ARE AT RISK OF A NEAR-FATAL ASTHMA ATTACK?

After initial stabilization of asthma death rates in the United States, mortality has now decreased since 1998 to 1.6 per 100,000 in the general population. This decrease is most likely a result of improved asthma management in combination with recent decreases in asthma prevalence. Presumably there are more near-fatal asthma episodes than fatal attacks, but no incidence data are available. This might be partly because there is no uniform definition of near-fatal asthma. In research studies near-fatal episodes of asthma usually concern patients who require intubation and mechanical ventilation, but sometimes also attacks associated with hypercapnia and respiratory acidosis are considered near fatal.

Clinical Features

From a clinical perspective it is extremely important to identify patients who are at risk of a near-fatal asthma attack in order to prevent such attacks in the future. Case-control studies have shown that multiple risk factors are likely to be involved. Asthma mortality seems to be increased in women, African Americans, and patients with a lower socioeconomic status. Further risk factors include a history of previous mechanical ventilation and admission to the intensive care unit because of an asthma attack and more severe uncontrolled disease. Furthermore, patients with near-fatal attacks report more food allergies and are more likely to have emotional or social events as the trigger for their attack. In women at reproductive age, menstruation might act as a contributing factor in the development of near-fatal asthma episodes.

Pathophysiologic Conditions

As in patients with frequent, less severe exacerbations, patients with near-fatal asthma attacks have a blunted perception of dyspnea at rest as well as at peak exercise. In addition, asthmatic patients with a low perception of dyspnea who were followed for 2 years had more emergency department visits, hospitalizations, near-fatal asthma attacks, and asthma deaths. Accurate recognition of asthma worsening is essential for prompting individuals to increase medication or seek medical help and prevent (near-) fatal attacks. Lung function measurements in patients before and after a life-threatening asthma attack showed that persistent airway obstruction, loss of elastic recoil pressure, and hyperinflation at total lung capacity (TLC) are risk factors for near fatal attacks.

Pathology

Fatal asthma is pathologically characterized by airway occlusion due to mucus accumulation, thickening of all compartments of the airway wall, neutrophilic and eosinophilic cell infiltration, and smooth muscle shortening. Lung tissue from fatal asthma cases shows loss of alveolar attachments and decreased elastic fiber content as compared to controls. These structural changes might contribute to the functional abnormalities observed in patients with severe asthma such as enhanced airway closure and loss of deep breath bronchodilator effect. It seems that different pathological changes account for differences in the course of fatal attacks. Asthma attacks that lead to sudden death (within 3 hours after onset of symptoms) are characterized by smooth muscle shortening and neutrophilic cell infiltration of the airway wall. Long-course cases tend to have more mucus accumulation in the airway lumen. Different triggers might be responsible for causing short- and long-course near-fatalities. Studies comparing rapid- and slow-onset asthma attacks showed in rapid-onset asthma a lower rate of suspected respiratory infection, higher rates of fume/irritant inhalation, and a higher intake of nonsteroidal anti-inflammatory drugs (NSAIDs). Furthermore, patients with rapid-onset asthma had a more severe presentation, but also a quicker response to treatment, with a faster recovery.

APPROACH OF THE PATIENT WITH DIFFICULT-TO-TREAT ASTHMA

The practical approach of a patient with suspected difficult-to-treat asthma should consist of a systematic analysis focused on a correct diagnosis, treatment adherence, and detection of endogenous and exogenous triggers and aggravating factors. An

algorithm for such an approach is given in Figure 36-1. The first crucial step is to confirm that the patient really has asthma, to exclude alternative diagnoses and to ensure proper inhalation technique and treatment adherence. Detailed history taking, physical examination, and diagnostic tests are needed to guarantee a thorough evaluation of the patient to identify factors that offer room for therapeutic intervention in order to improve asthma control.

History

A thorough history taking is the most important part of the evaluation of a patient with difficult-to-treat asthma since this provides valuable information about the clinical asthma phenotype. The past medical history should be questioned in detail with respect to age of asthma onset (at childhood versus adulthood) and duration of asthma. In case of childhood asthma, information about symptoms, medication, frequency of asthma attacks, treatment, and nonattendance at school will give an idea about asthma severity at that time. To evaluate present asthma severity, the number of exacerbations and

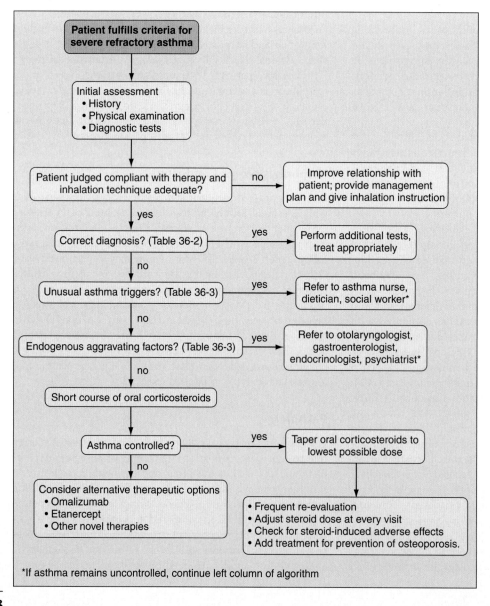

Figure 36-1 Algorithm for the approach to asthma management.

prednisone and antibiotic courses in the past few years, as well as the number of attacks resulting in admissions at an intensive care unit and/or mechanical ventilation, need to be estimated. Attention should be paid to current quality of life, possible limitations of daily activities, and daytime and night-time symptoms despite current treatment. Evaluation of past and current asthma treatment (and response to this) can give insight into already tried or missed treatment options.

Possible endogenous and exogenous risk factors need to be examined. Possible exogenous triggers include sensitization and exposure to allergens (inhalation allergens, food allergens, occupational triggers) and influence of drugs that can interfere with asthma control or induce asthma attacks (NSAIDs, beta-blockers, angiotensin-converting-enzyme-inhibitors, estrogens). The search for exogenous risk factors should focus on signs of gastroesophageal reflux, chronic rhinosinusitis, psychosocial problems, recurrent bacterial infections, symptoms of sleep apnea, and hormonal influences (perimenstrual asthma, asthma during pregnancy, thyroid problems). Especially chronic rhinosinusitis and psychosocial problems have been associated with frequent asthma exacerbations. Current and past smoking habits as well as passive smoking at home or at work need to be questioned, since (ex-) smoking has been associated with relative steroid resistance.

Physical Examination

The physical examination should be part of the systemic evaluation of a patient with severe asthma. It can particularly reveal signs that point toward alternative or additional diagnoses. Stridor can fit in with the diagnosis of vocal cord dysfunction or tracheal abnormalities. Dullness on percussion, crackles, squeaks, or pleural rub can reveal other diagnoses such as pleural fluid, heart failure, infections, bronchiectasis, and pulmonary embolism. Signs of systemic diseases might be present as well as signs of endocrine disorders (e.g., goiter). Furthermore, one may observe signs of chronic rhinosinusitis (e.g., postnasal drip) and signs of side effects of steroids (cushingoid appearance, hypertension, skin bruising, kyphosis due to osteoporosis).

Diagnostic Tests

Several diagnostic tests can be helpful to evaluate asthma diagnosis, severity of airway obstruction, and to obtain information about endogenous and exogenous risk factors. Attempts should be made to re-evaluate the diagnosis of asthma by performing spirometry showing reversible airway obstruction or by demonstrating bronchial hyperreactivity by provocation testing. Spirometry is also used to evaluate current lung function impairment and the presence of persistent airflow limitation. Additional lung volume measurements and measurement of diffusion capacity may be required to exclude diffuse parenchymal disorders and abnormalities pointing toward COPD or emphysema. To exclude other pulmonary diagnoses, a chest x-ray is mandatory in all patients. High-resolution CT scanning of the lung can be performed on indication, e.g., when pulmonary fibrosis or bronchiectasis is suspected.

Routine blood tests should be performed mainly to exclude additional diagnoses. A high erythrocyte sedimentation rate (ESR), for example, can point toward a systemic disease such as Churg-Strauss vasculitis. Peripheral blood eosinophilia can reveal hypereosinophilic syndromes. Atopy can be evaluated with serology or skin prick testing. Patients should be checked for signs of chronic rhinosinusitis. Since a considerable number of patients have extensive sinus disease without symptoms, sinus-CT scanning is recommended in all patients. Evaluation by an ear-nose-throat (ENT) specialist is often needed to determine whether surgical intervention is needed. Furthermore, the presence of gastroesophageal reflux can be checked by performing a 24-hour pH measurement of the esophagus. Alternatively, when patients cannot support this procedure, a 4- to 8-week trial with proton-pump inhibitors can be considered. If obstructive sleep apnea syndrome is suspected, a polysomnography should be performed. Patients who are on long-term oral steroid treatment need to be evaluated for osteoporosis, one of the major side effects of this treatment with bone densitometry.

After this diagnostic work-up, when the diagnosis of severe asthma is confirmed and alternative diagnoses are ruled out, the first step is to address possible aggravating factors. This includes the avoidance of allergens and occupational sensitizers; discontinuation or replacement of drugs that interfere with asthma control; and treatment of chronic rhinosinusitis, gastroesophageal reflux, and obstructive sleep apnea syndrome. Psychosocial problems should be addressed and when indicated the patient should be referred to a psychologist or psychiatrist.

HOW ABOUT NONINVASIVE MEASUREMENTS OF AIRWAY INFLAMMATION?

Noninvasive measures of airway inflammation that can be used in the clinic include the assessment of sputum cell counts and exhaled nitric oxide (FE_{NO}). Induced-sputum cell counts are particularly well validated, and normal ranges from large adult populations have been published. Sputum induction is a well-tolerated, safe procedure even in those with severe disease and during exacerbations. In two large prospective studies, therapy directed at normalizing sputum eosinophil counts markedly reduced asthma exacerbations. Both of these studies included severe asthma patients and the greatest benefit was observed in them. Management strategies that incorporated measures of FE_{NO} have not led to a reduction in asthma exacerbations in adults or children, although these studies were performed in patients with milder disease. Thus, to date, sputum induction is the most robust measure of airway inflammation in asthma, but simpler assessment tools are needed.

Some patients with asthma show elevated numbers of eosinophils and high levels of FE_{NO} in their sputum despite intensive high-dose steroid therapy. These patients seem to represent an asthma phenotype with more severe disease characterized by near-fatal attacks, more severe symptoms, adult onset of asthma, and persistent airflow limitation.

Other patients seem to be characterized by predominant neutrophilic inflammation. Neutrophilia can occur in patients with noneosinophilic asthma of varying severity but can also coexist with eosinophilic inflammation in severe asthma. The mechanisms of this neutrophilic inflammation are not clear. Possible mechanisms include an inflammatory response directed toward an as yet unidentified respiratory pathogen, or a defense mechanism against noxious stimuli including cigarette smoke, environmental pollutants, or occupational sensitizers. In any case, neutrophilic inflammation in asthma is associated with a markedly reduced response to inhaled and oral corticosteroids.

Finally, a small subgroup of patients with asthmatic symptoms hardly show any sign of inflammation in induced sputum. This might be the case in patients who have symptoms that mimic asthma (e.g., VCD, hyperventilation), but do not have asthma after all. An alternative explanation in patients with long-standing asthma might be that inhaled or oral steroids have abolished the airway inflammatory component of asthma but not the residual airway hyperresponsiveness.

Thus, noninvasive assessment of airway inflammation can assist in phenotyping the patient with difficult-to-treat asthma, which will ultimately lead to better-targeted treatment regimens.

MANAGEMENT OF THE PATIENT WITH DIFFICULT-TO-TREAT ASTHMA

The management of patients with difficult-to-treat asthma should ideally be undertaken in a multidisciplinary asthma center with extensive expertise in evaluating and treating these patients. Specialized centers have access to tests that are not routinely available, such as measurement of nitric oxide in exhaled air, analysis of induced sputum cells and supernatant, and examination of bronchial biopsies that will add to the medical evaluation. It may take several months to complete a full diagnostic and management protocol, and to eliminate the exogenous and endogenous factors that aggravate asthma. In some patients, admission to hospital may even be required to exclude environmental exposure to hidden allergens, sensitizers, or trigger factors; to explore the influence of psychosocial factors; or to check compliance with therapy. By paying attention to these factors, the control of refractory asthma can often be improved substantially.

Education

Education of patients to improve self-care is another element of the integrated management process of patients with difficult-to-treat asthma. Studies have suggested that a lack of self-management coupled with medical nonadherence is an important factor in hospitalization and asthma death. A good dialogue between patients and care providers is strongly encouraged. Intensive education might help these patients to better self-manage their asthma.

Rehabilitation Programs

Rehabilitation programs are highly recommended for patients with difficult-to-treat asthma. Many patients are debilitated by their condition, by inactivity and sedentary lifestyle, or by the side effects of systemic corticosteroid therapy. Exercise programs have proved to have health-related benefits, to improve quality of life, and to increase exercise performance and fitness.

Pharmacotherapy

Pharmacotherapy of severe asthma is based primarily on the combined use of high-dose inhaled corticosteroids (more than $1600\,\mu g$ per day of beclomethasone dipropionate) and long-acting inhaled beta$_2$-agonists, as outlined in the guidelines.[8] Higher doses of inhaled steroids are not likely to give more benefit since the dose-effect relationship of these drugs clearly shows a maximum. However, dose-response curves may vary among patients and some patients may thus respond to higher doses, which makes a trial with high doses of inhaled steroids worth trying. Sometimes, change of inhalation device such as switching to a dose aerosol administered via an inhalation chamber in case of poor inhalation technique might be helpful. In case of insufficient response to a combination of inhaled corticosteroids and long-acting beta$_2$-agonists, and after evaluation and treatment of environmental and comorbid aggravating factors, additional treatments can be tried: inhaled extra-fine aerosol corticosteroids might benefit the patient with peripheral airway inflammation; patients with chronic rhinosinusitis may improve with nasal corticosteroids; those with aspirin sensitivity may respond to leukotriene modifiers; and, in cases of evident allergic symptoms and frequent exacerbations, anti-IgE therapy may be effective.[9]

To date, there is no approved treatment for intervention in nonatopic patients who remain uncontrolled with recurrent exacerbations and chronically impaired lung function despite intensive multidrug treatments. Many of these patients require continuous systemic corticosteroid treatment to keep their asthma under control and to prevent irreversible loss of lung function. Systemic steroid therapy is, however, associated with serious side effects including osteoporosis, skin thinning, diabetes, hypertension, cataract formation, and myopathy, and every effort should be undertaken to minimize the dosage of these drugs. In this context, it is important for physicians to be aware that patients may have different ideas from doctors regarding optimal asthma control or optimal dosing of systemic steroids. With continuous high-dose systemic steroid therapy, the goal must be to find the optimal balance between therapeutic efficacy and short- and long-term side effects of the drug.

Although initial reports with treatments such as oral gold, methotrexate, and cyclosporin were encouraging, experience over the past decades has been disappointing. Meta-analyses have shown that there is insufficient evidence to support the use of these drugs in the routine treatment of severe asthma as steroid-sparing agents. In most cases, the limited steroid-sparing efficacy of these drugs appeared to be insufficient to offset the serious side effects.

Promising new asthma therapies include humanized monoclonal antibodies against tumor necrosis factor (TNF)-α.[10] These drugs have been shown to produce remarkable clinical responses in chronic inflammatory diseases such as rheumatoid arthritis and Crohn disease. Recent evidence suggests that patients with refractory asthma also show clinical benefit. Three clinical trials, an open-label study with etanercept in 17 patients, a double-blind placebo-controlled trial with etanercept in 10 patients, and a double-blind parallel trial with infliximab in 38 patients with severe asthma have shown improvements in symptoms, lung function, airway hyperresponsiveness, and the number of asthma exacerbations. Large-scale studies are now under way to confirm these promising findings.

FUTURE PERSPECTIVES

Since existing therapies for asthma offer only partial relief for chronic severe asthmatic patients, there remains an unmet medical need for these patients, and innovative therapeutic agents are required. Such therapies need to be developed to target not only the steroid-resistant inflammatory component of asthma, but also the remodeling aspects of these diseases. New treatments in development for asthma include inhibitors of the pro-inflammatory enzymes, such as phosphodiesterase-4 (PDE4), p38 mitogen-activated protein (MAP) kinase, and nuclear-factor (NF)-κB activating kinase. PDE4 inhibitors have a broad spectrum of anti-inflammatory effects in asthma. They inhibit the recruitment and activation of key inflammatory cells, including mast cells, eosinophils, T lymphocytes, macrophages, and neutrophils, as well as the hyperplasia and hypertrophy of structural cells, including airway smooth-muscle cells, epithelial cells, and sensory and cholinergic nerves. P38 MAP kinase has received particular attention, because of its involvement in the expression of several inflammatory proteins and its role in corticosteroid resistance in asthma. Inhibitors of p38 MAP kinase do not only inhibit the synthesis of many inflammatory cytokines, but also decrease eosinophil survival. Several inhibitors of p38 MAP kinase are now under development. Whether this new class of anti-inflammatory drugs will be safe in long-term studies remains to be established.

It is likely that such a broad-spectrum anti-inflammatory drug will have some toxicity, but inhalation might be a feasible therapeutic approach.

Transcription factor inhibitors such as the inhibitor of NF-κB have also shown promising anti-inflammatory properties and these drugs are currently in development. However, one concern about long-term NF-κB inhibition is that it could result in immune suppression and impaired host defense.

More specific approaches include inhibiting chemokine receptors on eosinophils and T lymphocytes, inhibiting adhesion molecules that recruit key inflammatory cells, and inhibiting mast cells with Syk kinase inhibitors.

SUMMARY AND CONCLUSIONS

Not all patients with "difficult-to-treat" asthma have "severe" asthma. A diagnosis of severe asthma requires confirmation of asthma by objective means, removal of causal and aggravating factors, and adequate education of the patient. In most patients with severe asthma, oral steroids remain the mainstay of treatment, while steroid-sparing immune suppressant drugs have shown disappointing efficacy. Severe asthma is a heterogeneous condition, and conscientious clinical phenotyping of patients is essential for a better understanding of the underlying mechanisms and the development of novel therapies.

REFERENCES

1. Chung KF, Godard P, Adelroth E, et al: Difficult/therapy-resistant asthma: the need for an integrated approach to define clinical phenotypes, evaluate risk factors, understand pathophysiology and find novel therapies. ERS Task Force on Difficult/Therapy-Resistant Asthma. European Respiratory Society. Eur Respir J 1999;13:1198–1208.
2. Proceedings of the ATS workshop on refractory asthma: current understanding, recommendations, and unanswered questions. American Thoracic Society. Am J Respir Crit Care Med 2000; 162(6):2341–2351.
3. Chanez P, Wenzel S, Anderson G, et al: Severe asthma: what are the important questions? J Allergy Clin Immunol 2007;119:1337–1348.
4. Wenzel SE: Asthma: defining of the persistent adult phenotypes. Lancet 2006;368(9537):804–813.
5. Robinson DS, Campbell DA, Durham SR, et al: Systematic assessment of difficult-to-treat asthma. Eur Respir J 2003;22(3):478–483.
6. ten Brinke A, Sterk PJ, Masclee AA, et al: Risk factors of frequent exacerbations in difficult-to-treat asthma. Eur Respir J 2005;26(5):812–818.
7. Holgate ST, Polosa R: The mechanisms, diagnosis, and management of severe asthma in adults. Lancet 2006;368(9537):780–793.
8. National Institutes of Health, National Heart, Lung, and Blood Institute. Global Initiative for Asthma. Global strategy for asthma management and prevention. NHLBI/WHO Workshop Report Number 95–3695, 1995. Update 2006, available at www.ginasthma.org.
9. Humbert M, Beasley R, Ayres J, et al: Benefits of omalizumab as add-on therapy in patients with severe persistent asthma who are inadequately controlled despite best available therapy (GINA 2002 step 4 treatment): INNOVATE. Allergy 2005;60(3):309–316.
10. Berry MA, Hargadon B, Shelley M, et al: Evidence of a role of tumor necrosis factor alpha in refractory asthma. N Engl J Med 2006;354(7):697–708.

Chronic Sinusitis

CHAPTER
37

John W. Steinke and Larry Borish

CLINICAL PEARLS

- Chronic sinusitis comprises numerous disorders including those characterized by chronic inflammation with mucous gland hyperplasia, chronic hyperplastic eosinophilic sinusitis, and allergic fungal sinusitis. Only very rarely is chronic sinusitis *primarily* an infectious disorder.

- Chronic hyperplastic eosinophilic sinusitis (CHES) is characterized by unrestrained proliferation of eosinophils, T-helper lymphocytes, fibroblasts, goblet cells, and mast cells. The pathological appearance of CHES is very similar to that of asthma and is frequently diagnosed in association with asthma.

- Exacerbations of CHES occur temporally with worsening of asthma. In the absence of well-controlled studies this linkage at present remains unproven, as precipitants of asthma exacerbations are capable of concomitantly producing sinusitis episodes.

- Many mechanisms have been ascribed for the putative linkage of sinusitis to asthma. These include a sinus-bronchial neural reflex, the harmful effects of mouth breathing and inhaling unconditioned air into the lungs, and aspiration of sinus contents into the lungs. The best explanation for an association of CHES with asthma is that the activation of T-helper lymphocytes in the sinuses leads to the differentiation and activation of immune cells including eosinophils and basophils in the bone marrow. In subjects with preexisting asthma, the presence in the inflamed lungs of specific adhesion and chemotactic molecules will promote the recruitment of these newly generated cells from the circulation.

- Pharmacological and surgical interventions that act to reduce the systemic effects of CHES, including topical corticosteroids, leukotriene modifiers, and aspirin desensitization could modulate the severity of asthma, although clinical trials with appropriate outcome measures are needed.

The term sinusitis refers to the presence of inflammation within any of the four pairs of paranasal sinuses (Fig. 37-1). Disease within the sinuses produces one of the most common health care problems in the United States, affecting approximately 16% of the population and having a significant adverse impact on quality of life and daily functioning.[1,2] The diagnosis and management of sinusitis have been challenging and, to a great extent, unsatisfactory. Sinusitis comprises many distinct conditions and recognition of this has led to an increased appreciation of the importance of categorizing the unique presentations of sinusitis, with the expectation that this will lead to improved, disease-specific treatments.

Sinusitis historically has been divided into three categories, acute, subacute, and chronic, based on disease duration (Table 37-1). Patients whose sinus symptoms are of less than 4 weeks duration are considered to have *acute sinusitis. Subacute sinusitis* comprises patients whose disease is of 4 to 8 weeks' duration, and, when the condition persists beyond 8 weeks, it is termed *chronic sinusitis* (CS). Acute and subacute sinusitis are typically infectious processes caused by respiratory viruses and pyogenic bacteria (*Streptococcus pneumoniae, Haemophilus influenzae,* and *Moraxella catarrhalis*). Chronic sinusitis, historically, has primarily been approached as an infectious disease caused by anaerobic bacteria, gram-negative organisms, *Staphylococcus aureus,* and other unusual bacteria. This concept led to the use of antibiotics and surgical drainage as treatment. It is becoming apparent that most patients with chronic sinusitis do not *primarily* have an infectious disorder. Patients with chronic sinusitis lose mucociliary clearance and other mechanisms that act to maintain the relative sterility of healthy sinuses and thereby become colonized with numerous bacteria. When sinus cultures are performed well these studies have demonstrated polymicrobial and nonvirulent organisms present at low titer. In combination with the

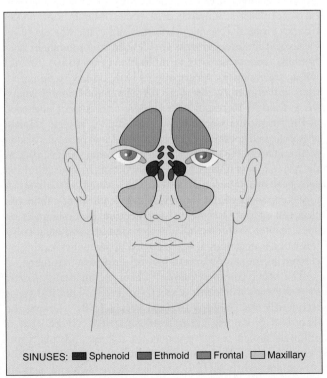

SINUSES: ■ Sphenoid ■ Ethmoid ■ Frontal □ Maxillary

Figure 37-1 Normal sinuses. The four pairs of paranasal sinuses are displayed.

Table 37-1
CLASSIFICATION OF SINUSITIS

Categories	Grouping	Etiology
Acute sinusitis	Viral sinusitis	Rhinovirus, metapneumovirus, influenza A/B
	Acute bacterial sinusitis	*Streptococcus pneumoniae,. Moraxella catarrhalis, Haemophilus influenzae*
Subacute sinusitis	Bacterial sinusitis	*S. pneumoniae. M. catarrhalis, H. influenzae*
Chronic sinusitis	Chronic infectious sinusitis	Immune deficiency, CF, anatomical abnormalities. Secondary infections with anaerobes, gram-negative organisms, *Staphylococcus aureus*
	Chronic inflammatory sinusitis	Anatomical abnormalities, allergic rhinitis, bacteria biofilms
	Chronic hyperplastic eosinophilic sinusitis	Aspirin-tolerant
		Aspirin-exacerbated respiratory disease
	Allergic fungal sinusitis	*Bipolaris spicifera, Curvularia lunata, Aspergillus fumigatus, Fusarium* sp.

absence of neutrophils[3] and the failure to respond to broad-spectrum antibiotics, these observations support the increasing recognition that most patients with CS do not have an infectious disease. It remains plausible that this bacterial colonization is not completely benign. Bacterial-derived microfilms could contribute to the severity of the chronic inflammation, and bacterial by-products such as endotoxin, superantigens, and other immune adjuvants can exacerbate the immune mechanisms that underlie CS. Finally, while most patients with CS do not *primarily* have an infectious disorder, it is important to appreciate that the development of CS predisposes the patient to recurrent episodes of acute sinusitis. However, the acute sinusitis that complicates CS is produced by the same spectrum of pyogenic organisms that affects patients without CS.

The recognition that most chronic sinusitis is not infectious has instigated efforts to better categorize these disorders (see Table 37-1). A small subset of patients with chronic sinusitis does, in fact, have *chronic infectious sinusitis*. This group typically consists of patients with underlying anatomical abnormalities, immune deficiencies, human immunodeficiency virus, Kartaganer syndrome, and cystic fibrosis (CF). Pathologically these patients are identified by prominent neutrophilia and intense bacterial infiltration ($>10^5$ to 10^6 cfu/mL) within their sinuses. Most patients with CS have a noninfectious inflammatory disorder. *Chronic inflammatory sinusitis* is thought to result from chronic or recurrent occlusion of the sinus ostia secondary to viral rhinitis, allergic rhinitis, anatomic predisposition, or other causes. These processes lead to recurrent acute (or subacute) bacterial infections and damage to the respiratory epithelium, ciliary destruction, mucous gland and goblet cell hyperplasia, and bacterial colonization. The inflammatory component of this form of sinusitis consists of a mononuclear cell infiltrate with few, if any, neutrophils. Eosinophils are not a feature of chronic inflammatory sinusitis and nasal polyp formation is uncommon. When caused by anatomical occlusion, chronic inflammatory sinusitis may be responsive to surgery.

The other common cause of chronic sinusitis is *chronic hyperplastic eosinophilic sinusitis* (CHES). This disease is frequently associated with nasal polyps (NP).[1] Among the disorders producing chronic sinusitis, it is CHES that is uniquely linked to the presence of asthma and this disorder will be the focus of this chapter. Up to 20% to 30% of patients with CHES who also have NP and asthma demonstrate exacerbation of their upper and lower airway symptoms with exposure to aspirin and other nonsteroidal

anti-inflammatory drugs. This has led to the recognition of a distinct subset of patients who have *aspirin-exacerbation respiratory disease* (AERD, or Samter' triad). In contrast to chronic inflammatory sinusitis, CHES is self-propagating and does not respond well to surgery. The final condition associated with chronic sinusitis is *allergic fungal sinusitis* (AFS). AFS represents a severe variant of CHES associated with the colonization of fungi within the sinus cavities and the presence of an immunoglobulin E (IgE)- and T-helper lymphocyte–mediated allergic inflammation. The remainder of this chapter will focus on CHES, its association with asthma, its role in contributing to the presence, severity, and exacerbations of asthma, and evidence that attenuation of CHES might have therapeutic utility in asthma.

PATHOGENESIS: IMMUNE MECHANISMS OF CHRONIC HYPERPLASTIC EOSINOPHILIC SINUSITIS

CHES is an inflammatory disease characterized by the accumulation of eosinophils, fibroblasts, mast cells, goblet cells, and T-helper lymphocytes. It is the prominent accumulation of eosinophils, however, which is the diagnostic feature of this condition (Fig. 37-2).[3,4] The diagnosis of CHES can only be unambiguously established upon pathological examination of tissue taken from the disease site with staining for eosinophils or eosinophil-derived mediators (such as eosinophil cationic protein or major basic protein).[3,4] However, while nasal polyposis frequently occurs with cystic fibrosis and less commonly can occur with chronic inflammatory sinusitis, the presence of nasal polyposis (and also asthma) may be used in practice as presumptive evidence for CHES.[1,5]

In CHES, the sinus tissue demonstrates a marked increase in cells, including lymphocytes, fibroblasts, and eosinophils themselves, that express cytokines, chemokines, and pro-inflammatory lipid mediators (especially the cysteinyl leukotrienes [CysLTs]) that are responsible for the development of eosinophilia. Eosinophilic inflammation is a complex process reflecting the need to synthesize these cells, recruit them into the sinus tissue, and activate them to release their toxic cationic granule proteins and other mediators that are responsible for sinus inflammation. Eosinophil synthesis reflects primarily the biological activity of the cytokine interleukin (IL)-5. Other cytokines including IL-3, and granulocyte-macrophage colony-stimulating factor (GM-CSF) and the CysLTs synergize with IL-5 in this process. Eosinophil precursors are increased in numbers in both

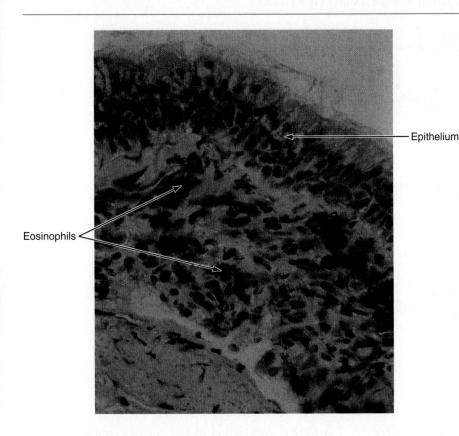

Epithelium

Eosinophils

Figure 37-2 Immunohistochemical analysis of a sinus biopsy from a patient with sinusitis and chronic allergic rhinitis. Eosinophils were labeled with an antibody to eosinophil cationic protein and were localized as aggregates within and beneath the epithelium (original magnification ×400). *(From Demoly P, Crampette L, Mondain M, et al: Assessment of inflammation in noninfectious chronic maxillary sinusitis. J Allergy Clin Immunol 1994;94:95–108.)*

the blood and bone marrow of patients with CHES and asthma. Recruitment of eosinophils into the sinus tissue reflects the influences of cellular adhesion and chemotaxis. Important to adhesion are the induction on endothelium of selectins by cytokines and CysLTs and vascular cell adhesion molecule (VCAM)-1 by IL-4, IL-13, and tumor necrosis factor (TNF)-α. Important chemotactic factors include CCL11 (eotaxin), platelet-activating factor (PAF), and CysLTs. Newly synthesized eosinophils display a limited ability to degranulate in response to inflammatory stimuli. In order for degranulation to occur, the cells need to be "primed," an effect mediated primarily by IL-3, IL-4, IL-5, and GM-CSF. Within the sinus tissue, eosinophils are activated by many compounds including CCL5 (RANTES), CCL11, IL-1, IL-3, IL-5, GM-CSF, TNF-α, PAF, and the CysLTs. Although normally short-lived, many of these factors including IL-3, IL-5, and GM-CSF inhibit eosinophil apoptosis and permit the cells to survive for days or even weeks within the inflamed sinuses. Finally, in CHES, the sinuses contain eosinophil- (and basophil-) specific progenitor cells. These eosinophil/basophil progenitors allow the bone marrow–independent perpetuation of sinus inflammation. That eosinophils are a prominent source of many of these cytokines and lipid mediators suggests that CHES is a disease of unrestrained inflammation in which eosinophils, once recruited, can provide the growth factors necessary for their further recruitment, proliferation, activation, and survival.

THE ROLE OF BACTERIA AND BACTERIAL-DERIVED IMMUNE ADJUVANTS IN CHES

Patients with CHES routinely become colonized with numerous bacteria and are prone to recurrent bacterial infections. Bacteria may be relevant to the pathophysiology of CHES through their ability to provide antigens and immune adjuvants (such as endotoxin). *Staphylococcus aureus* colonizing the sinuses is thought to play a particularly important role in exacerbating CHES through their ability to generate *superantigens*. *S. aureus*-derived superantigens non-specifically activate nearby T-helper lymphocytes that express targeted T-cell receptors (up to 30% of all T cells). Staph colonization is present in 66.7% of subjects with CHES and, among aspirin-sensitive subjects, this frequency increases to 87.5%. Reducing the volume of bacteria in the sinuses, and thereby the concentration of superantigen, could explain the anecdotal benefits ascribed to antibiotics in CHES.

ASPIRIN-EXACERBATED RESPIRATORY DISEASE

Aspirin-exacerbated respiratory disease reflects a distinct subset of CHES. These patients develop upper respiratory symptoms of nasal congestion, rhinorrhea, and paroxysmal sneezing, typically with severe exacerbations of their asthma after taking aspirin or other nonsteroidal anti-inflammatory drugs (NSAIDs) that are nonspecific cyclooxygenase (COX) inhibitors. Ingestion of these agents leads to a shift in arachidonic acid metabolism from cyclooxygenase products (prostaglandins) to the CysLTs (Figs. 37-3 and 37-4). CysLTs are produced by activated eosinophils, basophils, mast cells, and to a lesser extent by monocytes, dendritic cells, and T cells. CysLTs are metabolites of arachidonic acid, which is liberated from membrane phospholipids in response to cytosolic phospholipase A_2 (see Fig. 37-3). For CysLT generation, 5-lipoxygenase (5-LO) acts in concert with the 5-LO-activating protein (FLAP) to convert arachidonic acid to LTA_4. LTA_4 is conjugated to glutathione by LTC_4 synthase (LTC_4S) to form LTC_4. LTC_4 is released and further metabolized by the removal of glutamate to LTD_4 and then by removal of glycine to form LTE_4.

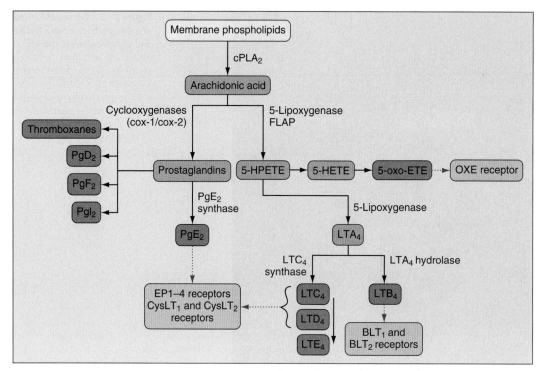

Figure 37-3 Arachidonate metabolic pathway.

AERD was originally defined by the triad of nasal polyps, aspirin sensitivity, and asthma (Samter triad). Other features of this disorder are its association with severe CHES, tissue and circulating eosinophilia, and the frequent absence of allergy.[6] Aspirin intolerance occurs in as many as 20% of asthmatic adults and up to 30% of asthmatic patients with chronic sinusitis and nasal polyposis. In many patients, asthma is not present; thus the current preference for the term AERD rather than aspirin-intolerant asthma or "triad" asthma.

AERD is explained in part by the overproduction of and overresponsiveness to the CysLTs. AERD subjects display dramatic upregulation of two essential enzymes involved in CysLT synthesis, 5-LO and LTC_4S (Fig. 37-5).[5,6] This overexpression leads to the constitutive overproduction of the CysLTs and the life-threatening surge in CysLTs that occurs following ingestion of aspirin or other NSAIDs (see Fig. 37-4). CysLTs have important pro-inflammatory and fibrotic effects that contribute both to the extensive hyperplastic sinusitis and nasal polyposis that characterize this disorder and to the severity

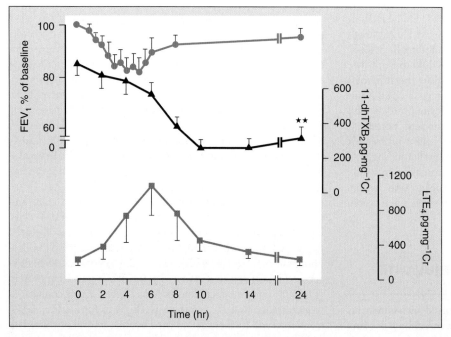

Figure 37-4 In AERD, aspirin challenge produces a depression of prostaglandin metabolites (the thromboxane B_2 metabolite 11-dhTXB$_2$) and an increase in the cysteinyl leukotriene metabolite LTE_4 appearing in the urine. The surge in cysteinyl leukotrienes occurs temporally in association with the decline in lung function (FEV_1 % of baseline). *(Data from Sladek K, Szczeklik A: Cysteinyl leukotrienes overproduction and mast cell activation in aspirin-provoked bronchospasm in asthma. Eur Respir J 1993;6:391–399.)*

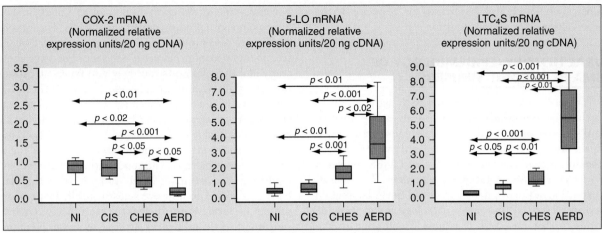

Figure 37-5   Increased 5-LO and LTC₄S expression and diminished COX-2 expression in AERD. Relative mRNA expression of COX-2, 5-LO, and LTC₄S measured in cDNA equivalent to 20 ng of RNA extracted from sinus tissue of patients with chronic sinusitis (CS) without nasal polyps (chronic inflammatory sinusitis [CIS]), CS with nasal polyps (CHES), CHES with nasal polyps and aspirin sensitivity (AERD), and inferior turbinate tissue (normal mucosa) from healthy subjects (NI). *P* values after the unpaired Wilcoxon test are shown. *(Data from Perez-Novo CA, Watelet JB, Claeys C, et al: Prostaglandin, leukotriene, and lipoxin balance in chronic rhinosinusitis with and without nasal polyposis. J Allergy Clin Immunol 2005;115(6):1189–1196.)*

of these patients' asthma.[7] Prostaglandin E_2 (PgE_2) inhibits mast cell and eosinophil activation. It is hypothesized that PgE_2 prevents activation of these allergic inflammatory cells and that when PgE_2 concentrations are reduced by NSAIDs the cells become activated. Support for this concept is derived from the observation that inhaled PgE_2 prevents this response from developing. The robust expression of 5-LO and LTC₄S leads to the subsequent surge in CysLT secretion. Aspirin tolerant subjects have much lower expression of 5-LO and LTC₄S and therefore cannot have this surge in CysLT secretion. In general, selective COX-2 inhibitors are well tolerated in these subjects suggesting that it is constitutive, COX-1-derived PgE_2 that is necessary for this protective effect.

CysLTs function through their ability to interact with two homologous receptors. The CysLT type 1 receptor is prominently expressed on airway smooth muscle, eosinophils, and other immune cells and these receptors mediate CysLT-induced bronchospasm. CysLT2 receptors are prominently expressed in the heart, prostate, brain, adrenal cells, endothelium, and lung but are also expressed on eosinophils, monocytes, T and B lymphocytes, and mast cells. The precise function of CysLT2 receptors in allergic disease and immunity is not known, although they are thought to play a greater role in remodeling and fibrosis. Subjects with AERD demonstrate enhanced responsiveness to CysLTs related to impressive overexpression of CysLT receptors on their sinus and NP tissue (Fig. 37-6).[8]

In addition to modulation of CysLTs and their receptors, the pathophysiology of AERD also involves dysregulation of the prostaglandin synthesis pathway. The expression of COX-2 and PgE_2 are both diminished in AERD (see Fig. 37-5).[5] This baseline deficiency in PgE_2 renders AERD patients

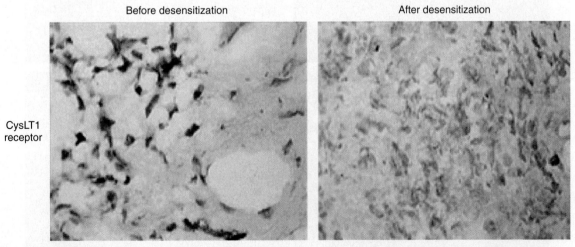

Figure 37-6   Upregulation of cysteinyl leukotriene 1 receptor expression on nasal mucosal inflammatory cells in AERD and decrease after aspirin desensitization. Nasal biopsy specimens immunostained for CysLT1 before and after desensitization with topical lysine aspirin (×1000). *(From Sousa AR, Parikh A, Scadding G, et al: Leukotriene-receptor expression on nasal mucosal inflammatory cells in aspirin-sensitive rhinosinusitis. New Engl J Med 2002;347(19):1493–1499.)*

increasingly susceptible to anaphylaxis in response to its further reduction after aspirin ingestion.

NATURAL HISTORY/EPIDEMIOLOGY OF ASTHMA IN CHRONIC SINUSITIS

CHES frequently coexists in patients with asthma. When adult asthmatics are evaluated by CT scan, approximately 74% to 90% have some degree of mucosal hyperplasia. Most individuals diagnosed with CHES have asthma and, among nonasthmatic individuals, the presence of CHES defines a cohort at high risk for its future development. The sinuses are an extension of the respiratory tract and the inflammation observed in CHES/NP has many pathological and immune similarities to that observed in asthma. In addition to the shared eosinophilia and inflammatory mediators, these similarities extend to the same prominent basement membrane thickening (Fig. 37-7).[4] It is these shared features that support the view that CHES and asthma represent different manifestations of the same disease process involving both the upper and lower respiratory tracts.

It is generally accepted doctrine that sinusitis contributes to the presence and severity of asthma. This is largely based on anecdotal association studies demonstrating worsening of sinusitis concomitantly with asthma exacerbations and intervention studies alleging that surgical or medical treatment of sinusitis improves asthma. The problem with this argument is that precipitants of asthma are generally also precipitants of sinusitis. For example, allergen exposure and respiratory viruses are the most important precipitants of asthma exacerbations and both produce or worsen sinusitis. The intervention studies are also problematic insofar as the effect of sinusitis treatment on asthma has *never* been addressed in a controlled study and these patients routinely also receive treatments to improve their asthma. In addition to the absence of a controlled study, many of the interventions used to establish this dogma are unproven in CS (antibiotics), largely ineffective for CS (Caldwell-Luc surgery), or are likely to mediate their beneficial effects through direct effects on the airway (macrolide antibiotics). The concept that treatment of CHES might improve asthma is based on treatments that have not been established to improve sinusitis itself. In summary, the present literature is insufficient to categorically conclude that sinusitis directly influences asthma severity and it remains quite plausible that these are merely similar disease processes effecting the upper and lower respiratory tract and sharing similar natural histories. A national effort is under way to define effective therapies for chronic sinusitis.[1] It should, therefore, become possible to perform definitive studies to address this important question.

While it is important to appreciate that the concept regarding a linkage of sinusitis to asthma has yet to be proven, there is some evidence to support such a linkage and the concept remains plausible. What follows is a discussion of current theories regarding the basis for a connection by which sinusitis could worsen asthma and, by extension, through which sinusitis treatment could ameliorate asthma severity (Table 37-2).

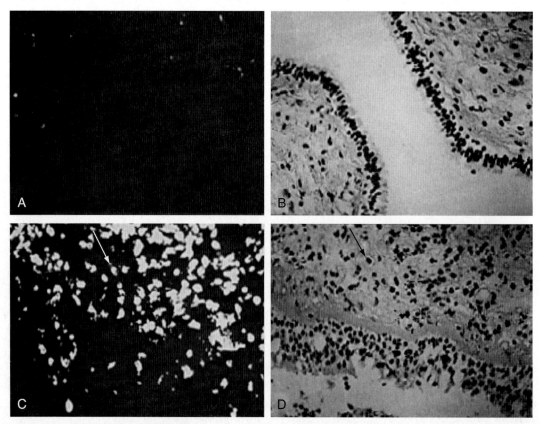

Figure 37-7 Basement membrane thickening in CHES. Histological analysis of sinus tissue. **A** and **C,** Stained for major basic protein by immunofluorescence. **B** and **D,** Same fields were counterstained with hematoxylin and eosin. *Arrows* depict an eosinophil. *(From Harlin SL, Ansel DG, Lane SR, et al: A clinical and pathologic study of chronic sinusitis: the role of the eosinophil. J Allergy Clin Immunol 1988;81:867–875.)*

Table 37-2
MECHANISMS OF SINUSITIS EXACERBATION OF ASTHMA

Coincidental association of similar pathological processes in upper and lower airways	In the absence of controlled studies, there may not be a causal interplay between sinusitis and asthma.
Sinus-bronchial reflex	Some evidence; however, the distinct innervation of the lungs (vagus) and sinuses (trigeminal) is inconsistent with typical reflexes or axonal loops.
Mouth breathing	Inhaling unconditioned air could cause bronchospasm but would not exacerbate inflammation
Aspiration	Well performed studies with *instillation* of isotope into the sinuses (as opposed to intranasal application) eliminates this as an etiology in conscious subjects
Vocal cord dysfunction (see Chapter 38)	In contrast to aspiration, mucopurulent posterior pharyngeal drainage could cause laryngeal irritation and produce VCD. Studies connecting sinusitis and asthma may have failed to address confounding effects of VCD.
Humoral recirculation of cytokines and immune cells (T-helper lymphocytes, eosinophils, and eosinophil precursors) from the upper airway and sinuses to the lungs	The currently accepted model (Fig. 37-8)

PROPOSED MECHANISMS LINKING CHRONIC SINUSITIS TO ASTHMA

Neurologic Reflex

A sinus-bronchial reflex mediated by the cholinergic neural pathway is supported by some data. However, the distinct innervation of the lungs (vagus nerve) and sinuses (trigeminal nerve) is inconsistent with typical reflexes or axonal loops.

Mouth Breathing

The nose exists in large part to condition air being inhaled into the lungs. This involves providing a tortuous surface over which inhaled air is humidified and warmed and on which large particles impact and are removed. Nasal congestion developing with CHES could force the patient into mouth breathing. Inhaling unconditioned (cold, dry) air is a known cause of bronchospasm in asthmatic individuals. Again, however, this is unlikely to be a cause of worsening airway *inflammation* as occurs with the concomitant flares of sinusitis and asthma.

ASPIRATION

This is the concept that sinus-derived posterior pharyngeal drainage, enriched in inflammatory cells, their secreted by-products, and other irritants could be aspirated into the airways and thereby exacerbate asthma. However, when studies were performed with instillation of radioisotopes directly into the sinuses, no evidence for aspiration could be discerned. Conflicting studies showing apparent aspiration of sinus contents into the lungs used nasal sprays and this approach may have allowed direct access of the spray into the airway. While significant aspiration below the larynx is not likely to occur in alert subjects, posterior pharyngeal drainage is a characteristic feature of CS and this is likely to function as a laryngeal irritant. CS could contribute to the paradoxical closure of the vocal cords that is responsible for *vocal cord dysfunction* (VCD or "paradoxical laryngospasm"; see Chapter 38). Many of the studies linking CS to asthma may have failed to address the confounding effects of including patients who actually had VCD.

Humoral Recirculation

A link between sinusitis and asthma can best be ascribed to a systemic inflammatory process. The cytokines associated with allergic inflammation do not function hormonally. Thus, T-helper lymphocyte–associated cytokines such as IL-4, IL-5, and IL-13 cannot be identified in serum samples and certainly are unlikely to access the bone marrow at a concentration sufficient to drive hematopoietic differentiation. In contrast, T-helper lymphocytes activated within the sinus tissue are capable of migrating to the bone marrow. This is analogous to the migration of T lymphocytes from the asthmatic airway to the bone marrow, which has been described. It is this ability of activated cytokine-expressing cells to circulate that allows cytokines to function at a distance. Once delivered to the bone marrow, these T-helper cells stimulate the production of inflammatory cells including basophils, eosinophils, and mast cell precursors. Cells activated in the sinuses also include locally produced eosinophil/basophil precursors and these will also be released into the circulation.[9] Eosinophils (and other inflammatory cells) generated through these mechanisms will be selectively recruited back into the sinus tissue. However, these cells will also migrate into the lungs of susceptible individuals, specifically, individuals with preexisting asthma. Newly generated eosinophils (and other cells) produced through these mechanisms express adhesion molecules that will direct their migration and adherence to inflamed tissue displaying relevant counter-ligands. For example, very late antigen (VLA)-4 on eosinophils will interact and adhere to endothelial cells expressing the counter-ligand VCAM-1. This will lead to the further influx of eosinophils into the sinuses. However, in the presence of *established* asthma, vascular endothelium in the lungs will also express VCAM-1, leading to eosinophil adherence in the lung. These inflamed organs are also rich in CCL11, PAF, and CysLTs, which will drive the chemotaxis of these cells into the sinuses and lungs.[7] Through these systemic mechanisms, inflammation in the sinuses can produce increased inflammation in the lungs including eosinophil influx.[9] Nonasthmatic individuals do not express the necessary adhesion molecules and chemotactic mediators in their airways and thus do not have the machinery necessary to recruit inflammatory cells into their lungs during exacerbations of sinusitis. This model is summarized in Figure 37-8.

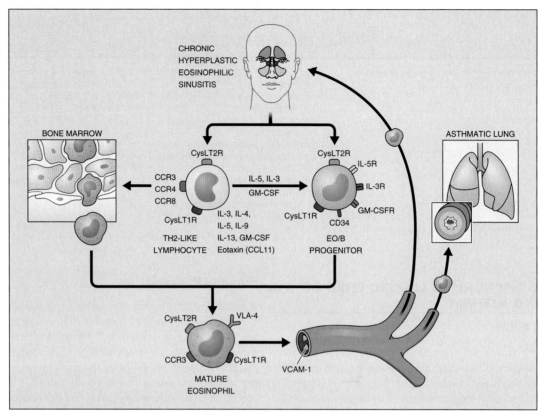

Figure 37-8 **Model giving overview of mechanism by which allergen immune activation can induce inflammation in sinus tissue.** See text for details.

While this model has never been specifically studied, the concept that CHES could contribute to asthma severity is supported by studies linking CHES to systemic and airway inflammation. Several studies have shown that severity of CHES directly influences circulating eosinophilia and CHES may have a stronger influence upon absolute eosinophil counts than does asthma. In the most intriguing study, subjects with CHES were divided into cohorts with limited and more severe disease according to a volumetric measure of hyperplastic tissue content in their sinuses. More severe sinus disease linked not only to increased absolute eosinophil counts (440/μL versus 170/μL) but, more impressively, appeared to influence airway inflammation as shown by eosinophilia in induced sputum samples (7.3% versus 0.7%). This circumstantial evidence supports a linkage between CHES and asthma. At present, however, the concept that sinusitis directly influences the development or severity of asthma and that sinusitis treatment will improve asthma has not been categorically established. Treatment of CHES may be warranted as part of a treatment plan for the refractory asthmatic and certainly is essential at reducing the morbidity directly ascribable to this disorder. The remainder of this chapter will address current approaches to the treatment of CS.

CLINICAL COURSE: THERAPEUTIC IMPLICATIONS

The management of CS has been disappointing and at present there is not a single treatment approved by the Food and Drug Administration (FDA) for this disorder. A problem confounding the evaluation of clinical interventions of sinusitis has been the absence of validated criteria to assess the

presence and severity of sinusitis. Traditionally, studies have used clinical criteria to evaluate the sinuses including presence of such symptoms as purulent anterior or posterior nasal drainage, nasal congestion, frontal headaches, cough, and so forth. However, none of these criteria is at all specific for the sinuses, but largely reflects the presence of either nasal disease (purulent drainage) or lower respiratory tract disease (cough). The relevance of headaches to sinus disease is unclear as compelling data suggest that most patients with "sinus headaches" actually suffer from atypical migraines. As a result, clinical studies that have compared sinusitis symptom scores with computed tomography (CT) scans show that clinical scores are often little better than random in predicting the presence and severity of sinusitis. The absence of validated objective criteria for assessing presence of CHES or responsiveness to therapeutic interventions has rendered meaningless most sinusitis studies.

Ancillary Therapies

Many ancillary therapies are routinely recommended for CS and are similar to those used for acute sinusitis (Table 37-3). Interventions designed to increase sinus openings into the nasal passages are based on the hypothesis that reducing obstruction should help in the expulsion of retained mucous and infectious materials—mechanisms of dubious benefit in CHES. This approach includes the use of systemic decongestants such as pseudoephedrine. While decongestants reduce nasal resistance, the only study of a systemic decongestant on sinus function was performed with phenylpropanolamine and this agent produced an *insignificant* increase in maxillary sinus opening. No controlled study with systemic decongestants in CS has

Table 37-3
TREATMENT OF CHRONIC HYPERPLASTIC EOSINOPHILIC SINUSITIS

Category	Proposed Mechanism	Role in CHES
Nasal saline irrigation	Diminish viscosity of inspissated secretions—improve mucociliary clearance	Useful adjunct therapy
Decongestants (pseudoephedrine, phenylephrine	Reduce sinus ostial obstruction; promote expulsion of mucous and infectious materials	Unproven. Proposed mechanism is of dubious benefit in CHES
Antihistamines (loratadine, fexofenadine, cetirizine)	Reduce edema and mucus secretion caused by histamine	Ineffective. CHES is not an established allergic disease and histamine is not a prominent mediator
Expectorants: guaifenesin, potassium iodide, acetyl cysteine	Ease clearance of tenacious, viscous mucous	Unproven. Limited efficacy in COPD; this has never been extended to CS
Allergy avoidance/Immunotherapy	A role for allergy in CHES is unproven and inconsistent with inability of aeroallergens to access the sinus cavities	Unproven
Systemic corticosteroids	Corticosteroids have potent anti-inflammatory and especially anti-eosinophil efficacy	Effective therapy but inappropriate in the face of long-term treatment requirements
Topical corticosteroids	Reduce eosinophils and cytokines	Reduce size and recurrence of NP. Unproven for CHES; efficacy is limited by ability to access sinus cavities
Leukotriene modifiers	Cysteinyl leukotrienes are important pro-inflammatory mediators highly expressed in CHES tissue	LT receptor antagonists are unproven. 5-LO inhibitor zileuton associated with diminished polyp size and reversal of anosmia
Aspirin desensitization	Associated with diminished cysteinyl leukotriene production and responsiveness (CysLT receptor expression)	Reduce frequency of acute sinusitis complications of CHES, polyp recurrence, and anosmia. Only effective in aspirin intolerant patients
Surgery	Provide drainage of inspissated mucous and inflammatory tissue	Produce instant reduction in CHES biomass. Without follow-up medical therapy disease is likely to recur. Useful adjunct to medical therapies.

been performed and the only controlled study in acute sinusitis demonstrated no clinical benefit. Improved mucociliary clearance can be accomplished by reducing the viscosity of secretions, such as with nasal saline irrigation. Saline irrigation must be performed with large volumes of saline, which can be administered with a bulb syringe or other device. Various mucolytics and expectorants have also been recommended in CS based on the hypothesis that they should ease clearance of tenacious, viscous mucous. While these agents, including iodinated glycerol, guaifenesin, and acetyl cysteine have some efficacy in chronic obstructive pulmonary disease (COPD), there have been no studies demonstrating efficacy in CS.

Allergy Avoidance/Immunotherapy: The Role of Allergy in CHES

A role for allergen avoidance or allergen desensitization immunotherapy is contingent on the extent to which CHES is an allergic disorder. In support of this, chronic sinusitis has been linked to the increased expression of allergic (IgE) sensitization. Thus, allergic rhinitis was seen in 56% of 200 consecutive patients with CS. Similarly, 50% of children with "recalcitrant" sinusitis were skin test positive as were 78% of patients with "severe" sinus disease. In another study, slightly less than half of patients with CHES/NP had allergies. The significance of these observations is unclear insofar as the prevalence of allergic rhinitis or positive skin tests in well-matched control populations was not reported and can be highly variable, reflecting variables in how the skin testing is performed. In fact, a recent extensive National Health Survey reported the prevalence of positive prick skin tests to be 54.3% in healthy adults, not impressively different from what is reported in CS. The presence of a positive skin test in a patient with CHES cannot be interpreted as signifying an allergic etiology. An additional argument against a

role for allergy in CHES is the lack of evidence that inhalant allergens access the sinus cavities. In one study, radiolabeled allergen did not access the sinuses. Using a much smaller radioisotope placed on the nasal mucosa, it was shown that isotope could access the sinuses with nose blowing, but not with nasal breathing, sneezing, or coughing. These studies were performed in healthy volunteers and this limited potential access of allergens into the sinuses is likely to be further reduced with the onset of sinus disease and the occlusion of the sinus openings. Ironically, this natural protection of sinus tissue from inhalant allergens is likely be reversed by sinus surgery.

Despite the unlikelihood that allergens directly access the sinuses, there is intriguing evidence that still supports a role for allergy in CHES. Thus, insufflation of ragweed pollen in sensitive subjects was associated with increased blood flow and metabolic activity in the maxillary sinus and similar changes were observed during the ragweed season that became inactive post-seasonally. In a different study, either radiographic changes in the maxillary sinuses or symptoms referable to the sinuses were seen in approximately half of the subjects undergoing allergen provocation challenges. The strongest evidence that inhalant allergens could have a role in CHES is derived from studies in which catheters were inserted into both maxillary sinuses. Nasal challenges were performed with grass or ragweed extracts instilled into one nostril after which bilateral sinus lavages were performed. In these studies, nasal allergen challenges triggered eosinophil influx into the ipsilateral—but more impressively, this also occurred in the contralateral—maxillary sinus. These data support a role for inhalant allergens in the pathophysiology of CHES, but also suggest that this does *not* necessarily require direct allergen access into the sinuses. Allergic rhinitis activates T-helper lymphocytes in the nose with subsequent mast cell recruitment and eosinophil activation.

It is reasonable to speculate that a systemic inflammatory mechanism similar to that described for the link between sinusitis and asthma could develop between the nose and the sinuses. At present, however, a role for allergies in the etiology or severity of CHES remains unproven. No clinical studies have shown that either allergy avoidance or immunotherapy has clinical benefit in CHES using validated sinus-specific outcome parameters. Recommendations for allergen avoidance and immunotherapy should be primarily focused on achieving benefit for the underlying allergic rhinitis or asthma.

Systemic Corticosteroids

Systemic corticosteroids benefit CHES through their ability to directly attenuate eosinophilia and other components of the inflammation of this disorder. The ability of topical corticosteroids (CCS) to locally reduce cytokine production (including IL-4, IL-5, GM-CSF and TNF-α), inhibit T-helper lymphocyte function, and inhibit activation of both eosinophils and eosinophil precursors supports the concept that these agents could provide efficacy in CHES. In contrast to allergic rhinitis and asthma, however, it is unlikely that *intranasal* CCS can directly access the sinus cavities in order to achieve that efficacy. Although various maneuvers have been proposed to promote the drainage of nasal corticosteroids into the sinuses, the likely presence of occlusion of the ostiomeatal complex precludes their direct access, although this may be partially achieved in subjects who have undergone FESS. In contrast to their lack of proven efficacy for CHES, intranasal CCSs can reduce nasal polyps, reflecting their ability to directly access the polyp tissue. The role of intranasal CCS in CHES has not been adequately addressed in a properly performed controlled clinical trial with validated outcome criteria.

Leukotriene Modifiers

CHES tissue demonstrates increased presence of CysLTs and metabolic enzymes involved in LT synthesis.[5,7] CysLTs have important pro-inflammatory capabilities including primarily their ability to promote eosinophilic inflammation. Other activities of leukotrienes relevant to CHES include their ability to increase vascular permeability, stimulate mucus secretion, decrease mucociliary clearance, and promote tissue remodeling.[7] Clinical trials of leukotriene modifiers in asthma and allergic rhinitis have shown reductions in both circulating absolute eosinophil counts and tissue eosinophilia. Leukotriene modifiers could therefore provide benefit in CHES through direct reduction of eosinophil recruitment and activation in the sinuses. CysLT1 receptor antagonists (zafirlukast and montelukast) have been suggested to have efficacy in CHES in uncontrolled trials. In the only placebo-controlled trial of an LT modifier in CHES, the 5-LO inhibitor, zileuton, was shown to reduce polyp size and restore sense of smell. The efficacy of zileuton is intriguing as inhibition of 5-LO has broader implications than use of one of the CysLT1 receptor antagonists. In addition to blocking the LTB_4 pathway, reduced synthesis of CysLTs will thereby block inflammation mediated through CysLT2 as well as CysLT1 receptor.

Aspirin Desensitization

Aspirin desensitization is a proven therapy in patients with AERD. This technique involves successive ingestion of increasing doses of aspirin over several days, until a therapeutic dose is achieved (generally 650 mg two times per day). This technique is risky and must be done cautiously, ideally in a hospital setting. The use of a leukotriene modifier reduces, but does not eliminate, the risks of aspirin desensitization. Successful aspirin desensitization decreases basal and aspirin-stimulated leukotriene synthesis as well as decreasing sensitivity to cysteinyl leukotrienes by dramatically down-regulating CysLT receptor expression (see Fig. 37-6).[8] Aspirin desensitization decreases symptoms of sinus disease, reduces courses of antibiotics reflecting reduced numbers of secondary acute sinusitis episodes, decreases the need for sinus surgeries, and restores the sense of smell. These beneficial results are tempered, however, by the risks of desensitization and long-term aspirin administration. Aspirin desensitization can also be indicated in patients with AERD who require aspirin treatment for an unrelated medical condition. While selective COX-2 inhibitors can generally be safely administered to individuals with AERD, these agents do not provide benefit for the sinus disease.

Surgery

No controlled trial of functional endoscopic sinus surgery (FESS) has been performed; however, FESS has been associated with high reported rates of clinical improvement (up to 97.5% at 2 years). Patients with extensive disease, multiple sinus involvement, nasal polyposis, asthma, or aspirin-intolerance have a poor outcome. These observations suggest that FESS may be uniquely useful in patients with chronic inflammatory sinusitis in whom anatomical defects are present that are predisposing the patient to recurrent acute or subacute infections with the subsequent mucociliary damage, remodeling, and chronic inflammation. With CHES, FESS is less likely to be curative for what is primarily an immune-mediated hyperplastic disease of the sinuses. In the absence of postsurgical medical management, the immune mechanisms underlying CHES are still in place and the disease is likely to recur. FESS remains a valuable adjunct to the treatment of this disorder, as medical approaches are likely to be more effective in preventing recurrence of CHES and NP than in ameliorating well-established disease.

Newer Biotechnology Approaches

Given the pathophysiological similarities between CHES and asthma and the likelihood that these are similar or perhaps even identical disease processes affecting the upper and lower airways, respectively, it seems likely that newer biotechnology-derived therapies designed to treat severe asthma are likely to produce similar benefits for CHES. Clinical experience with *humanized anti-IgE* (omalizumab) in asthma (see Chapter 31) shows that it lessens allergen-induced IgE-mediated activation of mast cells and basophils and thereby attenuates acute allergic reactions. The efficacy of omalizumab in CHES is obviously limited by the extent to which CHES is an IgE-mediated disease. As previously discussed, allergen-specific mechanisms may produce a systemic inflammatory milieu that could contribute to the severity of CHES. It seems less likely, however, that inhaled aeroallergens directly access the sinus cavities and exacerbate CHES in an IgE-dependent fashion that is likely to be ameliorated by omalizumab. It is also plausible, however, that IgE-dependent reactions could develop in CHES to locally produced allergens. For example, allergic fungal sinusitis is associated with IgE-mediated allergic reactions to fungi colonizing the sinuses and similarly, specific IgE is known to develop to Staph-derived antigens in patients colonized with that microorganism. At present no clinical data exist to support the use of humanized anti-IgE as a specific treatment for CHES.

Another treatment intervention showing some promise in asthma is the neutralization of TNF with either *soluble TNF receptor* (etanercept) or *humanized anti-TNF* (infliximab) or neutralization of IL-1β with human *anti-IL-1β antibodies* (remicade). TNF is present in CHES and is likely to be important in both initiating immune responses to allergens and in promoting the recruitment and activation of inflammatory cells. Etanercept was recently shown to improve lung function and to reduce bronchial hyperreactivity, suggestive of an anti-inflammatory influence that could extend to chronic sinusitis. These are intriguing candidates as therapeutic interventions in CHES.

Insofar as CHES is defined by the accumulation of activated eosinophils, it seems likely that interventions designed to attenuate eosinophilic inflammation will be particularly beneficial in this disorder. There is convincing evidence regarding the role of eosinophilia in fibrosis and airway remodeling in allergic disease. IL-5–deficient mice have markedly diminished eosinophil numbers and suppression of remodeling. More specifically, mice genetically engineered to lack eosinophils continue to display airway hyperreactivity and increased mucus secretion but do not develop fibrosis and remodeling. The production of transforming growth factor-β and other growth factors by activated eosinophils contributes to the proliferation of fibroblasts and deposition of the connective tissue observed in asthma and CHES. The experience with *humanized anti-IL-5* (mepolizumab) in asthma supports the ability of this intervention to greatly attenuate both the bone marrow eosinophilopoietic response associated with asthma and airway eosinophilia. Similar to what was observed in the murine model, anti-IL-5 treatment, while markedly reducing eosinophil numbers, had no significant effect on lung function or bronchial hyperreactivity in human studies. However, anti-IL-5 is associated with diminished deposition of matrix proteins. As a disease characterized by exuberant remodeling and deposition of matrix proteins, CHES could be uniquely responsive to eosinophil-directed therapies, such as with anti-IL-5.

That significant residual tissue eosinophilia was observed in the anti-IL-5 studies suggests that single target interventions may insufficiently reduce tissue eosinophilia to produce adequate therapeutic benefit in CHES (or asthma). Further attenuation of tissue eosinophilia could be accomplished by using either inhibitors of eosinophil-specific chemokines (e.g., inhibition of CCL11 [eotaxin] using a *chemokine receptor CCR3 antagonist*) or inhibition of eosinophil-specific adhesion molecules (e.g., through the use of *VLA-4 antagonists*). Arguably no single agent is likely to be effective for CHES and it will be necessary to synergistically block both the systemic bone marrow component of CHES as well as local factors critical for inflammatory cell recruitment. The shared pathology of CHES with asthma suggests that as newer agents become established for asthma they may subsequently prove to have utility in CHES.

SUMMARY

Our understanding of sinusitis has advanced in recent years, due in part to the recognition that this is not just one disease, but many different conditions affecting the sinus tissue. Further characterization is still needed, however. Asthmatic patients usually present with concomitant CHES, a condition that has a similar pathophysiology to asthma. As such, it has been proposed that there is a link between the upper and lower airways and exacerbation of sinusitis can lead to worsening of asthma. The link between the upper and lower airways is believed to be a result of T-cell activation at one site leading to stimulation of hematopoiesis in the bone marrow. Newly formed eosinophils, basophils, mast cells, and others can traffic to either the lung or sinus cavity, resulting in worsening of disease at both sites. Recognition of this link should lead to new therapeutic approaches aimed at breaking this cycle of T-cell activation and trafficking.

REFERENCES

1. Meltzer EO, Hamilos DL, Hadley JA, et al: Rhinosinusitis: establishing definitions for clinical research and patient care. J Allergy Clin Immunol 2004;114(6 Suppl):S155–S212.
2. Slavin RG, Spector SL, Bernstein IL, et al: The diagnosis and management of sinusitis: a practice parameter update. J Allergy Clin Immunol 2005;116(6 Suppl):S13–S47.
3. Demoly P, Crampette L, Mondain M, et al: Assessment of inflammation in noninfectious chronic maxillary sinusitis. J Allergy Clin Immunol 1994;94:95–108.
4. Harlin SL, Ansel DG, Lane SR, et al: A clinical and pathologic study of chronic sinusitis: The role of the eosinophil. J Allergy Clin Immunol 1988;81:867–875.
5. Perez-Novo CA, Watelet JB, Claeys C, et al: Prostaglandin, leukotriene, and lipoxin balance in chronic rhinosinusitis with and without nasal polyposis. J Allergy Clin Immunol 2005;115(6):1189–1196.
6. Cowburn AS, Sladek K, Soja J, et al: Overexpression of leukotriene C4 synthase in bronchial biopsies from patients with aspirin-intolerant asthma. J Clin Invest 1998;101:834–846.
7. Steinke JW, Bradley D, Arango P, et al: Cysteinyl leukotriene expression in chronic hyperplastic sinusitis-nasal polyposis: importance to eosinophilia and asthma. J Allergy Clin Immunol 2003;111(2):342–349.
8. Sousa AR, Parikh A, Scadding G, et al: Leukotriene-receptor expression on nasal mucosal inflammatory cells in aspirin-sensitive rhinosinusitis. New Engl J Med 2002;347(19):1493–1499.
9. Steinke JW, Borish L: The role of allergy in chronic rhinosinusitis. Immunol Allergy Clin North Am 2004;24(1):45–57.

Vocal Cord Dysfunction

Frederick S. Wamboldt and Ronald C. Balkissoon

CLINICAL PEARLS

- With intense or repeated stimulation, central nervous system reflexes devoted to protecting respiration can sometimes become hyperresponsive and dysfunctional, producing breathing disorders via a process called "central sensitization."

- Vocal cord dysfunction (VCD) likely arises from central sensitization of reflexes designed to protect the glottis.

- Central sensitization also underlies a number of other conditions that often overlap with VCD, such as panic anxiety and idiopathic chronic cough.

- Although patients with VCD often have comorbid psychological problems or overt psychiatric disorders, these should be considered associated features, not primary causal factors.

- With prompt recognition and appropriate diagnosis, patients with VCD usually respond well to simple, targeted treatments that improve respiratory symptoms and quality of life and decrease excess health care utilization.

- Unfortunately, due to misdiagnosis and misguided treatment, many patients with VCD suffer considerable iatrogenic harm.

Paradoxical vocal cord dysfunction (VCD) is a common but poorly understood condition in which the vocal cords close during inspiration and/or early to mid-expiration, thereby producing airflow obstruction at the larynx and audible wheeze or stridor. VCD most frequently is diagnosed as a mimic or confounder in patients with difficult-to-treat asthma or some other chronic respiratory disorder. However, it increasingly is reported in other settings including seemingly healthy, young individuals (e.g., "perfectionistic" teenagers, elite athletes, active duty military) and in patients with other allergic and/or inflammatory disorders that involve the upper airway (e.g., gastroesophageal reflux disorder [GERD], sinusitis, occupational irritant exposures, and post–upper respiratory infection [URI]). Typical clinical episodes range from transient, mild asthma-like symptoms (i.e., chest tightness, shortness of breath, wheezing, and cough) to total upper airway occlusion. The clinical presentation of acute VCD is often quite dramatic. Hence, VCD frequently is misdiagnosed as acute severe asthma, anaphylaxis or angioedema, leading to unnecessary treatment with high doses of corticosteroids, intubation, or tracheotomy, often resulting ultimately in iatrogenic complications.[1,2]

NATURAL HISTORY/EPIDEMIOLOGY

While the true prevalence of VCD is unknown, it does not appear to be rare. There are a plethora of case reports describing VCD-like clinical conditions in disparate and nonoverlapping literatures (e.g., anesthesia, otolaryngology, emergency medicine, psychiatry, pulmonology, and pediatrics), typically with names evoking psychiatric causality such as "Munchausen stridor," "factitious asthma," and "emotional laryngeal wheeze." Newman and colleagues[1] reported that nearly 40% of adult patients presenting to a national pulmonary referral center with difficult-to-control asthma were diagnosed with VCD, with roughly half ultimately being diagnosed solely with VCD and half with VCD plus chronic asthma. The patients with VCD alone had been misdiagnosed with asthma for 4.8 years on average, and at intake were taking a mean prednisone dose of approximately 30 mg. In the prior year they averaged nearly 10 emergency room visits and six hospital admissions. Young adults, females, health care workers, and individuals with stressful life circumstances and/or psychiatric illness appeared most likely to receive a diagnosis of VCD. The presence of inspiratory stridor during exercise challenge (presumed to be VCD) has been reported in 5% of elite athletes training at the Lake Placid United States Olympic Training Center.[3] The inspiratory stridor was reported to begin quickly after onset of intense physical performance, resolve within 5 minutes after cessation, and not respond to inhaled beta₂-agonist. Females competing in outdoor sports predominated. Half also had coexistent exercise-induced bronchospasm. Similarly, VCD confirmed by laryngoscopy has been reported as the cause of nearly 10% of children and adolescents presenting with exercise-induced dyspnea.[4]

PATHOGENESIS

The etiology and pathophysiology of VCD remain largely unknown. It is widely recognized, however, that one of the primary physiological functions of the larynx is protection of the airway via the cough, glottic closure, and other central nervous system (CNS) reflexes. Hence, VCD is increasingly thought to be caused by hyperresponsiveness of the intricate set of monitors and protective reflexes that link the control of breathing not only to the upper and lower airways, but also to higher-level CNS affective, anxiety, and cognitive centers.

The key dynamics of respiration, such as rate and rhythm, are controlled primarily by medullary and pontine brainstem centers. These same centers not only monitor the status of respiration, but also other associated systems, such as the status of the airway from the nose into the bronchi. When respiratory function is endangered (e.g., smoke inhalation), various protective reflexes (e.g., cough, glottic closure, and "fight or flight" panic anxiety) are employed to protect the individual until the source of respiratory danger has ended. Considerable evidence has accrued that these CNS respiratory control centers can become sensitized so that these short-term protective reflexes become hyperactive, leading to a family of related clinical syndromes in which the CNS directly contributes to common respiratory symptoms, such as chest tightness, cough, dyspnea, and wheezing.

Solid support for this hypothesis comes from animal models in which early exposure to various lung irritants (e.g., capsaicin, environmental tobacco smoke, upper respiratory viruses) can cause "central sensitization" of CNS respiratory centers resulting in persistent hyperactivity of respiratory reflexes. For example, Bonham and colleagues[5] exposed juvenile guinea pigs to environmental tobacco smoke for 5 weeks and demonstrated that this exposure activated vagal C-fiber afferents to the nucleus tractus solitarius (NTS) causing increased responsiveness of caudomedial NTS neurons to subsequent respiratory irritant exposure. As a result of this relatively brief early exposure, these animals displayed lifelong CNS hyperactivity to subsequent irritant exposure, including more rapid and shallow breathing, lowered cough threshold, increased mucus production, and increased bronchial hyperresponsiveness.

Morrison and colleagues[6] have proposed a similar model of CNS "neural plasticity" as causing an "irritable larynx syndrome" (ILS). Specifically, they hypothesized that the ILS arises from "CNS changes that leaves sensorimotor pathways in a hyperexcitable state" with the presumptive causal mechanisms being either an adaptive response to "nerve or tissue injury" or "repeated noxious stimulation." In a clinical series of 39 patients, onset of ILS was associated with GERD, recent viral URI, "psychogenic" factors, and chronic respiratory disorder. Once such factors place the larynx in a "spasm-ready state," they observed that a wide variety of nonspecific triggers can produce subsequent symptoms with odors (e.g., perfumes and cleaning products), GERD, foods, emotions, voice use, coughing, and exertion most frequently reported.

Morrison and colleagues' "irritable larynx syndrome" provides a clinically useful model of pathways whereby various "threats" to breathing which are of sufficient intensity and/or sustained over time could cause the CNS reflexes that normally defend the airway to become sensitized, hyperresponsive, and dysfunctional.[6] Subsequent research is needed to better delineate the role of such CNS processes in VCD.

"SUBTYPES" OF VCD

Clinicians can approach the various populations in which VCD occurs as representing different "threats" to breathing that sensitize the normally protective CNS reflexes and lead to VCD.

Respiratory Irritants, Inflammation, and Allergy

Support for the role of irritant and inflammatory processes in VCD comes from Bucca and colleagues[7,8] who have described a VCD-like syndrome of extrathoracic hyperresponsiveness (ETHR) in over 500 patients with asthma-like symptoms. Following histamine challenge when asymptomatic, the vast majority of patients exhibited some type of airway hyperresponsiveness: approximately 25% of patients had only ETHR, as defined by a provocative concentration of histamine less than 8 mg/mL producing a 25% drop in maximal mid-inspiratory flow rate from baseline ($PC_{25}MIF_{50}$); around 10% had only lower airway reactivity, as defined by a provocative concentration of histamine of less than 8 mg/mL producing a 20% drop in forced expiratory volume in 1 second ($PC_{20}FEV_1$); and the remaining 40% of patients showed both. Using laryngoscopy they showed that although laryngeal exams were normal in all patients at baseline, following the histamine challenge mucosal edema, pharyngoconstriction, and inspiratory vocal cord adduction were seen in the patients showing ETHR, but not in those showing only bronchial hyperreactivity. ETHR was associated with postnasal drip, dysphonia, and sinusitis, suggesting a role of chronic irritation and/or inflammatory processes. Over 75% of subjects with ETHR were female. Similar findings have also recently been reported in children.[9] With aggressive treatment of coexistent rhinosinusitis and GERD, ETHR improves.[8,9] ETHR likely occurs across a spectrum, with severe VCD residing at one extreme endpoint.

The onset of VCD has been reported in 11 patients within 24 hours of a single, albeit typically intense, exposure to occupational respiratory irritants.[10] All cases were confirmed by laryngoscopy to have VCD even though these exams were performed weeks to months after the occupational exposure. Our experience with such patients suggests that sometimes the initial exposure results in permanent damage to the airway that leads to direct, ongoing activation of the glottic closure and/or cough reflexes, thereby generating and perpetuating the symptoms of VCD. However, more often the initial exposure and airway injury set up a "vicious cycle" of cough, mucus drainage, inflammation, and vocal cord sensitivity that interfere with resolution of the original injury. Similar mechanisms likely explain the reports of VCD onset after viral URIs and during postsurgical recovery.

VCD during Intense Athletic Competition and Military Experience

A second set of "threats" to breathing is suggested by reports of VCD occurring in healthy, physically fit individuals stressed by intense, peak-level physical performance.

McFadden and Zawadski[11] described seven elite athletes in whom acute exercise-induced dyspnea was ultimately diagnosed as VCD based on spirometric and/or laryngoscopic testing during bronchoprovocation. Interestingly, exercise-induced VCD could be differentiated from exercise-induced bronchospasm (EIB) by the clinical history of the attacks, with VCD episodes (1) coming on during rather than after intense exercise; (2) not consistently recurring with exposure to similar stimuli; and (3) not responding to prophylactic or rescue asthma treatments. These athletes were described as "highly competitive, success oriented, and either personally intolerant of failure or . . . the offspring of parents so inclined." The authors attributed the cause of these VCD episodes to "psychological stress" leading to "choking" during competition, in both the medical and sports connotations. The pathway(s) whereby stress leads to VCD was not well articulated.

The prevalence of exercise-induced inspiratory stridor (confirmed only by laryngeal auscultation) in a cohort of 370 elite athletes training at the U.S. Olympic program in Lake Placid, New York, was slightly greater than 5%.[3] These authors also reported that that inspiratory stridor attributed to VCD could be differentiated from EIB by (1) onset during, not after exercise; (2) rapid resolution following cessation of exercise; and (3) lack of response to bronchodilator treatments. Female athletes participating in outdoor sports were most likely to demonstrate inspiratory stridor. Although the authors mentioned that Olympic-level competition is "psychologically stressful," they made no specific causal attributions about why inspiratory stridor occurred in these elite athletes.

Morris and colleagues[12] reported that 15% of a cohort of young U.S. Army soldiers who were unable to pass the required physical fitness task (a 2-mile run) during basic training due to exertional dyspnea had VCD by laryngoscopy. They, too, note that Army basic training is "a time of great emotional, psychological, and physical stress" and cite reports in the literature that VCD represents a conversion reaction, or another form of psychopathology, but do not report any direct data concerning psychiatric distress and/or disease in these cases.

The best (albeit weak) evidence that exercise-induced VCD may arise from psychological stress or psychiatric disorder is that such episodes, in contrast to asthma, are not reliably provoked by hyperventilation or bronchoprovocative challenges; rather variable responses to differing challenges typically are observed both within and across subjects.[11-13] On the other hand, several other observations argue against this. First, brief, simple speech therapy and breathing retraining interventions are extremely effective for exercise-induced VCD, with the vast majority of those affected being able to return to baseline performance during competition.[14,15] Although effective treatments exist for many psychiatric disorders, such interventions are usually more time and effort intensive, and in most cases less effective. Second, VCD-like episodes have been observed in thoroughbred race horses exhibiting stridorous breath sounds during competition, and as a side effect in patients treated with vagal nerve stimulation for intractable seizure disorders, again suggesting that VCD arises in the context of CNS reflex dysfunction, rather than from psychodynamic processes. It is important to remember that many body reflexes are augmented by both psychosocial stress and increased muscle tension, so the observed association of VCD with stress may simply reflect reflex facilitation rather than direct causation. Consistent with this supposition are the clinical observations that patients with VCD typically focus their attention on the larynx and airway, and indeed, have palpable tension of the laryngeal musculature.[6]

Psychiatric Disorders and Vocal Cord Disorder

Given that VCD is frequently labeled a "functional" or "psychogenic" disorder in the literature, we will examine the evidence around two key questions: are any specific psychiatric conditions associated with VCD and causally related to VCD?

A very wide range of different psychiatric diagnoses have been reported in association with VCD including anxiety disorder, depression, conversion and factitious disorder, family conflict, personality disorders, and posttraumatic stress disorder. Several studies have compared patients with VCD to patients with moderate to severe asthma and reported no group differences in overall rates of psychopathology.[1,16] Rates of psychopathology in these studies ranged up to 73%

in the Newman and associates[1] study, but VCD clearly also occurs in patients without psychopathology, arguing against a causal role of psychiatric factors in VCD. Virtually all prior reports of psychiatric issues and VCD are limited by their reliance on retrospective chart reviews, and their use of self-report or clinical interview assessments of psychopathology rather than research-grade measures.

One important exception is the report of Gavin and colleagues[17] who prospectively examined psychiatric symptoms in adolescents admitted to an inpatient pulmonary rehabilitation program with a diagnosis of severe, chronic asthma. Twelve patients whose primary discharge diagnosis was changed to VCD were matched to patients whose discharge diagnosis remained severe, chronic asthma with no evidence of VCD. Medical records for the adolescents were reviewed by a pediatric pulmonologist to ensure that all patients in both groups had been appropriately studied to rule in or rule out VCD. Research-grade psychiatric assessments were conducted before the diagnoses of VCD were established. Patients ultimately diagnosed with VCD were found to have higher levels of self-reported and parent-reported panic anxiety and received a higher number of panic anxiety diagnoses during a structured psychiatric interview. Two thirds of patients with VCD (i.e., 8/12) received such diagnoses, versus only 2 asthma controls. In addition, the vast majority of the VCD patients had onset of their panic anxiety symptoms before their respiratory problems began, whereas this was not true for any asthma controls. Given that panic disorder, like VCD, may also arise from protective CNS respiratory reflexes gone awry, the findings of this study deserve replication and extension.

In summary, although psychological problems and overt psychiatric disorders are frequently associated with VCD, there is essentially no evidence that these factors directly cause VCD. Panic anxiety is the one psychiatric syndrome that deserves further scrutiny as possibly being causally related to VCD. Nonetheless, clinicians are wise to recognize and address psychiatric factors in the context of VCD, even if they are not causally related, as their presence does make a difference in the course and outcome of managing VCD.

CLINICAL COURSE

Making the Diagnosis of VCD

Vocal cord dysfunction can cause stridor, shortness of breath, wheezing, chest tightness, and cough (Table 38-1). Patients often will report throat tightness or voice changes during an acute attack. VCD should be suspected when a patient with recurrent cough or wheeze does not have a clear cause of upper airway obstruction or does not respond to standard asthma therapy. VCD symptoms often start and cease abruptly. Patients usually are asymptomatic between attacks, although some report more chronic air hunger, anticipatory anxiety (e.g., "I worry about when my next attack will occur"), cough, throat tightness, or voice changes outside of overt VCD episodes. Patients who have "pure" VCD may indicate that bronchodilators do not help, and often worsen their breathing. On physical exam, many patients will have palpable tension of the laryngeal musculature. Although stridorous wheezing can sometimes be heard over the larynx, these sounds are also transmitted to the

Table 38-1
IS IT VCD OR ASTHMA?

When You Have Trouble Breathing:	Answer Suggestive of:	
	VCD	Asthma
Where do you feel tight?	Throat; upper, midline chest	Lower, distal chest
What is more difficult, breathing in or out?	Breathing in	Breathing out
When do you make noise, breathing in or out?	Breathing in (stridor)	Breathing out (wheeze)
Does your voice change or do you get hoarse?	Yes	No, may lose voice during severe attack
Can you hold your breath or pant?	Yes	No
Did it start during exercise or soon after?	During	After
Does your rescue inhaler help?	No to maybe	Yes

lower airways; hence, it can be difficult to differentiate a VCD attack from an asthma episode by physical examination alone. However, if during acute symptoms the patient can hold his or her breath or pant, this is suggestive of VCD because most patients having an acute asthma attack will be unable to comply. When asymptomatic, patients with pure VCD have normal pulmonary function tests. This can help distinguish them from patients with more severe asthma, who often have increased residual volumes, due to air trapping from chronic small airways closure. During episodes, patients with VCD often show variable flattening or truncation of the inspiratory portion of their flow-volume loop, with the ratio of expiratory flow to inspiratory flow at 50% of forced vital capacity often being greater than 1.5 (Fig. 38-1). During an acute VCD attack, the alveolar-arterial oxygen difference is usually normal. It is important (and usually relatively easy) to exclude other conditions that can cause acute stridor and wheezing, including foreign bodies, epiglottitis and croup, and hereditary angioedema.[2]

The diagnosis of VCD is definitively established by direct visualization of the vocal cords while the patient is having symptoms (Fig. 38-2). "Classic" vocal cord dysfunction is characterized by adduction of the anterior two thirds of the vocal cords with a characteristic "posterior chink" observed during inspiration. Wood and Milgrom[2] provide a detailed description of diagnostic laryngoscopy, including recommendations of how to differentiate true VCD from vocal cord movement induced by the procedure itself (e.g., via the cough or gag reflex or through inadequate anaesthesia). A normal laryngoscopy in the absence of acute symptoms does not exclude the diagnosis of VCD, as approximately half of the laryngoscopies done without first provoking VCD symptoms were normal in patients ultimately diagnosed with VCD.[1] Accordingly, various challenge procedures have been recommended before laryngoscopy, including methacholine or histamine, specific irritant, and exercise.[2,13] If vocal cord adduction is not seen in a symptomatic patient, the diagnosis of VCD should be questioned.

Treatment of Vocal Cord Disorder

Many patients who ultimately are diagnosed with VCD first present for urgent or emergency care in respiratory crisis. In such a context, until a diagnosis of VCD is established, management is that for acute airway compromise of unclear etiology, with the key objectives being to ensure adequate oxygenation and gas exchange. Many acute episodes of laryngeal dysfunction can be controlled and managed with sedation and/or heliox (80% helium/20% oxygen). Topical lidocaine applied to the larynx may also be useful during acute episodes in select patients. In certain patients visualization of the larynx during acute episodes can be reassuring to the patient (and physician) as to the nature of the problem and increase patient acceptance of the diagnosis and treatment recommendations. Intubation is rarely if ever necessary as it is commonly accepted that most patients will have relaxation of the vocal cords if they lose consciousness. Intubation should be reserved for only the most extreme circumstances in which patients are highly distressed *and* show blood gas abnormalities, such as severe hypoxemia or hypercarbia.

Once the diagnosis of VCD is established, most authorities emphasize the role of a multidisciplinary team (pulmonologist, otolaryngologist, psychiatrist/psychologist, and speech therapist). For most patients, receiving the diagnosis of VCD

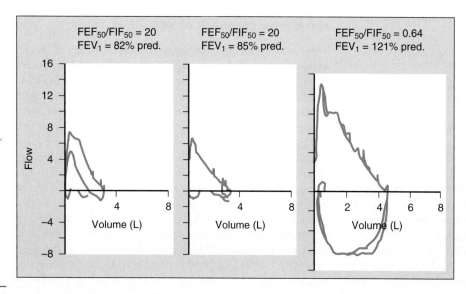

Figure 38-1 Characteristic spirometric abnormalities seen in VCD. Variable flattening and truncation of the inspiratory portion of the flow-volume loop when symptomatic.

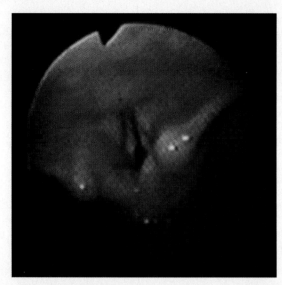

Figure 38-2 Photograph of vocal cord adduction during inspiration with the "classic" posterior chink.

requires them to change the beliefs they have about their illness arising from their prior medical diagnosis and treatment,[15] including a sizable number of patients who have suffered iatrogenic harm from misdiagnosis. In general, patients who are pleased and respond well to being informed about the true nature of their condition usually are more accepting of appropriate therapy and have a better outcome. Therefore, clinicians should take great care in explaining the diagnosis of VCD to the patient. For example, with patients who have a prior asthma diagnosis, they should be told whether or not they still have asthma and given the appropriate action plan for their particular clinical situation, be it "pure" VCD or coexistent VCD and asthma. Viewing the videotape of their own or another patient's vocal cords closing on inspiration is often a powerful aid in explaining how their symptoms arise. We specifically tell patients that the main pathophysiologic mechanism underlying VCD can be viewed as a reflex designed to protect their breathing that now has become hyperactive and dysfunctional; although we acknowledge that this is just a reigning hypothesis, not an established fact.

Based on the results of the diagnostic work-up, treatment should be initiated or maximized for all associated medical conditions, such as rhinosinusitis or GERD. The mainstay, however, of outpatient VCD therapy is various speech exercises, focused on two key goals.[2,15] First, a set of "rescue" techniques are taught so that the patient can open the cords during acute episodes and regain control over their symptoms. These techniques involve substituting a voluntary and competing behavior, such as panting or sibilant breathing, whenever the vocal cords start to adduct. When employed whenever VCD symptoms are triggered, and coached by supportive persons, these techniques usually are very effective in taking the "acute"

out of the patient's experience of VCD. Second, patients are coached in other techniques (e.g., slow, relaxed, abdominal breathing) to change their breathing outside of episodes (i.e., throughout the day) to (1) refocus their breathing efforts away from the larynx and airway thereby reducing laryngeal tension, and (2) possibly decrease feedback to the CNS that drives and maintains the hyperactive reflexes underlying VCD.

Some evidence exists that biofeedback, relaxation, and hypnosis also can be effective. However, since they are not as specific and efficient as the speech therapy exercises, they probably are best reserved for patients requiring additional tools to recover. For patients who have associated psychiatric problems (e.g., panic disorder or depression), or whose VCD symptoms have become incorporated into their self-image or entangled in interpersonal conflicts (e.g., in the context of workplace injury), consultation with a psychiatrist or psychologist experienced in the management of VCD is often very helpful to both the patient and the primary clinician. Antidepressant/antipanic medications are useful in cases when depression and/or panic anxiety are present, and may be helpful more generally. One group has found that pretreatment with an anticholinergic inhaler (ipratropium) helped all six pediatric patients with exercise-induced VCD control their episodes and continue their sports activities.[14] In severe cases, superior laryngeal blocks with clostridium botulinum toxin have been attempted with variable success, although this treatment appears more successful for muscle tension dysphonia than for VCD. Tracheotomy has been used for some patients with severe VCD refractory to conventional therapy, but it is rarely (if ever) indicated.

The literature suggests that the vast majority (more than 70%) of patients with VCD have a good outcome with some combination of education and reassurance, speech or breathing exercises, and psychosocial interventions, including two recent reports of longer term outcomes.[14,15]

CONCLUSION

The current best approach to the diagnosis and treatment of VCD is a collaborative and, whenever possible, multidisciplinary effort targeting (1) the likely pathophysiologic importance of CNS reflexes gone awry; (2) the importance of getting the patient to understand and accept the diagnosis of VCD and the recommended speech therapy treatment; and (3) the frequent confounding role of psychological stress and psychiatric disorders in the course and prognosis of VCD. Given the high prevalence rates, frequency of misdiagnosis and iatrogenic harm, significant degree of preventable morbidity, and availability of effective treatments for VCD, more widespread understanding of the pathophysiology and treatment of VCD will help health care providers succeed with what otherwise can be a difficult and frustrating group of patients to understand and treat.

REFERENCES

1. Newman KB, Mason UG, Schmaling KB: Clinical features of vocal cord dysfunction. Am J Respir Crit Care Med 1995; 152: 1382–1386.
2. Wood RP, Milgrom H: Vocal cord dysfunction. J Allergy Clin Immunol 1996;98:481–485.
3. Rundell KW, Spiering BA: Inspiratory stridor in elite athletes. Chest 2003;123:468–474.
4. Abu-Hasan M, Tannous B, Weinberger M: Exercise-induced dyspnea in children and adolescents: if not asthma then what? Ann Allergy Asthma Immunol 2005;94:366–371.

5. Bonham AC, Chen CY, Mutoh T, et al: Lung C–fiber CNS reflex: role in the respiratory consequences of extended environmental tobacco smoke exposure in young guinea pigs. Environ Health Perspect 2001;109(Suppl 4):573–578.

6. Morrison M, Rammage L, Emami AJ: The irritable larynx syndrome. J Voice 1999;13:447–455.

7. Bucca C, Rolla G, Brussino L, et al: Are asthma-like symptoms due to bronchial or extrathoracic airway dysfunction? Lancet 1995; 346(8978):791–795.

8. Bucca C, Rolla G, Scappaticci E, et al: Extrathoracic and intrathoracic airway responsiveness in sinusitis. J Allergy Clin Immunol 1995;95:52–59.

9. Turktas I, Dalgic N, Bostanci I, et al: Extrathoracic airway responsiveness in children with asthma-like symptoms, including chronic persistent cough. Pediatr Pulmonol 2002;34:172–180.

10. Perkner JJ, Fennelly KP, Balkissoon R, et al: Irritant-associated vocal cord dysfunction. J Occup Environ Med 1998;40:136–143.

11. McFadden ER, Zawadski DK: Vocal cord dysfunction masquerading as exercise-induced asthma: a physiologic cause for "choking" during athletic activities. Am J Respir Crit Care Med 1996;153:942–947.

12. Morris MJ, Deal LE, Bean DR, et al: Vocal cord dysfunction in patients with exertional dyspnea. Chest 1999;116:1676–1682.

13. Perkins PJ, Morris MJ: Vocal cord dysfunction induced by methacholine challenge testing. Chest 2002;122:1988–1993.

14. Doshi DR, Weinberger MM: Long-term outcome of vocal cord dysfunction. Ann Allergy Asthma Immunol 2006;96:794–799.

15. Sullivan MD, Heywood BM, Beukelman DR: A treatment for vocal cord dysfunction in female athletes: an outcome study. Laryngoscope 2001;111:1751–1755.

16. Ramirez J, Leon I, Rivera LM: Episodic laryngeal dyskinesia—clinical and psychiatric characterization. Chest 1986;90:716–721.

17. Gavin LA, Wamboldt MZ, Brugman SM, et al: Psychological and family characteristics of adolescents with vocal cord dysfunction. J Asthma 1998;35:409–417.

CLINICAL PEARLS

- Gastroesophageal reflux (GER) occurs in approximately 70% of asthmatic individuals. Furthermore, 65% of asthmatic individuals who do not have typical GER symptoms have esophageal pH tests consistent with GER, so their GER is clinically silent.

- Predisposing factors for GER development in asthmatic individuals include autonomic dysregulation, an increased pressure gradient between the thorax and the abdomen, obesity, hiatal hernia, and airflow obstruction. Some asthma medications may also induce reflux events.

- Esophageal acid alters airway function through a vagally mediated reflex, heightened airway reactivity, and/or microaspiration. Neuroinflammation is also activated with esophageal acid.

- Reflux therapy improves asthma outcomes in selected asthmatic individuals. Potential predictors of asthma response include difficult-to-control asthma, the use of long-acting beta-agonists (LABAs), and the presence of nighttime asthma symptoms.

- A 3-month empiric trial using GER lifestyle modifications along with a proton pump inhibitor (PPI) can help identify individual asthmatic individuals with GER-triggered asthma. Currently, no clinical test reliably identifies asthmatic individuals with GER-triggered asthma.

Asthma is a disease in which many triggers and/or contributing conditions lead to bronchospasm and inflammation in the lung. Controlling potential contributing conditions or triggers improves asthma control.[1] Asthmatic individuals are a heterogeneous group with respect to triggers and sensitivity to their triggers. Gastroesophageal reflux (GER) is a potential trigger or contributing factor in many asthmatic individuals. Even in the 19th century, Sir William Osler spoke of the association: "attacks may be due to direct irritation of the bronchial mucosa or . . . indirectly, too, by reflex influences of the stomach. . . ."[2]

The relationship between GER and asthma remains controversial. Esophageal acid alters airway inflammation through a vagally mediated reflex, heightened airway reactivity, and/or microaspiration.[3] Neuroinflammatory mediators also play a role.

Both GER and asthma are common diseases in the U.S. population. About one third of American adults have GER. Gastroesophageal reflux symptom prevalence in asthmatic individuals approximates 75% and abnormal esophageal acid contact times are present in up to 82% of asthmatic

individuals.[4] Asthmatic individuals with GER have a higher rate of future asthma hospitalizations compared with asthmatic individuals without GER.[5] Despite multiple outcome studies, there is still much controversy about the association between asthma and GER.

DEFINITIONS

Gastroesophageal Reflux

Gastroesophageal reflux can be defined by symptoms or by objective testing. According to updated guidelines from the American College of Gastroenterology, GER is defined by symptoms or by mucosal damage produced by the abnormal reflux of gastric contents into the esophagus.[6] Gastric contents flow in a retrograde direction across the gastroesophageal junction and the lower esophageal sphincter (LES) into the esophagus. Gastric contents are commonly acidic in nature; however, nonacid GER also occurs, especially in patients who are on acid suppressive therapy. In asthmatic individuals, nonacid GER has not been extensively investigated; however in patients with chronic cough, nonacid GER can elicit cough.[7] In these patients, cough resolution occurs with surgical fundoplication.

Gastroesophageal reflux can also be defined by means of esophageal pH testing. In this test, the distal pH probe is placed in the esophagus 5 cm above the LES. Oftentimes a proximal esophageal pH probe is also placed just below the upper esophageal sphincter (UES) or even in the hypopharynx. A GER event occurs when the pH is less than 4. Normal esophageal pH values (or esophageal acid contact times) are displayed in Table 39-1.[8] Note that upright values are taken during awake times and supine values are taken during sleep times as recorded by the patient in a diary. Nonacid GER can be identified by combining esophageal impedance with pH monitoring. A nonacid liquid GER event is defined by the presence of a drop in esophageal impedance without a drop in pH (<4).[9]

GER-Triggered Asthma

GER-triggered asthma can be defined by several means. One way is to note whether patients temporally associate respiratory symptoms with GER events. A more definitive way is to show that asthma outcomes improve with GER-directed therapy. Since asthmatic individuals have multiple asthma triggers and asthma is a complex inflammatory disorder, elimination of one comorbid condition or trigger would not be expected to eliminate the disease.

Table 39-1
NORMAL 24-HOUR ESOPHAGEAL pH VALUES (% TIME pH < 4)

Distal Probe (5 CM Above the LES)*	Proximal Probe (Just Below UES)†
Total < 5.5%	<1.1%
Upright < 8.1%	<1.7%
Supine < 3.0%	<0.6%

Data from Harding SM, Richter JE, Guzzo MR, et al: Asthma and gastroesophageal reflux: acid suppressive therapy improves asthma outcome. Am J Med 1996;100:395–405.
*Distal based on 110 normal controls
†Proximal based on 20 normal controls

NATURAL HISTORY/EPIDEMIOLOGY

Natural History with GER Treatment

If asthmatic individuals have GER-triggered asthma, then treating their GER should improve their asthma symptoms. Asthma and GER are both common diseases in our population, so some asthmatic individuals may have GER, but their GER may not impact or be a trigger of their asthma. Different investigators observed that aggressive GER therapy including lifestyle modifications, medical therapy (PPI, prokinetic agents, and H_2 receptor antagonists), and/or surgical therapy improve asthma in selected patients. Reflux therapy requires significant time to have an impact on asthma outcomes. Only one study examined this carefully. In asthmatic individuals with GER-triggered asthma, 1 month of acid suppressive therapy resulted in a 30% reduction in asthma symptoms, at 2 months a 43% reduction, and at 3 months a 57% reduction.[8] A minimum of 3 months of acid suppressive therapy is needed before making an assessment as to whether asthma is improved in individual asthmatic patients.[8] Long-term follow-up for up to 19 years is available in 16 surgically treated patients.[10] There was a sustained improvement in nocturnal asthma symptoms noted within months.

Gastroesophageal reflux may also be more difficult to treat in asthmatic individuals compared with GER subjects without asthma. Approximately 30% of asthmatic individuals with GER required more than 20 mg of omeprazole a day to normalize esophageal acid contact times.[8] If an empiric GER medical therapy trial is initiated, a high-dose PPI regimen should be initiated along with lifestyle modifications for at least 3 months.[1]

GER Population Studies

Population studies are one way to explore the potential interaction between asthma and GER. A case-controlled study involving 101,366 veterans discharged from 172 Veterans Administration hospitals noted that veterans with esophageal disease were more likely to have asthma than veterans without esophageal disease, with an odds ratio of 1.15.[11] There are also data examining incidence of GER and asthma over a mean follow-up period of 3 years in over 15,000 patients having a first diagnosis of asthma or GER, and in more than 17,000 matched controls.[12] Patients with a first diagnosis of asthma had a significant increased risk of subsequent GER development even when controlling for confounding factors.

GER Prevalence Studies

GER SYMPTOMS

Gastroesophageal reflux symptom prevalence in adult asthmatic individuals is estimated to be between 33% and 89%. Perrin-Fayolle noted GER symptoms in 65% of 150 consecutive asthmatic individuals.[13] Sontag and colleagues noted that 72% of 189 consecutive asthmatic individuals had heartburn and that approximately 50% had nighttime heartburn with 18% reporting nocturnal burning in the throat.[4] Field and associates examined GER symptoms in 109 asthmatic individuals and 135 controls by questionnaire in a cross-sectional study. Of the asthmatic individuals, 77% had heartburn, 55% had regurgitation, and 24% had difficulty swallowing.[14] Forty-one percent had GER-associated respiratory symptoms and 28% used their inhalers while experiencing GER symptoms. Other investigators have also noted a high prevalence of GER symptoms in asthmatic individuals. Kiljander and colleagues selected every 14th patient from a multicenter group of 2225 asthmatic individuals, of which 51% had GER symptoms.[15] In combining all reported prevalence studies to date, including 538 asthmatic individuals, 68% had GER symptoms.

Not all asthmatic individuals with GER have esophageal GER symptoms, so GER can be "clinically silent." In asthmatic individuals without GER symptoms, 62% of them had abnormal esophageal acid contact times consistent with GER.[16]

ABNORMAL ESOPHAGEAL MANOMETRY

Gastroesophageal reflux is an esophageal motility disorder and investigators found that many asthmatic individuals have esophageal dysmotility and/or low LES pressures on esophageal manometry. For instance, in 97 consecutive asthmatic individuals, 38% had esophageal dysmotility and 27% had LES hypotension.[17] Another report showed that 68% of asthmatic individuals had esophageal dysmotility.[18] Asthmatic individuals, therefore, compared with control subjects, have significantly lower LES pressures, predisposing them to GER.

ABNORMAL ESOPHAGEAL ACID CONTACT TIMES ON ESOPHAGEAL PH TESTING

Esophageal pH testing in asthmatic individuals reveals a high prevalence of abnormal esophageal acid contact times. In 90 randomly selected asthmatic individuals, abnormal esophageal acid contact times were found in 36%.[15] In 104 consecutive asthmatic individuals in a Veterans Administration health care system, 82% had abnormal esophageal acid contact times.[4] In another study of 199 asthmatic individuals referred for 24-hour esophageal pH testing, 119 (79%) of 151 reported respiratory symptoms were temporally associated with esophageal acid.[19] Respiratory symptom correlation with esophageal acid events supports the hypothesis that GER may trigger asthma. In eight studies performed in five countries totaling 718 patients, 63% had abnormal amounts of esophageal acid on esophageal pH testing.

ESOPHAGITIS

Furthermore, in a prospective study of consecutive asthmatic individuals referred for upper endoscopy, 39% had esophagitis, with 13% having Barrett esophagus.[20]

Table 39-2
GER PREVALENCE IN ASTHMATIC ADULTS*

GER symptoms	77%
GER-associated respiratory symptoms	41%
Asthma inhaler use with GER symptoms	28%
Abnormal esophageal acid contact times	82%
Abnormal esophageal acid contact times in the absence of GER symptoms	62%
Esophageal dysmotility	38%
Lower esophageal sphincter hypotension	27%
Esophagitis	39%

*Data from Harding SM: Gastroesophageal reflux: A potential asthma trigger. J Immunol Allergy Clin N Am 2005;25:131–148.

Table 39–3
PREDISPOSING FACTORS FOR GER DEVELOPMENT IN ASTHMATIC INDIVIDUALS

Intrinsic Factors	Extrinsic Factors
Autonomic dysregulation	Eating before bedtime
Increased pressure gradient	Medications
Hyperinflation	Theophylline
Airway obstruction	Albuterol
Obesity	Oral corticosteroids
Hiatal hernia	

CONCLUSIONS

Even though many prevalence studies had selection bias, and the large population-based incidence studies included biases of physician-based diagnoses and their knowledge of the relationship between asthma and GER, evidence supports previous suppositions that GER prevalence is much greater in asthmatic individuals than in the general population. Table 39-2 summarizes important prevalence findings in asthmatic individuals.

Predisposing Factors for GER Development in Asthmatic Individuals

There are many predisposing factors for GER development in asthmatic individuals. Autonomic dysregulation, an increased pressure gradient between the thorax and the abdomen, obesity, hiatal hernia, airflow obstruction, and certain asthma medications may promote GER.

Asthmatic individuals with GER have a heightened vagal responsiveness on autonomic function testing.[21] Autonomic dysregulation may result in decreased LES pressure and trigger transient LES relaxations that promote GER.

Furthermore, with increased work of breathing, the thorax generates negative pressure swings, leading to an increased pressure gradient between the thorax and abdomen that overrides LES pressure.[3]

Airway obstruction also triggers transient LES relaxations and GER episodes. Altered crural diaphragm function may also be present. The crural diaphragm contributes to LES pressure generation. Hyperinflation associated with airflow obstruction leads to geometric flattening of the diaphragm, placing it at functional disadvantage.[3]

Furthermore, asthmatic individuals have a high prevalence of hiatal hernia (58% to 64%).[1] Transient LES relaxations are more likely to be followed by GER episodes if a hiatal hernia is present.

Pulmonary medications may also promote GER. Theophylline, for instance, increases gastric acid secretion and decreases LES pressure. In a placebo-controlled trial, GER symptoms increased 170% and daytime acid episodes increased 24% with theophylline.[22] However, other studies found no differences in 24-hour esophageal pH variables.[23] Inhaled beta-agonists caused dose-dependent decreases in LES pressure and in the amplitude of esophageal contractions.[24] In a randomized double-blind placebo-controlled

crossover study, oral corticosteroids (prednisone 60 mg daily) increased esophageal acid contact times at both the proximal and distal esophagus.[25]

Lifestyle issues may also predispose some asthmatic individuals to GER. Sixty percent of asthmatic individuals eat right before bedtime.[26] This habit was associated with nocturnal awakening from heartburn, suffocation, cough, and/or wheezing preceded by heartburn or regurgitation during sleep. Obesity is associated with an increased relative risk of asthma and predisposal to GER development.[27] Table 39-3 reviews predisposing factors for GER development in asthmatic individuals.

PATHOGENESIS OF GER-INDUCED AIRWAY RESPONSES

Many pathophysiologic mechanisms can elicit esophageal acid-induced airway responses and are shown in Table 39-4. Mechanisms include a vagally mediated reflex, local axonal reflexes, heightened bronchial reactivity, microaspiration, increased minute ventilation, and airway inflammation. The vagus nerve is involved in the vagally mediated reflex mechanism, the heightened bronchial reactivity mechanism, and the microaspiration mechanism.

Vagal Reflex

The tracheobronchial tree and the esophagus share common embryonic foregut origins and autonomic innervation through the vagus nerve. Animal models and human studies show that esophageal acid causes respiratory responses that are vagally mediated. In an animal model, esophageal acid caused a 10% increase in total respiratory resistance that was ablated with bilateral vagotomy.[28] In humans, esophageal

Table 39–4
MECHANISMS OF GER-INDUCED PULMONARY RESPONSES

- Vagal reflex
- Local axonal reflexes
- Heightened bronchial reactivity
- Microaspiration
- Increase in minute ventilation
- Inflammation:
  Substance P
  Tachykinins
  Interleukin-8

acid caused a decrease in peak expiratory flow (PEF) rates and increases in respiratory resistance.[29] Atropine pretreatment reduced these findings. Neural mechanisms underlying this pathway appear to involve the release of substance P. Harding et al found evidence of autonomic dysfunction in asthmatic individuals with GER with hypervagal responses noted during deep breathing, Valsalva, and tilt test maneuvers.[21] This prominence of hypervagal tone can trigger transient LES relaxations and thus GER. Hypervagal tone predisposes to airflow obstruction.

Local Axonal Reflexes

Local axonal reflexes also play a role. In this mechanism, central nervous system (CNS) intervention is not required for airway responses. Anatomical neuronal connections exist in animal models between the esophagus and the lung with nitric oxide–containing neurons.[30] In a guinea pig model, esophageal acid caused marked airway edema, and tachykinin receptor (NK-1 and NK-2) antagonists prevented this airway response.[31] This verifies that nonvagal peripheral pathways acting through the autonomic ganglia are active.

Heightened Bronchial Reactivity

Heightened bronchial reactivity from esophageal acid priming the lung allows asthmatic individuals exposed to another trigger to have a heightened response. For instance, esophageal acid infusions increased the bronchoconstrictive effects of isocapnic hyperventilation and methacholine provocation tests, as compared to esophageal saline infusions. Furthermore, atropine pretreatment abolished this effect, so that the vagus nerve is involved in the heightened bronchial activity mechanism. In 105 consecutive asthmatic individuals, PD_{20} correlated with the number of GER events during 24-hour esophageal pH testing.[33] Heightened bronchial reactivity also occurs during sleep. Acid GER episodes were associated with increases in lower airway resistance in seven asthmatic individuals with GER during sleep.[34]

Microaspiration

Microaspiration of esophageal contents also elicits significant airway responses. In humans, tracheal microaspiration is associated with more significant pulmonary function deterioration compared to esophageal acid.[35] In a cat model, 10 μL of esophageal acid caused a 1.5-fold increase in total lung resistance compared to 5.0-fold increase when 50 μL was instilled into the trachea.[36] Interestingly, in the microaspiration model, these respiratory effects were abolished with cervical vagotomy.

Minute Ventilation

Esophageal acid increases minute ventilation and respiratory rate without bronchoconstriction in healthy subjects.[37] Esophageal acid clearance normalized the minute ventilation. Chest discomfort correlated with this increase in minute ventilation. This increase in minute ventilation may explain why GER worsens respiratory symptoms without necessarily changing pulmonary function test results. This study needs to be repeated in asthmatic individuals with GER.

Airway Inflammation

Esophageal acid also induces airway inflammation. In a guinea pig model, esophageal acid caused the release of substance P, which was associated with airway edema.[31] Tachykinins, including substance P and neurokinins, contract airway smooth muscle, increase bronchial gland secretion, increase vascular permeability, and induce cough. Tachykinins are released from the lung by capsaicin, histamine, bradykinins, prostaglandin F, allergic responses, and antidromic electrical stimulation of the vagus nerve. These neuro-inflammatory mechanisms are active in acid-induced models. Inhaled citric acid in a guinea pig model caused a dose-dependent increase in total pulmonary resistance mediated by activation of sensory nerves and release of tachykinins from peripheral nerve terminals.[38] This bronchoconstriction was reversed by giving tachykinin NK-1 receptor antagonists. Nitric oxide was also released, which may explain why esophageal acid does not always result in bronchoconstriction. Nitric oxide is also a marker of airway inflammation. In children with allergic asthma, exhaled nitric oxide levels were lower in asthmatic children with GER compared with asthmatic children without GER.[39] Inhalation of gastric acid contents may interfere with nitric oxide production in the airways.

Esophageal acid, especially with proximal migration, may result in inhalation or aspiration of acid material, which in turn alters airway homeostasis. Esophageal contents may also damage upper airway epithelium, resulting in the release of cytokines and adhesion molecules and initiating other inflammatory pathways.[40] For instance, children with GER and respiratory symptoms have higher numbers of neutrophils, lipid-laden macrophages, and higher levels of interleukin (IL)-8, myeloperoxidase, and elastase in bronchoalveolar lavage (BAL) fluid compared with asthmatic children without GER.[41]

Nonacid GER may also induce respiratory changes. Esophageal fluid osmolality can initiate local axonal reflexes.[31] Esophageal distention alone can also initiate vagal reflexes.[3] Future research will further delineate mechanisms of these esophageal pulmonary interactions.

CLINICAL COURSE

Recognition of GER in Asthmatic Individuals

Clinical features of GER-related asthma are very similar to clinical features of asthma. Since GER is a potential asthma trigger, all asthmatic individuals should be questioned about GER symptoms.

Patients should be asked about dysphagia, heartburn frequency and severity, regurgitation, and cough. Patients may experience worsening bronchospasm after consuming foods that lower LES pressure.[42] Use of rescue inhalers when patients are experiencing GER symptoms should also alert physicians. If asthmatic individuals are obese, they are at increased risk for developing GER. Nocturnal GER and obesity are independent risk factors for asthma onset, wheeze, and nighttime symptoms. Some asthmatic individuals may develop GER symptoms only during acute asthma exacerbations. Patients may also present with other extraesophageal manifestations of GER including laryngitis, sore throat, globus, upper airway cough syndrome (UACS), and/or hoarseness. Physicians should also pay special attention to sleep time awakenings due to bronchospasm that may point to GER-triggered asthma. Symptoms that occur while lying in the supine position or after consuming a large meal prior to bedtime can be a clue to prompt a suspicion of GER. Sontag and co-workers showed that 50% of asthmatic individuals had nocturnal awakenings from heartburn with 33% noticing suffocation, cough, or wheezing preceded by heartburn or regurgitation that awakened them from sleep.[26] Some asthmatic individuals with GER do not have typical GER symptoms and their GER is clinically silent.

Diagnostic Evaluation of GER

Most helpful diagnostic tools for GER include an empiric trial of medical GER therapy (to see if asthma symptoms improve), esophageal pH testing, and esophageal manometry.

If GER is suspected clinically or if asthma is difficult to control, an empiric trial of a PPI should be considered. A PPI should be given two times a day, 30 minutes to an hour before breakfast and dinner, for a period of 3 months. Recommendations from the ATS Workshop on Refractory Asthma suggest that GER should be investigated in cases of refractory asthma.[43] An empiric trial should also be considered in those patients with moderate to severe-persistent asthma requiring oral corticosteroid treatment.[44] Asthma symptoms, PEF rates, and use of asthma medications should be monitored during this trial. After three months, if improvement in asthma symptoms is evident, then the PPI dose can be tapered to once a day before breakfast.[1] Patients should also be counseled about foods that promote GER symptoms, and about lifestyle changes that should also be implemented. Esophageal pH testing should be considered in the asthma nonresponders to see if esophageal acid is controlled on GER therapy. If acid is controlled on pH testing, then two possibilities should be considered. First, the asthmatic has GER, but it does not have a significant impact on their asthma. The other possibility is that nonacid reflux may be present, which is not controlled on medical therapy. This is a rare theoretical possibility. Prospective studies are needed to assess the diagnostic accuracy of the empiric trial.

Esophageal pH testing allows correlation of asthma symptoms with esophageal acid events, and assessment regarding the adequacy of GER therapy. It is also useful in diagnosing GER in asthmatic individuals who do not have GER symptoms. Esophageal pH testing has a sensitivity and specificity of approximately 90% in diagnosing GER in asthmatic individuals.[45] Many published reports of esophageal pH testing may underestimate the amount of GER. Esophageal testing does not reliably predict which asthmatic individuals have improvement in asthma outcomes with GER therapy.[46]

Other diagnostic tests may be useful in asthmatic individuals; however, they are problematic because they have poor sensitivities.[46-48] Esophageal manometry is useful in documenting motility disorders in asthmatic individuals. Upper endoscopy is useful in detecting esophageal mucosal injury—such as esophagitis, strictures, webs, Barrett esophagus, and esophageal carcinoma. Barium esophagram, radio-labeled technetium sulfur colloid, and the Bernstein test are also used but have low sensitivities. Inspection of sputum for lipid-laden

macrophages (to document lipids in lung from gastric aspiration) has low specificity. Scintigraphic monitoring using technetium 99m is also useful in documenting pulmonary aspiration of gastric contents directly into the lung; however, false negative scans are possible. These methods support the diagnosis of GER-related lung disease; however, none have proven reliable in predicting which patients have GER-triggered or GER-associated respiratory disease.[1]

Esophageal impedance combined with pH testing detects the presence of nonacid GER. It detects liquid, gas, and liquid-gas boluses.[9] Minimal data is available in asthmatic individuals using this technique.

GER Management in Asthmatic individuals

All asthmatic individuals should be screened for GER symptoms. If a 3-month empiric trial of PPI along with GER lifestyle modifications shows subjective and/or objective asthma improvement, then chronic GER therapy is indicated.[1]

LIFESTYLE MODIFICATION
The cornerstone of GER management is GER lifestyle modifications. Weight loss (if obese) and avoidance of tight-fitting clothes that increase abdominal pressure and predispose to GER, are helpful modifications. Patients should avoid high-fat meals since this delays gastric emptying. They should also avoid eating within 3 hours of bedtime, and avoid foods that decrease LES pressure including peppermint, chocolate, alcohol, and caffeine.[1] Nicotine also lowers LES pressure; thus, smoking should be avoided. Acidic foods (including carbonated beverages, citrus foods, and tomatoes) may also worsen GER. Elevating the head of the bed with blocks or using a mattress wedge may improve nighttime GER. Furthermore, improved asthma control may prevent GER episodes. If clinically appropriate, avoidance of medications that worsen GER may be indicated, especially theophylline at high doses.

MEDICAL THERAPY
Along with GER lifestyle modifications, decrease the PPI dose to once daily (before breakfast) and continue monitoring asthma response. Proton pump inhibitors have been safely used for GER treatment for more than 18 years.[49] Prokinetic agents can be helpful; however, metoclopramide is the only available agent in the United States approved by the Food and Drug Administration. Agents that control transient LES relaxations, a key cause of GER events, are currently in development, but only baclofen is currently available.[1] Baclofen has many side effects. Nasal continuous positive airway pressure (CPAP) decreases GER during sleep and is useful in asthmatic individuals with GER and obstructive sleep apnea.[50]

SURGICAL THERAPY
Surgical fundoplication can be considered in asthmatic individuals whose asthma improved with medical GER therapy, especially in patients with normal esophageal motility and reduced LES pressures.[1] Surgery is not recommended for an asthma indication in the asthma nonresponders. Before surgery, esophageal testing including esophageal manometry, endoscopy, and esophageal pH testing off GER medications are indicated. Effective laparoscopic fundoplication has a learning curve, so ensure that the surgeon can document good

outcomes. Also, inform the potential surgical candidate that fundoplication does not ensure that GER medications will no longer be required.[51]

WHEN TO REFER

Referral to a gastroenterologist is recommended if a patient has long-term GER symptoms (especially in white males over age 40) that may require endoscopic screening for Barrett esophagus.[6] Patients presenting with GER complications such as bleeding, dysphagia, or continued GER symptoms despite medication should also be referred to a gastroenterologist. A gastroenterologist should also evaluate patients who are considering fundoplication.

Asthma Outcomes with GER Therapy

If GER triggers asthma, then GER therapy should improve asthma outcomes in selected asthmatic individuals. There have been multiple studies investigating the efficacy of medical or surgical GER therapy on asthma outcomes. Many asthmatic individuals with GER show improvement in asthma symptoms and/or other measures of disease activity. However, the data are inconsistent. Many studies have design flaws including small patient populations, lack of a placebo arm, and inadequate treatment duration. These studies examined multiple outcome parameters, but not in a uniform manner, making outcomes difficult to generalize in the general asthma population. Furthermore, asthma populations between trials are heterogeneous, further limiting their usefulness. Many trials used antacids, alginates, and H_2 receptor antagonists at standard doses, and reported mixed results. However, PPIs suppress gastric acid more effectively than other medical GER therapies currently available. A Cochrane dataset review of all randomized controlled trials of GER therapy in asthmatic individuals concluded that the published literature does not consistently support treatment of GER as a means of controlling asthma, and that additional larger randomized trials of longer duration are needed.[52] Most trials reviewed did not utilize PPIs. Asthma improvement was noted in certain asthma subgroups.

MEDICAL THERAPY

Prior to the routine use of PPIs, Field et al reviewed 12 medical therapy trials that evaluated asthma outcomes.[53] In 326 treated subjects, asthma symptoms improved in 69% of subjects, asthma medications were reduced in 62% of subjects, and evening PEF improved in 26% of subjects. Pulmonary function test variables did not improve.

Table 39-5 reviews nine placebo-controlled trials that examined asthma outcomes with PPI therapies.[54–62] Six of these studies (Meier and colleagues, Ford and colleagues, Teichtahl and colleagues, Kiljander and colleagues, Harmanci and colleagues, and Levin and colleagues) did not have adequate treatment durations.[54–56,58,59] Even so, some studies noted reduction of nighttime asthma symptoms, improved quality of life, and mild PEF improvement. Boeree and associates performed a double-blind, randomized, placebo-controlled, parallel trial in 36 asthmatic individuals with GER, and noted improvements in nocturnal cough without improvement in pulmonary function variables.

Overcoming the problem of inadequate treatment duration, two recent multicentered, placebo-controlled studies by Littner and co-workers and Kiljander and co-workers have employed adequate treatment duration and a PPI dose that would adequately suppress acid in most subjects.[61,62] Both studies noted marked asthma symptom improvement in both

Table 39-5
PLACEBO-CONTROLLED TRIALS EXAMINING ASTHMA OUTCOMES WITH PROTON PUMP INHIBITOR THERAPY

Study	Design	NBR	Medication	Duration	Outcome
Meier JH et al, Dig Dis Sci 1994;39:2127[54]	Double-blind, randomized, crossover, placebo-controlled	16	Omeprazole 20 mg bid	6 weeks	29% increased FEV$_1$ by 20%
Ford GA et al, Postgrad J Med 1994; 70:350[55]	Double-blind, randomized, crossover, placebo-controlled	11	Omeprazole 20 mg bid	4 weeks	No improvement in PEF
Teichtahl H et al, Aust NZ Med 1996;26:671[56]	Double-blind, randomized, crossover, placebo-controlled	20	Omeprazole 40 mg qd	4 weeks	Mild improvement in PEF
Boeree MJ et al, Eur Respir J 1998;11:1070[57]	Double-blind, randomized, placebo-controlled, parallel	36	Omeprazole 40 mg bid	3 months	Improvement in nocturnal cough, no change in PFTs
Kiljander TO et al, Chest 1999; 116:1257[58]	Double-blind, randomized, crossover, placebo-controlled	69	Omeprazole 40 mg qd	8 weeks	Reduction in nighttime asthma symptoms
Harmanci E et al, Allergol Immunopathol (Madr) 2001;29:123[59]	Prospective, single-blinded, crossover, placebo-controlled	5	Omeprazole 40 mg qd	4 weeks	No improvement in PFTs
Levin TR et al, Am J Gastroenterol 1998; 93:1060[60]	Double-blind, randomized, crossover, placebo-controlled	9	Omeprazole 20 mg qd	8 weeks	Morning and evening PEF improvement, improved quality of life, trend toward FEV$_1$
Kiljander TO et al, Am J Respir Crit Care Med 2006;173:1091–1097[61]	Double blind, randomized, placebo-controlled	770	Esomeprazole 40 mg bid	16 weeks	Improved PEF in those with GER and nocturnal asthma symptoms
Littner MR et al, Chest 2005;128:1128[62]	Multicenter, double-blind, randomized, placebo-controlled	207	Lansoprazole 30 mg bid	24 weeks	Decreased exacerbations and improved quality of life. No improvement in asthma symptoms, pulmonary function, or albuterol use

NBR, number of subjects; PFT, pulmonary function test.

the placebo and treatment groups, showing a significant placebo response. However, asthma symptoms in the PPI-treated group showed no improvement over the placebo group. Both studies did show that *selected* asthmatic individuals are more likely to improve. Littner and co-workers noted that the PPI-treated group had quality of life improvement and had fewer asthma exacerbations compared to the control group. A post-hoc analysis showed that asthmatic individuals receiving one or more asthma control medications in addition to inhaled corticosteroids were more likely to improve.[62] Kiljander and co-workers noted that asthmatic individuals on long-acting beta-agonists with GER symptoms and nighttime asthma symptoms had improvement in PEF rates.[61] Future investigations should carefully evaluate predictors for asthma response.

SURGICAL THERAPY

Uncontrolled surgical trials have also examined asthma outcomes. Of 110 carefully selected asthmatic individuals with GER undergoing fundoplication in combined trials, 34% were free of asthma symptoms and 42% of subjects had asthma symptom improvement.[63] Open versus laparoscopic fundoplication showed similar results in controlling asthma symptoms.

Two placebo-controlled trials examined surgical versus medical GER therapy in asthmatic individuals with GER. Both studies were performed before the availability of PPIs. Larrain and colleagues examined 81 nonallergic asthmatic individuals with GER, with a minimum follow-up of 6 months. Asthma symptoms improved by 74% in the medically treated group (cimetidine 300 mg four times a day) and by 77% in the surgically treated group, compared to controls.[64] Sontag and associates reported long-term follow-up in 73 asthmatic individuals with GER randomized to receive either antacids, ranitidine 150 mg three times a day, or fundoplication.[10] Only the surgically treated group had significant improvement in asthma symptoms, asthma medication use, and pulmonary function.

Conclusion

Treatment of GER does not improve asthma outcomes in the general asthma population, but may improve asthma outcomes in selected patients. Asthma symptoms are more likely than pulmonary function to improve with GER therapy. In placebo-controlled trials, there was a marked improvement in the placebo group, so uncontrolled trial outcomes are suspect for showing a significant asthma response.

On the other hand, the trials noted that subgroups of asthmatic individuals are more likely to respond to GER therapy. Table 39-6 illustrates these potential predictors of asthma response. These potential predictors need to be validated in prospective trials.

CONTROVERSIES

The Association between GER and Asthma

There are many remaining controversies about the association between GER and asthma. Data suggest that GER is more prevalent in asthmatic individuals compared with healthy control populations. Furthermore, esophageal acid

Table 39–6
POTENTIAL PREDICTORS FOR ASTHMA RESPONSE WITH GER THERAPY

Asthma Variables	GER Variables
Nonallergic asthma	Proximal acid on esophageal pH test
Oral corticosteroid use	Regurgitation
Long-acting beta-agonist use	
Nighttime asthma symptoms	
Reflux-associated asthma symptoms	

can elicit airway responses through at least three pathophysiologic mechanisms. Controlled studies to date do not show significant improvement with GER therapy, although selected asthmatic individuals had a significant response. Although esophageal acid can precipitate asthma symptoms, there are many difficulties involved in establishing a definite cause and effect relationship between GER and asthma. Currently, there is no diagnostic test that identifies patients with GER-triggered asthma, specifically those who would respond to GER therapy. Preliminary work is being done with exhaled breath condensate as a potential diagnostic test.

Empiric PPI Trials in Asthmatic individuals without GER Symptoms

Another controversy is whether an empiric PPI trial should be considered in asthmatic individuals who do not have GER symptoms. Kiljander and co-workers' careful placebo-controlled trial showed that asthmatic individuals without GER symptoms did not have improvement in asthma outcomes.[61] Other investigators have shown that asthmatic individuals on oral corticosteroids who do not have reflux symptoms improve with GER therapy.[44] Hopefully, carefully designed prospective trials will answer this controversy.

Long-term GER Management in Asthmatic Individuals

There is minimal data concerning long-term medical management of GER in asthmatic individuals, with the longest study being 6 months in duration. Long-term surgical outcomes have been more carefully evaluated. There is minimal data regarding the most cost-effective way to manage GER in asthmatic individuals both acutely and long-term. The availability of generic omeprazole has decreased the cost of GER medical therapy significantly.

Nonacid GER

Another controversy is whether nonacid GER triggers asthma. In chronic cough studies, nonacid GER was temporally associated with cough when combined esophageal impedance and pH testing were utilized.[65] Surgical fundoplication resulted in cough resolution. If nonacid GER triggers asthma, then fundoplication may be necessary to adequately treat these patients.

Endoscopic GER Therapies in Asthmatic Individuals

New endoscopic GER therapies are being utilized in GER management. Currently, there are no studies using these therapies in asthmatic individuals. Their use should be considered experimental at this time.

Further investigations will offer guidance on these controversies and allow effective diagnosis and management in patients with GER-triggered asthma.

REFERENCES

1. Harding SM: Gastroesophageal reflux: A potential asthma trigger. J Immunol Allergy Clin N Am 2005;25:131–148.
2. Osler WB: The Principles and Practice of Medicine, 8th ed. New York, D. Appleton, 1912, pp 1148–1156.
3. Harding SM: GERD, airway disease, and the mechanisms of interaction. In Stein MR (ed): Lung Biology in Health and Disease, Vol. 129, Gastroesophageal Disease and Airway Disease. New York, Marcel Dekker; 1999, pp 139–178.
4. Sontag SJ, O'Connell S, Khandelwal S, et al: Most asthmatics have gastroesophageal reflux with or without bronchodilator therapy. Gastroenterology 1990;991:613–620.
5. Shireman TI, Heaton PC, Gay WE, et al: Relationship between asthma drug therapy patterns and healthcare utilization. Ann Pharmacother 2002;36:557–564.
6. DeVault KR, Castell DO: American College of Gastroenterology. Updated guidelines for the diagnosis and treatment of gastroesophageal reflux disease. Am J Gastroenterol 2005;100:190–200.
7. Irwin RS, Zawacki JK, Wilson MM, et al: Chronic cough due to gastroesophageal reflux disease: Failure to resolve despite total/near-total elimination of esophageal acid. Chest 2002;121:1132–1140.
8. Harding SM, Richter JE, Guzzo MR, et al: Asthma and gastroesophageal reflux: Acid suppressive therapy improves asthma outcomes. Am J Med 1996;100:395–405.
9. Shay S, Tutuian R, Sifrim D, et al: Twenty-four hour ambulatory simultaneous impedance and pH monitoring: A multicenter report of normal values from 60 healthy volunteers. Am J Gastroenterol 2004;99:1037–1043.
10. Sontag SJ, O'Connell S, Khandelwal S, et al: Asthmatics with gastroesophageal reflux: Long term results of a randomized trial of medical and surgical anti-reflux therapies. Am J Gastroenterol 2004;98:987–999.
11. el-Serag HB, Sonnenberg A: Comorbid occurrence of laryngeal or pulmonary disease with esophagitis in United States military veterans. Gastroenterology 1997;113:755–760.
12. Ruigómez A, Rodriquez LA, Wallander MA, et al: Gastroesophageal reflux disease and asthma: A longitudinal study in UK general practice. Chest 2005;128:85–93.
13. Perrin-Fayolle M, Bel A, Kofman J, et al: Asthma and gastro-esophageal reflux. Results of a survey of over 150 cases. Poumon Coeur 1980;36:225–230.
14. Field SK, Underwood M, Brant R, et al: Prevalence of gastroesophageal reflux symptoms in asthma. Chest 1996;109:316–322.
15. Kiljander TO, Laitinen JO: The prevalence of gastroesophageal reflux disease in adult asthmatics. Chest 2004;126:1490–1944.
16. Harding SM, Guzzo MR, Richter JE: The prevalence of gastroesophageal reflux in asthma patients without reflux symptoms. Am J Respir Crit Care Med 2000;162:34–39.
17. Kjellen G, Brundin A, Tibbling L, et al: Oesophageal function in asthmatics. Eur J Respir Dis 1981;62:87–94.
18. Campo S, Morini S, Re MA, et al: Esophageal dysmotility and gastroesophageal reflux in intrinsic asthma. Dig Dis Sci 1997;42:1184–1188.
19. Harding SM, Guzzo MR, Richter JE: 24-h esophageal pH testing in asthmatics: respiratory symptom correlation with esophageal acid events. Chest 1999;115:654–659.
20. Sontag SJ, Schnell TG, Miller TQ, et al: Prevalence of oesophagitis in asthmatics. Gut 1992;33:872–876.
21. Lodi U, Harding SM, Coghlan HC, et al: Autonomic regulation in asthmatics with gastroesophageal reflux. Chest 1997;111:65–70.
22. Ekström T, Tibbling L: Influence of theophylline on gastro-oesophageal reflux and asthma. Eur J Clin Pharmacol 1988;35:353–356.
23. Hubert D, Gaudric M, Guerre J, et al: Effect of theophylline on gastroesophageal reflux in patients with asthma. J Allergy Clin Immunol 1988;81:1168–1174.
24. Crowell MD, Zayat EN, Lacy BE, et al: The effects of an inhaled beta(2)-adrenergic agonist on lower esophageal function: A dose-response study. Chest 2001;120:1184–1189.
25. Lazenby JP, Guzzo MR, Harding SM, et al: Oral corticosteroids increase esophageal acid contact times in patients with stable asthma. Chest 2002;121:625–634.
26. Sontag SJ, O'Connell S, Miller TQ, et al: Asthmatics have more nocturnal gasping and reflux symptoms than nonasthmatics, and they are related to bedtime eating. Am J Gastroenterol 2004;99:789–796.
27. Gislason T, Janson C, Vermeire P, et al: Respiratory symptoms and nocturnal gastroesophageal reflux: A population-based study of young adults in three European countries. Chest 2002;121:158–163.
28. Mansfield LE, Hameister HH, Spaulding HS, et al: The role of the vagus nerve in airway narrowing caused by intraesophageal hydrochloric acid provocation and esophageal distention. Ann Allergy 1981;47:431–434.
29. Harding SM, Schan CA, Guzzo MR, et al: Gastroesophageal reflux-induced bronchoconstriction: Is microaspiration a factor? Chest 1995;108:1220–1227.
30. Fischer A, Canning JB, Undem BJ, et al: Evidence for an esophageal origin of VIP-IR and NO synthase-IR nerves innervating the guinea pig trachealis: A retrograde neuronal tracing and immunohistochemical analysis. J Comp Neurology 1998;394:326–334.
31. Hamamoto J, Kohrogi H, Kawano O, et al: Esophageal stimulation by hydrochloric acid causes neurogenic inflammation in the airways in guinea pigs. J Appl Physiol 1997;82:738–745.
32. Herve P, Denjean A, Jian R, et al: Intraesophageal perfusion of acid increases the bronchomotor response to methacholine and to isocapnic hyperventilation in asthmatic subjects. Am Rev Respir Dis 1986;134:986–989.
33. Vincent D, Cohen-Jonathan AM, Leport J, et al: Gastro-oesophageal reflux prevalence and relationship with bronchial reactivity in asthma. Eur Respir J 1997; 10:2255–2259.
34. Cuttitta G, Cibella F, Visconti A, et al: Spontaneous gastroesophageal reflux and airway patency during the night in adult asthmatics. Am J Respir Crit Care Med 2000;161:177–181.
35. Jack CIA, Calverley PMA, Donnelly RJ, et al: Simultaneous tracheal and oesophageal pH measurements in asthmatic patients with gastro-oesophageal reflux. Thorax 1995;50:201–204.
36. Tuchman DN, Boyle JT, Pack AI, et al: Comparison of airway responses following tracheal or esophageal acidification in the cat. Gastroenterology 1984;87:872–881.
37. Field SK, Evans JA, Price LM: The effects of acid perfusion of the esophagus on ventilation and respiratory sensation. Am J Respir Crit Care Med 1998;157:1058–1062.
38. Ricciardolo FLM, Gaston B, Hunt J: Acid stress in the pathology of asthma. J Allergy Clin Immunol 2004; 113;610–619.
39. Silvestri M, Mattioli G, Defilippi AC, et al: Correlations between exhaled nitric oxide levels and pH-metry data in asthmatics with gastro-oesophageal reflux. Respiration 2004;71:329–335.
40. Stein MR: Advances in the approach to gastroesophageal reflux (GER) and asthma. J Asthma 1999;36:309–314.

41. Sacco O, Silvestri M, Sabatini F, et al: IL-8 and airway neutrophilia in children with gastroesophageal reflux and asthma-like symptoms. Respir Med 2006;100:307–315.

42. Sontag SJ, Harding SM: Gastroesophageal reflux-triggered asthma. GI Motility online. Chapter 47A (Pulmonary Complications of GERD). Available at www.nature.com/gimo, accessed January 7, 2008.

43. Proceedings of the ATS workshop on refractory asthma: Current understanding, recommendations, and unanswered questions. American Thoracic Society. Am J Respir Crit Care Med 2000;162:2341–2351.

44. Irwin RS, Curley FJ, French CL: Difficult-to-control asthma: contributing factors and outcome of a systematic management protocol. Chest 1993;103:1662–1669.

45. Kahrilas PJ, Quigley EM: Clinical esophageal pH recording: A technical review for practice guideline development. Gastroenterology 1996;110:1982–1996.

46. Harding SM: Gastroesophageal reflux and asthma: Insight into the association. J Allergy Clin Immunol 1999;104:251–259.

47. Richter JE: Diagnostic tests for gastroesophageal reflux disease. Am J Med Sci 2003;326:300–308.

48. DeVault KR, Castell DO: Updated guideline for the diagnosis and treatment of gastroesophageal reflux disease. The Practice Parameters Committee of the American College of Gastroenterology. Am J Gastroenterol 1999;94:1434–1442.

49. Klinkenberg-Knol EC, Nelis F, Dent J, et al: Long-term omeprazole treatment in resistant gastroesophageal reflux disease: Efficacy, safety, and influence on gastric mucosa. Gastroenterology 2000;118:795–798.

50. Tawk M, Goodrich S. Kinasewitz G, Orr W: The effect of 1 week of continuous positive airway pressure treatment in obstructive sleep apnea patients with concomitant gastroesophageal reflux. Chest 2006;130:1003–1008.

51. Spechler SJ, Lee E, Ahnen D, et al: Long-term outcome of medical and surgical therapies for gastroesophageal reflux disease: Follow-up of a randomized control trial. JAMA 2001;285:2331–2338.

52. Coughlan JL, Gibson PG, Henry RC: Medical treatment for reflux oesophagitis does not consistently improve asthma control: A systematic review. Thorax 2001;56:198–204.

53. Field SK, Sutherland LR: Does medical anti-reflux therapy improve asthma in asthmatics with gastroesophageal reflux? A critical review of the literature. Chest 1998; 114:274–283.

54. Meier JH, McNally PR, Punja M, et al: Does omeprazole (Prilosec) improve respiratory function in asthmatics with gastroesophageal reflux? A double-blind placebo-controlled crossover study. Dig Dis Sci 1994; 39:2127–2133.

55. Ford GA, Oliver PS, Prior JS, et al: Omeprazole in the treatment of asthmatics with nocturnal symptoms and gastro-oesophageal reflux: A placebo-controlled cross-over study. Postgrad Med J 1994;70:350–354.

56. Teichtahl H, Kronborg IJ, Yeomans ND, et al: Adult asthma a gastro-oesophageal reflux: The effects of omeprazole therapy on asthma. Aust NZ J Med 1996;26:671–676.

57. Boeree MJ, Peters FTM, Postma DS, et al: No effects of high-dose omeprazole in patients with severe airway hyperresponsiveness and (a)symptomatic gastro-oesophageal reflux. Eur Respir J 1998;11:1070–1074.

58. Kiljander TO, Salomaa ER, Hietanen EK, et al: Gastroesophageal reflux in asthmatics: A double-blind, placebo-controlled crossover study with omeprazole. Chest 1999; 116:1257–1264.

59. Harmanci E, Entok E, Metintas M, et al: Gastroesophageal reflux in patents with asthma. Allergol Immunopathol (Madr) 2001;29:123–128.

60. Levin TR, Sperling RM, McQuaid KR: Omeprazole improves peak expiratory flow rate and quality of life in asthmatics with gastroesophageal reflux. Am J Gastroenterol 1998;93:1060–1063.

61. Kiljander TO, Harding SM, Field SK, et al: Effects of esomeprazole 40 mg twice daily on asthma: A randomized placebo-controlled trial. Am J Respir Crit Care Med 2006;173:1091–1097.

62. Littner MR, Leung FW, Ballard ED 2nd, et al: Effects of 24 weeks of lansoprazole therapy on asthma symptoms, exacerbations, quality of life, and pulmonary function in adult asthmatic patients with acid reflux symptoms. Chest 2005;128:1128–1135.

63. Harding SM, Richter JE: The role of gastroesophageal reflux in chronic cough and asthma. Chest 1997;111:1389–1402.

64. Larrain A, Carrasco E, Galleguillos F, et al: Medical and surgical treatment of nonallergic asthma associated with gastroesophageal reflux. Chest 1991;99:1330–1335.

65. Sifrim D, Dupont L. Blondeau K, et al: Weakly acidic reflux in patients with chronic unexplained cough during 24 hour pressure, pH, and impedance monitoring. Gut 2005;54:449–454.

Exercise-Induced Asthma

Jeremy D. Bufford and Robert F. Lemanske, Jr.

CLINICAL PEARLS

- Exercise-induced asthma/exercise-induced bronchoconstriction (EIB) is the transient airway narrowing associated with exercise, which can occur in patients with and without chronic asthma.

- The following factors influence the propensity to develop EIB: ambient conditions, type of exercise, and baseline level of airway hyperresponsiveness.

- EIB is due to effects of airway cooling/rewarming, dehydration, hyperosmolarity, and mediator release (histamine, leukotrienes, and prostaglandins).

- Diagnosis requires the demonstration of a decline in lung function following an exercise challenge or bronchoprovocation. The gold standard for diagnosis is eucapnic voluntary hyperventilation.

- The goal of treatment is prevention. Treatment includes prophylactic medication before exercise or daily controller medication for persistent asthma.

Exercise-induced asthma (EIA) or, perhaps more appropriately termed, exercise-induced bronchoconstriction (EIB), is defined as acute transient airway narrowing or obstruction that occurs after, or less commonly during, vigorous bouts of exercise or exertion. EIB represents a form of airway hyperresponsiveness that is most frequently manifested as coughing, wheezing, shortness of breath, and chest tightness during, or immediately following, exercise or exertion. EIA/EIB occurs in children and adults of all ages at all levels of athletic prowess, from participants in recreational sports to elite athletes. In addition, EIA/EIB occurs in patients both with and without underlying symptoms of persistent asthma. While the pathophysiology of EIA/EIB remains the topic of much debate, it likely occurs as a result of changes in airway temperature and osmolarity. Factors contributing to airway narrowing may include vasodilation or hyperemia of the bronchial vasculature, as well as bronchoconstriction due to the release of inflammatory mediators including histamine, prostaglandins, and leukotrienes. Numerous modalities exist to diagnose EIA/EIB including pre-/postbronchodilator spirometry, exercise challenge, hyperosmolar challenge, and eucapnic voluntary hyperventilation (EVH). The goal of treatment of EIB is to prevent symptoms and reduce airway hyperresponsiveness that increases the propensity for EIA/EIB. Medications currently available for the treatment and prevention of EIA/EIB include beta-agonists, leukotriene modifiers, and inhaled corticosteroids, among others. Effective prevention allows patients to live normal lives and engage in physical activities without limitation.

EIA/EIB is underrecognized by patients, coaches, and trainers. It is frequently both under- and overdiagnosed by physicians in all patient populations. Failure to diagnose this condition may result in the unnecessary avoidance of sports, imposed limitations on physical activity, or submaximal performance. Overdiagnosis may lead to the unnecessary use of medications or the failure to recognize other clinically relevant disorders. Asthma deaths related to sports participation have been reported; however, it is unclear whether these outcomes represent the most severe cases of EIA/EIB, poorly controlled chronic asthma, or some unrecognized cardiac disorder that is aggravated by physical activity.

NATURAL HISTORY/EPIDEMIOLOGY

The natural physiologic airway response to exercise includes an initial bronchodilation and the recruitment of additional generations of airways. Even in healthy individuals without EIB, there may be a decline in FEV_1 (forced expiratory volume in 1 second) up to 5% following exercise; however, this drop in FEV_1 is usually asymptomatic. The diagnosis of EIB requires demonstration of a fall in FEV_1 of more than 10% following exercise or a surrogate challenge (e.g., eucapnic hyperventilation) (Fig. 40-1). The symptoms of EIB include coughing, wheezing, shortness of breath, chest tightness/discomfort, mucus production, and the subjective perception of a decrease in physical endurance (Table 40-1). Hypoxemia has also been reported. These symptoms usually occur within 5 to 10 minutes following exercise and usually resolve within 30 to 60 minutes following the completion of exercise, with or without the use of bronchodilator medications for rescue.

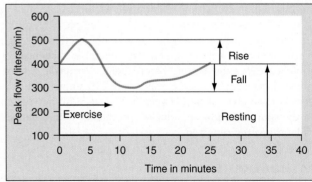

Figure 40-1   Typical response to exercise in exercise-induced bronchoconstriction. The initial response to exercise includes bronchodilation with improvement in airflow. Following exercise, there is a decline in airflow, which may be measured by FEV_1 or peak flow. Airflow obstruction and symptoms usually peak 5 to 10 minutes following exercise, and usually resolve within 30 to 60 minutes after exercise completion.

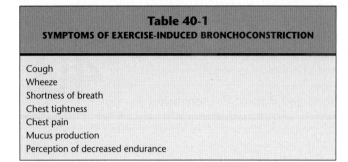

Table 40-1
SYMPTOMS OF EXERCISE-INDUCED BRONCHOCONSTRICTION

Cough
Wheeze
Shortness of breath
Chest tightness
Chest pain
Mucus production
Perception of decreased endurance

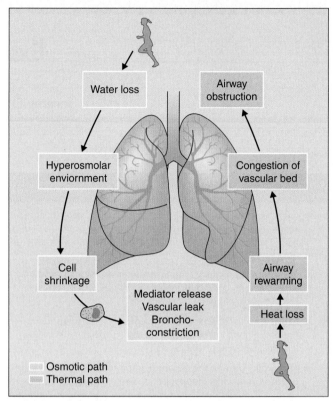

Figure 40-2 Pathophysiology of exercise-induced bronchoconstriction. The precise pathophysiology of EIB remains unclear, but may involve heat and water loss from the airway. The osmotic hypothesis proposes that this water loss leads to dehydration and hyperosmolarity of the airway surface liquid causing the release of water from airway cells. This water loss results in cell shrinkage, vascular leak and the release of mediators, which cause airway smooth muscle contraction, edema, and bronchoconstriction. This shift in water from the cells and the subsequent regulatory volume increase most likely involve alterations in ion channels and signaling pathways. The thermal hypothesis proposes that the rapid rewarming of the airway following heat loss during exercise is associated with a reactive hyperemia of the bronchial vasculature, which results in congestion of the vascular bed and airway obstruction.

The initial exercise stimulus has been reported to induce a refractory period occurring up to 2 hours following exercise in some patients. During this period, bronchoconstriction and the resulting symptoms are attenuated during and following subsequent exercise. The mechanism(s) behind the refractory period are unknown, but increases in catecholamines and prostaglandins have been proposed, as well as depletion of mediators of bronchoconstriction.

EIA/EIB is common among patients with underlying asthma, and exercise is the second-leading trigger for asthma symptoms next to viral upper respiratory infections. However, EIB can also exist in patients with no prior history of asthma who remain asymptomatic in between bouts of exercise, even when exposed to common asthma triggers including upper respiratory infections, cold air, and airborne allergens and irritants. EIA is commonly referred to as exercise-induced bronchoconstriction in patients with isolated exercise-related symptoms, and may represent the first phenotypic expression of asthma. For the remainder of this chapter, the term EIB will refer to both EIA and EIB collectively.

The prevalence of EIB has been estimated to be 40% to 90% among asthmatic individuals and 5% to 20% in the general population. EIB occurs in patients of all ages and at all levels of athletic ability, ranging from usual child's play and recreational sports to competitive sports at international levels. The prevalence has been shown to be higher among elite athletes and has been increasing in this population over the past several years. This is demonstrated by the increase in the reported use of bronchodilator medications by Olympic athletes over the past 20 years. As a result, the International Olympic Committee Medical Commission (IOC-MC) recently started requiring Olympic athletes to provide evidence of reversible airway obstruction through pre-/post-bronchodilator spirometry, exercise challenge, or bronchoprovocation testing before being permitted to use inhaled beta-agonists. The prevalence of EIB among elite athletes is estimated to be between 10% and 50%, depending on the sport. In addition, a higher prevalence among female athletes is often reported.

PATHOGENESIS

The pathophysiology surrounding the airway narrowing seen in EIB remains controversial. It most likely involves the physiologic process of warming and conditioning inspired air, which may be overwhelmed during exercise or exertion due to high demands for ventilation. There are currently two working hypotheses, and there is evidence to support both of them, indicating that the pathophysiology of this phenomenon may actually be a combination of both schools of thought (Fig. 40-2).

The first hypothesis, known as the osmotic hypothesis, proposes that the trigger for the airway narrowing seen in exercise is due to dehydration or water loss from the airways that occurs during the process of conditioning the inspired air. This water loss results in hyperosmolarity of the airway surface liquid. As a result, there is subsequent water loss from the airway cells in order to correct this osmotic imbalance. This is accompanied by the release of mediators such as histamine, leukotrienes, prostaglandins, and neuropeptides from local airway cells such as mast cells and epithelial cells due to cell shrinkage or the regulatory changes in cell volume involving shifts in ions, ion channels, and other signaling pathways. These mediators, accompanied by vascular leak, cause inflammation, edema, airway smooth muscle contraction, mucus production, and bronchoconstriction that result in the symptoms of EIB. In support of the osmotic hypothesis, humidification of inspired air has been shown to reduce the severity of EIB.

The second hypothesis is known as the thermal hypothesis and proposes that changes in airway temperature result in airway narrowing or obstruction. During exercise and the associated hyperventilation, there is a loss of heat in the airways because of the physiologic need to warm the inspired air. Thermal losses increase as ventilation increases, in part because there is less time for warming of the air by the upper airway, including the nose. Since airway cooling alone is not an adequate stimulus to induce EIB, the thermal hypothesis proposes that the rewarming of the airways immediately following exercise results in a reactive hyperemia of the bronchial circulation with vascular engorgement, vasodilation, and edema contributing to airway narrowing. These vascular changes may be augmented by nitric oxide production. In addition, the role of an airway cooling-rewarming gradient and the rate of temperature change have also been proposed as contributing factors. Removal of the rewarming stimulus by inspiring cold air after exercise has been shown to attenuate the EIB response. There is no role for airway smooth muscle contraction and the resulting bronchoconstriction in the thermal hypothesis.

The controversy surrounding the pathogenesis of EIB also includes debate on whether or not inflammation plays a role in EIB. Early studies analyzing bronchoalveolar lavage fluid following exercise challenge failed to demonstrate evidence of airway inflammation or mast cell activation. However, recent studies have demonstrated an increase in inflammatory cells and airway epithelial cells, as well as increases in mediators such as cysteinyl leukotrienes, tryptase, and histamine in induced sputum from asthmatic patients with EIB either at baseline or following an exercise challenge. Reductions in prostaglandin E_2 have also been demonstrated among patients with EIB. These studies have implicated a role for the activation of mast cells and airway epithelial cells, airway epithelial cell injury, and the release of mediators including histamine and leukotrienes in the pathogenesis of EIB. Most studies looking into the inflammatory basis of EIB have included subjects with chronic asthma with EIB symptoms; however, some researchers have suggested that the pathogenesis of EIB in patients with isolated EIB may be different from EIB in patients with underlying asthma. An inflammatory basis for isolated EIB has not been established.

CLINICAL COURSE

Exacerbating Factors

Factors influencing EIB include the type of exercise (duration and intensity); ambient conditions including temperature, humidity, air quality, and aeroallergen exposure; and the baseline level of airway hyperresponsiveness. EIB is most likely to occur during exercise or sports with high levels of intensity of sufficient duration. As a result, some sports or activities are certainly more prone to trigger symptoms of EIB. Sports requiring high intensity for sustained periods of time such as distance running and cycling are the most asthmagenic. Other highly asthmagenic sports include swimming, basketball, soccer, track/sprinting, ice hockey, figure skating, and cross-country skiing. The asthma trigger in these sports, and for EIB in general, is thought to be due to the demand for increased ventilation. The severity of EIB

correlates with ventilation, which is a reflection of intensity. Sports with brief, interrupted periods of high intensity such as baseball, football, and tennis are less likely to induce EIB; however, symptoms may occur in the middle of these activities due to fluctuations in demand for ventilation. Less asthmagenic sports or exercise include golf and walking.

Patients with EIB may be able to participate in some sports or activities, but not others, depending on the intensity and ventilatory requirements. Importantly, however, there are no specific activities that should be avoided by patients with asthma or EIB. In addition, patients may be able to participate in a particular sport under certain conditions but not others. It is clear that the environment plays a role in EIB. The most potent stimulus for EIB is exercise in cold, dry air. Exercising in cold weather conditions is known to induce EIB more than in warm, temperate environments. As a result, the prevalence of EIB among participants in cold weather sports such as cross-country skiing, ice hockey, and figure skating is higher than summer athletes. In cross-country skiers, the prevalence of EIB is estimated to be around 50%. Exposure to irritants and allergens and viral upper respiratory infections are known to increase airway hyperresponsiveness in asthmatic individuals, and positive correlations have been demonstrated between the intensity and severity of EIB and airway hyperresponsiveness. Therefore, pollutants, particulate matter, and gases in the air such as carbon dioxide, nitrogen dioxide, and sulfur dioxide, may also contribute to EIB, especially in athletes who compete in indoor venues such as ice arenas. Chlorine exposure encountered by swimmers is also known to trigger symptoms of EIB. Allergic sensitization may predispose an individual to an increased tendency to develop EIB during relevant allergy seasons due to alterations in airway responsiveness known to occur as a result of aeroallergen exposure. As a result, seasonal fluctuations in EIB may be seen in this population. Distance runners and other outdoor athletes are most affected by exposure to aeroallergens. EIB in patients with sensitization to seasonal aeroallergens may be attenuated by exercising indoors or avoiding exercise or other activities when pollen and mold spore counts are highest.

Differential Diagnosis

As the saying goes, "not all that wheezes is asthma." This saying also applies to EIB, especially in patients who fail to meet the diagnostic criteria for EIB or patients who have isolated EIB with no evidence for underlying asthma. EIB is both under- and overdiagnosed, especially if the diagnosis is based on history, physical exam, and baseline spirometry alone. Other conditions, such as physical deconditioning, vocal cord dysfunction (paradoxical movement of vocal cords), laryngomalacia, gastroesophageal reflux, exercise-induced hyperventilation, and cardiac abnormalities or dysfunction can mimic the symptoms of EIB (Table 40-2). Alternatively, these symptoms may represent normal physiologic exercise limitation. Just as in EIB, symptoms associated with these conditions are often absent at rest or present only at low level, and they are also triggered or exacerbated by exercise or exertion. Additionally, some of these conditions may coexist in patients with EIB and influence the frequency, intensity, or severity of symptoms.

Table 40-2
DIFFERENTIAL DIAGNOSIS OF EIB
Physical deconditioning Vocal cord dysfunction Laryngomalacia Underlying pulmonary disease Other airway obstruction Gastroesophageal reflux Exercise-induced hyperventilation Cardiac abnormalities or dysfunction Neuromuscular disorders

Table 40-3
THE DIAGNOSTIC WORK-UP OF EIB

Pre-/postbronchodilator spirometry
Direct bronchoprovocation:
   Methacholine challenge
   Histamine challenge
Indirect bronchoprovocation:
   Exercise challenge (field or laboratory challenge)
   Hypertonic challenge
     Hypertonic saline
     Mannitol
Eucapnic voluntary hyperventilation

Diagnostic work-up for these other conditions is necessary in patients with normal lung function at baseline or following bronchoprovocation, including exercise. In addition, these other diagnoses must be entertained in patients who have breakthrough symptoms despite bronchodilator prophylaxis or who fail to respond to bronchodilators for rescue use. Other conditions to rule out include neuromuscular disorders and airway obstruction from other underlying pulmonary diseases, including those with restrictive abnormalities. Work-up of the extensive differential diagnosis for EIB may include, but is not limited to, direct visualization of the upper airway and vocal cords by laryngoscopy, pH probe, esophagogastroduodenoscopy, electrocardiogram, echocardiogram, cardiac stress test, chest radiography, or exercise physiology testing.

Diagnosis

While a history consistent with EIB can be elicited from a thorough patient history, history alone is neither sensitive nor specific enough to use as the sole diagnostic tool. The diagnosis of EIB requires the objective demonstration of airflow obstruction through a decline in lung function. Patients who report symptoms of EIB may not demonstrate abnormal lung function, and patients with abnormal lung function may not report symptoms of EIB. The diagnostic criteria for EIB include a greater than 10% drop in FEV_1 or drop in peak expiratory flow rate ratio (PEFR) of more than 15% following an exercise challenge or a surrogate challenge. Some authors advocate the use of the 10% cut-off in laboratory challenges and reserve a higher threshold of more than 15% for field studies. The diagnostic criteria used for the general population and non-elite athletes may not be representative of EIB in elite athletes. Therefore, criteria of a greater than 7% drop in FEV_1 and a drop in PEFR of more than 18% has been proposed for this population. Declines in lung function meeting the diagnostic criteria for EIB have been identified in patients with no prior history or symptoms of EIB. The converse is also true.

Pre- and postbronchodilator spirometry may be performed to demonstrate the presence or lack of airway obstruction and reversibility; however, there is no relationship between either baseline lung function or bronchodilator response and the severity of EIB. Since not all patients with EIB have underlying asthma, normal pre- and postbronchodilator spirometry does not rule out EIB. Further evaluation with a bronchoprovocation study is necessary to make the diagnosis of EIB.

EIB may be diagnosed through an exercise challenge or some other method of bronchoprovocation testing with pre- and postchallenge measures of lung function with the use of spirometry or peak flow monitoring (Table 40-3). Postchallenge measurements of lung function should be obtained at frequent intervals for at least 30 minutes following bronchoprovocation. Exercise challenges may be performed using a free-running exercise field test or an exercise challenge that places the athlete in their natural setting performing the exact exercise and maneuvers that have triggered symptoms in the past. However, it is difficult to control for environmental conditions in these situations. As a result, laboratory exercise challenges using a cycle ergometer or treadmill are preferred. Treadmills may be more asthmagenic due to an increased minute ventilation rate for the same level of work. Laboratory exercise challenges should be performed for 6 to 8 minutes at 80% to 85% of the age-appropriate maximum heart rate. Since cold, dry air is known to be a potent stimulus for EIB, these exercise challenges may be augmented by the inhalation of cold, dry air. A decline in FEV_1 of 10% or less following an exercise challenge represents a negative challenge and a low likelihood of EIB. Peak flow meters are often used during these field challenges because they are a more convenient measure of pulmonary function than spirometry. However, spirometric measurement of FEV_1 is more reliable and reproducible than measurements of PEFR.

Direct bronchoprovocation testing using pharmacologic agents such as methacholine or histamine that act directly on airway smooth muscle receptors can also be performed. While these procedures are not specific to EIB, they are a good marker for airway hyperresponsiveness. Some authors argue that these direct bronchoprovocation challenges have no role in the diagnosis of EIB; however, they may be helpful in the diagnosis of other asthma phenotypes.

Indirect bronchoprovocation challenges, which have a high sensitivity and specificity to EIB, may also be performed. These challenges include exercise, eucapnic voluntary hyperpnea, and challenge with hyperosmolar stimuli such as hypertonic saline or mannitol. The gold standard for the diagnosis of EIB is the eucapnic voluntary hyperpnea (EVH); however, it is not widely available. During this test, the patient inhales air at a set temperature, humidity, and CO_2 level (5%) for approximately 6 minutes at increased levels of respiration, usually 60% to 85% of the maximal ventilation rate. The maximum voluntary ventilation (MVV) is calculated as 20 to $35 \times FEV_1$. EVH with escalating levels of MVV have also been described. EVH is a useful surrogate for exercise since it reproduces the hyperventilation that results from the exercise stimulus as well as the symptoms of EIB. The test is performed in the eucapnic state in order to avoid the physiologic vasoconstriction associated with hypocapnea.

Hyperosmolar challenges with hypertonic saline or escalating doses of mannitol can be used in the evaluation of EIB since these challenges induce the state of hyperosmolarity of the airway surface liquid that has been proposed as the basis of EIB in the osmotic hypothesis. The use of mannitol in the diagnosis of EIB remains experimental at this time. Both of these challenge methods have a high sensitivity and specificity to exercise.

Treatment

The primary goal of treatment of EIB is prevention of the airflow obstruction and associated symptoms that are triggered by exercise or exertion. Patients with EIB should be able to perform exercise with no limitation and to their maximum ability. There are several treatment options available to achieve these goals, including both pharmacologic and nonpharmacologic therapy (Table 40-4). Therapy may differ among patients with isolated EIB and those with chronic asthma and EIB. The general principles in the treatment of EIB include targeting the specific symptoms of EIB and maximizing asthma control in patients with underlying asthma.

Short-acting beta-agonists (SABAs) are first-line treatment of acute symptoms associated with EIB. In addition, they are also the first-line prophylactic agents for the prevention of EIB. Two to four puffs of albuterol or another SABA 5 to 15 minutes before exercise is effective at preventing the symptoms of EIB for a majority of patients through bronchodilation. Second-line prophylactic agents include sodium cromoglycate. This mast cell stabilizer used before exercise or exertion is also effective in preventing the symptoms of EIB in a majority of patients. The mechanism of action of sodium cromoglycate involves ion transport channels, and its ability to inhibit the bronchoconstriction of EIB provides support for the osmotic hypothesis. Unlike SABAs, these medications have no role in the management of acute symptoms of EIB. SABAs have a duration of action of approximately 4 hours, while cromolyn has a duration of action of about 1 to 2 hours. Therefore, these medications should be repeated if the duration of exercise or the sports activity lasts longer than the duration of action of these medications. In addition, SABA

and cromolyn may be used in combination for treating symptoms inadequately prevented with SABAs alone.

Recent studies have demonstrated a protective effect of long-acting beta-agonists (LABAs) such as salmeterol on EIB. This medication should be given 30 to 60 minutes before exercise; the protective effect lasts up to 12 hours (8 to 10). These medications, like SABAs, attenuate the smooth muscle contraction that contributes to the bronchoconstriction associated with EIB. Some authors have suggested using LABA only intermittently for treatment of EIB since loss of the bronchoprotective effect (i.e., duration of time the drug prevents EIB following administration) has been demonstrated with the regular use of these medications.

Leukotrienes, potent bronchoconstrictors, have been implicated in EIB, and several studies have demonstrated the protective effect of montelukast, a leukotriene receptor antagonist, on EIB. Some of these studies have evaluated the effects of a single dose of montelukast prior to exercise, whereas others have investigated the daily use of montelukast. In both cases, montelukast reduced the post-exercise drop in FEV_1 in patients with EIB. Tolerance to the daily use of this medication has not been demonstrated. The daily use of montelukast or other leukotriene modifiers may be more practical than the use of prophylaxis inhalers in children with EIB, since they often engage in unscheduled periods of exercise or exertion during play.

Treatment of patients with EIB and chronic asthma should initially be directed at maintaining control of the chronic asthma. This can be achieved through the use of daily anti-inflammatory controller medications like inhaled corticosteroids (ICSs). Studies have demonstrated improvements in baseline airway hyperresponsiveness and smaller declines in FEV_1 following exercise in patients with EIB who used ICSs regularly for short periods of time. ICSs lessen the severity of EIB in a dose-dependent manner in most patients with chronic asthma, and completely eliminate the symptoms of EIB in some. For those patients and athletes with break-through symptoms, treatment with ICSs may be combined with LABA, or preexercise prophylaxis with SABA or cromolyn. Unlike SABA, LABA, cromolyn, and leukotriene modifiers, there is no role for single dose ICS as preexercise prophylaxis.

Nonconventional medications including inhaled furosemide and heparin have also been proposed as possible treatments of EIB, although the use of these medications is certainly not standard of care. The mechanisms of action of these drugs in the treatment of EIB remain unclear; however, they are likely to involve alternations in ion channels and signaling pathways. The use of inhaled anticholinergic medications like ipratropium bromide has been shown to provide some degree of protection against EIB; however, this medication has a slow onset of action and the protective effect is inconsistent.

Prior to, or in conjunction with, the use of pharmacotherapy to prevent or reduce signs and symptoms of EIB, it is appropriate to consider the use of nonpharmacologic measures. These measures include cardiovascular training/conditioning, use of a warm-up period, airway barrier protection, and altering environmental exposures or ambient conditions. Improvements in cardiovascular fitness through training or a conditioning program have been associated with reductions in the severity of EIB; however, while these programs may

Table 40-4
TREATMENT OF EIB

Pharmacologic
Inhaled short-acting beta-agonists
Inhaled cromolyn
Long-acting beta-agonists
Leukotriene modifiers
Inhaled corticosteroids
Inhaled furosemide
Inhaled heparin
Nonpharmacologic
Warm-up period (induce refractory period)
Conditioning/training
Mask/barrier protection
Nose breathing

improve overall fitness, the protection against EIB has not been demonstrated in all studies. The use of a warm-up period prior to full exercise or exertion has been shown to result in attenuation or reduced severity of EIB. During this warm-up period, the patient or athlete performs exercise at a submaximal effort and at an intensity below the threshold for inducing EIB. This may be performed with continuous low-intensity exercise or with short sprints or bursts of activity. This warm-up period may induce a period up to 40 minutes during which time the airways become refractory to EIB with subsequent exercise. This is, in a sense, a refractory period; however, the refractory period following a warm-up is of shorter duration than the refractory period induced after the resolution of acute EIB symptoms. The protective mechanisms associated with the warm-up period are unknown, but an increase in bronchial blood flow and the associated increase in water delivery to the airway surface have been proposed. Masks or other coverings placed over the mouth and nose help capture heat and water on expiration and minimize the water and heat loss associated with exercise. These barrier devices also protect against the inhalation of gases, particulate matter and aeroallergens that are known to exacerbate EIB. The use of these devices has been shown to reduce the severity of EIB. Inhalation through the nose instead of the mouth is known to warm and condition the air more effectively than mouth breathing. Therefore, breathing though the nose is another nonpharmacologic method to reduce EIB. However, the ability of nose breathing alone to provide the appropriate ventilation required during vigorous exercise is often overwhelmed due to increases in nasal resistance. Mouth breathing becomes necessary at this point. Dietary changes, including salt restriction and increases in omega fatty acids, have also been associated with improvements in EIB.

CONTROVERSIES

In addition to the controversy surrounding the pathogenesis of EIB in general, it remains unclear if the mechanisms leading to EIB are the same in patients with persistent asthma and those with isolated EIB. In addition, some researchers have suggested that EIB in certain cold-weather athletes, specifically cross-country skiers, may represent a distinct asthma phenotype. Evaluations into these subjects have demonstrated different pathophysiology, pathology, and response to medications in this group. Evidence of airway remodeling has been discovered and the symptoms and signs of EIB are more difficult to control in this population. Additional studies aimed at enhancing our understanding of the pathophysiology of EIB are needed, especially in the case of the elite athlete where precise diagnosis and proper treatment are necessary to effectively and appropriately improve performance in these highly competitive individuals.

SUGGESTED READING

Anderson SD, Daviskas E: The mechanism of exercise-induced asthma is . . . J Allergy Clin Immunol 2000;106:453–459.

Anderson SD, Holzer K: Exercise-induced asthma: Is it the right diagnosis in elite athletes? J Allergy Clin Immunol 2000;106:419–428.

Anderson SD, Kippelen P: Exercise-induced broncho constriction: pathogenesis. Curr Allergy Asthma Rep 2005;5:116–122.

Becker JM, Rogers J, Rossini G, et al: Asthma deaths during sports: report of a 7-year experience. J Allergy Clin Immunol 2004;113:264–267.

Gotshall RW: Exercise-induced bronchoconstriction. Drugs 2002;62:1725–1739.

Hallstrand TS, Moody MW, Aitken ML, Henderson WR Jr: Airway immunopathology of asthma with exercise-induced bronchoconstriction. J Allergy Clin Immunol 2005;116:586–593.

Hallstrand TS, Moody MW, Wurfel MM, et al: Inflammatory basis of exercise-induced bronchoconstriction. Am J Respir Crit Care Med 2005;172:679–686.

Holzer K, Brukner P, Douglass J: Evidence-based management of exercise-induced asthma. Curr Sports Med Rep 2002;1:86–92.

McFadden ER Jr: Exercise-induced airway narrowing. In Adkinson NF Jr, Yunginger JW, Busse WW, et al (eds): Middleton's Allergy. Principles and Practice. 6th ed. Philadelphia, Mosby, 2003, pp 1323–1331.

Rundell KW, Jenkinson DM: Exercise-induced bronchospasm in the elite athlete. Sports Med 2002;32:583–600.

Rundell KW, Wilber RL, Lemanske RF Jr (eds.): Exercise-Induced Asthma: Pathophysiology and Treatment. Champaign, Ill: Human Kinetics, 2002.

Singh AM, McGregor RS: Differential diagnosis of chest symptoms in the athlete. Clin Rev Allergy Immunol 2005;29:87–96.

Tan RA, Spector SL: Exercise-induced asthma: diagnosis and management. Ann Allergy Asthma Immunol 2002;89:226–235.

Weiler JM: Exercise-induced asthma: a practical guide to definitions, diagnosis, prevalence, and treatment. Allergy Asthma Proc 1996;17:315–325.

Nocturnal Asthma and Obstructive Sleep Apnea

CHAPTER

41

Jonathan P. Parsons and John G. Mastronarde

CLINICAL PEARLS

- Asthma often worsens at night secondary to circadian and noncircadian factors.

- Asthmatic individuals have impaired sleep quality compared to people with many other chronic diseases.

- There is a significant relationship between asthma and obstructive sleep apnea.

- Sleep histories are an important facet of the clinical evaluation of asthmatic individuals.

- Pharmacokinetics is an important consideration when treating patients with nocturnal asthma.

Nocturnal asthma is a variable exacerbation of the asthmatic condition occurring at night. Nocturnal asthma is associated with increases in symptoms, worsening of lung function, and a greater need for medication. Nocturnal symptoms of asthma are extremely common. In addition, nocturnal asthma results in considerable morbidity and mortality, because the symptoms are often severe. Patients with asthma are more likely to have a fatal asthma attack at night than any other time of the day. Furthermore, proportionally, asthmatic individuals are more likely to die at night than when compared to the general population.

Asthma symptoms may worsen during sleep for many reasons including circadian variations in pulmonary function, inflammation, secretion of hormones, and influences from other concomitant health problems such as gastroesophageal reflux disease (GERD).

It also appears that there is a correlation between sleep quality and nocturnal asthma. Asthmatic individuals have been shown to have worse sleep quality and more sleep-related problems when compared to patients with other chronic health problems. Sleep fragmentation and resultant sleep deprivation can lead to excessive daytime sleepiness and contribute to poor daytime cognitive function leading to social and mental problems. It has also been suggested that there is a causal relationship between obstructive sleep apnea (OSA) and asthma.

For all these reasons, it is important for the clinician to address nocturnal symptoms in the evaluation of asthmatic individuals. Nocturnal asthma is often used as a marker for asthma control and can help guide physician assessment of asthma severity and treatment decisions. Furthermore, given the correlation between sleep quality and nocturnal asthma, it is recommended that clinicians elicit sleep histories from their asthma patients.

EPIDEMIOLOGY

Up to 90% of asthmatic individuals experience nocturnal symptoms at least once in their lifetimes and a significant proportion suffer from them routinely. Turner-Warwick surveyed 7729 patients with asthma and found that 74% of respondents experience nocturnal cough and wheeze at least once a week, 64% complained of nocturnal awakenings with asthma symptoms at least 3 times per week, and 40% awaken nightly. Other studies have shown that patients with asthma symptoms are more likely to present to the emergency department between midnight and 8 AM.

Sleep-disordered breathing (SDB) and specifically OSA have become increasingly recognized as significant public health problems. The prevalence of sleep-disordered breathing, defined as an apnea-hypopnea score of 5 or higher, has been shown in one study to be 9% for women and 24% for men. Furthermore, it is estimated 2% of women and 4% of men in the middle-aged work force meet the minimal diagnostic criteria for the sleep apnea syndrome (an apnea-hypopnea score of 5 or higher and daytime hypersomnolence). Up to 40 million patients with OSA may exist in the United States alone. Despite the severe morbidity and mortality associated with OSA, it likely remains undiagnosed in most men and women afflicted with the syndrome.

PATHOGENESIS

Why Might Asthma Worsen at Night?

Many physiologic changes that occur normally in sleep may promote nocturnal worsening of asthma (Fig. 41-1). Several hypotheses have been proposed to explain why asthma symptoms often worsen at night.

CIRCADIAN VARIATIONS IN LUNG FUNCTION

Several studies have demonstrated that there is a circadian variation in objective measurements of lung function as measured by spirometry or peak expiratory flow rate (PEFR) (Fig. 41-2). One study found that both asthmatic and healthy subjects reliably demonstrate their lowest PEFR in the early morning hours; however the asthmatic subjects have much lower PEFR values indicating more severe bronchospasm. The peak-to-trough swings in peak expiratory flow rate in that study were only 5% to 8% in healthy controls compared to 50% or more in asthmatic individuals.

In another study, asthmatic and healthy patients were studied on three occasions: during one night of normal sleep, one night awake, and one night after they were sleep deprived. During the normal sleep session, asthmatic subjects were found

367

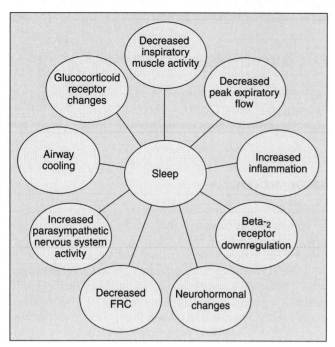

Figure 41-1 Physiologic variables that may influence nocturnal asthma. Many factors have been hypothesized to contribute to the worsening of asthma symptoms at night. FRC, functional residual capacity.

to have a much higher airway resistance than healthy controls. Interestingly, the asthmatic individuals were found to have 50% less airway resistance on the sleep prevention night when compared to the normal sleep night but still higher airway resistance than the healthy controls. The study concluded that in asthmatic patients with nocturnal worsening, airway resistance increases and forced expiratory volume in 1 second (FEV_1) falls overnight regardless of sleep state, but, more importantly, sleep accentuates the overnight increases in airway resistance.

The exact mechanism of the circadian variability in PEFR and airway resistance remains an unanswered question. Some

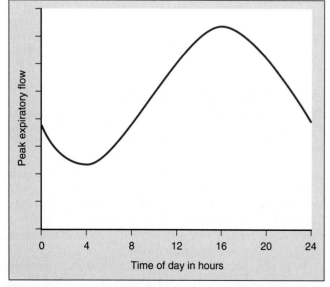

Figure 41-2 Diurnal variation in peak expiratory flow rates. Peak flow rates can vary widely in asthmatic patients and often reach their nadir at night during sleep.

have theorized that as the body cools normally during sleep, the cooling contributes to nocturnal bronchospasm. Studies have shown that breathing warm, humidified air can ameliorate the nocturnal worsening of lung function, even if the core body temperature is kept artificially lower, suggesting a direct effect of relatively cold air on the airway. Alternatively, it has been suggested nocturnal symptoms increase due to prolonged exposure to antigens such as dust mites that live in pillows and mattresses. However, a meta-analysis of studies that used physical barriers or chemical strategies to eliminate dust mites showed that such interventions had no significant effect on morning PEFR or symptom scores, suggesting there may be more than one antigen playing a role in nocturnal symptoms.

In addition to variations in PEFR, there is a decrease in functional residual capacity (FRC) that occurs during sleep in both normal patients and in patients with asthma. FRC is significantly reduced while supine and sleeping when compared to supine and awake, which suggests that sleep itself is important in the observed reduction in lung volumes. This decrease in FRC may have a significant influence on the increased lower airway resistance that occurs in patients with nocturnal asthma, as evidenced in a study demonstrating a twofold greater decrement in FRC in asthmatic individuals when compared to healthy controls. In addition to decreases in FRC, inspiratory muscle activity is reduced in sleep, which could further contribute to the reduction in lung volumes and increases in lower airway resistance.

BETA-$_2$ RECEPTOR REGULATION

The number and function of beta-$_2$ receptors differs among patients with or without nocturnal symptoms. One study compared asthmatic individuals with and without nocturnal symptoms to healthy controls and showed that at 4 AM compared with 4 PM, only patients with nocturnal asthma had a significant decrease in beta-adrenergic receptor density; however, there was no difference in binding affinity in all three groups. This downregulation in nocturnal asthmatic individuals may have a genetic basis in that glycine at position 16 (Gly16) on the coding sequence for the beta-$_2$ receptor is associated with an accelerated downregulation of the receptor when compared to arginine. The frequency for the Gly16 allele has been shown to be overrepresented in nocturnal asthma (80%) when compared to asthmatic individuals without nocturnal symptoms (52%) and may be an important genetic factor in the expression of this asthmatic phenotype.

INFLAMMATORY CHANGES AT NIGHT

Recent studies examining inflammation in nocturnal asthma have shown that the pattern and location of inflammation in nocturnal asthma are different compared to non-nocturnal asthma. Bronchoalveolar lavage (BAL) fluid from asthmatic individuals with nocturnal symptoms shows significantly more prominent inflammation in the airways. Nocturnal asthmatic individuals have been shown to have an increase in the total leukocyte count, neutrophils, and eosinophils from 4 PM to 4 AM; however, cellular components from a non-nocturnal asthma control group did not change. Further analysis showed that between groups, the 4 PM cell differentials were similar; however, at 4 AM, the nocturnal asthma group had significantly higher total leukocyte, neutrophil, eosinophil, lymphocyte, and epithelial cell counts. This study suggests that the nocturnal worsening of asthma has an associated cellular inflammatory response that is not seen in patients without overnight decrements in lung function.

The location of inflammation in the lung may also play a role in nocturnal asthma. In one study, asthmatic individuals with and without nocturnal symptoms underwent two bronchoscopies, one with proximal airway endobronchial biopsy and one with distal alveolar tissue transbronchial biopsy in a random order at 4 PM and 4 AM. Between-group comparisons showed that the number of eosinophils was greater in the alveolar tissue of the nocturnal asthma cohort at 4 AM compared with the subjects without nocturnal asthma. No difference in the inflammatory and epithelial cells between the two groups was seen at either time with respect to the proximal airway biopsies. Furthermore, the nocturnal asthma group exhibited greater eosinophils and macrophages in the alveolar tissue at 4 AM compared with 4 PM. Only alveolar tissue eosinophils, not proximal airway tissue eosinophils, correlated with a nocturnal decrement in lung function. These findings suggest that eosinophils accumulate to a greater extent in the alveolar tissue of subjects with nocturnal asthma and these changes contribute more to the variation in lung function compared with inflammation in the more proximal tissue.

Additional studies have further suggested that the inflammation in nocturnal asthma is localized in the alveolar space and is more significant than in asthmatic individuals without nocturnal symptoms. Alveolar nitric oxide (NO) concentration, a surrogate marker of inflammation, has been shown to be increased in asthmatic patients with nocturnal symptoms but is normal in asthmatic individuals without nocturnal symptoms. Furthermore, there does not appear to be a significant difference in the bronchial concentration of NO between the two groups, supporting the theory that inflammation in the alveolar compartment is important in the nocturnal asthma phenotype.

Inflammation in asthma is typically treated with corticosteroids. Studies suggest that glucocorticoid receptor binding affinity and steroid responsiveness also have circadian variation in subjects with nocturnal asthma. It has been suggested that this may contribute to nocturnal airway inflammation by inhibiting the anti-inflammatory effects of glucocorticoids.

VARIATION IN THE PARASYMPATHETIC NERVOUS SYSTEM

The parasympathetic nervous system has also been implicated in nocturnal asthma. Increased vagal tone during sleep could promote increased bronchoconstriction. There is a diurnal variation in vagal activity that has been demonstrated in asthmatic patients, with higher vagal activity occurring at night. Administration of intravenous atropine to patients in one study with nocturnal asthma produced improvement in the peak expiratory flow rate (PEFR) at 4 AM compared to 4 PM. That study also demonstrated a significant correlation between heart rate and PEFR, which further suggests increased vagal tone at night.

NEUROHORMONAL CHANGES

Just as there are variations in pulmonary function and parasympathetic nervous system tone, there are circadian variations in the levels of various neurotransmitters and hormones.

Histamine, which is a potent bronchoconstrictor, has been shown to be significantly lower in healthy individuals during sleep when compared with asthmatic individuals.

Melatonin, which is an endogenous sleep-inducing hormone, has been shown to be higher in asthmatic individuals with nocturnal symptoms as compared to healthy individuals. Melatonin also has been shown to be correlated inversely with lung function in nocturnal asthmatic individuals and to have pro-inflammatory properties.

GASTROESOPHAGEAL REFLUX

Several studies suggest there may be a significant association between GERD and asthma. Several mechanisms have been proposed to explain the potentially deleterious effects of GERD on asthma. GERD has been shown to be pro-inflammatory which adds to the inflammatory milieu in asthma. In addition to promoting inflammation, GERD may exacerbate asthma via exposure of the esophagus to acid, which has been shown in animal models to be associated with increased respiratory resistance. Microaspiration of gastric contents into the airway also has been shown to cause vagally mediated bronchospasm. Many patients have worse symptoms of GERD at night because they sleep in the supine position allowing stomach acid to more easily enter the esophagus and airway, which may subsequently exacerbate nocturnal asthma symptoms.

Relationship between Asthma and Obstructive Sleep Apnea

In addition to increased symptoms at night and impaired sleep quality, there appears to be a significant relationship between obstructive sleep apnea and nocturnal asthma (Figs. 41-3 and 41-4). Many studies have shown a positive association between obstructive sleep apnea (OSA) and occasional wheezing, persistent wheezing, snoring, and a history of asthma. In addition, several studies suggest a positive correlation between GERD and OSA, and the presence of both disorders may exert a synergistic negative effect on nocturnal asthma.

HOW NOCTURNAL ASTHMA MAY WORSEN OSA
Sleep Fragmentation
Asthmatic individuals have disrupted sleep architecture secondary to frequent arousals from sleep. Several small studies evaluating polysomnography in asthmatic individuals have reported increases in spontaneous arousals, decreases in sleep efficiency, and variable effects on sleep stage distribution. Furthermore, these studies also suggest that disrupted sleep

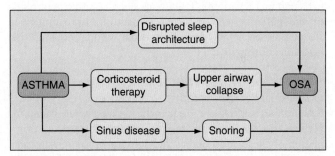

Figure 41-3 How asthma may potentiate OSA. Factors associated with asthma may exacerbate existing OSA or predispose patients to the subsequent development of OSA.

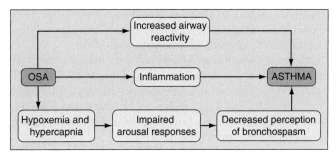

Figure 41-4 How OSA may worsen asthma. Factors associated with OSA can exacerbate existing asthma.

architecture may lay the foundation or predispose asthmatic individuals for the subsequent development of OSA. One study showed a significant association between fragmented sleep and increased airway collapsibility indicating that fragmented sleep may lead to early upper airway closure. Thus one can postulate that frequent arousals secondary to nocturnal asthma may unmask coexisting OSA by increasing the magnitude of airway collapse.

Corticosteroid Therapy

Corticosteroids are the recommended initial controller therapy for patients with persistent asthma symptoms, including nocturnal symptoms. However, steroid therapy may predispose patients to OSA. An unexpectedly high prevalence of OSA has been demonstrated among patients with unstable asthma receiving long-term chronic or frequent burst of oral corticosteroid therapy. It is possible that prolonged and especially continuous oral steroid therapy in asthma may increase upper airway collapsibility possibly via effects on upper airway muscle function and may play a role in the development of OSA.

Sinus Disease

Sinus and tonsillar inflammation and obstruction, which are extremely prevalent in asthmatic individuals, may also play a role in the development of sleep-disordered breathing and OSA. Nasal congestion from allergies or sinus disease has been suggested to be an independent predictor of snoring in some patients. Investigators studied 25 adults with a deviated nasal septum, who complained about excessive daytime sleepiness, chronic fatigue, and nocturnal insomnia. Polysomnography demonstrated disordered breathing during sleep in the form of hypopneas and arousals. Surgical treatment of the deviated septum in 14 patients resulted in a subjective improvement in the level of diurnal alertness and in the quality of nocturnal sleep in 12 patients. Follow-up sleep recordings in seven of the patients who reported subjective improvement in sleep disclosed notably less spontaneous waking and abnormal breathing during sleep.

HOW OSA MAY WORSEN NOCTURNAL ASTHMA
Increased Airway Hyperreactivity

Patients with OSA are frequently hypoxic while sleeping. Hypoxia can lead to reflex bronchoconstriction through stimulation of the carotid bodies and subsequent increased vagal tone. This increased frequency of bronchoconstriction can become dangerous as patients with asthma often have poor perception of the symptoms of bronchoconstriction. The

response to bronchoconstriction has been shown to be further impaired by sleep deprivation, which is also common in people with OSA. One study demonstrated that prior sleep deprivation significantly raised the arousal threshold in response to induced bronchoconstriction, that is, sleep-deprived asthmatic individuals were less likely to arouse in response to bronchoconstriction These results suggest that patients with OSA and disrupted sleep architecture and with concomitant asthma may not sense or perceive significant bronchoconstriction.

In addition to vagally mediated bronchoconstriction, patients with OSA can experience bronchoconstriction through other mechanisms. Patients with OSA typically snore, and snoring causes repetitive stimulation of the pharynx and glottic inlet. Repetitive stimulation of these areas during snoring and upper airway closures stimulates neural receptors that have been shown to mediate significant reflex bronchoconstriction.

Impaired Arousal Responses

Ventilatory responses to changes in blood gases and lung function are important defense mechanisms. Patients with OSA have significantly impaired arousal responses to alterations in blood gases. Specifically, OSA patients with hypercapnia and/or hypoxemia have reduced ventilatory responses to hypercapnic and hypoxic stimulation. In addition, many patients with asthma have blunted perception of bronchospasm. In patients with both OSA and asthma, the impaired responses to hypoxia and increased prevalence and decreased perception of bronchoconstriction may lead to a vicious cycle of worsening asthma and sleep deprivation and subsequently to increased morbidity and mortality (Fig. 41-5).

Inflammation

Inflammation is an essential component of asthma and recent data from several laboratories demonstrate that obstructive sleep apnea is characterized by an inflammatory response. Many of the cytokines that have been shown to be elevated in OSA such as interleukin (IL)-8, IL-6, and tumor necrosis factor (TNF)-α have also been implicated in the inflammatory pattern demonstrated in asthma. The similarities between the inflammatory patterns in asthma and OSA can also be seen histologically. Histologic changes with increased interstitial edema, mucous gland hypertrophy, and infiltration of the uvula lamina propria with T cells in the pharyngeal epithelium in patients with OSA are similar to changes in the bronchi of asthmatic individuals. Thus, the inflammatory response to OSA may be an important contributor to the vicious cycle of nocturnal asthma and OSA.

Relationship between Nocturnal Asthma and Sleep Quality

In addition to worsening of asthma symptoms at night, general sleep quality is impaired in asthmatic individuals. Specifically, patients with nocturnal asthma have disrupted sleep architecture and more frequent arousals and report overall worse sleep quality. Asthmatic individuals have been shown to have worse sleep quality as measured by the Pittsburgh Sleep Quality Index (PSQI) than patients with inflammatory bowel disease, end-stage renal disease, or cystic fibrosis. Studies have found

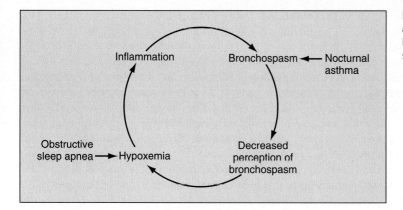

Figure 41-5 The vicious cycle of OSA and asthma. Concomitant OSA and asthma can lead to a cycle of continued OSA and increasingly severe asthma.

positive associations between physician-diagnosed asthma and difficulty initiating sleep, daytime sleepiness, snoring, and self-reported apneas. Patients in those studies were twice as likely to complain of difficulty initiating sleep and were more likely to have excessive daytime sleepiness. Others have shown that snoring and quality of sleep are positively associated with asthma, and asthmatic individuals are significantly more likely to report that their sleep is unrefreshing. The presence of impaired sleep quality in asthmatic individuals is clinically significant, because it has been correlated with impaired quality of life and impaired cognitive performance.

These studies illustrate that there is a significant relationship between asthma and sleep quality. Asthmatic individuals have decreased sleep quality, significant disruption of their sleep habits, and have impaired cognitive performance and quality of life. The results also suggest that patients with asthma have an increased prevalence of sleep disorders and impaired sleep quality that appears to be independent of asthma symptoms.

DIAGNOSTIC APPROACH AND CLINICAL MANAGEMENT

There are significant data to suggest that poor sleep quality and sleep-disordered breathing are common in asthmatic individuals and may play a role in asthma control. The evaluation of the patient with asthma should include a targeted sleep history in addition to investigation of control of nocturnal symptoms. Frequent wheezing, cough, and bronchodilator use at night are indicators that the patient may need more effective asthma control. In addition, presence and control of syndromes that can worsen nocturnal symptoms of asthma such as poor sleep hygiene, OSA, snoring, GERD, and allergic rhinitis should be addressed.

Accumulated data suggest that routine evaluation of the patient with nocturnal asthma should also include a comprehensive sleep history given the poor sleep quality in asthmatic individuals and overlap of OSA and nocturnal asthma. Current guidelines for management of asthma recommend asking about nocturnal asthma symptoms, but do not advise that clinicians take a global sleep history from their asthma patients. Detailed sleep histories (Table 41-1) should include time to sleep on a typical night, duration of sleep, sleep quality, whether snoring is present or absent, and whether the patient has excessive daytime sleepiness. In addition, body mass index and neck circumference are important to evaluate

as they are important risk factors for OSA. Other important issues to address include medications and caffeine and alcohol intake, which can lead to poor sleep hygiene. If screening questions suggest the possibility of a concomitant sleep disorder, then objective evaluation including instruments such as the Epworth Sleepiness Scale or the Pittsburgh Sleep Quality Index should be considered. If clinical suspicion of a sleep disorder such as OSA remains significant, then polysomnography may be required.

Treatment of patients with nocturnal asthma and OSA includes targeted therapy that is aimed at both diseases.

Treatment of Nocturnal Asthma

Medical treatment of nocturnal asthma includes control of contributing factors that can worsen asthma including specific environmental control measures based on individual antigen sensitization profiles, such as plastic covers on pillows and mattresses, and adequate ventilation and optimal humidity in the sleeping environment with minimization of dust for those with dust mite allergy. Other factors that are also important in the management of nocturnal asthma include diagnosis and treatment of coexistent poor sleep hygiene, OSA, gastroesophageal reflux, rhinitis, and sinusitis.

Direct pharmacologic interventions in the treatment of nocturnal asthma include medications that are routinely used in the management of asthma in general. However, applying what we know about the circadian biology of asthma, one may need to consider that optimal dosing levels and timing of administration may be important in the management of nocturnal symptoms.

Table 41-1
IMPORTANT ISSUES IN SLEEP HISTORIES

- Body mass index
- Neck circumference
- Time to fall asleep
- Total sleep time
- Presence of nocturnal awakening
- Presence of snoring
- Witnessed apneas
- Sleep quality
- Presence of excessive daytime sleepiness
- Medications
- Caffeine/alcohol intake

INHALED CORTICOSTEROIDS

Investigators demonstrated in one study that a single daily administration of inhaled triamcinolone at 3 PM produced similar improvement in lung function, bronchial hyperresponsiveness, and beta-agonist use compared to a standard regimen of triamcinolone given four times daily without any increase in systemic effects. The same authors performed a second study further evaluating single daily administration of inhaled steroids when they compared once-daily dosing at 8 AM versus once-daily dosing at 5:30 PM versus standard four times daily dosing. Results showed once-daily dosing of the inhaled steroid at 5:30 PM had no increased systemic effects and produced efficacy similar to standard four times a day dosing. Furthermore, dosing at 8 AM did not produce results consistently comparable to four times a day dosing. The authors concluded that optimal once-daily dosing of inhaled steroid may be between 3 PM and 5:30 PM.

LEUKOTRIENE MODIFIERS

The effect of administration of leukotriene modifiers on nocturnal asthma has been compared to placebo. Decreases in leukotriene levels, significant reductions in 4 AM BAL fluid and blood eosinophil percentages, and improvement in FEV_1 have been shown in patients receiving zileuton, an older generation leukotriene modifier, compared with placebo. Newer generations of leukotriene modifiers such as montelukast achieve mean peak plasma concentration in 3 to 4 hours and often are recommended to be taken at bedtime to take advantage of their efficacy in treating nocturnal asthma.

ORAL CORTICOSTEROIDS

The effect of a single dose of prednisone delivered to asthmatic patients at one of three specific times (8 AM, 3 PM, or 8 PM) has been studied. Only the 3 PM dose of prednisone resulted in overnight spirometric improvement and significant reduction in the level of inflammation in a 4 AM BAL sample. The circadian variation in lung function associated with the afternoon dose of prednisone was similar to the variation in lung function expected in healthy, non-asthmatic subjects. This study suggests that optimal dosing of oral corticosteroids is in late afternoon in patients with nocturnal asthma.

LONG-ACTING BETA-AGONISTS

Studies have shown that long-acting beta-agonists (LABAs) can lead to some improvement in nocturnal pulmonary function and improve sleep quality. One study of nocturnal asthmatic individuals showed that salmeterol significantly increased mean change from baseline in FEV_1, morning and evening PEF, percentage of nights with no awakenings due to asthma, and the percentage of nights with no supplemental albuterol use compared with placebo. Although LABAs may be effective in the management of nocturnal asthma, doses higher than 50 µg twice daily have been shown to decrease slow wave sleep. However, recent studies demonstrating a decrease in effectiveness of LABAs in patients with the gly-gly beta-agonist receptor variant coupled with decreased perception of bronchoconstriction during sleep suggest one should not use LABAs as monotherapy for nocturnal asthma symptoms. Indeed these nocturnal effects may play a role in the recently highlighted deleterious effects of LABAs used as monotherapy for asthma.

THEOPHYLLINE

Theophylline preparations are less commonly used in clinical practice now than in the past, but they may be of value in treating patients with nocturnal asthma. The pharmacokinetics of theophylline likely is important. Once-daily theophylline administration given at 7 PM has been compared to a typical twice-daily regimen. Results showed the serum theophylline levels were significantly higher at night with the once-daily regimen, and the awakening FEV_1 value was also improved. All polysomnographic variables were similar between the two dosing schedules, except that with the once-daily preparation there was a decreased number of hypopneas and fewer minutes below an oxygen saturation of 90%. Despite the findings of this study, other studies have shown that theophylline can reduce the quality of sleep in patients with asthma. More studies are needed investigating the utility and role of theophylline in the management of nocturnal asthma before it can be recommended as a standard therapy.

Treatment of Obstructive Sleep Apnea

A complete discussion of the treatment of OSA is beyond the scope of this chapter; however, just as the treatment of nocturnal asthma involves indirect and direct treatment approaches, the treatment of obstructive sleep apnea also is multifocal. Treatment of OSA begins with education about adequate sleep hygiene. Patients should spend time in bed only when sleeping, avoid daytime naps, avoid exercise, caffeine or alcohol before bedtime, and should have a comfortable, dark and quiet place to sleep.

Weight loss is another important aspect of treatment of OSA. Patients with OSA are often obese, and significant weight loss has been reported to result in varying degrees of improvement in sleep apnea, oxygen saturation, sleep architecture and daytime performance. Recent studies have also suggested obesity may play a role in worsening asthma control. It is not known if this is a primary effect or secondary to other obesity-related disorders such as OSA.

The mainstay for treatment of OSA is continuous positive airway pressure (CPAP). Several studies have demonstrated that CPAP therapy improves sleep quality, excessive daytime sleepiness and general health-related quality of life in patients with obstructive sleep apnea. Other studies have shown that CPAP therapy improves cognitive and functional status in patients with sleep apnea, with decreases in the incidence of motor vehicle crashes in these patients. Oral devices may be useful in select patients with mild OSA and/or those who are unable to tolerate CPAP. Surgical intervention for OSA is also an option, but current guidelines suggest it is a second-line therapy after CPAP. Treatment of obstructive sleep apnea in asthmatic individuals with significant nocturnal symptoms with CPAP has been shown to result in a marked improvement in nocturnal and daytime asthma symptoms and lung function, with an associated reduction in the use of bronchodilators.

CPAP has effects on the inflammatory cascade that may be important in the pathogenesis of nocturnal asthma and OSA. Treatment with CPAP has been shown to have significant effects on the severity of inflammation in patients with OSA. There is increased production of reactive oxygen species from inflammatory cells in patients with OSA. One study demonstrated elevated levels of C-reactive protein (CRP) and IL-6 in patients with OSA. These levels were higher than in control individuals without OSA and were decreased by treatment with CPAP. The anti-inflammatory effects of CPAP may help explain in part why many asthmatic individuals with OSA that are treated with CPAP have improvement in their asthma symptoms.

CONCLUSION

Asthma and sleep disorders are both common conditions with a complex intertwined relationship. There is significant overlap in the clinical manifestations of OSA and asthma as hypoxemia, inflammation, and airway hyperreactivity often are significant consequences of both diseases. In addition, both asthma and OSA result in disrupted sleep architecture and decreased sleep quality. It is important as a clinician to recognize that management of the patient with nocturnal asthma should include a comprehensive sleep history including inadequate sleep hygiene, symptoms of GERD, sinus disease, and OSA. Knowledge of how OSA and nocturnal asthma are related will assist clinicians in the management of their patients with nocturnal asthma, allowing for improved asthma- and sleep-related quality of life.

SUGGESTED READING

Busse WW: Pathogenesis and pathophysiology of nocturnal asthma. Am J Med 1988;85(1B):24–29.

D'Ambrosio CM, Mohsenin V: Sleep in asthma. Clin Chest Med 1998;19(1):127–137.

Douglas NJ: Nocturnal asthma. Q J Med 1989;71(264):279–289.

Fitzpatrick MF, Engleman H, Whyte KF, et al: Morbidity in nocturnal asthma: sleep quality and daytime cognitive performance. Thorax 1991;46(8):569–573.

Sutherland ER, Ellison MC, Kraft M, Martin RJ: Altered pituitary-adrenal interaction in nocturnal asthma. J Allergy Clin Immunol 2003;112(1):52–57.

Turner-Warwick M: Epidemiology of nocturnal asthma. Am J Med 1988;85(1B):6–8.

Wenzel S: Severe asthma in adults. Am J Respir Crit Care Med 2005;172(2):149–160.

White J, Cates C, Wright J: Continuous positive airways pressure for obstructive sleep apnea. Cochrane Database Syst Rev 2002;(2):CD001106.

Yigla M, Tov N, Solomonov A, et al: Difficult-to-control asthma and obstructive sleep apnea. J Asthma 2003;40(8):865–871.

Young T, Palta M, Dempsey J, et al: The occurrence of sleep-disordered breathing among middle-aged adults. N Engl J Med 1993;328(17):1230–1235.

Occupational Asthma

Anthony J. Frew

CLINICAL PEARLS

- Occupational asthma is common and underdiagnosed.

- Occupational causes should be considered in all adults presenting with asthma.

- Several different mechanisms appear to operate.

- Diagnosis is based on history, including exposure assessment, and supported by lung function assessments.

- Formal occupational challenges may help where doubt remains.

- Optimal outcome requires early diagnosis and removal from exposure.

- Inhaled steroids may help accelerate remission/resolution.

- Doctors need to know the compensation rules and advise patients appropriately.

The association of respiratory problems and the workplace has been recognized for many centuries. In past centuries, occupational dust exposure was the main concern, leading to fibrosis of the lung, as found in silicosis, and coal-worker's pneumoconiosis. With improving industrial hygiene, and recognition of the employer's responsibility for the health of the workforce, dust diseases have become less common. In the mid- and late 20th century asthma emerged as the most common form of occupational lung disease. Occupational asthma varies in its presentation and course, but has been linked to a large number of different products and processes. Partly for the purposes of industrial compensation schemes, and partly for clinical practice, it has become necessary to define occupational asthma quite precisely. Most authorities now restrict the term occupational asthma to patients whose asthma is caused by sensitization to a substance encountered in the workplace. Patients with coincidental or preexisting asthma may well develop exacerbation of their symptoms when exposed to dusts, fumes, or solvents. While this is clearly work related, it does not meet the definitions of occupational asthma that are used to determine compensation, and so it is probably best to call this *work-related asthma*. Equally, some patients develop nonspecific wheezing and asthma-like symptoms after exposure to high levels of irritant or corrosive vapors. Since they are not sensitized to the offending agent, this does not meet the definition of occupational asthma either, and is best termed *irritant-induced asthma*.

Once established, asthma can often be triggered or exacerbated by exposure to relatively low concentrations of nonspecific irritants. This enhanced bronchial irritability can be demonstrated by nonspecific bronchial inhalation challenges with histamine or methacholine, and is termed *nonspecific bronchial hyperresponsiveness* (NSBHR). NSBHR is a characteristic feature of asthma, but is also found in a proportion of people who appear completely healthy. In a small proportion of cases, patients with symptomatic occupational asthma show NSBHR without any other evidence of asthma.

Thus for practical purposes occupational asthma may be defined as "a disorder characterised by variable airflow limitation and/or airway hyperresponsiveness, due to causes and conditions attributable to a particular working environment and not to stimuli encountered outside the workplace" (Chan-Yeung et al).

Clinically, the patient presents with asthma in the workplace, and diagnostic pathways need to start there, rather than with etiological definitions. Patients whose preexisting asthma is worsened through occupational exposure need expert assessment and counseling, just as much as those whose asthma is due to occupational sensitization. Unfortunately the desire of the patient for compensation, and sometimes for punishment of the employer, can lead to conflicts of understanding among patients, trade union officials, employers, and physicians. Asthma in the workplace is thus an area in which medicine and the law sit uncomfortably beside one another.

A recurring theme throughout this discussion of occupational asthma will be the difficulty of making an accurate diagnosis. Ultimately, the diagnosis is a matter of medical judgment, and has two key components: (1) a willingness to consider the possibility that adult-onset asthma may be driven by workplace exposure, and (2) a sober assessment of whether the individual's personal exposure history and clinical data are sufficient to support a diagnosis of true occupational asthma.

HISTORICAL BACKGROUND

Asthma was recognized in antiquity, and within the discourses of Hippocrates one may find reference to asthma in metal workers, tailors, farmers, and fishermen, among others. Early discussion of occupational lung disease focused on mining and smelting. In 1713, Ramazzini published his treatise on occupational disease, and describes what we would now recognize as extrinsic allergic alveolitis, as well as respiratory problems associated with baking. With the recognition that asthma was often caused by external factors such as dust and pollen, clinicians began to appreciate the importance of obtaining information on current and past occupations, and considering the possibility that illness (including asthma) might be related to occupational exposure. The first well-documented form of occupational asthma was described in 1923, in workers handling castor beans. Over the next 30 years this was followed by a steady stream of new agents identified as causes of asthma, including dusts, insects, metals, and a variety of chemicals. From 1960 onward, an increasing number of low-molecular weight chemicals were identified as causes of occupational asthma. In part this reflected an increasing awareness of occupational asthma, but this period also saw an ever-increasing number of chemicals used in industry, and a shift in developed economies from heavy industries (e.g., steelworking, shipbuilding) toward light industries, electronics, and plastics manufacturing, which often involved the use of reactive chemicals, such as isocyanates and acid anhydrides.

EPIDEMIOLOGY

Assessing the prevalence of occupational asthma is always difficult. Cross-sectional surveys of individual industries suffer from several inbuilt biases. First, the definition of cases is variable. In industries known to carry a high risk of occupational asthma, overdiagnosis can easily occur, as anybody with respiratory symptoms may report they have asthma. Conversely if awareness is low, patients may not be aware that their asthma is in fact work related. On the survey date, those with asthma are more likely to be off sick and therefore fail to appear in the statistics. Once diagnosed, patients may leave the industry, leaving behind a cohort of workers that are relatively resistant to developing asthma. Moreover, if the industry is known to carry a risk of asthma, people with mild asthma or a family history of asthma may avoid joining the workforce. Taken together these lead to the impression that the workforce is in fact healthier than it really is (the so-called healthy worker effect).

SPECIFIC AGENTS

Isocyanates

The isocyanates (or polyisocyanates) are a group of low molecular weight organic compounds that readily form esters of substituted carbamic acid, also known as urethanes. Isocyanates are used to form plastics, adhesives and foam that can be used in the manufacture of furnishings. They are also used in a wide range of molding and core processes in steel foundries, and as insulating materials in the building industry. One of their most widespread uses is as hardening agents for paints, especially those used for spraying cars. Other applications in the automobile industry include production of dashboards, body parts, and upholstery. Consequently, a large number of workers in a variety of industries may be exposed to isocyanates.

Medical problems associated with isocyanates were described in the 1950s, connected to with the use of toluene diisocyanate (TDI) to manufacture polyurethane foam. TDI remains the commonest isocyanate to cause sensitization and occupational asthma, although cases have been reported with other isocyanates, including methylene diphenyl-diisocyanate (MDI) and hexamethylene diisocyanate (HDI). Both TDI and HDI are volatile at room temperature but MDI has to be heated above 60°C before significant quantities are vaporized. Isocyanates can also cause contact sensitization and occupational dermatitis, especially when present in glues.

Various animal models have been developed to mimic isocyanate sensitivity. Antibodies detected in experimental animals and exposed workers suggest that some individuals can form immunoglobulin G (IgG) antibodies to conjugates of TDI and human serum albumin. Immunoglobulin E (IgE) antibodies have not been convincingly demonstrated in TDI asthma. Generally speaking, workers who develop TDI asthma will have a period of exposure without symptoms following which they become sensitive to relatively small levels of TDI exposure. This latent period and subsequent heightened sensitivity are indicative of an immunological process rather than simple irritant-induced asthma. It should be noted that isocyanates are also irritants; at high levels of exposure, humans experience acute inflammation of the eyes and nose with associated tears, coughing, and burning sensation in the throat and chest. The higher the level of exposure, the quicker an individual is likely to become sensitized. Once individuals have developed asthma, extremely low levels of diisocyanate in the region of 1 part per billion can trigger reactions. Proper attention to occupational hygiene substantially reduces the risk of sensitization but once an individual has become sensitized, they may develop asthma even on exposure at levels below the threshold for sensitization. Consequently, once somebody has developed isocyanate asthma, it is usually necessary for them to become completely withdrawn from the workplace and they may not be safe at levels that are regarded as nonhazardous in terms of sensitization.

Once isocyanate asthma develops, a proportion (perhaps 30% to 35%) will lose their asthma altogether if withdrawn from the workplace but the remainder will have persistent asthma, despite ceasing exposure to isocyanates. Most individuals will also have NSBHR although there are individual case reports of diisocyanate asthma without NSBHR.

In cases where there is doubt about the diagnosis, challenge procedures may demonstrate bronchospasm after exposure to low levels of diisocyanates. In common with other low molecular weight antigens, late-phase asthmatic reactions are common, and some individuals may have isolated late-phase reactions (without any sign of acute response to challenge). This makes challenges time-consuming, as only one dose of isocyanate can be given on any one day. In most countries, workers who develop asthma while working with isocyanates will generally be regarded as having developed occupational asthma without requiring specific challenge tests, provided that they did not have asthma in childhood or before entering the workplace. The diagnosis should be confirmed by taking an accurate exposure history and, where possible, obtaining records of routine monitoring of isocyanates within the workplace environment.

Acid Anhydrides

Acid anhydrides are used in a variety of chemical processes but particularly in epoxy resins. Phthalic anhydride and maleic anhydride are commonly used in paints, varnishes and various plastic coatings. Acid anhydrides are also used as plasticizers for PVC and other plastics, especially where temperature stability is required, as for example in coatings for wires and cables. Acid anhydrides have direct irritant effects and also can sensitize individuals, leading to occupational asthma. Strict exposure limits are in place for most anhydrides with relatively low threshold limit values. Direct toxicity of acid anhydrides includes irritation and burns of the skin and conjunctiva, cough, pulmonary edema and transient changes in airflow resistance. In contrast to isocyanates, immune reactions against acid anhydrides appear to involve IgE antibodies and, therefore, occupational asthma to acid anhydrides is more common in those who are predisposed to make IgE. In addition to asthma, acid anhydrides can cause a hypersensitivity pneumonitis.

The development of IgE antibodies to acid anhydrides is enhanced by concurrent smoking. In workplace surveys, smoking appears to enhance the risk of developing IgE antibody by five- to sixfold compared with nonsmokers. Consequently, most patients with occupational asthma to acid anhydrides will have some background tendency toward allergy and asthma as well as being current smokers. As with isocyanates, accurate diagnosis requires assessment of occupational exposure hazards and working practices, as well as conventional investigation of asthma.

Metals

Inhalation of metals can cause acute pulmonary toxicity, chronic fibrosis, or occupational asthma. In the western world, the commonest metals for workers to be exposed to (in descending order) are zinc, aluminum, chromium, nickel, cobalt, vanadium, and platinum. Usually the metals are encountered in the form of oxides or other salts such as sulfides, halides, carbides, or hydrides. The bioavailability of metal salts depends on their solubility. Insoluble compounds will be deposited in the airways and cleared by the mucociliary escalator, whereas soluble salts are more likely to dissolve and enter the lung in the form of ionic metals. Generally speaking, workers in metal industries will be aware of the potential for lung toxicity, including metal fume fever and occupational asthma. In addition, metal salts may cause asthma in people exposed to paint pigments (especially chromates), plastics, or catalysts.

In absolute terms, the largest number of metal-induced asthma cases have been reported with aluminum and platinum. Aluminum-associated asthma was first reported as an occupational health hazard in aluminum smelters and is sometimes termed *potroom asthma*. This condition was originally attributed to fluoride in the smelter environment. The latent period from first exposure to onset of asthma can vary widely from a matter of weeks to about 10 years. Allergy is not a feature of this condition. It has been suggested that this condition may overlap with irritant-induced asthma (discussed later in this chapter).

Platinum is widely used in the chemical industry but the heaviest occupational exposures occur during the refining process. Secondary refining involves the recycling of precious metals from scrap metal and catalytic converters. The process involves burning to remove combustible components followed by solution in acid and subsequent separation of the various metal salts. This process includes exposure to chlorine, formaldehyde, nitric acid, sulfur dioxide and other irritant chemicals as well as the metal salts. Platinum salts have a strong tendency to induce IgE antibodies, even in workers who have no history of atopy. Platinum-induced occupational asthma was recognized before World War I and even with good industrial hygiene, up to 10% of workers may have to leave the industry each year. Skin tests with platinum salts are a reliable indicator of sensitization and are generally positive in affected workers.

Zinc is widely used in industry and most often causes metal fume fever, a flu-like illness starting 4 to 12 hours after exposure to zinc oxide. A few cases of occupational asthma have been described with zinc exposure, but given the wide use of zinc in industry, it seems that zinc is much less able to induce asthma than other metals listed here. Chromate and nickel generally cause contact hypersensitivity but a few case reports exist of occupational asthma for both these metals and also for vanadium. Cobalt asthma has been documented in hard metal workers and is thought to be driven by sensitized lymphocytes rather than antibodies.

Wood Dust

Exposure to wood dust is common and occurs both in the sawmill industry and a variety of jobs involving carpentry (e.g., furniture and cabinet making). Several respiratory illnesses are associated with wood dust including hypersensitivity pneumonitis, asthma, and chronic bronchitis. Wood-induced asthma is the commonest medical picture and is usually associated with occupational exposure but can also occur with hobby-associated exposure. Many different types of wood dust have been implicated but as we know little about the amount and extent of wood use within the furniture and construction industry, it is difficult to establish relative risks for particular woods. In sensitized individuals, positive skin tests can often be demonstrated with aqueous extracts of relevant wood dusts. However, some woods that clearly cause asthma do not seem to induce IgE antibodies. The best understood of these is Western red cedar (*Thuja plicata*).

Western red cedar is an economically important timber of the Pacific Northwest, growing widely on the coasts of Oregon, Washington, and British Columbia. The tree has a very straight grain with few knots and is highly resistant to rot. Consequently, it has been used to form native totem poles and cabins, and also for external constructions such as roof tiles, garden sheds, decking, and so forth. Western red cedar wood contains large amounts of chemicals that are responsible for its resistance to fungal rot. About 90% by weight of the nonvolatile components of cedar resin is an organic acid, plicatic acid (PA). PA is a low-molecular-weight compound that induces immediate and delayed asthmatic reactions, similar to those that can be induced by inhaling aqueous extracts of Western red cedar dust. Patients with nonoccupational asthma do not react to PA, indicating that PA is probably the main causative agent of Western red cedar asthma (WRCA). In contrast to ordinary allergic asthma (to pollen, dust mite, cat, and so forth), about 40% of patients with WRCA show isolated late-phase reactions after inhaling PA. Cedar asthma is no commoner in smokers than nonsmokers and is not particularly associated with atopy. Early studies reported IgE antibodies against conjugates of PA and human serum albumin but subsequent work has cast doubt on their relevance. When WRCA patients inhale PA, both histamine and leukotrienes are released into their airways and they develop increased bronchial hyperresponsiveness. Bronchial biopsies from WRCA patients show the typical eosinophilic inflammation seen in other types of asthma, and this increases after inhalation challenge. WRCA is diagnosed like all other types of occupational asthma, on a combination of history and objective evidence of asthma after exposure to cedar dust. Specific challenge tests may be useful in cases where there is doubt or where medicolegal consequences are expected.

Cotton Dust

Several early studies found increased rates of respiratory morbidity and mortality among cotton workers. *Byssinosis* is a term applied to the acute and chronic respiratory diseases associated with occupational exposure to cotton and related dusts. Typically patients report chest tightness when they go back to exposure after a period away from regular attendance at work. Pathologically there is chronic bronchitis, and, in many series, emphysema is also present. Smoking appears to be a significant risk factor for byssinosis and of course there are difficulties in distinguishing between the pathology induced by cigarette smoking and those attributable to vegetable dusts. Clinically, there is acute decline in lung function across shifts and also a gradual decline in lung function with restriction in those with long-term exposure. The precise component in cotton that is responsible for this condition has been disputed. Some believe that endotoxin is the principal agent while others suggest that there must be a specific response to the vegetable matter. New entrants to the industry may experience acute fever and malaise about 8 to 12 hours after their initial exposures to heavy levels of dust but these symptoms resolve within a few days. Atopy is not a risk factor for developing symptoms but does seem to predict a greater degree of decline in FEV_1 (forced expiratory volume in 1 second) over time.

Grain Dust

Several different clinical syndromes can be caused by exposure to grain dust, including acute asthma, nonspecific bronchoconstriction, chronic reduction in lung function, grain fever, and hypersensitivity pneumonitis. Grain dusts contain a variety of allergens including the grain itself, mites, and insects, as well as endotoxin. Occupational health surveys suggest that people with asthma or NSBHR are unlikely to remain in employment where there is chronic exposure to grain dust. This leads to a healthy worker effect as the people working with grain are generally selected for people who are tolerant of dust exposure.

Several patterns of airways response have been reported after inhalation of grain dust in patients reporting grain-induced asthma, including single immediate, dual, and isolated late reactions. The degree of response is related to the underlying bronchial reactivity but is not clearly related to grain allergens: Skin tests to grain extracts are generally negative. The role of sensitization to storage mites is the subject of ongoing research. Field studies have demonstrated acute changes in lung function over the course of working shifts among grain workers. These decrements in lung function are related to the amount of exposure to dust and are similar clinically to byssinosis rather than acute asthma. Chronic lung disease certainly occurs in people working with grain dust but the link between the exposure and the disease remains controversial. Rates of lung function decline are accelerated in grain workers suggesting that there is a chronic effect on the conducting airways, over and above any acute asthmatic effect.

Grain fever is an acute illness related to exposure to high levels of grain dust. As with other acute pulmonary fevers, the illness is characterized by myalgia, fever, malaise, cough, and chest tightness. Acute episodes are often associated with increased neutrophil counts in peripheral blood.

Laboratory Animals

Many people who work with laboratory animals become sensitized to them. Most cases involve rats and mice since these are the animals most commonly used in research and industry. However, those working with rabbits, guinea pigs and other small rodents can also become sensitized in the workplace. Allergenic proteins are aerosolized by the movement of the animals and are inhaled by the worker. In both rats and mice, urine proteins are an important source of allergenic proteins. These dry in the bedding material and are then aerosolized. The risk of sensitization is greater in those with other preexisting allergic problems. Sensitization is more likely in those who have higher levels of exposure. Once sensitized, personal protective equipment may enable the sufferer to continue working with animals but in most cases, a change of career or experimental focus may be required.

Other Agents

A wide variety of high molecular weight agents have been implicated in occupational asthma. These include cereal proteins and alpha amylase (baker's asthma), detergent enzymes used in washing powders, and various enzymes and gums used in the pharmaceutical industry (e.g., papain, ipecacuanha, psyllium). Many different vegetable products have been implicated including coffee, flax, linseed, tea, garlic, castor bean, egg proteins, and latex. Occupational asthma can also be induced by fish and shellfish processing.

PATHOPHYSIOLOGY

Sensitization to high molecular weight (HMW) agents occurs via the same mechanisms that are thought to lead to sensitization with pollens, molds, dust mite, animal dander, and so forth. The HMW agent is processed through antigen-presenting cells, most likely dendritic cells from the lung, and presented to T cells in the regional lymph nodes. In people who are predisposed to atopic allergy, these T cells may be biased towards the Th2 phenotype. Activation of allergen-specific Th2 cells leads to the induction of IgE antibodies that then sensitize the respiratory mucosal mast cells. Subsequent exposure to the HMW agent causes typical immediate and late-phase bronchoconstriction and increased bronchial hyperreactivity.

In contrast, low molecular weight (LMW) agents are usually incomplete antigens and are thought to need to bind to carrier proteins such as albumin, in order to be seen by the immune system. This may explain why many LMW occupational allergens are highly reactive compounds capable of binding to proteins. Some LMW agents mainly cause sensitization in atopic individuals. This group of compounds can induce IgE antibodies and, presumably, the mechanism of responsiveness is similar to that found with HMW agents. Other agents, particularly isocyanates and plicatic acid, do not seem to induce IgE antibodies and there is no particular risk for atopic subjects compared to nonatopic individuals. Despite the absence of IgE antibodies, the typical mediators of asthma are released including histamine and leukotrienes when sensitized patients are exposed to the inducing LMW agents. Basophils and bronchial mast cells obtained from patients with occupational asthma will respond in vitro to the inciting agent with the release of histamines but it is thought that T cell responses may be more important in LMW asthma. Immediate asthmatic responses are seen on challenge but it is not unusual to experience an isolated late-phase reaction. Care must therefore be taken during challenge tests since the absence of an immediate reaction does not allow the investigator to proceed to the next dose of allergen until it is clear that there is no prospect of an isolated late-phase response. Attempts to demonstrate T cell responses in vitro have been frustrating. There is clearly some MHC haplotype association for certain LMW agents, indicating that T cell responses are important but we do not yet have reliable in vitro tests which discriminate the sensitized from nonsensitized individuals.

CLINICAL CONTEXT

The diagnosis of occupational asthma requires the physician to have a high index of suspicion, while at the same time avoiding paranoia. Since about 10% of adult cases presenting with asthma are thought to have occupational causes, it is important to consider occupation and occupational exposure in every patient who presents with asthma in adulthood. Patients who have asthma in childhood and have recurrence as adults will most often have an intrinsic form of asthma, but it is possible for them to become sensitized to occupational allergens and have true occupational disease. However, for medicolegal purposes, it is generally considered that when asthma recurs in people who have had asthma in childhood, this represents recurrence of their underlying disease rather than true occupational asthma. Challenge tests may help to discriminate between these two possibilities, but are not foolproof.

The other important clinical context is someone working in a "high-risk" industry who becomes breathless. Most people working in bakeries, paint shops, electronics factories, and so forth are aware of the possibility of occupational asthma and may therefore present quite early when they have respiratory symptoms. Alternatively, they may be picked up on health screening with early signs of obstructive airways disease. In both settings, it is quite common for people with spontaneous asthma or chronic obstructive pulmonary disease (COPD) to be mislabeled as having occupational asthma. A detailed and comprehensive history is essential, including the timing of symptoms in relation to exposure. Special consideration should be given to working practices that may lead to inadvertent or accidental exposure above the levels that are normally expected for that job. Baseline investigations will include lung function tests, serial peak flow measurements, and chest x-rays. Formal challenge tests are not always necessary. When people working in high-risk industries appear to have developed occupational asthma, the diagnosis will generally be accepted without argument, but when there is no clear history of exposure or the subject has been exposed to

agents that are not normally thought to cause occupational asthma, it may be appropriate to proceed to formal challenge. In some cases, formal occupational challenge may be necessary to allow the worker to continue in employment if a diagnosis of unrelated COPD is made.

IMPORTANT DIAGNOSTIC ISSUES

- When occupational asthma is suspected, try to get the patient to make serial peak flow recordings for 2 weeks at work, and 2 weeks while off work. Three values should be recorded each time, every 2 hours if possible, but at a minimum on rising and on retiring to bed, and also before and after shifts. The sooner this can be done the better, as many employers will put the patient off work once they know this diagnosis is suspected.
- As far as possible try not to tell the patient what will be looked for in the peak flow records. Patients can and do fabricate data so it is best not to guide them on patterns that will lead to a compensatable diagnosis.
- Make sure the patient marks on the graph which days they were at work and which shift they were working.
- Review the patient's records for evidence of previous symptoms that might represent asthma (if not previously diagnosed as asthmatic). Prior asthma does not exclude the development of occupational asthma, but may alter compensation status.
- Consider the possibility of alternative causes of breathlessness.
- Obtain a detailed history of chemicals and dusts to which the patient is exposed at work.
- Ask the patient to obtain safety data sheets on all products and processes in the workplace.
- If the initial tests suggest occupational asthma, do tell the patient that they should take legal advice on their compensation status and document this in the medical records. Strict time limits often apply to making a claim. Failure to inform the patient may lead to claims being made against the physician.
- Obtain a specialist's opinion if there is any doubt about the diagnosis, and also before advising a patient to leave his or her employment.

NATURAL HISTORY

In broad general terms, about one third of patients with occupational asthma will resolve completely if they are withdrawn from the workplace. Of the remainder, half will have some improvement on withdrawal from the workplace while the other half will have persistent symptoms with no improvement despite withdrawal from the workplace. In this latter group, it is obviously difficult to distinguish whether the occupational exposure was really important in causing their symptoms. There is nothing on lung function or investigation that will allow one to distinguish between nonimproving occupational asthma and unrelated intrinsic disease. For diagnostic purposes the important issue is to make an initial diagnosis that the disease was brought on by exposure to agents in the workplace and may have shown exacerbation on reexposure, even though at a later date the symptoms appeared to be more persistent.

Factors that influence the likelihood of improvement or resolution include age (with those getting asthma later in life more likely to persist), duration of exposure (with those exposed for the longest periods prior to diagnosis more likely to retain their asthma), and severity (with those more seriously affected more likely to have persistent symptoms). It is not known whether inhaled steroids and other anti-inflammatory drugs influence the long-term outcome of occupational asthma but these agents are likely to be given for symptom control and there is a widespread belief that the use of inhaled steroids improves the likelihood of resolution. A limited number of biopsy studies have been performed, indicating that when patients with occupational asthma do improve, there is resolution both of the eosinophilic inflammation and also of the sub-basement membrane collagen deposition that is normally associated with asthma. This resolution of the remodeling process is not seen in other forms of asthma and offers an interesting model in which one might study the processes associated with resolution. Excess expression of tumor necrosis factor (TNF)-α has been linked to persistence of occupational asthma but intervention studies with TNF-receptor antagonists have not yet been performed.

IRRITANT-INDUCED ASTHMA

Some patients develop an asthma-like syndrome after acute exposure to high levels of irritant vapors. This condition is distinct from occupational asthma in that the symptoms come on immediately or very quickly after exposure and do not involve specific sensitization to the inciting substance. A wide range of materials has been indicated, including acidic and alkaline vapors, ammonia, chlorine, and smoke. In the initial phase, it may be difficult to distinguish irritant-induced asthma (IIA) from acute chemical pneumonitis. However, whereas pneumonitis causes fever and resolves within a few days, IIA is less likely to cause fever and will tend to persist. Lung function tests may be normal but there will be evidence of bronchial irritability as shown by histamine or methacholine challenge. Histologically, IIA is characterized by neutrophilic inflammation although some eosinophils may be present. Strictly speaking, a diagnosis of IIA should not be made in somebody who has a history of childhood asthma or preexisting airflow obstruction. Since IIA does not involved sensitization, there are no specific diagnostic tests relating to the inciting agents. It is generally believed that this condition will resolve more quickly if treated with inhaled steroids but cases are relatively few and far between and there has not been any symptomatic study of treatment. Some authorities believe that chronic sequential exposure to lower levels of irritant vapors may also cause IIA although the initial definition of IIA was for acute onset following massive exposure.

WORKERS COMPENSATION ISSUES

Occupational asthma is a prescribed occupational disease in many countries. Definitions vary between countries and between states within federal countries such as the USA. Most jurisdictions define an occupational disease as illness caused by and exacerbated by substances encountered within the workplace. Aggravation of preexisting asthma is often excluded from the definition of occupational asthma for compensation purposes but synergistic effects of a patient's atopy and occupational exposure are usually judged to be work-related even though the subject is at increased risk of the disease as a result of their own constitution.

A detailed discussion of workers compensation schemes is beyond the scope of this chapter. In some systems, low levels of compensation are available on a no-fault basis but larger levels of compensation can only be obtained by proving negligence by the employer. The existence of different standards of proof for these levels of compensation can lead to considerable anxiety and dissatisfaction among patients.

In many workplaces, it is difficult to identify the causative factors for the disease and even when clearly identifiable hazards are present, it may be difficult to undertake challenge tests due to the hazardous nature of the material. Diagnosis of occupational asthma can be straightforward if patients have normal lung function while away from work but in many cases there is persisting disability while away from the workplace and it may take several weeks before a plateau is reached. Irritant substances are encountered in many workplaces, which can trigger attacks of preexisting asthma. These can easily be mistaken for true occupational asthma. It follows that accurate diagnosis and assessment by someone familiar with the issues surrounding the diagnosis and compensation of occupational asthma will be needed in most cases. Patients with preexisting asthma have a duty to disclose this to employers or their occupational health advisors. In some cases this will preclude them from taking up employment in certain industries (e.g., baking, paint spraying, armed services).

Some countries have lists of agents that are recognized as causing occupational asthma and anyone who works with these and develops asthma can expect to achieve some level of compensation. Those who develop occupational asthma from other substances may have more difficulty in proving that they have true occupational disease. However, recent changes to European regulations have made it easier for workers to establish that their disease is due to occupational exposure and to achieve compensation.

SUGGESTED READING

Burge SP: New guidelines for the management of occupational asthma in primary care and occupational health. Prim Care Respir J 2004;13:131–132.

Chan-Yeung M, Malo J-L, Bernstein IL: Asthma in the Workplace, 3rd ed. New York, Taylor & Francis, 2006.

Cullinan P, Tarlo S, Nemery B: The prevention of occupational asthma. Eur Respir J 2003;22:853–860.

Mapp CE, Boschetto P, Maestrelli P, Fabbri LM: Occupational asthma. Am J Respir Crit Care Med 2005;172:280–305.

Genetics

Kim SH, Oh HB, Lee KW, et al: HLA DRB1*15-DPB1*05 haplotype: a susceptible gene marker for isocyanate-induced occupational asthma? Allergy 2006;61:891–894.

Mapp CE: The role of genetic factors in occupational asthma. Eur Respir J 2003;22(1):173–178.

Risk Factors

McDonald JC, Chen Y, Zekveld C, Cherry NM: Incidence by occupation and industry of acute work related respiratory diseases in the UK, 1992-2001. Occup Environ Med 2005;62:836–842.

Siracusa A, Marabini A, Folletti I, Moscato G: Smoking and occupational asthma. Clin Exp Allergy 2006;36:577–584

Tarlo SM, Malo JL, ATS/ERS: An ATS/ERS report: 100 key questions and needs in occupational asthma. Eur Respir J 2006;27:607–614.

Mechanisms

Jones MG, Floyd A, Nouri-Aria KT, et al: Is occupational asthma to diisocyanates a non-IgE-mediated disease? J Allergy Clin Immunol 2006;117:663–669.

Sastre J, Vandenplas O, Park HS: Pathogenesis of occupational asthma. Eur Respir J 2003;22:364–373.

Allergic Bronchopulmonary Aspergillosis

Raymond G. Slavin

The inclusion of allergic bronchopulmonary aspergillosis (ABPA) in a text on clinical asthma is quite appropriate. ABPA can be viewed as a complication of bronchial asthma in that it occurs exclusively in asthmatics or in cystic fibrosis (CF) patients who have asthma. It represents a condition in which a basic immunologic disease, bronchial asthma, is complicated by the introduction of another immune response resulting in a different disease entity. The diagnostic index of suspicion of ABPA should remain high, for appropriate therapy must be instituted early enough to prevent irreparable tissue damage.

Aspergillus, the responsible antigen or allergen, is a ubiquitous organism that has been found in air, fertile soil, decayed vegetation and swimming pool water. It is commonly cultured from basements, crawl spaces, bedding, and dust from homes. The specimen of *Aspergillus* that most commonly affects man is *fumigatus*. Pulmonary disease caused by *A. fumigatus* is varied and illustrates how the same organism can elicit different clinical responses, depending on the degree of exposure and the nature of the host. The five types of aspergillus lung disease are:

1. Invasive or septicemic aspergillosis. This condition occurs in individuals with a compromised immune response and is associated with invasion of the bronchial wall resulting in a definite bronchitis. Pneumonia, mycotic abscesses, chronic granuloma, and systemic spread are often seen.
2. Saprophytic aspergillosis or aspergilloma. This is the most common form of aspergillosis and consists of superficial invasion of an anatomic abnormality such as a bronchogenic cyst or a bronchiectatic cavity.
3. Bronchial asthma. *Aspergillus* is one of many molds that can cause immunoglobulin E (IgE)-mediated allergic asthma.
4. Extrinsic allergic alveolitis. This condition is known as malt workers' lung, a form of hypersensitivity pneumonitis due to *Aspergillus clavus* growing in the barley on the floors of breweries.
5. Allergic bronchopulmonary aspergillosis. This condition, described first in 1952, is an example of pulmonary infiltrates with eosinophilia (PIE) syndrome, that is, pulmonary infiltrates with peripheral blood and sputum eosinophilia. Initially thought to be rare in the United States, it is being increasingly reported in this country.[1]

CLINICAL CHARACTERISTICS

History and Physical Examination

Patients with allergic aspergillosis are almost always atopic and have a history of bronchial asthma. Patients complain of anorexia, headache, general aches and pains, loss of energy, temperature elevation, production of solid sputum plugs, and acute attacks of wheezing dyspnea. The disease tends to affect the younger age group, with most cases occurring under the age of 40. Several children have developed the disease before 2 years of age. Most often, no clear relationship can be established between a history of exposure to moldy vegetative matter and the onset of symptoms.

In most patients, there are general signs of airway obstruction, with crepitant rales localized over areas of pulmonary infiltration.

Eosinophilia

Peripheral blood eosinophils are generally over 1000/mm^3, and levels greater than 3000/mm^3 are common.

Sputum

On direct examination of sputum plugs, fungal mycelia are frequently seen with large numbers of eosinophils (Fig. 43-1). A cardinal feature of ABPA is that the organism can actively grow at body temperature shedding antigens and enzymes into the surrounding tissue. The preservation of cytoplasm as seen in Figure 43-1 indicates active growth of the fungus. This is in contrast to the dead mycelia that are devoid of cytoplasmic content as seen in aspergilloma.

A positive sputum culture is not diagnostic of aspergillosis, as aspergillus is commonly inhaled and expectorated by the population at large. By the same token, patients with allergic

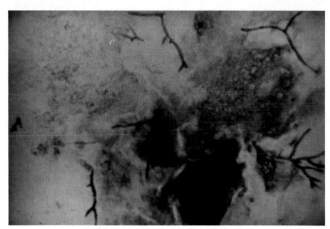

Figure 43-1   Sputum smear of patient with ABPA showing eosinophils with good preservation of cytoplasm, Gomorimethenamine silver stain. *(From Slavin RG: Allergic bronchopulmonary aspergillosis. In Fireman P, Slavin RG [eds]: Atlas of Allergies, 2nd ed. London, Mosby-Wolfe, 1996, pp 131–139.)*

aspergillosis frequently have negative sputum culture during episodes of pulmonary infiltration. The organism can best be grown in Sabouraud's glucose peptone broth or Czapek-Dox medium.

Skin Tests

The presence of a positive immediate wheal and erythema reaction to an aspergillus skin test is a necessary finding in allergic aspergillosis. A negative skin test for all intents and purposes rules out the diagnosis. On the other hand, a positive skin test indicates only the presence of immunoglobulin E (IgE) antibodies to aspergillus and is not diagnostic of allergic aspergillosis. Twenty-five percent of bronchial asthmatic individuals are skin test positive to *A. fumigatus*.

Precipitins

Precipitating antibody of the IgG type to *A. fumigatus* is present in the serum of 69% of patients with allergic aspergillosis. When the serum is concentrated three- to fourfold, the percentage of positive precipitin reactions increases to well over 90%. As in the case of immediate skin reactivity, the presence of precipitating antibody to *A. fumigatus* is not diagnostic of allergic aspergillosis, for it has been demonstrated in 9% of hospitalized patients, 3% of healthy office workers, 12% of allergic asthmatic patients, 27% of patients with farmer's lung, and practically all patients with aspergilloma.

IgE

Serum IgE levels in allergic aspergillosis are generally markedly elevated, being significantly higher than in uncomplicated bronchial asthma. A recent Cystic Fibrosis Consensus Document recommends IgE levels higher than 417 IU/mL or higher than 1000 ng/mL as being consistent with ABPA.

Studies using absorption of serum with *A. fumigatus* antigens indicate that the majority of the total serum IgE in ABPA is not specific for *A. fumigatus*. This nonspecific elevation of total serum IgE is probably due to production of interleukin

(IL)-4 by ABPA lymphocytes when they are incubated with *A. fumigatus* in vitro.

The Cystic Fibrosis Foundation has recently suggested that all CF patients have yearly determination of serum IgE.

Imaging Studies

A variety of radiographic abnormalities are present in allergic bronchopulmonary aspergillosis. Most commonly seen is a massive homogeneous shadow without fissure displacement that usually appears in the upper lobes. The shadow may be patchy, triangular, lobar, or oblong, and it frequently shifts from one site to another (Fig. 43-2). A recurrence in the same area suggests previous bronchial damage that may predispose locally to further episodes.

Another frequently seen abnormality is "tramline" shadows, which consist of two parallel hairline shadows extending out from the hilum in the direction of the bronchi. This is thought to represent bronchial wall edema. Parallel line shadows are similar to tramline shadows, but the width of the transparent zone is wider. They appear to be caused by bronchial damage and often appear in areas where homogeneous shadows had previously been observed and then resolved. A bandlike or "toothpaste" shadow represents secretions in a dilated bronchus. After a mucous plug is expectorated, a toothpaste shadow often reverts to a tubular shadow. A gloved ring shadow represents secretions in a dilated bronchus with an occluded distal end, and ring shadows, consisting of a hairlike ring, indicate cavities.

A commonly seen radiographic finding in allergic aspergillosis is atelectasis of a segment, a lobe, or total collapse of the whole lung due to mucous plug occlusion.

It is important to realize that an inconspicuous radiographic appearance can represent extensive tissue damage. The diagnosis of ABPA can be suspected from such a modest finding as a tramline shadow or by residual damage, such as a shrunken upper lobe.

The imaging features described thus far are best identified with computed tomography (CT). CT is far more sensitive than chest radiography for the detection of bronchiectasis. Mucous plugging in large bronchi can be seen on plain radiographs but is more frequently identified by CT. Centrilobular nodules and high-attenuation mucous plugs can be identified only by CT.[2]

Pulmonary Function

In allergic aspergillosis, pulmonary function testing during clinical flares shows significant decline in total lung capacity, vital capacity, forced expiratory volume in 1 second (FEV_1), and carbon monoxide diffusion (DLCO). The decrease in DLCO is probably due to the presence of bronchiectasis and is an extremely important index of disease severity, as uncomplicated bronchial asthma is associated with a normal DLCO. The abnormal pulmonary function tests return toward baseline with remission, and in most patients, no significant functional deterioration occurs with proper treatment after diagnosis.

Bronchial Challenge

The patient with allergic aspergillosis will respond to a bronchial challenge of *A. fumigatus* in a dual fashion.

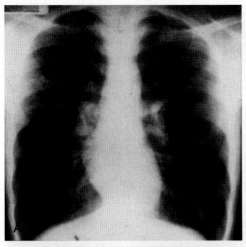
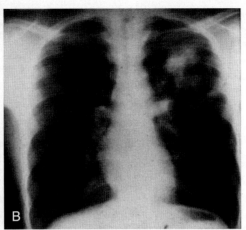
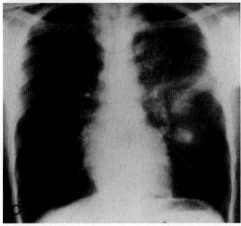

Figure 43-2 Chest radiographs demonstrating fleeting infiltrates in the case of ABPA. A, Soft nodular infiltrates in the right upper lobe suggest tuberculosis. **B,** Fourteen days later, there is some clearing on the right with a new infiltrate present in the left midlung field. **C,** Ten days later, the left midlung has cleared but a new infiltrate is present in the upper lobe. *(From Slavin RG: Allergic bronchopulmonary aspergillosis. In Fireman P, Slavin RG [eds]: Atlas of Allergies, 2nd ed. London, Mosby-Wolfe, 1996, pp 131–139.)*

After an immediate decrease in FEV_1, with subsequent clearing, a late asthmatic reaction occurs at 4 to 6 hours that is associated with fever and leukocytosis. The immediate reaction can be blocked by a beta-agonist. Corticosteroids will prevent the late reaction, and cromolyn blocks both the immediate and late responses.

Lung Biopsy

In an earlier study of lung biopsy in ABPA, the bronchial wall demonstrated infiltration with mixed inflammatory cells, primarily mononuclear cells and eosinophils. Some bronchi were dilated and filled with inspissated mucus and exudate. Fungal hyphae were identified with the exudates but there was no invasion of bronchial wall and lung parenchyma. In areas of lung parenchyma that were extensively consolidated, there were chronic inflammatory cells and large numbers of granulomas, most of which displayed central necrosis, multinucleated giant cells, and a prominent eosinophil infiltrate.

In a later study using newly available immunohistologic techniques, new insights were gained into the pathogenesis of ABPA. Light microscopy revealed a marked inflammatory process that was largely bronchocentric. Elastin layers were intact in blood vessels and markedly disrupted in bronchioles. By immunofluorescence, major basic protein was demonstrated in eosinophils (Fig. 43-3), was freely deposited outside of eosinophils especially in the interlobular septum, and was taken up by macrophages. A number of lymphocytes

stained positively for IgE. A significant increase in IL-2 positive staining T cells was observed with an approximate 2:1 ratio of helper to suppressor cells. The most significant finding, demonstrated through an immunoperoxidase stain, was the presence of septate hyphae of aspergillus in the lung parenchyma.[3]

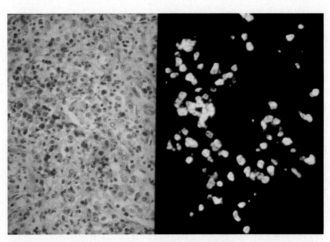

Figure 43-3 Lung biopsy of a patient with ABPA. Hematoxylin and eosin stain is on the left. On the right, the same section is stained with fluorescein-labeled, anti-major basic protein antibody. Positive staining corresponds to eosinophils ($\times 400$). *(From Slavin RG, Bedrossian CW, Hutcheson PS, et al: A pathologic study of allergic bronchopulmonary aspergillosis. J Allergy Clin Immunol 1988;81:718–725.)*

DIAGNOSIS

The diagnostic criteria for allergic aspergillosis are shown in Table 43-1. It has been suggested that the presence of the first seven major criteria makes the diagnosis of allergic aspergillosis highly likely, whereas all eight make it certain.[1]

A practical approach to the diagnosis of allergic aspergillosis is seen in Figure 43-4. First, evaluate any patient with a history of pulmonary infiltrates and asthma with an aspergillus skin test. If this is positive, then serum should be checked for a total IgE level and precipitins to *A. fumigatus*.

If the total serum IgE is less than 500 IU/mL, ABPA is highly unlikely. If the IgE is higher than 500 IU/mL then anti-aspergillus IgE and IgG should be determined irrespective of precipitins. If these are elevated, then a high-resolution CT of the chest should be obtained to determine the extent of lung involvement.

Asthmatic individuals who require corticosteroids for management might well be a group with underlying allergic aspergillosis. In a study of 42 such patients, 12 were found who were suspect. Of these, three had definite and three had probable allergic aspergillosis. This subgroup is more likely to be younger, to require larger corticosteroid doses, to have a higher incidence of positive skin test to *A. fumigatus* and other antigens, and to have elevated serum IgE levels. It is now recognized that species of aspergillus other than *fumigatus* may be responsible for allergic aspergillosis. In suspected patients whose serum is negative to a battery of *A. fumigatus* antigens, it may be necessary to isolate and extract the strain or species of aspergillus in the patient's sputum to elicit precipitin reactivity. Both *Aspergillus ochraceus* and *Aspergillus terreus* have been shown to cause allergic aspergillosis.

It has been suggested that a staging system can be used for ABPA. Stage I is the acute stage associated with all of the clinical and serologic characteristics of the disease. Stage II is clinical remission in which there are no chest infiltrates or need for prednisone for at least 6 months. Stage III is recurrent exacerbation similar to clinical and x-ray presentation with stage I. Stage IV is steroid-dependent asthma in which there

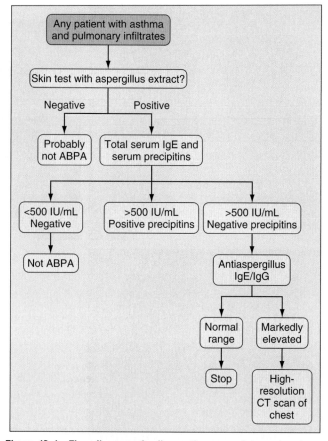

Figure 43-4   Flow diagram of a diagnostic approach to allergic bronchopulmonary aspergillosis. *(From Slavin RG: Allergic bronchopulmonary aspergillosis. In Fireman P, Slavin RG [eds]: Atlas of Allergies, 2nd ed. London, Mosby-Wolfe, 1996, pp 131–139.)*

may or may not be subsequent roentgenography infiltrate. Stage IV is end-stage fibrotic disease with irreversible impairment of pulmonary function.[4]

DIFFERENTIAL DIAGNOSIS

A number of medical conditions may be associated with asthma and pulmonary infiltrates. The primary diagnostic considerations are bacterial pneumonia, carcinoma, and tuberculosis. The frequently seen radiographic findings in allergic aspergillosis of upper lobe shrinkage and cavitation are particularly suggestive of tuberculosis. Appropriate bacterial study should rule this out.

Mucoid impaction of bronchi is associated with obstruction of proximal bronchi, with large plugs of inspissated mucus and exudates. Fungal hyphae are generally not identified in mucus plugs, and there is usually no evidence of aspergillus hypersensitivity. In contrast to the favorable response seen in allergic aspergillosis, corticosteroids are rarely of benefit in mucoid impaction.

Eosinophilic pneumonia consists of migratory pulmonary infiltrates that are usually accompanied by an excess of eosinophils in the peripheral blood. Cough, anorexia, and weight loss are noted. A characteristic radiographic finding is a peripheral density adjacent to the pleura of pulmonary edema. Lung biopsy shows the alveoli to be filled with eosinophils and large mononuclear cells with an interstitial infiltrate of

Table 43-1 DIAGNOSTIC CRITERIA FOR ALLERGIC ASPERGILLOSIS	
Major Criteria	**Minor Criteria**
1. Episodic bronchial obstruction	1. *Aspergillus fumigatus* positive sputum culture
2. Peripheral blood eosinophilia	2. History of expectorating brown plugs or flecks
3. Positive immediate skin reactivity	3. Arthus (late) skin reactivity
4. Serum-precipitating antibodies	
5. Elevated serum IgE	
6. Elevated IgG and IgE anti-Aspergillus antibodies	
7. History of pulmonary infiltrates	
8. Central bronchiectasis	

Data from Slavin RG: Allergic bronchopulmonary aspergillosis. In Fireman P, Slavin RG (eds): Atlas of Allergies, 2nd ed. London, Mosby-Wolfe, 1996, pp 131–139.

eosinophils, lymphocytes, and plasma cells. Etiologic factors include chemicals, helminths, and fungi. When an etiologic diagnosis is not found, the condition is termed cryptogenic or idiopathic pulmonary eosinophilia. Characteristics include marked eosinophilia, predominance in females, with less cough and sputum and less airway obstruction. Chest x-ray shows diffuse bilateral low-density shadows, with no atelectasis, bronchiectasis, or lobar shrinkage. Corticosteroids are quite effective treatment.

Bronchocentric granulomatosis is associated with asthma, mucoid impaction, and presence of noninvasive fungi. The distinctive pathologic lesion is replacement of bronchial epithelium by granulation tissue. Radiologic findings include atelectasis, pneumonic consolidation, bronchiectasis, and bronchiolectasis. Although no sensitizing agent has been identified, an allergic pathogenesis is strongly suspected.

PATHOGENESIS

There is generally no clear relationship between exposure to an environment rich in aspergillus spores and the development of allergic aspergillosis. To be sure, isolated cases have been reported, such as ABPA occurring in a habitual marijuana user whose stock supply of drugs contained a heavy growth of aspergillus. However, the incidence of allergic aspergillosis in urban dwellers with little exposure to moldy hay or grain is every bit as high as that in rural inhabitants. A careful survey of patients with diagnosed allergic aspergillosis shows no higher spore exposure than atopic control subjects. In a study of 131 sugar cane workers who were heavily exposed to *A. fumigatus*, only 2 (1.5%) developed allergic aspergillosis. Thus, a high exposure to aspergillus spores is not necessarily important in the development of allergic aspergillosis, and persistent exposure to high concentrations of the organism may not lead to development of the disease. These studies would tend to indicate that specific host susceptibility is more important to the development of allergic aspergillosis than the extent of exposure to the organism.

The disease process begins with the inhalation and trapping of the short chain spores of *A. fumigatus* in viscid secretions contained in the constricted airways of the asthmatic patient. The size of the spores and the broad range of temperatures at which *A. fumigatus* grows makes this organism uniquely suited for colonization of the human bronchial tree. Most other fungal spores will not survive at human body temperature, but *A. fumigatus* germinates and forms mycelia in the bronchi. Allergic aspergillosis is clearly distinguished from other hypersensitivity responses to inhaled allergens in that the organism grows in the respiratory tract and continually sheds antigens into the tissues. Antigens released from the mycelia combine with the previously mentioned IgE and IgG antibodies to set in motion a chain of immunologic reactions culminating in bronchial wall damage and the surrounding pulmonary eosinophilic consolidation.

Aspergillus itself has profound deleterious effects on defense mechanisms. These include decrease in ciliary beat frequency, impairment of fungicidal proteins, inactivation of complement, interference with phagocytic and killing capacity of phagocytic cells, and release of proteolytic enzymes with elastolytic and collagenolytic activities.

The importance of T lymphocytes in orchestrating the immune response is clearly seen in ABPA. Supernatants obtained from aspergillus-stimulated T cells of CF patients with ABPA cause in vitro allogeneic B cell IgE synthesis. Consistent with these findings, peripheral blood B cells from CF patients with ABPA spontaneously synthesized large amounts of IgE in vitro, which is evidence for polyclonal in vivo IgE B-cell differentiation. CD4+ T cell lines derived from ABPA patients and specific for the immunodominant antigen of aspergillus, Asp f1, revealed that the majority of the lines were of the Th2 phenotype. T cell clones (TCC) specific to the Asp f1 antigen were established from the peripheral blood of ABPA patients and all proliferated in response to Asp f1.[5]

Flow cytometric analysis demonstrated that all of the Asp f1-specific clones were CD3+, CD4+, CD8-, and expressed the αβ T-cell receptor. Measurements of cytokine levels after specific stimulation with Asp f1 revealed a high interleukin 4 (IL-4)/interferon γ (IFN-γ) ratio indicative of a Th2-like pattern of cytokine production.

Following up on the previously stated specific host susceptibility, human leukocyte antigen (HLA) typing of ABPA patients has shown a high incidence of HLA-DR2 with allelic predominance of *1501 and *1503. In addition, the HLA-DQ2 allele appears to confer protection.[6]

ASSOCIATION WITH CYSTIC FIBROSIS

The incidence of allergic aspergillosis appears to be markedly increased in patients with cystic fibrosis. Making the diagnosis of ABPA in these patients is particularly difficult because of the similarities of the two diseases (Table 43-2). In cystic fibrosis, there is an increased frequency of all of the following: atopy (46%), positive skin test to *A. fumigatus* (53%), positive sputum culture and precipitins to *A. fumigatus* (51%), and increased IgE (22%). In addition, the radiographic findings are similar, with hyperinflation, peribronchial inflammatory changes, nodular and branching densities of mucous impaction, atelectasis, predominant upper lobe infiltrates, and bronchiectasis being common to both. The diagnosis of ABPA may be suggested if peripheral blood eosinophils are markedly increased, if the serum IgE is greatly elevated to levels above 1000 IU/mL, and if pulmonary infiltrates do not respond to antibiotics, are transient, and resolve with corticosteroids.[7]

One study explored the hypothesis that the cystic fibrosis transmembrane regulator (CFTR) gene plays a role in ABPA. In 11 individuals who met strict criteria for the diagnosis of

Table 43-2
SIMILARITIES OF ALLERGIC BRONCHOPULMONARY ASPERGILLOSIS AND CYSTIC FIBROSIS
Atopy
Asthma
Positive skin test to *Aspergillus fumigatus*
Positive precipitin to *A. fumigatus*
Elevated IgE
Pulmonary infiltrates
Bronchiectasis

ABPA and had normal sweat electrolytes, one carried two CF mutations and five carried one CF mutation.

PROGNOSIS

In a long-term study of 50 patients with untreated ABPA, all patients followed a chronic course with airway obstruction, recurrent pulmonary consolidation, and in many instances, severe lung destruction. Interestingly, one third of these patients with recurrent pulmonary infiltrates were asymptomatic. Therefore, symptoms may bear no relationship to disease severity and cannot be used as a guide to therapy. The majority of patients with allergic aspergillosis who have early diagnosis and proper treatment will show no significant functional deterioration, as determined by pulmonary function testing.

TREATMENT

The basic aim of therapy in ABPA is to break the vicious cycle in which fungus, trapped in viscid secretions contained in the constricted asthmatic airway, continues to provide large quantities of antigenic and enzymatic material. The clinical presentation of ABPA may be quite subtle and a paucity of symptoms may be associated with quite profound tissue damage. Therefore, early and vigorous treatment is important to prevent the inexorable consequences of bronchiectasis, pulmonary fibrosis, and cor pulmonale.

The cornerstone of treatment is systemic corticosteroids. Once the diagnosis of ABPA is made, corticosteroids must be given in a large enough quantity over a sufficient period of time. A daily dose of prednisone, 60 mg/kg body weight in divided doses, is frequently required to clear the chest radiograph completely in the adult. After radiographic clearing, a single daily dose of 0.5 mg/kg of body weight is given for 2 weeks. At this point, there is a gradual taper to 0.25 mg/kg body weight over a 6-week period. The dose is then switched to 0.5 mg/kg body weight every other day for another

6 weeks and then gradually tapered over a 3-month period. In total, the steroid treatment is given over approximately a 7-month period. During this period, monthly serum IgE levels are obtained. A decrease from the initial, markedly elevated level is always seen. A rise in the serial IgE level, subsequently tested on a monthly basis, should prompt an increase in steroid therapy.

Because of the known beneficial effects of corticosteroids, other important aspects of therapy are often forgotten. Effective removal of fungus from the airway is vital and, therefore, attention to bronchial toilet is extremely important. Bronchodilator therapy must be continued throughout the course of therapy. Particularly in the acute phase, effort should be made to remove the viscid secretions with oral fluids, to avoid ice that may cause reflex bronchospasm, to use expectorants such as potassium iodide or guaifenesin, and to employ aggressive physical therapy and postural drainage. In stubborn cases, bronchial lavage may have to be used. Removal of the nidus of infection will hopefully prevent permanent anatomical, bronchial damage. The majority of patients who receive an early diagnosis and proper treatment will show no significant functional deterioration.

There have been promising reports on the effectiveness of itraconazole, an oral antifungal agent, on decreasing the fungal burden in ABPA. In one study of nine patients treated with prednisone, the addition of itraconazole at a dose of 400 mg daily resulted in a decrease in recurrence of radiographic shadows and a reduction in oral steroid requirement. An open study showed that this approach reduced recurrence of flare-ups, reduced IgE levels and blood eosinophils, and improved FEV_1. In a study of clinically stable ABPA patients, 400 mg daily of itraconazole alone resulted in reduction in sputum eosinophils and eosinophilic cationic protein, total serum IgE, specific IgG to aspergillus, and requirement of oral steroids for respiratory symptoms.[8] At present, itraconazole should be considered add-on therapy to prednisone. Patients should be under a specialist's care for the treatment of ABPA.

REFERENCES

1. Rosenberg M, Patterson R, Mintzer R, et al: Clinical and immunologic criteria for the diagnosis of allergic bronchopulmonary aspergillosis. Ann Intern Med 1977;86:405–414.
2. Malo J, Pepys J, Simon G: Studies in chronic allergic bronchopulmonary aspergillosis. 2. Radiologic findings. Thorax 1977;32:262–268.
3. Slavin RG, Bedrossian CW, Hutcheson PS, et al: A pathologic study of allergic bronchopulmonary aspergillosis. J Allergy Clin Immunol 1988;81:718–725.
4. Patterson R, Greenberger PA, Radin RD: Allergic bronchopulmonary aspergillosis: staging as an aid to management. Ann Intern Med 1982;96:286–291.
5. Slavin RG, Hutcheson PS, Chauhan B: New insights into the pathogenesis of allergic bronchopulmonary aspergillosis. ACI International 2003;15:79–81.
6. Chauhan B, Santiago L, Kirschmann DA, et al: The association of HLA-DR alleles and T cell activation with allergic bronchopulmonary aspergillosis. J Immunol 1997;159:4072–4076.
7. Stevens DA, Moss RB, Kurup VA, et al: Allergic bronchopulmonary aspergillosis in cystic fibrosis—state of the art: Cystic Fibrosis Foundation Consensus Conference. Clin Inf Diseases 2003;37 (suppl 3):S225–264.
8. Wark PAB, Hensley MJ, Saltos N, et al: Anti-inflammatory effect of itraconazole in stable allergic bronchopulmonary aspergillosis: a randomized controlled trial. J Allergy Clin Immunol 2003;111:952–957.

Churg-Strauss Syndrome

CHAPTER

44

Michael E. Wechsler

CLINICAL PEARLS

- Churg-Strauss syndrome is characterized by asthma and eosinophilia in conjunction with sinusitis, pulmonary infiltrates, neuropathy, and eosinophilic vasculitis that may involve the heart, kidneys, gastrointestinal tract, skin, or nervous system.

- Churg-Strauss syndrome must be differentiated from other eosinophilic lung conditions (e.g., eosinophilic pneumonia), vasculitides (e.g., Wegener granulomatosis), infections (e.g., helminthic infestation), other myeloproliferative and lymphoproliferative hypereosinophilic syndromes, and drug reactions.

- In addition to standard asthma therapies, oral corticosteroids are the cornerstone of Churg-Strauss syndrome management.

- Cytotoxic therapy with cyclophosphamide, azathioprine, or methotrexate should be considered for severe systemic involvement or disease that is refractory to corticosteroids.

- Patients with Churg-Strauss syndrome should be monitored on a regular basis utilizing pulmonary function testing, measurement of blood eosinophils, C-reactive protein, erythrocyte sedimentation rate, and radiologic studies including chest x-ray, computed tomography scan, or echocardiography.

In the management of patients with difficult to control asthma, one special situation that one must consider is the case of those individuals with asthma and eosinophilia who fulfill the diagnostic criteria of Churg-Strauss syndrome (CSS). CSS is a relatively rare multisystem disorder that is manifested by airway obstruction, pulmonary infiltrates, systemic eosinophilia, sinusitis, neuropathy, constitutional symptoms and eosinophilic vasculitis of several organs including the lungs, heart, gastrointestinal (GI) tract, and kidneys. Untreated, CSS may have a dire prognosis, but treatment with corticosteroids and/or other cytotoxic agents usually results in clinical remission of the disease. Thus, it is important to establish a tissue diagnosis and exclude other diseases in the differential diagnosis as treatment options differ significantly from other eosinophilic lung diseases. While the eosinophil is felt to play a central role in CSS pathogenesis, the etiology of this syndrome remains unknown. First described in the 1950s, CSS was perceived to be quite rare. While there has been an increase in reporting of CSS cases in association with various asthma therapies since the late 1990s, it does not appear that any particular agent plays a causative role in CSS pathogenesis.

DEFINITIONS

In 1951, Churg and Strauss first described this clinical disorder in patients who had severe asthma and rhinitis and developed hypereosinophilia, pneumonia, and eosinophilic arteritis and granulomas in multiple organs. They distinguished these subjects with necrotizing vasculitis, extravascular granulomas, and eosinophilic tissue invasion from others with polyarteritis nodosa by virtue of their history of asthma and allergies and were the first to call this distinct syndrome "allergic granulomatosis and angiitis." It is now referred to as *Churg-Strauss syndrome*, although Osler described a case consistent with CSS at the turn of the century.

The clinical description of syndrome has evolved significantly since Churg and Strauss described its pathologic findings. Several sets of criteria have been used to define this condition, resulting in some difficulty in clinicians' establishing the diagnosis if they adhered strictly to any one set of criteria (Table 44-1). In 1984, Lanham and colleagues noted that not all cases have the extravascular granulomas, necrotizing vasculitis, or eosinophilic tissue infiltration that characterized the original cohort, and emphasized a more clinical approach to this disease. According to the so-called Lanham

Table 44-1
CRITERIA USED IN DIAGNOSIS OF CHURG-STRAUSS SYNDROME

Churg and Strauss, 1951	1. Asthma 2. Necrotizing vasculitis of small and medium arteries and veins 3. Eosinophil infiltration around involved vessels and tissues 4. Extravascular granulomas 5. Fibrinoid necrosis of involved tissues
Lanham, 1984	1. Asthma 2. Eosinophilia > 1.5×10^7 3. Systemic vasculitis involving 2 or more organs
American College of Rheumatology, 1990	1. Asthma 2. Eosinophilia > 10% 3. Neuropathy 4. Pulmonary infiltrates 5. Paranasal sinus abnormality 6. Extravascular eosinophil infiltration on biopsy
Chapel Hill, 1994	1. Asthma 2. Eosinophilia 3. Eosinophil-rich granulomatous inflammation involving the respiratory tract 4. Necrotizing vasculitis affecting small- to medium-sized vessels

criteria, CSS is defined by asthma, peripheral eosinophilia, and systemic vasculitis involving two or more organ systems. In 1994, an international conference on vasculitis nomenclature at Chapel Hill developed a set of CSS criteria defined more by pathologic criteria. According to the Chapel Hill criteria, CSS is defined as asthma and eosinophilia in association with eosinophil-rich and granulomatous inflammation involving the respiratory tract, with necrotizing vasculitis affecting small- to medium-sized vessels. Today, the most commonly used criteria are the vasculitis classification criteria adopted by the American College of Rheumatology (ACR) in 1990, which include both clinical and pathologic features. By these criteria, CSS is defined as the presence of four of the following six features: asthma, eosinophilia, neuropathy, pulmonary infiltrates, paranasal sinus abnormality, and presence of eosinophilic vasculitis.

NATURAL HISTORY/EPIDEMIOLOGY

Although it has an incidence in the general population of 3 to 6 cases per million per year, the incidence of CSS in asthma patients is approximately 20 times higher. CSS occurs with equal frequency in men and women and the mean age at time of diagnosis is 48 years. Pediatric cases occur but are extremely rare. CSS typically occurs in several phases (Table 44-2), with the most common presenting manifestation being asthma. In these patients, asthma often arises later in life, with a mean age at onset of 35 years, and often occurs in the absence of family history of atopy. The asthma can often be severe and oral steroids are often required to control symptoms, but may lead to suppression of vasculitis. Following the prodromal asthma and allergic rhinitis phase, the second phase is characterized by peripheral eosinophilia and eosinophilic tissue infiltration of various organs including the lungs and GI tract (Table 44-3). The third phase is the vasculitic phase and may be associated with constitutional signs and symptoms including fever, weight loss, malaise and fatigue. The average length of time between diagnosis of asthma and vasculitis is 9 years.

Table 44-2
CLINICAL PHASES OF CHURG-STRAUSS SYNDROME

Prodromal phase: Asthma, allergic rhinitis, sinusitis
Eosinophilic phase: Peripheral eosinophilia, eosinophilic tissue infiltration
Vasculitic phase: End-organ vasculitis accompanied by constitutional symptoms (fever, weight loss, malaise, fatigue)

Table 44-3
ORGAN SYSTEMS INVOLVED BY CHURG-STRAUSS SYNDROME

Respiratory tract: Asthma, pulmonary infiltrates, alveolar hemorrhage, sinusitis
Nervous system: Mononeuritis multiplex, polyneuropathy, cerebral hemorrhage, stroke
Skin: Palpable purpura, skin nodules, urticaria, livedo
Heart: Cardiomyopathy, myocarditis, heart failure, arrhythmia
Kidney: Glomerulonephritis, renal insufficiency, renal infarct
Gastrointestinal tract: Ischemic bowel, pancreatitis, cholecystitis

---

CLINICAL FEATURES OF CHURG-STRAUSS SYNDROME

Presentation

As CSS develops in patients with a history of upper airway disease and asthma, patients with CSS will most often present to internists, general practitioners, allergists/immunologists, pulmonologists, and otolaryngologists. The syndrome may go unrecognized and be difficult to distinguish from asthma, however, unless other organ systems become involved or unless lab and radiologic testing are undertaken.

In addition to lung involvement, which can be manifested by cough, dyspnea, alveolar hemorrhage, and hemoptysis, CSS involves many organ systems including the sinuses, skin, nerves, heart, GI tract, and kidneys. Sinusitis can be insidious and often requires multiple courses of antibiotics and surgeries for what may be perceived as infection, before eosinophilic involvement is uncovered. While the allergic features of CSS are often but not always dominant, patients with CSS may be seen by neurologists, dermatologists, cardiologists, hematologists, and nephrologists for the extra pulmonary manifestations. Neurologic involvement occurs in approximately 78% of patients, with mononeuritis multiplex commonly affecting the peroneal, ulnar, radial, internal popliteal, and, occasionally, cranial nerves. Polyneuropathy may develop in the absence of treatment, and may be symmetric or asymmetric. Cerebral hemorrhage and infarction may also occur and are important causes of death. Despite treatment, neurologic sequelae often do not completely resolve.

Approximately half of CSS patients develop dermatologic manifestations. These include palpable purpura, skin nodules, urticarial rashes, and livedo. The heart is a primary target organ in CSS and often portends a worse prognosis. Granulomas, vasculitis, and widespread myocardial damage may be found on biopsy or at autopsy, and cardiomyopathy and heart failure may be seen in up to half of all patients, but are often at least partially reversible. Acute pericarditis, constrictive pericarditis, myocardial infarction, and other electrocardiographic changes all may occur. Gastrointestinal symptoms are also common in CSS and likely represent an eosinophilic gastroenteritis characterized by abdominal pain, diarrhea, GI bleeding, and colitis. Ischemic bowel, pancreatitis, and cholecystitis have also been reported in association with CSS and usually portend a worse prognosis. Renal involvement is more common than once thought and approximately 25% of patients may demonstrate proteinuria, glomerulonephritis, renal insufficiency, and, rarely, renal infarct. Constitutional symptoms are very common in CSS and include weight loss of 10 to 20 pounds, fevers, and diffuse myalgias and migratory polyarthralgias. Myositis may be present with evidence of vasculitis on muscle biopsies.

Laboratory and Radiologic Abnormalities

Systemic eosinophilia is the hallmark laboratory finding in patients with CSS and reflects the likely pathogenic role that the eosinophil plays in this disease. Eosinophilia greater than 10% is one of the defining features of this illness and may be as high as 75% of the peripheral white blood cell count. It is present at the time of diagnosis in over 80% of subjects but may respond quickly (often within 24 hours) to initiation of systemic corticosteroid therapy. Even in the absence of systemic eosinophilia, tissue eosinophilia may be present.

While not specific to CSS, antineutrophil cytoplasmic antibodies (ANCAs) are present in up to two thirds of patients, mostly with a perinuclear staining pattern. Other nonspecific lab abnormalities that may be present in patients with CSS include an elevated erythrocyte sedimentation rate (ESR), anemia, elevated immunoglobulin E (IgE), and positive rheumatoid factor and antinuclear antibody. While bronchoalveolar lavage often reveals significant eosinophilia, this may be seen in other eosinophilic lung diseases. Similarly, pulmonary function testing often reveals an obstructive defect similar to asthma.

Chest x-ray abnormalities are extremely common in CSS and consist of bilateral nonsegmental, patchy infiltrates that often migrate and may be interstitial or alveolar in appearance. Reticulonodular and nodular disease without cavitation can be seen, as can pleural effusions and hilar adenopathy. The most common thin-section CT findings include bilateral ground-glass opacity and airspace consolidation that is predominantly subpleural and surrounded by the ground-glass opacity. Other CT findings include bronchial wall thickening, hyperinflation, interlobular septal thickening, lymph node enlargement and pericardial and pleural effusions.

PATHOGENESIS

Like other vasculitides, the etiology and pathogenesis of CSS remain unknown and very few studies have addressed potential pathophysiological mechanisms of CSS. As ANCAs are present in many patients with CSS, some have speculated that the binding of ANCAs to vascular walls contributes to vascular inflammation and injury as well as chemotaxis of inflammatory cells. It is also felt that this syndrome likely represents an autoimmune process because of the prominence of allergic features and the presence of immune complexes, heightened T-cell immunity, and altered humoral immunity, as evidenced by elevated IgE, ANCA, and rheumatoid factor. However, a component of eosinophil regulation is clearly aberrant in this population as CSS is distinguished from asthma and other entities by virtue of the peripheral eosinophilia and significant tissue infiltration by eosinophils resulting in necrotizing vasculitis and extravascular granulomas (Fig. 44-1). These may occur in isolation or may coexist, and are commonly found in the lungs, heart, skin, muscle, liver, spleen and kidneys. The eosinophilic vasculitis predominantly affects small and medium-sized arteries and veins, and may include fibrinoid necrosis and thrombosis.

There is evidence of a perturbation in various cytokines in this syndrome. CSS is associated with markedly increased levels of circulating soluble interleukin (IL)-2 receptor, eosinophil cationic protein, and thrombomodulin, indicating that activation of eosinophils and T cells may be important in CSS pathogenesis. CSS is also characterized by increased production of IL-4, IL-13, and interferon-gamma relative to that in healthy controls, suggesting an important role for type 2 cytokine production. Others have shown that among the cytokines, only IL-10 is able to discriminate between CSS and Wegener granulomatosis or microscopic polyangiitis.

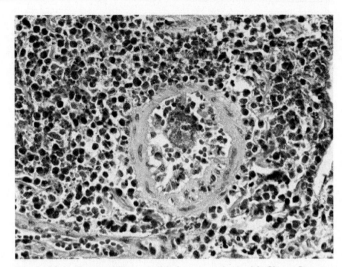

Figure 44-1 **Eosinophilic vasculitis from a patient with Churg-Strauss syndrome.** Abundant eosinophils are appreciated within the blood vessel wall and within the vascular lumen (hematoxylin and eosin, ×400, original photo).

More recently, it was observed that vascular endothelial growth factor (VEGF) levels were elevated in CSS patients; this suggested that VEGF released from eosinophils might contribute to the recruitment of inflammatory cells, including T cells and eosinophils, by increasing vascular permeability in the development of CSS. Another hypothesis suggested that CSS results from an impairment of CD95 ligand-mediated killing of lymphocytes and eosinophils in CSS and is also thought to result from variation in the expression of the CD95 receptor isoform. Because of the potential association between CSS and the use of leukotriene modifiers, it has been hypothesized that CSS results from an imbalance of leukotrienes in the setting of cysteinyl leukotriene receptor blockade. To date, this theory has not been tested. In summary, while each of these molecular entities may play a role in CSS pathogenesis, it is not clear exactly how eosinophils mediate the pathophysiology of CSS and which specific mediators are most important in the development of this disease.

While there has been an abundance of active research in the genetics of asthma, to date no specific studies of the genetics or heritability of CSS have been reported. There has been one report describing the familial clustering of CSS and a related ANCA-associated vasculitis, Wegener granulomatosis, in first-degree relatives who shared a common human leukocytes antigen (HLA) haplotype. There have been a number of reports of other ANCA-associated vasculitides clustered within families. However, while there has been some association between ANCA-associated vasculitides and genes encoding for proteinase 3 (PR3, a target of ANCA) and its inhibitor, alpha-1 antitrypsin, no specific genes involved in ANCA-related disease induction or expression have yet been identified.

CLINICAL COURSE

While the natural clinical course of CSS is modified by systemic corticosteroids and other therapies, the clinical course of CSS is variable and prognosis depends substantially on early establishment of a CSS diagnosis, early implementation of therapy, and close clinical follow-up with vigilance for relapse.

Establishing a Diagnosis

One must use a combination of clinical, laboratory, pathologic, and radiographic criteria to establish a diagnosis of CSS. Generally, the presence of vasculitis and eosinophilia in an individual with airway obstruction is enough to make a diagnosis of CSS. While a biopsy specimen with eosinophilic vasculitis is desired in most cases, noninvasive surrogates of CSS pathogenesis including electromyogram (EMG), nerve conduction studies, or perinuclear ANCA (pANCA) can often be used to establish the diagnosis. The most common sites for biopsy include the skin, nerve and muscle, although pathologic specimens may be obtained from biopsy of any affected organ system including the lung (by open lung or thoracoscopic biopsy; transbronchial biopsy is generally not helpful), the heart (by endomyocardial biopsy), the GI tract (endoscopically), the liver, or the kidney. Angiography is often used diagnostically and may show signs of vasculitis in the coronary, central nervous system, and peripheral vasculature.

Although the onset of the vasculitis phase is often sudden, the duration of the prodromal phase can be difficult to precisely identify. Most patients appear to suddenly experience the development of the cardinal manifestations (such as foot drop, palpable purpura, or pulmonary infiltrates) without a perceptible prodrome. Most likely, blood and tissue eosinophilia develop over extended time but are unrecognized. Acute-phase reactants and ANCAs also probably become detectable during the preclinical phase, but for most patients, these tests are not routinely obtained for asthma treatment. Hence, the possibility of CSS should be considered early on, and difficult-to-treat asthmatics should be screened periodically for peripheral blood eosinophilia.

Even in the presence of asthma and significant eosinophilia, the diagnosis of CSS can be difficult and includes a broad differential. While it is generally best to satisfy at least four of the six ACR criteria, several other eosinophilic lung conditions may present with similar findings and constitutional symptoms (Table 44-4). For instance, patients with allergic bronchopulmonary aspergillosis (ABPA) or chronic eosinophilic pneumonia may present with airway obstruction, sinus disease, eosinophilia, and pulmonary infiltrates, but do not necessarily have end-organ evidence of vasculitis that would define them as having CSS. Other conditions in the differential diagnosis of CSS include other vasculitides

such as Wegener granulomatosis or microscopic polyangiitis; infections, including helminthic and fungal disease; drug reactions; bronchocentric granulomatosis; eosinophilic granuloma; malignancy; and both myeloproliferative and lymphocytic variants of the hypereosinophilic syndromes. While subjects with each of these disorders may meet ACR criteria, the treatment algorithm differs significantly for each of these entities; therefore, it is extremely important to make a tissue diagnosis before proceeding with therapy.

CSS Therapy and Prognosis

Most patients diagnosed with CSS have previously been diagnosed with asthma, rhinitis, and sinusitis, and have received treatment with inhaled or systemic corticosteroids. As these agents are also the initial treatment of choice for CSS patients, institution of these therapies in patients with CSS who are perceived to have severe asthma may delay the diagnosis of CSS as signs of vasculitis may be masked. Corticosteroids (starting at 1 mg/kg, and tapering over 3 to 6 months) dramatically alter the course of CSS: up to 50% of those who are untreated die within 3 months of diagnosis while treated subjects have a 6-year survival of over 70%. Common causes of death include heart failure, cerebral hemorrhage, renal failure, and GI bleeding, as well as sepsis due to immunosuppression. Recent data suggest that clinical remission may be obtained in over 90% of subjects treated; approximately 25% of those subjects may relapse, often due to corticosteroid tapering, with a rising eosinophil count heralding the relapse. Myocardial, GI, and renal involvement most often portends a poor prognosis. In such cases, treatment with higher doses of corticosteroids or the addition of cytotoxic agents such as cyclophosphamide is often warranted. Although survival does not differ between those treated or untreated with cyclophosphamide, it is associated with a reduced incidence of relapse and an improved clinical response to treatment. Other therapies that have been used successfully in the management of CSS include azathioprine, methotrexate, intravenous gamma globulin, and interferon alpha. Plasma exchange has not been shown to provide any additional benefit.

Monitoring of Disease Activity

Monitoring of disease activity is essential in order to prevent clinical relapses and to maximize therapeutic benefit while minimizing therapy-related toxicity. Assessment of treatment response in affected patients, however, is limited by the relatively poor understanding of the natural history of the disease. Although the essential pathophysiologic feature of CSS is tissue eosinophilia, repeated tissue biopsy is not practical and blood eosinophilia is not always a reliable marker of tissue eosinophilia. Nevertheless, the monitoring of blood eosinophil counts is generally a useful strategy to facilitate decision making for changes in therapy. Reductions in blood eosinophil counts coupled with the improvement of clinical findings (such as skin lesions, foot drop, and chest radiograph findings) provide reassurance that the treatment is effective. Monitoring of acute-phase reactants (erythrocyte sedimentation rate, C-reactive protein levels, or quantified ANCA) in conjunction with symptom assessment can also be important in guiding care.

Table 44-4
DIFFERENTIAL DIAGNOSIS OF CHURG-STRAUSS SYNDROME: DISEASE ENTITIES ASSOCIATED WITH PULMONARY INFILTRATES AND EOSINOPHILIA

Acute eosinophilic pneumonia
Allergic bronchopulmonary aspergillosis (ABPA)
Asthma
Bronchocentric granulomatosis
Chronic eosinophilic pneumonia
Drug reactions
Hypereosinophilic syndromes
Infections, including bacterial, fungal, mycobacterial, and parasitic
Malignancy, including lymphoma and leukemia
Sarcoidosis
Vasculitides, including Wegener granulomatosis and microscopic polyangiitis

The frequency of monitoring for any laboratory value depends on the clinical situation. A general recommendation is to assess blood eosinophil counts and acute phase reactants frequently during the initiation of therapy, weekly to monthly when the disease is stable, and every few months during long-term care. Repeat ANCA testing may be helpful when discordant laboratory or clinical findings occur or after clinical control of the disease (to establish a new baseline value). Increases in ANCAs, peripheral eosinophil counts, and/or acute-phase reactants may precede clinical exacerbation and increased vigilance is warranted. Increasing therapy before clinical worsening probably results in reduced morbidity and mortality rates and the total medication required for disease control. Exacerbation or relapse may occur after prolonged periods of apparent disease inactivity; therefore, extended clinical and laboratory monitoring are encouraged. The lack of detectable disease activity for more than 18 to 24 months would mitigate the value of ongoing laboratory follow-up, but relapse should be considered indefinitely. Clinical acumen and judicious use of the laboratory are essential in following CSS.

CONTROVERSIES

CSS Epidemiology and Relationship to Asthma Therapy: Do Asthma Therapies Cause CSS?

Although CSS has long been thought of as a rare disease, there has been a recent increase in case reports in association with different asthma therapies, raising the question of the true rarity of this entity. This has raised the question of whether recognition of the condition has improved or whether the incidence in association with various forms of asthma therapy has actually increased. Recognition of an association with asthma therapies first became apparent in the late 1990s when CSS was first reported in patients receiving zafirlukast. Since then, there have been several reports of the syndrome in association with both montelukast and pranlukast and with various inhaled steroids. In these cases, CSS occurred in patients with long histories of difficult-to-control asthma after patients had either tapered systemic or high doses of inhaled steroids or had advancing disease despite increasing doses of inhaled steroids. In many cases, CSS developed following steroid withdrawal as a result of, or concomitant with, leukotriene modifier or inhaled steroid use in patients who likely had what was perceived to be severe asthma but was likely CSS masked by steroids (forme fruste CSS).

While incidence estimates of CSS have ranged from two to four cases per million patient-years in the general population, recent studies have ascertained the incidence of CSS in asthma populations, the individuals who are at highest risk for developing this syndrome, to be approximately 60 cases per million patient-years. Thus, although current estimates of CSS incidence suggest it is indeed a rare disease in the general population, it is likely not as rare as once thought, especially when the asthma population inherently at risk for developing the syndrome is considered. It is likely that CSS incidence rates are actually higher, as many cases of CSS remain unreported or have yet to be recognized because of masking by systemic or high doses of inhaled steroids. CSS has been associated with various asthma therapies, including leukotriene modifiers and inhaled corticosteroids, but no causal

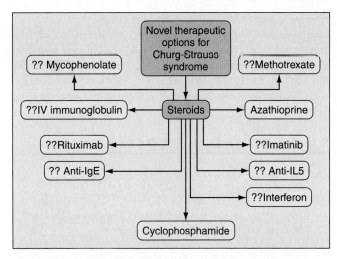

Figure 44-2   Novel therapeutic options for Churg-Strauss syndrome. Many different immunosuppressants have been tried in addition to corticosteroids. While data are scant for many of these options and few large trials exist, it is hoped that newer biologic therapies may be beneficial for the management of CSS.

link has been established. The relationship could be due to confounding, unmasking, or some causal relationship to drug treatment. This is an area of active ongoing research.

Can CSS Be Cured? What Are the Goals of Therapy?

A major question that CSS patients often ask is whether or not their disease can be cured. While in rare circumstances some CSS patients may be able to taper off both corticosteroid therapy and immunosuppressants, most patients who stop anti-inflammatory therapy develop clinical relapses consisting of worsening asthma or recurrence of vasculitis. Thus, the goal of therapy is to get the disease under control at the outset, to prevent any long-term damage, and to prevent relapses. While another goal of CSS management is to minimize adverse effects associated with these therapies, one must balance treatment-related toxicity with relapse-related long-term damage such as irreversible neuropathy. Thus, it is strongly recommended that patients be maintained on low levels of systemic corticosteroids or immunosuppressants until we learn more about what causes relapses, and what the underlying pathophysiology of CSS is. It is possible that newer therapies such as monoclonal antibodies directed against IL-5, tumor-necrosis factor, or B cells may address underlying pathology and hopefully result in a "cure" of this otherwise difficult-to-control disease (Fig. 44-2).

SUMMARY AND CONCLUSIONS

Churg-Strauss syndrome is a relatively rare multisystem disorder associated with asthma that is manifested by airway obstruction, pulmonary infiltrates, systemic eosinophilia, sinusitis, neuropathy, constitutional symptoms and eosinophilic vasculitis of several organs including the lungs, heart, GI tract, and kidneys. It is important to establish a tissue diagnosis and exclude other diseases in the differential diagnosis as treatment options differ significantly from other eosinophilic lung diseases. Untreated, CSS may have a dire prognosis, but treatment with corticosteroids and/or other cytotoxic agents usually results in clinical remission of the disease. While the eosinophil is felt to play a central role in CSS pathogenesis, the etiology of this syndrome remains unknown. While there has been an increase in reporting of CSS cases in association with leukotriene modifiers and inhaled corticosteroids, no causative role for these agents in CSS pathogenesis has been firmly established. It is hoped that newer biologic therapies targeted at the underlying biology of eosinophils and vasculitis will result in long-term beneficial effects for patients with this syndrome.

SUGGESTED READING

Churg J, Strauss L: Allergic granulomatosis, allergic angiitis, and periarteritis nodosa. Am J Pathol 1951;27:277–301.

Guillevin L, Cohen P, Gayraud M, et al: Churg-Strauss syndrome. Clinical study and long-term follow-up of 96 patients. Medicine (Baltimore) 1999;78:26–37.

Harrold LR, Andrade SE, Go AS, et al: Incidence of Churg-Strauss syndrome in asthma drug users: a population-based perspective. J Rheumatol 2005;32:1076–1080.

Hellmich B, Ehlers S, Csernok E, Gross WL: Update on the pathogenesis of Churg-Strauss syndrome. Clin Exp Rheumatol 2003; 21:S69–S77.

Klion AD, Bochner BS, Gleich GJ, et al: Approaches to the treatment of hypereosinophilic syndromes: a workshop summary report. J Allergy Clin Immunol 2006;117(6):1292–1302.

Lanham JG, Elkon KB, Pusey CD, Hughes GR: Systemic vasculitis with asthma and eosinophilia: a clinical approach to the Churg-Strauss syndrome. Medicine 1984;63:65.

Masi AT, Hunder GG, Lie JT, et al: The American College of Rheumatology 1990 criteria for the classification of Churg-Strauss syndrome (allergic granulomatosis and angiitis). Arthritis Rheum 1990; 33:1094–1100.

Noth I, Strek ME, Leff A: Churg-Strauss syndrome. Lancet 2003; 361:587–594.

Wechsler ME, Garpestad E, Flier SR, et al: Pulmonary infiltrates, eosinophilia, and cardiomyopathy following corticosteroid withdrawal in patients with asthma receiving zafirlukast. JAMA 1998; 279:455–457.

Weller PF, Plaut M, Taggart V, Trontell A: Relationship of asthma therapy and Churg-Strauss syndrome: NIH workshop summary report. J Allerg Clin Immunol 2001; 108(2):175–183.

Psychological Sequelae in Pediatric Asthma: Identification and Intervention

CHAPTER 45

Jane Robinson, Bruce G. Bender, and Kimberly Kelsay

CLINICAL PEARLS

- Psychological distress can appear in numerous forms, each impeding attempts to successfully treat the chronic illness.

- Health care professionals must assess psychosocial stressors among children with asthma.

- Observable behaviors may signal need for psychosocial intervention.

- The presence of a psychosocial clinician on the medical treatment team can significantly facilitate effective treatment of childhood asthma.

In 2001, an estimated 8.7% of all children in the United States, or nearly 6.3 million children,[1] had asthma. Included in the epidemiologic picture are significant psychosocial consequences from childhood asthma that impact family finances, restrict the child's physical activities, impair the child's development of social connections and adaptive resources, and cause general disruption in the family.[2] Psychological distress can result from childhood asthma, and it can in turn directly impact inflammatory processes and subsequently asthma symptoms.[3]

In the past decade, emerging asthma research has helped to identify cellular and molecular explanations for the underlying pathophysiology that is responsible for the exacerbations and persistence of asthma.[4] In addition to identification of key biological factors, there is growing body of evidence regarding the interface and reciprocal interaction between biology of asthma, behavior, stress and the immune system.[5,6] Wright and colleagues[6] identified three trends in medical research that have led both clinicians and investigators to reconsider the role of psychosocial stress in asthma: (1) rising worldwide incidence in the diagnosis of asthma; (2) evidence linking behavioral, neural, endocrine and immune processes; and (3) recognition of the substantial role of the social environment and social integration in health and disease. Collectively, these trends have resulted in a paradigm shift linking psychological stress to endocrine and immune functioning and provide a framework to explore the mind-body relationship in the presence of pediatric asthma. For clinicians who treat childhood asthma, the identification and amelioration of stressors that cause psychological distress and interfere with the management of asthma can be daunting. Health care professionals frequently identify barriers that preclude them from probing psychosocial concerns: (1) limited time during the medical appointment; (2) hesitation in identifying psychological concerns because of a lack of knowledge about how to intervene or where to refer the patient; (3) fear that asking about emotionally laden content will result in negative emotion that the health care professional may not be equipped to manage; (4) uncertainty about how to query psychosocial issues; and (5) concern that the family will think the health care professional is implying they are "crazy" if a referral to a psychosocial clinician is recommended.

This chapter provides a definition of stress, identifies behavioral observations that might guide health care professionals to identify areas of potential stress, and through two clinical case examples, illustrates approaches to treatment of the psychosocial effects of pediatric asthma.

WHAT IS "STRESS"?

When confronted with environmental demands, individuals cognitively appraise whether an event is threatening or potentially overwhelming to their existing coping resources.[7] Events that are judged to place demands on an individual are labeled as stressors. If the demands are found to be taxing or threatening, and at the same time coping resources are viewed to be inadequate, individuals will perceive themselves as under stress.[8] Cohen and colleagues[8] conceptualized stress within three primary categories: (1) objective characteristics, (2) subjective characteristics, and (3) physiologic responses. Each of these definitions also suggests specific approaches to assessment.

1. Objective characteristics. The most common approach to defining stress identifies the *events that create the stressful stimuli*. This approach typically uses self-report checklists derived from studies linking events and negative outcomes. Participants indicate whether specific events such as loss of employment, death of spouse, or incarceration have occurred within the past 6 or 12 months. In some cases, queries are made asking participants about the duration and intensity of the stress.

2. Subjective characteristics. The second approach to defining stress considers the importance of the individual's subjective reactions to the stressor. If demands are perceived as threatening and coping resources inadequate, this can result in negative mood states such as fear, anger, anxiety, and/or depression. Therefore, this approach asserts that the amount of stress experienced depends in large part on how an individual interprets the situation. The same objective event may cause different stress reactions in different individuals depending on their perceived ability to manage and cope with the stressor. Assessing the participants' subjective response to life stress entails querying their perceptions of stress. For example, questionnaires can measure general perceived

stress, and assess the degree to which subjects find life to be stressful. More specific questions can also be posed that query appraisals of specific life events.

3. Physiologic responses. The third approach incorporates attempts to detect a physiologic response to stress. The same stressor may cause different reactions in different individuals; assessment relies on understanding physiologic indicators of stress rather than an individual's self-report. Physiologic approaches to measuring stress responses include assessing stress responses of the autonomic nervous system, the neuroendocrine system, and the immune system.

Stress in sufficient intensity and duration may impact the onset and severity of chronic diseases including asthma. This possibility has been explored and assessed in many studies involving clinical observations, laboratory studies with animals and humans, and in epidemiologic and clinical studies. A range of stressors such as public disaster, performing mental arithmetic tasks, school examinations, public speaking, family conflict, neighborhood events, and exposure to violence have been documented to be related to asthma symptoms.[9] Stress may impact children and families through changes in health behavior or comorbid diseases, or may have more direct physiologic effects through the pathways impacting inflammation including neuroendocrine, immune, and oxidative systems.[5]

Stressful events and their impact on health and illness are determined, in part, by the intensity, duration and frequency of the stressor.[8] Life stressors can last for years or a few minutes. For example, ongoing unemployment, poverty, and living in a dangerous environment all represent chronic external stimuli that trigger the stress response and their biological concomitants. However, the potential for negative consequences of stress also depends on the long-term mitigation of individual coping resources. On the other hand, events that last a very short time but are significantly traumatic can have long-term stress effects and lasting physiological responses. In addition, several stressors can occur together with potential additive effects. Therefore, interventions must consider effects of recent stress, events that have occurred well in the past, co-occurring stress, and the individual's internalization of distant and ongoing events. Further complicating the relationship between stress and illness is the finding that illness itself can also act as a stressor.[10]

HOW CAN THE CLINICIAN IDENTIFY POTENTIALLY DANGEROUS LEVELS OF STRESS IN THE CHILD AND FAMILY?

Behaviors demonstrated in the office can be cues to psychosocial stress within the child, in the parent/child relationship, within the family system, and/or within a larger system (e.g., community, school, social support system). Table 45-1 describes some stressors that have been associated with negative outcomes for asthma, and behaviors that may be indicative of these problems.

The health care professional who identifies psychosocial stressors within the family may find the subject difficult to broach. A general statement regarding the stress of living with a chronic illness can open the door for further communication. For example, "We believe asthma can be a very stressful experience for everyone in the family. So, I would like to

Table 45-1
BEHAVIORS THAT MAY INDICATE PROBLEMS WITH FAMILY, CHILD, OR SCHOOL

Source of Stress	Example of Observable Behavior
Parent-child relationship problems	Bickering between child and parent, parent unable to set effective limits
Parent marital problems	One parent is rarely seen at appointments, is spoken about disparagingly
Parent/staff conflict	Parent is hostile with staff
Child psychopathology	Child is irritable or anxious
Parent psychopathology	Parent distracted, disorganized, distressed, or labile
Overwhelmed parent coping	Medications are not refilled, appointments are missed
Poor school functioning	Child is missing more school than physician would agree is indicated due to disease

ask you a few questions and then give you the opportunity to discuss concerns that are important to you." Providing the family an opportunity to discuss their concerns can open up more emotional content than the clinician is prepared to handle. The following statement is an example of how to graciously contain the discussion while also leaving the family with a sense of support: "Thank you for sharing your concerns. I see that this is a very distressing topic for you and appreciate that you trust me with this sensitive information. I have a colleague I would like to refer you to so you can discuss these concerns further." Importantly, the clinician must acknowledge the psychological distress identified by the family and offer a means of addressing the problem, often by referral to a mental health professional.

Table 45-2 includes examples of questions that can lead to more in-depth information about the child's and the family's functioning.

SUBJECTIVE REACTIONS AS SOURCES OF STRESS

Some children and families are able to discuss their feelings about asthma, while others may struggle to put their feelings into words. Mental health professionals often facilitate patients' expression of feelings through art. This technique can also be useful in the asthma clinic setting while patients are waiting for tests or appointments. This task can be framed in the context of understanding more about the illness, for example, "I treat lots of children with asthma, but I don't know what it is like to have asthma. Can you draw me a picture of what having asthma feels like to you?" Art can provide an enlightening window into the patient's subjective experience of the stress of their illness. Just as people vary considerably in their individual reactions to a stressor, children with chronic illness likewise may have quite different responses to their illness, and even those without life-threatening asthma may find their illness to be greatly distressing. The artwork presented in Figure 45-1 depicts an elephant sitting on a boy's chest, a clear communication from this child about his distress over asthma. Many children take delight in explaining their artwork, and in so doing often share important information about the subjective experience of their disease.

Table 45-2
QUESTIONS TO ELICIT PSYCHOSOCIAL CONCERNS

Coping	1. Chronic illness generally stresses everyone in the family. How are you managing all the responsibility and the worry? How about your spouse? child? other children?
	2. Children are often angry at their illness. Does your child ever express any anger? fear? panic?
	3. Do you have any concerns at all about your child's adjustment in other areas besides his/her illness?
	4. Do you think your child has been traumatized by any medical procedure or perceptions of his/her illness?
Medical Compliance	1. It must be difficult managing all your children, the household, and the asthma too. Do you have any help with giving your child medications? Do you ever skip doses because it is just too difficult?
	2. Do you have any struggles getting your child to take his/her medications? What is giving you the most difficulty? How do you handle it?
	3. If the patient is in charge of his/her medications: There is a lot to remember. What type of help does he/she want?
School/Social Activities	1. How is your child doing in school? Any recent changes?
	2. How many days of school has your child missed because of his/her asthma?
	3. How does he/she feel about taking medication in front of other children? Is it difficult for him/her to do this? Does your child try to hide symptoms from peers?
	4. Has your child missed a lot of activities with friends like sports, church activities, or social events? If so: Does your child ever talk about it?
Loss/Grief	1. Has your child had to give up activities because of asthma? If so: Has he/she expressed sadness about this loss?
	2. Have you or your spouse had to change jobs or quit your job to care for your child?
	3. Are you having financial stress because of your child's medical expenses?

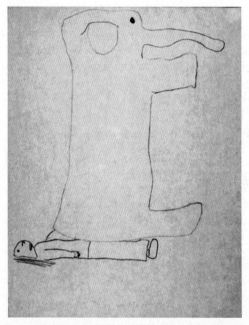

Figure 45-1 Child's drawing depicting his distress over asthma in the form of an elephant sitting on his chest.

BRIEF INTERVENTION STRATEGIES

In the National Jewish Medical and Research Center tertiary care setting, mental health services are available to all children with asthma and their families, most of whom are visiting our clinic for several days to 2 weeks. Patients generally present to this asthma clinic with diagnostic challenges or symptoms that are not controlled to the satisfaction of their referring physician or the patient's family. Children and families in these circumstances can generally benefit from a brief mental health intervention. Given time limits during hectic visits, often from out-of-state families, a very focused practical approach to providing intervention has been developed. The main goal is to assess needs and target intervention to these needs. The conceptualization of stress from outside

events and from the illness itself has been helpful in these assessments and interventions, leads to rapid identification of key problems, and is generally well-accepted by families.

The Stress of Illness

There are several tasks specific to illness. If patients and their families are struggling with these tasks, this may indicate that the illness is particularly stressful or that the family has inadequate resources to cope with the illness. Illness tasks include symptom recognition, formulating a plan to address symptoms, communicating with the health care professionals, complying with medications and medical recommendations, and managing emotions around illness. Tasks that are not specific to illness but are complicated by illness include many of the major tasks of childhood: achieving growth and developmental milestones, forming peer relationships, attending and succeeding at school, participating in other activities, maintaining good nutrition and fitness, maintaining good relationships within the family, avoiding substance abuse and other risk-taking behaviors, maintaining a good self-image. When framed within the context of living with asthma, patients and families are generally willing to share this information within a short intake interview. Intervention is focused first on any problems with illness-specific tasks and secondly on tasks made more difficult by asthma. For many families, psycho-educational intervention about coping with illness, normalization of problems when appropriate, and what to expect in the future can be helpful. The psycho-educational approach involves strategically sharing educational information with patients and families and guiding problem-solving discussion. For example, families are often relieved to hear that many adolescents have difficulty taking steroids because of side effects, and that noncompliance is not always an indication that a child wants to be sick. Compliance is generally approached through a family systems model emphasizing that most children and adolescents can benefit from some level of supervision and help, and fostering a working agreement within the family about how to share responsibilities for illness care. The level of supervision can be adjusted to the child's need and varies from a parent witnessing the child taking their medication to the parent monitoring a checkoff sheet. Some families may have needs around illness-specific tasks that cannot be met during a brief intervention. For example, panic or post-traumatic stress disorder (PTSD) around medical events can be identified but may need a referral for further treatment within the patient's community.

Interventions targeting difficulty mastering major tasks of childhood may be accomplished during the visit, or may also need further intervention and referral to mental health providers within the home community. For example, a child who is having difficulty in school because of illness absences may benefit from a school care plan letter or call to school administration staff. The letter may help the school track absences through medical documentation, provide structure for obtaining homework and completing catch-up work, and give the school a plan to manage symptoms that occur while the child is at school. A more complicated intervention may include a referral to mental health clinician for treatment of school avoidance brought on by absences due to illness.

Stressors That Can Affect Asthma

While relationship problems, mental illness, and coping difficulties can impact asthma as outlined above and in Table 45-1, some families may be less willing to discuss these areas. Families with limited insight or shame may have difficulty understanding how their psychopathology or marital distress might affect their child's asthma and may perceive probes into these topics as intrusive. The goal of our brief intervention with these families is to establish a model of mental health intervention that is tolerated by the family and may lead them to seek rather than to avoid working with mental health providers in the future. This entails following the family's lead regarding their comfort, gentle probing and interpretation, and modeling. For example, some families are not comfortable with their child or adolescent seeing the mental health provider alone. The team is careful to assess this and not overstep these boundaries set by the family. With resistant families, distress is often present, and through beginning to relieve this, the mental health clinician can begin to ally with the family and plant the seed for future intervention.

Other families are open and willing to work on areas of stress that may impact asthma. Surprisingly, often the family has not realized how stresses in other aspects of their lives can impact illness. Helping the family make this connection can often enable them to care for these aspects of their lives. For example, parents may be feeling overwhelmed and depressed, but have not allowed themselves the time and energy to address this as they feel their child's asthma should take precedence. After realizing that they can provide better care for their child if they care for themselves, they are more willing to address this issue. One of the goals of the brief intervention is then to identify problems and mobilize the family to address these problems, as they are likely affecting the asthma. Some problems may require longer interventions and referrals to local mental health clinicians.

Although not always possible, it is preferable to refer the child to a mental health professional with knowledge about the medical illness being treated. Although insurance plans will limit the choice of clinicians, many physicians develop a relationship with one or more mental health clinicians, including psychiatrists, psychologists, and social workers, which facilitates communication and ensures shared goals. Referrals to mental health clinicians who may or may not have expertise in working with children with chronic illness or asthma often entail more than setting up an appointment. Outside clinicians are often very appreciative of additional information regarding the child's illness. It is helpful for the receiving clinician to understand the level of severity of illness, optimum symptom control for this patient, medical regimen, and other information relevant to managing illness such as concerns about compliance. The receiving mental health provider should be provided a contact number from the medical team, and feedback as to ongoing asthma management. Our mental health team also provides a psycho-educational intervention to the receiving clinicians about any ongoing problems. For example, clinicians in the community may feel that a child with severe asthma is expected to be depressed and therefore the depression cannot be treated. Although depression may be more common in children with severe asthma, it is not expected, and treatment with an antidepressant can be effective.

CASE 1

The following case demonstrates how asthma can lead to stress and consequently anxiety. This family is also struggling with a basic task of asthma, understanding and supervising the child's medical regimen.

Initial Presentation and Symptoms

Patient B, a 10-year-old white male, was referred to the Pediatric Day Treatment Program by his physician for diagnostic evaluation of asthma and potential contributing food allergies. B arrived with his parents, who looked somewhat defensive and angry while they oriented to the unit. Although scheduled for a 2-week visit, the family immediately began asking if they could leave early, in part because this visit was a significant financial burden and B's mother was at risk for losing her job having already missed numerous days of work because of B's illnesses. During the intake procedure, both parents appeared somewhat perplexed as to why their home health care professional had referred them for an extensive evaluation. They provided an incomplete medical history, and it became apparent that B knew more about his food allergies and asthma than did his parents. Both parents continually deferred to B for specific information. B, on the other hand, was an astute medical historian capable of reporting specific incidents of vomiting that were associated with certain foods as well as the number of times he had used his inhaler in the past several weeks. B's parents were surprised to learn that he had been using his rescue inhaler 3 to 5 times a day. B's medical history was unremarkable until 15 months of age, when he began to experience vomiting and nausea. He was diagnosed with hypereosinophilia and atopic dermatitis and went on to develop asthma by 5 years of age. B had never experienced a severe anaphylaxis, cyanosis, emergency services, intubation, intensive care unit (ICU) admission, or any recent hospitalization due to his illnesses. Medical interventions and testing had consisted mainly of blood draws, x-rays, spirometery, and skin prick testing.

Identification of Psychosocial Risk Factors

Several psychosocial "red flags" were identified in the medical and psychological intakes.

1. The parents in this family had relinquished to their child the responsibility for managing his illness. B's parents inappropriately assumed he was capable of managing both his asthma and food allergies. Coupled with this assumption was the observation that neither of B's parents had a clear understanding of B's asthma or food allergies.

2. B presented with mild to moderate anxiety. This was in contrast to his initial attempts to present himself as a child who had mastered life's challenges. In fact, as would be discovered through individual and group therapy, B maintained some very serious misperceptions about his illness, which in turn contributed to significant anxiety and fear.

3. The family was financially strained and B's mother was at risk of job loss due to B's chronic illness. Moreover, B's mother maintained some guilt because B had consumed so much of her attention, thus taking from her other children who were becoming resentful and angry toward B.

Interventions

Despite their initial defensiveness, B's parents allowed him to participate in individual and creative arts therapy, and they participated in family therapy. During an art therapy session B began to reveal a major source of his anxiety. B and another child portrayed themselves in their art project as doctors. In this scenario, B and his doctor friend told a child that she needed surgery because there was something wrong with her heart. During the surgery the doctors failed to administer enough medicine and the patient bled to death during the surgery. The doctors could do nothing to stop her death. The scenario included a funeral (Figs. 45-2 and 45-3).

Over the course of several individual sessions, and in conjunction with the art therapist, B revealed significant

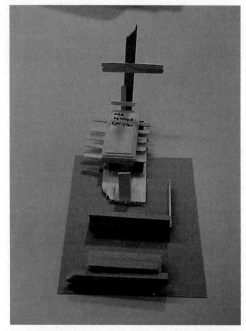

Figure 45-3 Child's artwork depicting a funeral scene and revealing his misperceptions that his illness would lead to his death.

perceptions and feelings. B's main fear was that he was "going to die." He was certain of this because he had heard a doctor say his high eosinophil count would cause heart damage. B also expressed his distrust of medical personnel, especially doctors: "Haven't you ever seen *ER*? Those doctors always mess up and kill people all the time! The doctors don't know what they are doing." B's misperceptions of illness and the psychological distress this was creating had until this point gone unrecognized.

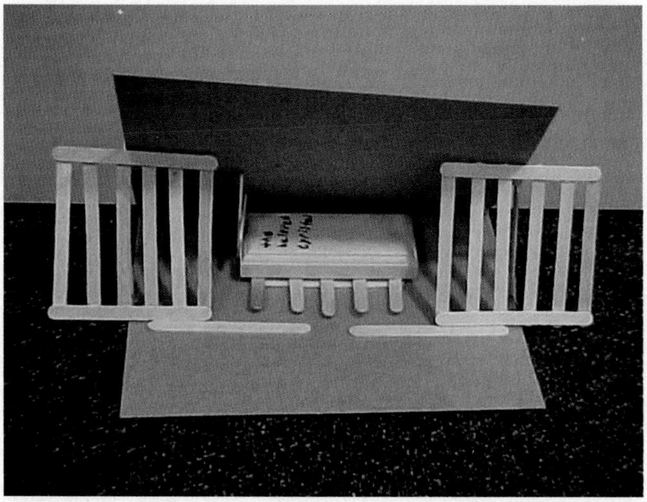

The consequent psycho-educational intervention with B and his family involved the medical team, including physician, nurse, and psychologist. The medical team was made aware that B had difficulty trusting the team because of having watched the television series *ER*, which helped them to understand some of B's distrust. B's attending physician explained eosinophils for the family, drawing pictures and adding detail that were appropriate for B and his parents. Meetings with the psychologist focused on helping B's parents understand how frightened B had become, particularly around his misperception of imminent death. B's parents were educated about how frightening managing an illness can be to a child if they feel they are doing this on their own. The psychologist also discussed the impact of having B watch *ER* and how the scenes portrayed in the television program had been traumatizing. B's mother agreed to avoid watching this program with B. In addition, through this intervention and education about asthma and food allergies, B's parents took an active role in managing B's asthma and food allergies.

Comment

This case points to several psychosocial problems that at first blush may not have been obvious in a short clinic visit. However, there were several evident red flags during the medical intake that could alert a health care professional this family would benefit from psychological services. The most

Figure 45-2 Child's artwork depicting a hospital scene and revealing his fears and anxieties about the doctors' treatment as insufficient to prevent his death.

evident indicator of psychosocial stress was B's inappropriate position as the family authority regarding his asthma and food allergies. At age 10 years, B was expected to manage an illness that most adults find challenging. When assessing psychosocial stressors in a child or family, the child's developmental stage is an essential factor for consideration. If a family requires too little or too much from their child, this should serve as an indication of need for further intervention.

This case example also illustrates that when coping resources are overwhelmed, fear and anxiety are more likely to result. Based on the intake information alone, B may have appeared a bit anxious but generally coping well with his illness. Although he had never experienced a traumatic medical event, his belief that he was close to death overwhelmed his coping abilities, resulting in anxiety. Once discovered, this belief could be addressed and corrected, and B's anxiety consequently was significantly reduced.

CASE 2

Unrecognized psychological distress may undermine good disease management. In the case that follows a mismatch between the adolescent symptoms and the parents' understanding of disease severity led to conflict and distress.

Initial Presentation and Symptoms

Patient J, a 15-year-old white female, was referred to National Jewish Medical and Research Center for treatment of moderate asthma. J was initially diagnosed with asthma at age 4 years and her symptoms were easily controlled until approximately 13 years of age when her asthma became progressively more difficult to control. In the 3 months before this encounter, J's medication had been intensively increased. Despite this, J reported daily and nearly constant symptoms. She would often wake in the night feeling chest tightness and requiring her albuterol. J reported increased use of her rescue medication at a rate of 10 to 20 puffs per day.

J had been an accomplished soccer player but was now unable to participate because of her asthma. Where previously J could play a 90-minute soccer match with pretreatment and some slight chest tightness, she now had difficulty running three quarters of a lap around the gym without becoming winded. Moreover, J had experienced a significant respiratory event while playing soccer. She had difficulty breathing, lost consciousness, and required emergency medical attention, leading to a hospitalization that included oxygen and IV steroids.

J and her mother were noted by the medical team to have significant conflict punctuated by yelling, screaming, and episodes of crying by both mother and daughter. The admitting physician indicated she would like some assistance in understanding if the conflict were "normal" adolescent behavior or something that needed further intervention.

During the intake, it became evident that J's soccer participation was of major importance to her parents. Engaging in soccer since an early age, J had developed friendships, and the team provided social connections for J's parents and reinforced the family value of success through hard work and perseverance. Conflict between J and her parents over her soccer participation was interpreted by her parents as an indication

that J was not sufficiently committed to her sport. Although J's resistance to continuing her soccer had led to several emotional outbursts, her parents also indicated their belief that this behavior as well as J's recent irritability and desire to seclude herself in her room was normal for an adolescent. J expressed anger and frustration with her parents' inability to understand her need to quit playing soccer. Through tears, J said she truly could not play soccer because she could not breathe and was fearful she could die. She thought her parents were insensitive and selfish for insisting she continue to play.

Identification of Psychosocial Risk Factors

Although irritability and changes in mood can be common in adolescence, the intensity and degree of J's behavior indicated reason for concern. Observations of J and her mother indicated open hostility towards each other. J's decision to stop playing soccer had created significant stress and conflict within the family. Not only were J's parents disappointed, they perceived J as shirking her responsibilities towards her team and the family, a behavior that was not well tolerated. The significant time and resources invested in J's soccer career created increased tension between J and her father, and subsequently had a negative impact on the marital relationship.

Questioning about J's level of distress revealed that J was upset about significant changes in her physical appearance, personal relationships, parental relationships, asthma symptoms, asthma management and the loss of soccer. J reported irritability, sadness, social isolation, and anhedonia. Augmenting the information obtained during the intake process were standardized behavior rating scales that compared J's behavior to that of her same-age peers. Overall, J was in the Clinically Significant range for depression and "At Risk" regarding her relationship with her parents.

Intervention

Therapeutic intervention with J and her family was very circumscribed, in large part because J's parents had difficulty accepting that she and her family required psychotherapeutic intervention. J's parents felt her depression was an affront to their parenting skills and signaled failure. However, they were willing to engage in a single family session with J's physician, which proved to be quite powerful, during which the physician shared data from a methacoline challenge and an exercise challenge indicating that J had a drastic reduction in lung function with limited provocation or exertion, especially when her inhaled steroid was withheld. Due to her pulmonary reactivity during these challenges, J was judged to be at great risk for a catastrophic outcome in the event that she exerted herself without pretreatment or when attempting to exercise with low lung function. Surprisingly, J's father began to cry upon hearing this information and apologized to J for pushing her to perform at soccer. J was also in tears and stated, "I have been trying to tell you this for a long time—I can't breathe!" J's parents agreed that they did not want J playing soccer if the results could potentially be fatal. The psychologist also discussed the importance of assisting J with her medication regimen and explained that her lung function would only improve if she was committed to taking her medications each day. Both parents were willing to explore ways of helping J with her asthma regimen and were open to hearing that adolescence is a difficult time to take on the responsibility of independent medication management.

Comment

This case highlights several psychosocial problems that were first expressed through parent/child conflict. While the treating health care provider was relatively certain J's behavior had crossed the threshold of "typical" adolescent behavior, she sought confirmation through a psychosocial referral. It was then revealed, through standardized self-report measures and a psychosocial intake interview, that the parent/child conflict was actually a symptom of other significant problems including a misunderstanding of asthma severity. Table 45-3 illustrates stress that can result from factors related to illness presentation and management. The family was not willing to continue the psychological intervention once they returned home. Nonetheless, through a brief psycho-educational intervention in the medical setting, the parents were capable of better

understanding their daughter and her need for medication supervision, acknowledged the grief associated with J's decision to temporarily stop playing soccer, and agreed to refrain from pushing her into sports activities that would place her physical health at risk.

SUMMARY

This chapter provides medical professionals with some understanding of how mental health interventions with children with asthma can be helpful, when to consider involving the mental health team, and how to broach this with families. It is important to remember that mental health interventions can be brief, targeted, and very helpful to families with chronic illness. Health care professionals must assess psychosocial stressors among children with asthma, be alert to red flags, and be prepared to involve a mental health professional in the child's treatment. The health care professional who identifies psychosocial stressors within the family may find the subject difficult to broach. However, when framed within the context of living with asthma, patients and families are generally willing to share this information about emotions and behaviors. The primary objective is to assess needs and target psycho-educational interventions to these needs. The psycho-educational approach involves strategically sharing educational information with patients and families and guiding problem-solving discussion, focusing on coping with illness, normalization of problems when appropriate, and clarifying what to expect in the future. Families are more accepting of such intervention in the medical setting when clinicians do not overstep boundaries set by the family. Compliance problems are generally approached by education and fostering a working agreement within the family about how to share responsibilities for illness care. Some families may have problems such as depression or chronic marital conflict that cannot be managed during a brief intervention in the medical setting and may need a referral for further mental health treatment within the patient's community. By communicating important aspects of the patient's medical care with the mental health provider, physicians caring for children with asthma can help care for a broader aspect of health.

Table 45-3
ILLNESS MANAGEMENT FACTORS CAN INCREASE THE RISK OF EMOTIONAL DISTRESS

Illness Management Factors	Potential Difficulties
Diagnostic uncertainty	Mistrust of medical team Anxiety
Change in diagnosis	Frustration with medical team Parental guilt
Mismatch between symptoms and expectations of either family or medical team	Anger, frustration, and mistrust
Change in illness severity	Anxiety, fear, frustration
New or unexpected diagnosis	Adjustment, anxiety
Life-threatening event	Anxiety, PTSD
Medical procedures	Anxiety, acting out, parental guilt

REFERENCES

1. Woodruff T, Axelrad D, Kyle A, et al: Trends in environmentally related childhood illnesses. Pediatrics 2004;113:1133–1140.
2. Klinnert M, Bender BG: Psychological implications of pediatric asthma. In Kaptein A, Creer T (eds): Behavioral Sciences and Respiratory Disorders. New York, Harwood Academic Publishers, 2002, pp 45–83.
3. Chen E, Hanson M, Paterson L, et al: Socioeconomic status and inflammatory processes in childhood asthma: the role of psychological stress. J Allergy Clin Immunol 2006;117(5):1014–1020.
4. Lemanske R, Busse W: Asthma: Factors underlying inception, exacerbation, and disease progression. J Allergy Clin Immunol 2006;117(2):S456–S461.
5. Wright R, Cohen R, Cohen S: The impact of stress on the development and expression of atopy. Curr Opin Allergy Clin Immunol 2005;5(1):23–29.
6. Wright RJ, Rodriguez M, Cohen S: Review of psychosocial stress and asthma: an integrated biopsychosocial approach. Thorax 1998;53(12):1066–1074.
7. Cohen S: Keynote Presentation at the Eight International Congress of Behavioral Medicine; the Pittsburgh common cold studies: Psychosocial predictors of susceptibility to respiratory infectious illness. Int J Behav Med 2005;12(3):123–131.
8. Cohen S, Kessler R, Gordon L: Strategies for measuring stress in studies of psychiatric and physical disorders. In Cohen S, Kessler R, Gordon L (ed): Measuring Stress: Again for Health and Social Scientists. New York, Oxford University Press, 1995, pp 3–26.
9. Bloomberg G, Chen E: The relationship of psychologic stress with childhood asthma. Immunol Allergy Clin N Am 2005;25:83–105.
10. Kean E, Kelsay K, Wamboldt F, Wamboldt M: Posttraumatic stress in adolescents with asthma and their parents. J Am Acad Child Adolesc 2006;45(1):78–85.

SUGGESTED READING

Bratton D, Price M, Gavin L, et al: Impact of a multidisciplinary day program on disease and healthcare costs in children and adolescents with severe asthma: A two-year follow-up study. Pediatr Pulmonol 2001;31(3):177–189.

Chen E, Hanson M, Paterson L, et al: Socioeconomic status and inflammatory processes in childhood asthma: the role of psychological stress. J Allergy Clin Immunol 2006;117(5):1014–1020.

Cohen S, Hamrick N: Stable individual differences in physiological response to stressors: Implications for stress-elicited changes in immune related health. Brain Behav Immun 2003;17(6):407–414.

Kaugars AS, Klinnert MD, Bender BG: Family influences on pediatric asthma. J Pediatr Psychol 2004;29(7):475–491.

Klinnert MD, Nelson HS, Price MR, et al: Onset and persistence of childhood asthma: predictors from infancy. Pediatrics 2001;108(4):E69.

McQuaid E, Walders N, Kopel S, et al: Pediatric asthma management in the family context: the family asthma management system scale. J Pediatr Psychol 2005;30(6):492–502.

Price M, Bratton D, Klinnert M: Caregiver negative affect is a primary determinant of caregiver report of pediatric asthma quality of life. Ann Allergy Asthma Immunol 2002;89(6):572–577.

Sandberg S, McCann DC, Ahola S, et al: Positive experiences and the relationship between stress and asthma in children. Acta Paediatr 2002;91(2):152–158.

Stevenson J: Relationship between behavior and asthma in children with atopic dermatitis. Psychosom Med 2003;65(6):971–975.

Wright R, Cohen R, Cohen S: The impact of stress on the development and expression of atopy. Curr Opin Allergy Clin Immunol 2005;5(1):23–29.

Managing the Pregnant Asthma Patient

Jennifer Altamura Namazy and Michael Schatz

CLINICAL PEARLS

- Asthma affects between 3.7% and 8.4% of pregnant women in the United States.

- Asthma course worsens in one third, improves in one third, or remains unchanged in one third of women during pregnancy.

- Pregnant asthmatic women have an increased risk of perinatal mortality, preeclampsia, low birth weight infants, and preterm births compared to non-asthmatic women.

- Uncontrolled asthma increases perinatal risks while controlled asthma reduces these risks.

- Objective assessments and monitoring, including pulmonary function testing (ideally spirometry), detailed symptom history, and physical examination should be performed on a monthly basis in pregnant asthmatic women with persistent asthma.

- In patients starting inhaled corticosteroids during pregnancy, budesonide has been recommended as the inhaled corticosteroid of choice.

- Current guidelines recommend a stepwise approach in achieving and maintaining asthma control with medications during pregnancy.

Asthma is the most common, potentially serious medical problem to complicate pregnancy. Studies have shown that pregnant asthmatic women have an increased risk of adverse perinatal outcomes, while controlled asthma is associated with reduced risks.

Managing asthma during pregnancy is unique because the effect of both the illness and the treatment on the developing fetus as well as the patient must be considered.

The two main goals of asthma management during pregnancy are to optimize maternal and fetal health. After reviewing pregnancy-associated changes in respiratory physiology, this chapter will discuss the effect of asthma on the course and outcome of pregnancy, the effect of pregnancy on the course of asthma, and review updated guidelines in regards to the optimal management of asthma during pregnancy.

PREVALENCE AND RACIAL DISPARITY OF ASTHMA DURING PREGNANCY

Previous estimates of asthma prevalence reported that between 4% and 7% of women suffer from asthma during their pregnancy; however, many of these reports were from retrospective data, rather than being based on a nationally representative sample. Recently, Kwon and colleagues

(reviewed in reference 1) reviewed United States national health surveys spanning 1997 to 2001. The aim was to more definitively determine the prevalence of asthma in pregnant women ages 18 to 44. Time trends were also examined using health surveys from 1976 to 1980 and 1988 to 1994. They found that asthma affected between 3.7% and 8.4% of pregnant women in the United States between 1997 and 2001. There was a twofold increase in the prevalence of asthma (from 2.9% to 5.8%) between 1976–1980 and 1988–1994. This study supports initial prevalence estimates but also suggests that they may, in fact, be a conservative estimate. More importantly, this study supports the observation that this is a disease affecting more pregnant women each year.

Two recent studies have also addressed racial and ethnic disparities in the rate and impact of asthma during pregnancy. Chung and associates[2] concluded that socioeconomic status explains much of the racial disparity. However, in a more recent cohort study, Carroll and co-workers[3] observed that in a low-income population of white and African American pregnant asthmatic patients, African American women were more likely to require oral corticosteroids, emergency room visits, and hospitalizations for asthma exacerbations.

MATERNAL RESPIRATORY PHYSIOLOGIC CHANGES DURING PREGNANCY

The various physiologic changes observed during pregnancy may alter the course of asthma in the pregnant asthmatic. Both the mechanical and hormonal changes of pregnancy can influence respiratory function (reviewed in reference 1). An increase in minute ventilation secondary to an increase in tidal volume has been observed as early as the first trimester, which appears to be predominantly progesterone-mediated. Pregnancy-induced hyperventilation leads to a compensated respiratory alkalosis with a mild increase in P_{O_2} and a decreased P_{CO_2}. The increase in pH secondary to alkalosis is usually blunted by an increase in renal excretion of bicarbonate. These alterations in the arterial blood gases (ABG) during pregnancy become important particularly in relation to acute asthma. The respiratory alkalosis of acute asthma will be superimposed on the "normal" respiratory alkalosis of pregnancy. As a result, lower P_{O_2} or higher P_{CO_2} in an ABG from a pregnant woman with acute asthma symptoms may represent a more severe respiratory compromise than a similar ABG in the nongravid state.

There are mechanical changes during pregnancy that can also influence respiratory function. For example, as the uterus enlarges during pregnancy there is secondary elevation of the diaphragm, decreased diameter of the chest, and an increase in abdominal pressure. These changes were thought to partially explain the decrease in expiratory reserve volume

(ERV), residual volume (RV), and functional residual capacity (FRC) observed in late pregnancy. However, these changes begin to occur before significant uterine enlargement, suggesting a metabolic cause. Despite the decrease in ERV and FRC during pregnancy, the fact that vital capacity (VC) and total lung capacity (TLC) do not change significantly is likely related to flaring of the ribs and unimpaired diaphragmatic excursion during pregnancy.

Physiologic tests of large airway function including forced expiratory volume in 1 second (FEV_1), forced vital capacity (FVC), FEV_1/FVC ratio, mean forced expiratory flow during middle half of forced vital capacity (FEF_{25-75}), and peak expiratory flow rate remain unaffected by pregnancy. Not only are these physiologic measures useful indicators of asthma control, but they are also helpful in differentiating dyspnea caused by asthma from dyspnea caused by hyperventilation or pressure on the diaphragm with late pregnancy.

Smooth muscle activity is reduced in many anatomic locations during pregnancy including the urethra, bowel, and gallbladder. This decreased tone is thought to be related to progesterone. Progesterone's effect on bronchial smooth muscle tone is less clear.

Around 30% to 40% of the women with asthma who visit outpatient clinics report perimenstrual worsening of symptoms.[4] The likelihood that female sex hormones influence asthma symptoms in this condition seems obvious, although the exact mechanisms remain to be determined. Because female sex hormones increase during pregnancy 100 to 1000 times over that in the nonpregnant female, their role in influencing asthma during pregnancy is also likely. Less clear are the underlying mechanisms through which these hormones influence asthma symptoms.

Progesterone, estrogens, or both are the most frequently implicated hormones but cortisol and prostaglandins may be important as well. Considerable evidence suggests that female sex hormones have effects on several cells and cytokines involved in inflammation.[4] Specifically attributed to estrogens are increases in B-cell differentiation, decreases in T-cell suppressor activity and numbers, and increases in antibody production (immunoglobulin G [IgG]). There is less documentation of the effects of progesterone on inflammation. Evidence suggests that progesterone can act as a partial glucocorticoid agonist and suppress histamine release from basophils. Both estrogen and progesterone are involved in eosinophilic infiltration in many organs including the uterus, and both can reduce the oxidative burst after phagocytic stimulus. Estradiol enhances eosinophilic adhesion to human mucosa microvascular endothelial cells and the combined effect with progesterone induces eosinophil degranulation.

There appears to be a cyclical variation in lymphocyte $beta_2$-adrenoreceptor density in healthy women with higher levels during the luteal phase. This up-regulation is most probably the result of progesterone rather than estrogen.[4] However, this pattern is not seen in asthmatic women; in fact, in these women there is a downregulation of $beta_2$-adrenoreceptor density when exposed to progesterone. Theoretically, as pregnancy progresses and progesterone levels increase, a similar effect may be seen causing worsening control of asthma in some pregnant asthmatic women.

Maternal plasma cortisol levels increase with pregnancy. This includes both free and total cortisol levels. Since more free cortisol is available during pregnancy one might expect both consistent improvement in asthma control and reduced steroid requirements in pregnant asthmatic women. However, it appears that cortisol's effects on asthma during pregnancy are more variable.

Several prostaglandins are involved in asthma, as bronchodilators (PGE2) and bronchoconstrictors (PGD2 and PGF2). During pregnancy, amniotic fluid contains a mixture of these prostaglandins. There is a 10- to 30-fold increase in PGF2-alpha during pregnancy and its levels have been found to correlate with estrogen levels. Asthmatic patients appear to be more sensitive to the bronchoconstrictive properties of aerosolized PGF2-alpha than normal persons. However, a relationship between increased levels of PGF2-alpha during pregnancy and asthma exacerbations in the pregnant patient has never been established.

One of the major concerns in managing the pregnant asthmatic patient is the maintenance of adequate fetal oxygenation. Data suggest that the combination of hypoxemia and respiratory alkalosis that may occur during acute airway obstruction in the asthmatic mother may have adverse effects on the fetus, and that alkalosis may be an important cause of depressed fetal oxygen level. Arterial oxygen tension (PaO_2) in the fetus is only about one fourth of the PaO_2 in the adult. Despite this, the fetus functions completely by aerobic metabolism. The fetus has made four major adaptations to compensate for low PaO_2. First, the rate of perfusion of fetal organs in sheep preparations (and presumably in humans) is 2.5-fold greater than blood flow to the same organs in the adult. Second, fetal hemoglobin has a higher affinity for oxygen than adult hemoglobin. Third, fetal hemoglobin levels are increased over adult values. Finally, a system of vascular shunts and streaming effects directs oxygenated blood to high-priority tissue in the liver, heart, and brain and guides deoxygenated blood back to the placenta. If fetal oxygenation is threatened, for example, from uncontrolled gestational asthma, the fetus can compensate for hypoxia by redistributing blood to vital organs, decreasing gross body movements, and increasing tissue oxygenation extraction. A common response to chronic hypoxia is deferment of growth needs which may lead to the small for gestational age infant (reviewed in reference 1).[15]

EFFECT OF PREGNANCY ON ASTHMA

Asthma course may worsen, improve, or remain unchanged during pregnancy, and the overall data suggest that these various courses occur with approximately equal frequency. In a prospective study (reviewed in reference 1) of 330 pregnant asthmatics followed up to 12 weeks postpartum, exacerbations appeared to be more frequent between 24 and 36 weeks' gestation, and general improvements in asthma symptoms were observed during the last 4 weeks of the pregnancy. Only about 10% of women in that study reported asthma symptoms during labor and delivery. Overall, asthma appeared to revert to the prepregnancy state by 3 months postpartum in most women. Some subjects were assessed in two successive pregnancies and 60% followed the same course of asthma in the second pregnancy as the first. However, a substantial minority did not follow the same course of asthma, suggesting that the course of an individual subject's asthma during pregnancy remains unpredictable.

Two observations may be mechanistically and clinically important regarding the course of asthma during pregnancy. First, more severe asthma tends to worsen during pregnancy while less severe asthma tends to remain unchanged or improved. Secondly, there is a significant concordance between rhinitis course and asthma course during pregnancy. One study (reviewed in reference 1) identified 568 pregnant women whose patient-reported asthma course during pregnancy was compared with the women's usual disease course. They found that those women who experienced improvement in asthma symptoms during pregnancy also had improvement in rhinitis symptoms. This suggests that the same mechanisms may influence both levels of the airway during pregnancy; that gestational rhinitis course may predict asthma course during pregnancy; and possibly, that rhinitis management during pregnancy may improve asthma.

The mechanisms responsible for the altered asthma course during pregnancy are unknown. There are multiple biochemical and physiologic changes during pregnancy that could potentially ameliorate or exacerbate gestational asthma. As discussed earlier, the myriad pregnancy-associated changes in levels of sex hormones, cortisol, and prostaglandins may contribute to changes in asthma course during pregnancy. In addition, exposure to fetal antigens, leading to alterations in immune function, may predispose some pregnant asthmatic women to worsening asthma. A recent article by Tamasi and colleagues [5] found that pregnant women with moderate to severe asthma had increased numbers of circulating IFN-gamma+ and IL-4+ T cells when compared with nonpregnant asthmatic women or healthy controls (pregnant and nonpregnant). Proliferation of these T lymphocytes may contribute to airway inflammation and may influence fetal development as well. Within the asthmatic pregnant group, significant negative correlations were revealed between the numbers of IFN-gamma+ and IL-4+ T cells and maternal expiratory flow as well as birth weight of newborns.

There is also the possible influence of fetal sex on maternal asthma during pregnancy. Several reports have suggested that asthma attacks or worsening asthma during pregnancy were associated with the presence of a female fetus (reviewed in reference 1). However, the mechanisms leading to changes in asthma during pregnancy in the presence of a female fetus require further investigation. An interesting hypothesis regarding the relationship between mother, placenta, and female fetus is that there may be abnormal levels of a placental enzyme that may lead to reduced fetal growth in female infants of pregnant asthmatic women.

EFFECT OF ASTHMA ON PREGNANCY

Controlled studies that have evaluated outcomes of pregnancy in asthmatic compared to nonasthmatic women have suggested that maternal asthma may increase the risk of perinatal mortality, preeclampsia, low birth weight infants, and preterm births compared to nonasthmatic women.

In a recent nested case control study by Sorensen and associates (reviewed in reference 1), the authors tried to determine the extent to which maternal asthma is associated with an increased risk of preterm labor and delivery. The study included women who delivered prior to the completion of 37 weeks' gestation in a cohort population of 3253 pregnant

women. In asthmatic women there was a twofold increased risk of preterm delivery as compared with women who had no history of asthma (odds ratio [OR] = 2.03; 95% confidence interval [CI] 1.01–4.09). While this study confirms previous reports, that have examined preterm labor and delivery in this population of patients, there exist several limitations. First, the number of asthmatic patients enrolled in the study is small and likely limits the ability to make inferences from the available data. For example, there were only 20 women with a positive history of asthma whose delivery classified as "preterm." Secondly, there is no detailed information regarding the severity of asthma during pregnancy or maternal use of asthma medication in study subjects. This is important information since these variables may contribute to adverse maternal and perinatal outcomes.

The observations that maternal asthma may increase the risk of perinatal complications is confirmed by one of the largest studies to date[6] which described the outcomes of pregnancy in 36,985 women identified as having asthma in either the Swedish Medical Birth Registry and/or the Swedish Hospital Discharge Registry. These outcomes were compared to the total of 1.32 million births that occurred in the Swedish population during the years of the study (1984–1995). Pregnancies in women with asthma were significantly more likely to be complicated by preeclampsia, perinatal mortality, preterm birth, and low birth weight (but not congenital malformations). This study also suggests that patients with more severe asthma are at a greater risk.

Mechanisms postulated to explain the possible increased perinatal risks in pregnant asthmatic women demonstrated in previous studies have included (1) hypoxia and other physiologic consequences of poorly controlled asthma, (2) medications used to treat asthma, and (3) pathogenic or demographic factors associated with asthma but actually not caused by the disease or its treatment, such as abnormal placental function.

Chronic hypoxia at high altitude is associated with lower birth weights in otherwise normal pregnancies. Therefore, hypoxia caused by uncontrolled asthma may be a plausible mechanism leading to adverse perinatal outcomes such as: low birth weight, preeclampsia, congenital malformations, spontaneous abortions, and placenta previa. However, maternal hypoxia during asthmatic pregnancies has never been directly investigated in relation to fetal outcome. Several observations do support the hypothesis that uncontrolled asthma increases perinatal risks while controlled asthma reduces these risks. For example, studies have shown that better controlled asthma (defined by lack of acute episodes or higher maternal pulmonary function) leads to improved intrauterine growth (measured by birth weight or ponderal indices), while more severe asthma symptoms can lead to intrauterine growth restriction.

In one of the first studies to determine pregnancy outcomes stratified by asthma severity (as classified by the National Asthma Education Program), Dombrowski and colleagues (reviewed in reference 1) conducted a multicenter, prospective, observational cohort study involving 16 centers between 1994 and 1999. Of all outcomes explored (including preterm delivery, gestational diabetes, preeclampsia, preterm labor, chorioamnionitis, oligohydramnios, caesarean delivery, low birth weight, small for gestational age, and congenital malformations), only caesarean delivery rates were increased in the group of moderate to severe asthmatic patients. This may be because study subjects underwent asthma severity classification upon enrollment and were followed by physicians familiar with asthma treatment guidelines, which may have led to more optimal asthma control and fewer observed complications.

In a separate study of the same cohort of patients, Schatz and associates (reviewed in reference 1) described the relationship between asthma morbidity during pregnancy and asthma severity classification. They observed that asthma morbidity (hospitalizations, office visits, oral corticosteroid use) correlated closely with asthma classification applied to the subjects at entry, that is, those subjects with mild asthma experienced fewer hospitalizations, unscheduled visits, oral corticosteroid courses and total exacerbations than those with moderate-severe asthma. An interesting finding was that about 30% of subjects whose asthma was classified as mild at entry "switched" categories during pregnancy to the moderate or severe groups. One of the most important conclusions to be made from this study is that pregnant asthmatic patients, even with initially mild or well-controlled disease, need to be closely monitored with pulmonary function testing during pregnancy. The existing data suggest that poor asthma control, by causing acute and/or chronic maternal hypoxia, may be the most remedial responsible factor for increased perinatal complication in pregnant asthmatic women. The data also support the important generalization that adequate asthma control during pregnancy is important in improving maternal fetal outcome.

Preplacental hypoxia as a result of smoking, high altitude, anemia, or asthma may directly affect fetal growth. As a result the placenta adapts by increasing capillary growth, trophoblast proliferation, and thinning of the placental barrier. One study examined how these vascular abnormalities might contribute to impaired fetal growth in the pregnant asthmatic woman (reviewed in reference 7). The authors found that placental vascular resistance may be prematurely decreased in the moderate to severe asthmatics. These individuals also demonstrated decreased placental responses to both dilator and constrictor agents. The authors concluded that altered placental blood flow may contribute to reduced fetal growth in moderate to severe asthmatic patients by reducing the supply of nutrients to the fetus.

Murphy and co-workers (reviewed in reference 7) observed that the birth weight of female neonates of mothers not using inhaled corticosteroids was significantly reduced compared with females in the control and corticosteroid-using groups. There were no similar effects on growth observed in the male neonates. They hypothesize that the mechanisms behind these observations are related to placental 11 beta-hydroxysteroid dehydrogenase type 2 activity. This enzyme prevents excess maternal cortisol from reaching the fetus by metabolizing cortisol to its inactive form, cortisone. Previous studies have demonstrated reduced enzyme activity in neonates with intrauterine growth retardation. In support of this, the authors measured fetal cortisol concentrations in the umbilical vein at delivery and found higher levels in female fetuses from mothers not using inhaled corticosteroids. This implies that the female fetus may have an adverse effect on maternal asthma and, when not treated with inhaled corticosteroids, can lead to reduced fetal growth via reduced 11 beta-hydroxysteroid dehydrogenase activity.

The association between some adverse pregnancy outcomes, such as preeclampsia and preterm labor or delivery, may be related to common pathogenetic factors that underlie both asthma and these perinatal complications. The common pathogenesis theory suggests that patients with bronchial hyperreactivity may also possess vascular hyperreactivity caused by the same mechanisms. These mechanisms could include vascular smooth muscle α-adrenergic hyperreactivity, beta-adrenergic hyporeactivity, or increased activity of, or sensitivity to, mediators, such as angiotensin and endothelin. However, it is difficult to distinguish the effects of these common pathogenetic factors from other factors such as medications used during pregnancy. This is particularly true for the moderate to severe asthmatic patient, who might possess more vascular hyperreactivity, while at the same time require more medication to control her asthma.

As mentioned earlier, another possible explanation for increased perinatal complications in the infants of asthmatic mothers is asthma medication use during pregnancy. As will be discussed later, except for oral corticosteroids, there are no data to suggest that commonly used asthma medications are responsible for the increased adverse perinatal outcomes observed in pregnant asthmatic women.

STUDYING MEDICATIONS DURING PREGNANCY

The choice of a specific medication for use during pregnancy is based on available human and animal data. Human studies exist in the form of case reports, cohort studies, and case control studies. The gold standard for medical human experimental studies is the randomized clinical trial. This type of study is generally not feasible to evaluate the safety of medications during pregnancy, partly because it would require a subset of pregnant women to be exposed to a medication that they did not need. While case control and cohort studies may suggest an association, they do not of themselves prove causation. These studies generally must be considered to suggest hypotheses requiring independent confirmation. Nonetheless, when effective alternatives are available, it seems advisable to avoid drugs implicated as causing adverse effects in cohort or case-control studies.

Animal teratology experiments can also be useful in evaluating human drug risks. Animal studies are designed to maximize the response of the system to potential toxic effects of the test agent by using large doses. There are no known human developmental toxicants that would not have been identified using current animal testing protocols. Negative data in animal studies for a developmental toxicant indicate a low potential for human developmental toxicity. However, positive animal data are less useful, because it is often not possible to know whether species differences, clinically irrelevant high doses used, or maternal toxicity was responsible for the adverse effects in the animal offspring.

The current pregnancy category system (i.e., the A, B, C, D, X system) adopted in 1979 by the Food and Drug Administration (FDA) is used in official labeling for drug products. This system was developed as a guide for drug selection best suited for the patient. Some problems associated with this form of labeling include (1) paucity of data on drug effects in human pregnancies, resulting in an emphasis on animal data, (2) an inability to interpret the C category clinically, and (3) difficulty assigning drugs to the A category. For a drug to be labeled as a category A, it must be proven safe when used in "adequate and controlled" studies in humans and cannot have shown adverse effects in animal studies. No asthma or allergy medication labeled to date meets the requirements for category A. Drugs in categories B, C, and D are almost always placed in these categories based on findings in animal studies alone because human data is not available. The FDA has elevated the classification of budesonide to a category B drug based on reassuring data from the population-based Swedish Medical Birth Registry (reviewed in reference 1).

UPDATED GUIDELINES FOR THE USE OF SPECIFIC ASTHMA MEDICATIONS DURING PREGNANCY

In 1993, the National Asthma Education and Prevention Program (NAEPP) published the *Report of the Working Group on Asthma and Pregnancy*, which reviewed the data from available studies and presented recommendations for the pharmacologic management of asthma during pregnancy. Since then there have been new developments including: the introduction of new medications, the availability of additional safety data, and revisions to severity classification and treatment guidelines in the general management of asthma. All of these developments led to an update of the 1993 report recently published: *NAEPP Working Group Report on Managing Asthma During Pregnancy: Recommendations for Pharmacologic Treatment—Update 2004.*[8] The focus of this update was to review new data regarding the safety and effectiveness of asthma medications taken during pregnancy and lactation. While this report presents an extensive review of the current literature with specific recommendations, the working group members do stress that these are guidelines meant to assist clinical decision making and should be used adjunctively when designing a treatment plan specifically tailored to the needs of an individual pregnant patient.

EFFICACY AND SAFETY OF ASTHMA TREATMENT DURING PREGNANCY

Inhaled Corticosteroids

Inhaled corticosteroids are well documented to prevent asthma exacerbations in nonpregnant patients. This is also true in the pregnant population as reported by Stenius-Aarniala and colleagues (reviewed in reference 1), who found a higher incidence of asthma exacerbations in pregnant women who were not initially treated with inhaled corticosteroid in comparison with patients who had been on an inhaled corticosteroid from the beginning of pregnancy. In addition, two randomized controlled trials during pregnancy support the efficacy of inhaled corticosteroids during pregnancy (reviewed in reference 1). First, in a prospective randomized controlled trial of 72 pregnant asthmatic patients presenting to an emergency department or prenatal clinic with an asthma exacerbation, the authors found there was a reduction of exacerbations and readmissions by 55% in women given inhaled beclometha-

sone dipropionate with oral corticosteroids and beta$_2$-agonists compared with women treated with oral corticosteroids and beta$_2$-agonists alone. Second, a prospective, double blind, double placebo-controlled randomized clinical trial compared the efficacy of inhaled beclomethasone dipropionate to oral theophylline for the prevention of asthma exacerbations during pregnancy. Results demonstrated that there was no significant difference in the proportion of asthma exacerbations among the 194 women in the beclomethasone cohort versus the 191 in the theophylline cohort. However, there were fewer reported side effects, less discontinuation of medication, and a lower proportion of women with FEV$_1$ less than 80% in the beclomethasone dipropionate treatment group. This study does support previous guidelines that inhaled corticosteroids are the therapy of choice for persistent asthma during pregnancy.

Concern has been raised regarding a possible adverse effect of inhaled corticosteroids on intrauterine growth because (1) oral corticosteroid use has been associated with reduced birth weight, and (2) inhaled steroids have been reported to reduce the growth rate in children, at least during the first year of exposure. Several studies since 1993 (reviewed in reference 1) have provided reassuring information regarding the lack of adverse effects of inhaled corticosteroids on perinatal outcomes.

In a prospectively followed cohort of 824 pregnant asthmatic patients, Schatz and colleagues[1] reported no significant relationship between congenital malformations, preeclampsia, preterm births, small for gestational age, or low birth weight infants and exposure to inhaled corticosteroids in the first trimester or at any gestational age (n = 158).

Bracken and associates provided reassuring information based on a prospective study (reviewed in reference 1) of 873 pregnant women with asthma. In the newborn infants of 176 women using inhaled corticosteroids, there was no increased risk of preterm delivery or intrauterine growth restriction.

Much of the information available regarding the safety of various asthma medications comes from large cohort studies. For instance, in the Registry for Allergic and Asthmatic Pregnant Patients (RAAPP) of the American College of Allergy Asthma and Immunology and the American Academy of Allergy Asthma and Immunology, pregnant asthmatic women treated with inhaled steroids were enrolled by the allergists managing their asthma. Namazy and colleagues (reviewed in reference 1) described the incidence of small for gestational age infants, an important measure of intrauterine growth retardation, in the offspring of 396 exposed mothers enrolled into the Registry. Beclomethasone was the most commonly used inhaled corticosteroid, and 20.2% of patients used more than one specific inhaled corticosteroid during pregnancy. The incidence of small for gestational age infants was 7.1% (95% CI 5.0%–10.1%) compared to the expected incidence of 10 %. There was no significant relationship identified between specific inhaled steroid use or the dose of inhaled steroid used and the incidence of small for gestational age infants or mean birth weight.

Schatz and associates (reviewed in reference 1) evaluated the relationship between a variety of asthma medications and adverse perinatal outcomes. This cohort included over 2000 subjects from 16 centers of the National Institute of Child Health and Human Developmental Maternal Fetal Medicine Units Network. No significant relationships were found between adverse perinatal outcomes and the use of inhaled beta-agonists, inhaled corticosteroids, theophylline, or cromolyn-nedocromil. There was an observed increased risk of preterm and low birth weight infants associated with oral corticosteroid use. Similar results were reported in a recent study by Bakhireva and co-workers[9] in which the authors compared mean birth weight, length, head circumference, and the incidence of small for gestational age in all infants born to asthmatic women who used (1) inhaled corticosteroids, (2) systemic corticosteroids, and (3) only beta$_2$-agonists to each other and to nonasthmatic control subjects. Although infants of the women taking inhaled corticosteroids during pregnancy did not have a lower birth weight compared with those of the control subjects, there was a significant decrease in birth weight in the pregnant women taking systemic corticosteroids compared to controls without asthma and exclusive beta$_2$-agonist users. It remains to be determined whether oral corticosteroids directly cause these outcomes, or rather, serve as a marker for asthma severe or uncontrolled enough to cause prematurity. One significant limitation of the study by Bakhireva and co-workers[9] was the lack of clinical assessment of asthma severity.

One of the largest cohorts of pregnant asthmatic patients comes from the Swedish Medical Birth Registry. In 1999, a report from Kallen and colleagues (reviewed in reference 1) found no increase in rate of congenital malformations, oral clefts, or cardiovascular malformations in infants of mothers exposed to inhaled budesonide during pregnancy. In a more recent report, Norjavaara and Gerhardsson de Verdier (reviewed in reference 1) searched for an association between inhaled budesonide use during pregnancy and other adverse perinatal outcomes. Data included information from 2968 pregnant women enrolled in the Swedish Medical Birth Registry who reported the use of inhaled budesonide. These women gave birth to infants of normal gestational age, birth weight, and length with no increased risk of stillbirths or multiple births.

Recent data from another large population-based case-control study in Canada[10] addressed the question of whether inhaled corticosteroids increased the risk of either pregnancy-induced hypertension or preeclampsia in asthmatic women. In a group of over 3000 women with asthma there were 302 cases of pregnancy-induced hypertension (6.6% of the study population). This included 165 cases of preeclampsia. The authors found that while oral corticosteroids were significantly associated with pregnancy-induced hypertension, using inhaled corticosteroids during pregnancy was not associated with either preeclampsia or pregnancy-induced hypertension. In addition, there was no observed dose-response relationship between inhaled corticosteroids and either of these conditions.

The data provided by these studies suggest that the currently available inhaled corticosteroids used at clinically relevant doses do not impair intrauterine growth or cause other adverse perinatal outcomes. These data suggest that inhaled corticosteroids should be used when indicated for the management of persistent asthma during pregnancy.

In 1993, the Working Group on Asthma and Pregnancy stated that corticosteroids are the most effective anti-inflammatory drugs for the treatment of asthma. At that time beclomethasone diproprionate, triamcinolone, and flunisolide were all recognized as treatment options, and, of the three, there was the most experience during pregnancy with beclomethasone dipropionate. Therefore, it was recommended as the inhaled corticosteroid of choice at that time. Since that time, review of recent publications support the overall safety of inhaled corticosteroid use in pregnancy, with the most data supporting the safety of inhaled budesonide. Thus, in the current guidelines,[8] budesonide is considered the inhaled steroid of choice during pregnancy.

However, the recent guidelines do emphasize that there are no data to suggest that other inhaled corticosteroids are less safe during pregnancy. Thus, if a pregnant asthmatic woman is using an alternative inhaled corticosteroid before pregnancy and her asthma is well controlled, it would not be unreasonable to continue it through the pregnancy.

Systemic Corticosteroids

Data regarding the use of systemic corticosteroids during pregnancy have not been totally reassuring. Recent available human studies include a meta-analysis of 6 cohort studies by Park-Wyllie and colleagues (reviewed in reference 1) evaluating the relationship between corticosteroid use during pregnancy and congenital malformations, and four case-control studies evaluating the potential relationship between systemic corticosteroid use during pregnancy and oral clefts. They found that while there was no definite increased risk of total congenital malformations, there was a statistically significant increased risk of oral clefts in infants of mothers treated with corticosteroids during the first trimester (summary OR = 3.35, 95% CI 1.97, 5.69).

Other adverse outcomes recently associated with systemic corticosteroid use during pregnancy include preeclampsia, prematurity, and low birth weight.[1] However, the available data make it difficult to separate the effects of the corticosteroids on these outcomes from the effects of severe or uncontrolled asthma. It must be stressed that the potential risks of oral corticosteroid use during pregnancy must be balanced against the risks to both the mother and infant of poorly managed disease. The current recommendations[8] continue to support the use of oral corticosteroids when indicated for the long-term management of severe asthma or for severe exacerbations during pregnancy.

Short-acting Bronchodilators

The 1993 guidelines did not make a specific recommendation regarding a specific inhaled agonist for use during pregnancy. Based on the data published since then, albuterol is recommended as the inhaled short-acting beta-agonist of choice during pregnancy.[8] Data from several human studies have been reassuring regarding the safety of short-acting beta-agonists in pregnancy (reviewed in reference 1). Schatz and associates in a prospective study found no relationship between major congenital malformations or other adverse perinatal outcomes and exposure to beta-agonist bronchodilators during pregnancy. Of note, metaproterenol and terbutaline were the most commonly used bronchodilators in that study with 129/667 using albuterol.

A more recent prospective study by Bracken and co-workers enrolled 873 pregnant women with a history of asthma, 529 of which were using short-acting bronchodilators (most commonly albuterol). The authors found no increased risk of short-acting bronchodilator use on primary outcome variables: preterm delivery and intrauterine growth retardation.

Recent data have demonstrated that the bronchodilatory effect of ipratropium may be additive to that of inhaled beta-agonists in the management of acute asthma. Although there are no available human data, animal studies are reassuring for ipratropium. Therefore nebulized ipratropium can be considered in women presenting with acute asthma who do not improve substantially with the first inhaled beta-agonist treatment or for those presenting with severe exacerbations.[8]

Long-acting Bronchodilators

Since 1993, two long-acting inhaled bronchodilators have become available: salmeterol and formoterol. According to current guidelines in the treatment of asthma in nonpregnant women, long-acting beta-agonists are considered add-on treatment of choice for those patients who are not well controlled on inhaled corticosteroids. There are few published data regarding the safety of these drugs during pregnancy. Wilton and colleagues (reviewed in reference 1) in a postmarketing surveillance study identified 65 women who took salmeterol during the first trimester of pregnancy. Of the 47 outcomes evaluated, one congenital anomaly occurred considered to have a genetic basis. There were also three reported premature singleton pregnancies in this group.

In terms of the safety of formoterol use during pregnancy, the data is even scarcer. In another post-marketing surveillance study (reviewed in reference 8) of 30 women who took formoterol during the first trimester of pregnancy there were 25 live births; of these, there were 5 premature births and 2 congenital malformations reported. It is difficult to make any conclusions regarding the safety of formoterol use during pregnancy since the numbers from the available data are so small.

Although the data are lacking, the recommendation for the use of long-acting beta-agonists during pregnancy is based on their efficacy, inhaled route, and chemical relationship to albuterol for which there are reassuring data. The new guidelines recommend salmeterol as the long-acting beta-agonist of choice during pregnancy due to longer availability in this country.[7]

Cromolyn Sodium

The 1993 report recommended that daily long-term controller therapy be initiated with cromolyn due to its safety profile. Two recent human studies have further demonstrated the safety of cromolyn (reviewed in reference 1). Schatz and associates found no significant relationship between cromolyn use during pregnancy and an increased incidence of congenital malformations, preeclampsia, preterm birth, low birth weight or small for gestational age infants. Bracken and associates found no relationship between preterm delivery and intrauterine growth restriction with cromolyn use among 22 pregnant women. Nevertheless, according to current guidelines, based on the superiority of inhaled corticosteroids over

cromolyn in the management of asthma symptoms, cromolyn is considered an alternative, but not preferred, treatment for mild persistent asthma during pregnancy.

Theophylline

Decades of theophylline use have supported its lack of teratogenicity. Since the 1993 report, additional studies have evaluated the risk of adverse perinatal outcomes associated with theophylline (reviewed in reference 1). One study demonstrated no increased risk of preeclampsia, preterm birth, low birth weight, or small for gestational age in infants of 429 exposed mothers. Another study found an increased risk of preeclampsia in 212 women using theophylline during their pregnancy, although that association may have been confounded by oral corticosteroid use. Bracken and associates found an increased risk of preterm delivery but not intrauterine growth restriction in 15 women using theophylline during pregnancy. The interpretation of those data is obviously limited by the number of patients using theophylline.

Dombrowski and colleagues (reviewed in reference 1) compared the efficacy of inhaled beclomethasone diproprionate to oral theophylline for the prevention of asthma exacerbations during pregnancy. While there was no significant difference in the proportion of asthma exacerbations in the beclomethasone cohort versus the theophylline cohort, significantly more women taking theophylline had an increased proportion of FEV_1 less than 80% predicted, and a greater proportion discontinued study medications because of side effects. Compared with beclomethasone dipropionate, theophylline has had the disadvantage of requiring serum level monitoring and has more frequent side effects.

According to the current recommendations,[8] theophylline may be used as alternative, but not preferred, medication for mild persistent asthma or as add-on therapy in addition to inhaled corticosteroid medication in those pregnant patients with moderate persistent asthma. It is important to note that the serum concentration of theophylline needs to be closely monitored and low-dose therapy is recommended with maintenance serum levels targeted at 5 to 12 µg/mL.[7]

Leukotriene Modifiers

A number of newer medications currently used in asthma management include the leukotriene modifier drugs (zileuton, zafirlukast, and montelukast). Animal studies have been reassuring for montelukast and zafirlukast while nonreassuring for zileuton. While leukotriene modifier drugs have been shown to be effective in the management of mild-moderate persistent asthma in nonpregnant patients, there are few human data regarding the use of these medications during pregnancy.

One recent study reported by Bracken and co-workers (reviewed in reference 1) followed 873 pregnant asthmatics using medications during pregnancy. Nine of these subjects used leukotriene modifiers. None of these patients had an increased risk of intrauterine growth restriction or preterm delivery. The small number of patients, however, limits inferences that may be made from these data. Current recommendations include consideration of zafirlukast or montelukast as alternative but not preferred drugs for mild persistent asthma or as add-on therapy for moderate asthma, especially in women with demonstrated efficacy of these drugs prior to pregnancy.[8]

PHARMACOLOGIC STEP THERAPY DURING PREGNANCY

Many pregnant asthmatic women require medications to control their asthma. Current guidelines[8] recommend a generalized stepwise approach in achieving and maintaining asthma control (Fig. 46-1). The number and dose of medications used are increased as necessary and decreased when possible. Decreasing doses should be performed carefully since this may lead to an exacerbation of symptoms. Current guidelines suggest that it may be prudent to postpone attempts at reducing therapy that is effectively controlling the patient's asthma until after the infant's birth.

MANAGEMENT OF ACUTE EXACERBATIONS OF ASTHMA DURING PREGNANCY

A recent large multicenter study reported that 20% of women with persistent asthma experience an unscheduled (emergency department or physician) visit for asthma during pregnancy and 8% required hospitalization (reviewed in reference 1). Such exacerbations can compromise fetal well-being; therefore, aggressive home management of acute symptoms needs to be reviewed with pregnant asthmatic patients. Above all, pregnant asthmatic patients should be taught to recognize the early signs and symptoms of exacerbations. The current recommendations[8] for home (Fig. 46-2) and emergency department (Fig. 46-3) management of asthma exacerbations in pregnant asthmatic women are not different than previously published Expert Panel Report 2 recommendations in nonpregnant asthmatic women except for the need for fetal monitoring.

Stepwise Approach for Managing Asthma During Pregnancy and Lactation: Treatment

Classify Severity: Clinical Features Before Treatment or Adequate Control			Medications Required to Maintain Long-Term Control
	Symptoms/ Day ___ Symptoms/ Night	PEF or FEV$_1$ ___ PEF Variability	Daily Medications
Step 4 **Severe** **Persistent**	Continual ___ Frequent	≤60% ___ >30%	• Preferred treatment • High-dose inhaled corticosteroid AND • Long-acting inhaled beta$_2$-agonist AND, if needed, • Corticosteroid tablets or syrup long term (2 mg/kg per day, generally not to exceed 60 mg per day.) (Make repeat attempts to reduce systemic corticosteroid and maintain control with high-dose inhaled corticosteroid.) • Alternative treatment: • High-dose inhaled corticosteroid AND • Sustained release thophylline to serum concentration of 5–12 μg/mL.
Step 3 **Moderate** **Persistent**	Daily ___ >1 night/week	>60%–<80% ___ >30%	• Preferred treatment EITHER • Low-dose inhaled corticosteroid and long-acting beta$_2$-agonist OR • Medium-dose inhaled corticosteroid If needed (particularly in patients with recurring severe exacerbations): • Medium-dose inhaled corticosteroid and long acting inhaled beta$_2$-agonist • Alternative treatment: • Low-dose inhaled corticosteroid and either theophylline or leukotriene receptor antagonist. If needed: • Medium-dose inhaled corticosteroid and either theophylline or leukotriene receptor antagonist.
Step 2 **Mild** **Persistent**	>2 days/week but <daily ___ >2 nights/month	≥80% ___ >20%–30%	• Preferred treatment: • Low-dose inhaled corticosteroid • Alternative treatment (listed alphabetically): cromolym, leukotriene receptor antagonist OR sustained-release theophylline to serum concentration of 5–12 μg/mL.
Step 1 **Mild** **Intermittent**	≤2 days/week ___ ≤2 nights/month	≥80% ___ <20%	• No daily medication needed. • Severe exacerbations may occur, separated by long periods of normal lung function and no symptoms. A course of systemic corticosteroid is recommended.

Figure 46-1 Stepwise approach for managing asthma during pregnancy and lactation: treatment.

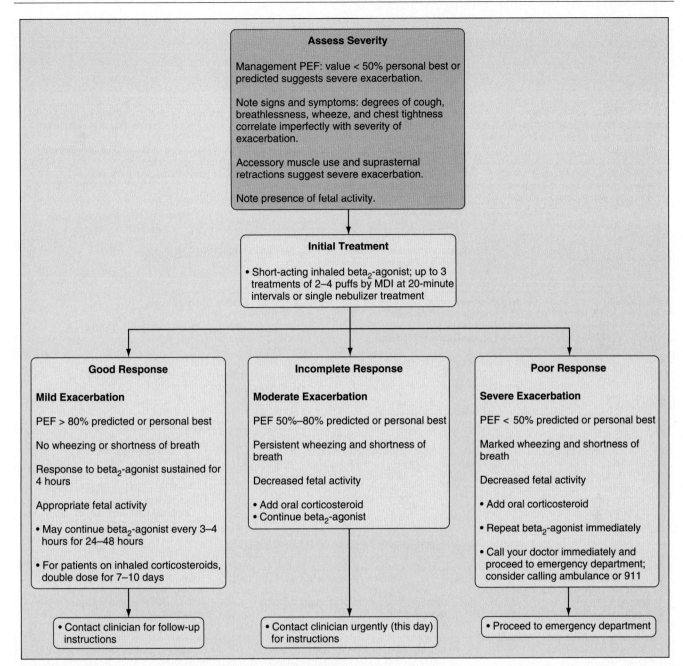

Figure 46-2   Management of asthma exacerbations: home treatment.

MANAGEMENT OF ASTHMA DURING LABOR AND DELIVERY

Only about 10% to 20% of women develop an exacerbation of asthma during labor and delivery. Nonetheless, asthma medications should be continued during labor and delivery. If a systemic steroid has been used in the previous month, then stress-dose steroid should be administered during labor to prevent maternal adrenal crisis. Practitioners should be aware of the potential adverse side effects that commonly used obstetric medications may have on asthma. For instance, PGF2-alpha and methylergonovine, used for postpartum hemorrhage, can induce bronchospasm. However, oxytocin, PGE2, and magnesium sulfate may be used safely in asthmatic patients. Maternal and fetal hypoxia due to asthma during labor and delivery can be managed medically, and rarely is it necessary to perform an emergency caesarean section for acute asthma during labor or delivery.

CONCLUSION

Over the past few years, much has been learned that is relevant to the management of asthma in pregnancy. While the studies reviewed here provide more insight in regards to the mechanisms involved and the treatment of asthma during pregnancy, there are still more questions to be answered. Hopefully, the updated guidelines, which address the safety of contemporary asthma medications during pregnancy, will be a helpful resource in the treatment of our pregnant asthmatic patients.

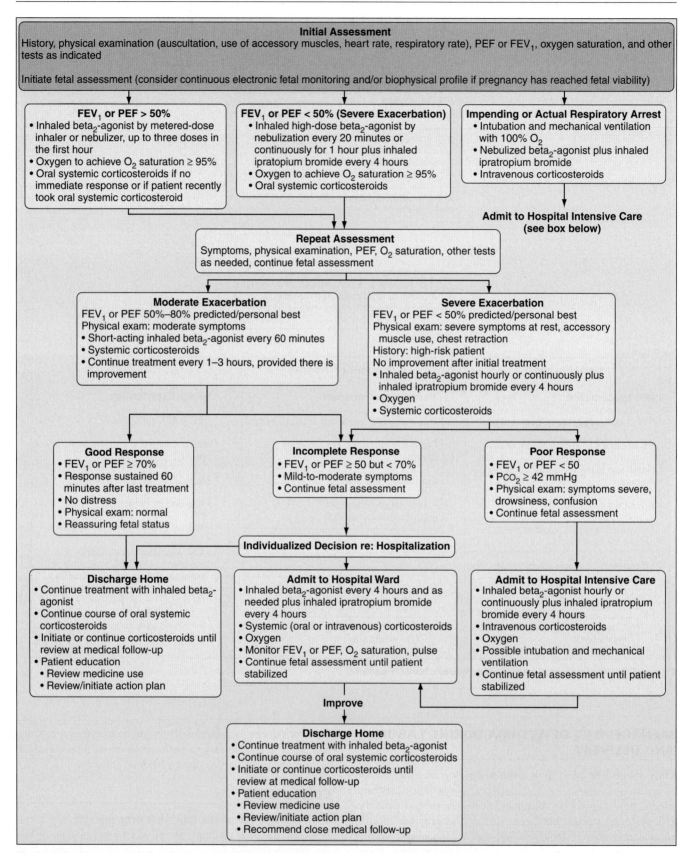

Initial Assessment

History, physical examination (auscultation, use of accessory muscles, heart rate, respiratory rate), PEF or FEV_1, oxygen saturation, and other tests as indicated

Initiate fetal assessment (consider continuous electronic fetal monitoring and/or biophysical profile if pregnancy has reached fetal viability)

FEV_1 or PEF > 50%
- Inhaled beta$_2$-agonist by metered-dose inhaler or nebulizer, up to three doses in the first hour
- Oxygen to achieve O_2 saturation ≥ 95%
- Oral systemic corticosteroids if no immediate response or if patient recently took oral systemic corticosteroid

FEV_1 or PEF < 50% (Severe Exacerbation)
- Inhaled high-dose beta$_2$-agonist by nebulization every 20 minutes or continuously for 1 hour plus inhaled ipratropium bromide every 4 hours
- Oxygen to achieve O_2 saturation ≥ 95%
- Oral systemic corticosteroids

Impending or Actual Respiratory Arrest
- Intubation and mechanical ventilation with 100% O_2
- Nebulized beta$_2$-agonist plus inhaled ipratropium bromide
- Intravenous corticosteroids

Admit to Hospital Intensive Care (see box below)

Repeat Assessment

Symptoms, physical examination, PEF, O_2 saturation, other tests as needed, continue fetal assessment

---

Moderate Exacerbation

FEV_1 or PEF 50%–80% predicted/personal best
Physical exam: moderate symptoms
- Short-acting inhaled beta$_2$-agonist every 60 minutes
- Systemic corticosteroids
- Continue treatment every 1–3 hours, provided there is improvement

Severe Exacerbation

FEV_1 or PEF < 50% predicted/personal best
Physical exam: severe symptoms at rest, accessory muscle use, chest retraction
History: high-risk patient
No improvement after initial treatment
- Inhaled beta$_2$-agonist hourly or continuously plus inhaled ipratropium bromide every 4 hours
- Oxygen
- Systemic corticosteroids

Good Response
- FEV_1 or PEF ≥ 70%
- Response sustained 60 minutes after last treatment
- No distress
- Physical exam: normal
- Reassuring fetal status

Incomplete Response
- FEV_1 or PEF ≥ 50 but < 70%
- Mild-to-moderate symptoms
- Continue fetal assessment

Poor Response
- FEV_1 or PEF < 50
- PCO_2 ≥ 42 mmHg
- Physical exam: symptoms severe, drowsiness, confusion
- Continue fetal assessment

Individualized Decision re: Hospitalization

Discharge Home
- Continue treatment with inhaled beta$_2$-agonist
- Continue course of oral systemic corticosteroids
- Initiate or continue corticosteroids until review at medical follow-up
- Patient education
  - Review medicine use
  - Review/initiate action plan

Admit to Hospital Ward
- Inhaled beta$_2$-agonist every 4 hours and as needed plus inhaled ipratropium bromide every 4 hours
- Systemic (oral or intravenous) corticosteroids
- Oxygen
- Monitor FEV_1 or PEF, O_2 saturation, pulse
- Continue fetal assessment until patient stabilized

Admit to Hospital Intensive Care
- Inhaled beta$_2$-agonist hourly or continuously plus inhaled ipratropium bromide every 4 hours
- Intravenous corticosteroids
- Oxygen
- Possible intubation and mechanical ventilation
- Continue fetal assessment until patient stabilized

Improve

Discharge Home
- Continue treatment with inhaled beta$_2$-agonist
- Continue course of oral systemic corticosteroids
- Initiate or continue corticosteroids until review at medical follow-up
- Patient education
  - Review medicine use
  - Review/initiate action plan
  - Recommend close medical follow-up

Figure 46-3 Management of asthma exacerbations: emergency department and hospital-based care.

REFERENCES

1. Schatz M, ed: Asthma and rhinitis during pregnancy. Immunol Allergy Clin N Am 2006;26:1–178.
2. Chung KD, Demissie K, Rhoads GG: Asthma in pregnancy—its relationship with race, insurance, maternal education, and prenatal care utilization. J Natl Med Assoc 2004;96:1414–1421.
3. Carroll KN, Griffin MR, Gebretsadik T, et al: Racial differences in asthma morbidity during pregnancy. Obstet Gynecol 2005;106:66–72.
4. Vrieze A, Postma D, Kerstjens H: Perimenstrual asthma: a syndrome without known cause or cure. J Allergy Clin Immunol 2003;112:271–282.
5. Tamasi L, Bohacs A, Pallinger E, et al: Increased interferon-gamma- and interleukin-4-synthesizing subsets of circulating T lymphocytes in pregnant asthmatics. Clin Exp Allergy 2005;35:1197–1203.
6. Kallen B, Rydhstroem H: Asthma during pregnancy—a population based study. Eur J Epidem 2000;16:167–171.
7. Murphy VE, Gibson PG, Smith R, et al: Asthma during pregnancy: mechanisms and treatment implications. Eur Respir J 2005;25:731–750.
8. NAEPP Expert Panel Report: Managing asthma during pregnancy: recommendations for pharmacologic treatment—2004 update. J Allergy Clin Immunol 2005;115:34–46.
9. Bakhireva LN, Jones KL, Schatz M, et al: The Organization of Teratology Information Services Research Group. Asthma medication use in pregnancy and fetal growth. J Allergy Clin Immunol 2005;116:503–509.
10. Martel M-J, Rey E, Beauchesne M-F, et al: Use of inhaled corticosteroids during pregnancy and risk of pregnancy-induced hypertension: nested case-control study. BMJ 2005;330:230–235.

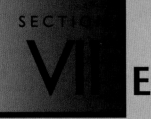

SECTION

VII EDUCATION

Assessing Educational Needs

Marianna M. Sockrider and Danita Czyzewski

CLINICAL PEARLS

- Perform a needs assessment with each clinical encounter to provide tailored education to the patient and family.

- Increase patients' confidence to control asthma by acknowledging past experiences and reinforcing successful efforts to self-manage.

- Have a plan among health care team members to share needs assessment tasks and to coordinate an intervention plan.

- Plan reassessment based on mutually negotiated educational goals.

- Help the caregiver(s) of children decide how they will be educated and coordinate asthma care.

Conducting an educational needs assessment is a classic methodological step in the design of an educational intervention or program for a population.[1] During a needs assessment, one identifies core knowledge, skills, and attitudes that are important to master, in this case, in order to become a successful collaborative self-manager of asthma. Identifying these needs is not only important when one is designing new educational material or intervention plan, but also when one selects an existing intervention for a new population. Even tested programs may require some adaptation for a new user group. On an individual basis, conducting a needs assessment is also a way of problem solving with an individual patient and team to improve asthma management. Identifying an issue of poor control or poor management and then identifying the possible causes (determinants) leads the clinician to a set of behavioral methods that address the determinants.

Assessing educational needs for individuals with chronic disease is not a one-time task, but an ongoing process. Even most patients who are newly diagnosed with asthma have some knowledge and experience at least with the symptoms that led to the diagnosis and perhaps with medications like albuterol. However, they have not organized the information and linked it to the decision making and skills to control the disease. For many patients, this will be their first experience with a chronic illness and with the necessity to use self-management skills in order to obtain optimal control and respond to changes in status over time. Those who have a diagnosis and have continued problems with control need reassessment to see what gaps in skills or applied knowledge or other barriers exist that might be addressed by tailored education.

One might ask, why is it important to explicitly assess educational needs? Some might assume that if patients have questions or barriers, they would mention them during the course of a clinical visit. While needs assessment may be done during the course of providing asthma education, one cannot assume that patients will recognize their own gaps in knowledge or skills and will initiate questions during a clinical visit. Patients may not have enough knowledge to recognize their gaps. Alternatively they may be embarrassed to admit not having mastered a skill or remembered information that they have been taught, or loath to admit to their own lack of confidence about the diagnosis or treatment. Repeated assessment of their educational needs using direct, noncritical questioning or other methods, will, over time, help patients feel safe to raise these concerns. In addition, by assessing patients and families' educational needs and current self-management abilities, one can tailor the messages provided, thereby optimizing the time spent. Patients will be more attentive and have greater satisfaction with the visit if they feel a clinician recognizes what they already know and helps them build on that without undue redundancy.

In this chapter, we discuss needs assessment in the context of clinical care with individuals with asthma and their families. The task of needs assessment is one that is shared by various members of the health care team just as delivery of education is shared by the entire team.

DETERMINANTS OF SELF-MANAGEMENT

Core skills and knowledge are required to optimally manage asthma. Practical knowledge that directly applies to asthma control should be stressed. One must distinguish between information that one "needs to know" versus information that is "nice to know." Does an individual need to understand cellular pathophysiology and pharmacokinetics to manage asthma? Focusing on the information that will lead directly to self-management behavior is advantageous in order to make the most of the limited time that one has to educate patients and to assure the patients don't get overwhelmed with too much information.

Typically when making educational goals, one focuses on core *behavioral capability* and *skills*.[1] *Behavioral capability* includes applied knowledge of what to do and how to do it. *Skills* are the demonstrated competence to perform self-management actions. Skills for asthma self-management include drug delivery and environmental control behaviors as well as symptom-monitoring and decision-making skills. Most basic asthma education programs include key knowledge and skills for both preventive behaviors as well as acute management behaviors. As discussed later in this chapter, the definition of *expert asthma self-management* includes a set of advanced cognitive skills that all patients cannot be expected to acquire, nor are they necessary for less complex asthma management.[2]

A clinician provides an individual or caregiver with basic practical knowledge and asthma management skills and assesses asthma management over time, with a focus on identifying factors that interfere with the patient's ability to carry out effective self-management. Knowing which factors are most relevant to a given patient will guide tailoring of further interventions. We identified a number of factors that have been theoretically or empirically related to asthma management. We organized these factors or determinants into categories.[3] Systematically considering each determinant category will help the clinician organize the needs assessment and assure that significant factors are not overlooked (Table 47-1).

Individuals may have issues related to more than one determinant. Start with a question such as, "What is keeping you from taking your asthma medicine as it is prescribed?" As determinants are identified and clarified, ask the question, "If *the problem* is addressed, will you then be able to take your medication?" to determine whether there are other obstacles.

Typically determinants that relate to *beliefs and goals* will need to be addressed before determinants that relate to the process of self-management (scheduling, skills, cooperation, finances). If one does not accept the diagnosis, lacks confidence to control asthma, or doubts that there will be benefit from a given therapy, it is less likely that the individual will take medications regularly.

BELIEFS ABOUT ASTHMA

The first step in becoming an effective self-manager in chronic disease is to accept the diagnosis. An asthma diagnosis is typically based on clinical judgment. A patient needs to trust the clinician's assessment and share any doubts or uncertainty. In addition, patients have to accept that asthma is a *chronic* disease that is likely to have recurring symptoms. This is particularly important for those patients who meet criteria for persistent disease since these individuals often need daily controller therapy for an indefinite period. Patients who have reduced lung function and poor perception of airflow obstruction are a particularly important group in which to assess beliefs about asthma and asthma control. Because their perception of "disease" is blunted, controlling this dangerous situation is dependent upon beliefs—not feelings—about asthma.

In addition to accepting the diagnosis, the approach to managing asthma may be affected by the patient's or family's beliefs about the causes of asthma or its symptoms. If it is thought that symptoms are due to an emotional reaction or as a means of avoiding exercise, school, or work, the patient's symptoms may be dismissed. Sometimes cultural beliefs such as theories related to hot and cold temperature or the passing of asthma to a Chihuahua may play a role in self-management practices. Patients may not accept an asthma diagnosis because they believe they will outgrow it. National asthma guidelines advise active monitoring of pulmonary function as well as regular follow-up care, so-called "well asthma" visits. Patients have to believe that there is benefit in taking time to make clinic visits when they are asymptomatic and that it is worth the expense and effort to assess pulmonary

Table 47-1	
DETERMINANTS OF ASTHMA SELF-MANAGEMENT BEHAVIOR	
Determinant Category	**Examples**
Beliefs about asthma	Acceptance of the diagnosis
	Beliefs about causes of asthma
	Knowledge and acceptance of chronic inflammatory nature and need for ongoing care
	Confidence to manage asthma in specific situations
	Perceived benefit of "well asthma visits"
Beliefs about medicines and other control strategies	Expectations regarding response to medications
	Concerns about medication dependence or tolerance
	Fear of side effects/complications from medications
	Expectations about strategies to avoid or eliminate triggers in the environment
	Confidence to control trigger exposure
Goals	Expectations regarding optimal function possible with good asthma control
	Perceived need to limit physical activity to avoid symptoms
	Value of exercise and physical fitness
Scheduling	Possesses basic organization skills
	Lifestyle allows for organization
	Takes medications at times prescribed
	Gets timely prescription refills
	Makes and keeps scheduled asthma follow-up appointments
	Obtains preventive care such as annual influenza vaccination
	Uses reminders
Cognitive skills	Has basic asthma knowledge of personal symptoms, triggers, control strategies
	Recognizes a change in symptoms
	Uses problem solving to manage obstacles and acute episodes
	Communicates effectively with others about asthma
Hands-on skills	Identifies medications
	Drug-delivery technique is effective
	Spirometry or peak flow technique is effective
Child cooperation	Refusal to take medication correctly
	Reluctance to report symptoms
	Participation in avoiding triggers
	Hand hygiene
Finances	Cost of medications
	Medical insurance coverage
	Indirect costs
	Transportation issue

function. Clinicians should explore patients' opinions about how often they think visits are needed and discuss the benefit of periodic assessments.

Self-efficacy has been shown to be important in the performance of self-management behaviors.[1,4] Self-efficacy is the expressed confidence to perform a behavior in a specific situation; thus asking a person directly how confident they are that they can perform a specific task is a good way to assess if they will do the task. Self-efficacy is task specific; thus one's confidence to perform some actions may differ from one's perceived ability to do other behaviors.

For example, one may feel able to monitor a child's trigger exposures at home but not in the school.

Example probes:

Do you believe that you have asthma?

Do you believe that asthma episodes can be prevented or that they will occur no matter what you do?

How confident are you that you can prevent an asthma episode at work?

Do you expect asthma to limit your activities?

BELIEFS ABOUT MEDICINES AND OTHER CONTROL STRATEGIES

The individual's beliefs, both positive and negative, about asthma medications and control strategies are an important determinant of asthma management. To begin to establish reasonable expectations for these asthma interventions, the clinician should clearly outline for the patient a time frame and markers to judge medication benefit. Patient concerns should be explored over time and issues addressed.

Outcome expectations are beliefs that the treatments will improve the symptoms of asthma.[1] Those with persistent disease who are prescribed anti-inflammatory controller therapy must develop appropriate outcome expectations regarding the benefit of daily treatments. Because a person does not feel immediate benefit from a dose of controller medication, appropriate outcome expectation and consistent symptom monitoring will determine that patient's long-term adherence to the controller.

Negative beliefs about medicine may interfere with appropriate use. A bronchodilator may be underused because of fear of developing tolerance resulting in a lack of benefit when really needed. Patients may also be concerned about becoming "addicted" or dependent on a medication over time. They may worry that regular use of a medication may make the lungs weak. Despite education to the contrary, some patients may underuse controllers because they do not appear to "work" like bronchodilator medications do.

Patients also modify use of medication based on concerns about side effects. They have experienced side effects and stopped the medication rather than checked to see if a dose adjustment or change in delivery technique would help. Some worry about the potential for side effects such as growth suppression, osteoporosis, or cataracts from inhaled corticosteroids. Risks and benefits should be discussed openly. A plan for reducing controller medication in the future with good control should be discussed in the context of self-regulation and planned in relation to the individual's triggers, time of year, and personal experience.

Environmental control to avoid or eliminate triggers is another core component of asthma therapy. Individuals may not know the best control strategies to use for specific triggers, they may have low expectations regarding the likely benefit of taking action to change the environment in improving asthma control, or they may have beliefs about ineffective strategies and do those without positive effect.[5] While it may be true that there are limits to the effectiveness and the feasibility of environmental control for asthma, a discussion about what a person believes may be helpful, what they can do and how they can recognize the expected benefit in asthma control is of value.

Example probes:

How do you understand that controller medications work differently from rescue medications?

What medication side effects are you concerned about?

What is the main reason you are not taking your daily medication?

Why did you delay using albuterol when you started coughing?

How would it make a difference in your asthma if you stopped smoking?

What exposures have you tried to avoid to prevent asthma episodes?

GOALS

Identifying patient/family goals or expectations may be a key to understanding less-than-optimal asthma management in some patients.[6] Unrealistically high goals are an issue for some ("I will never need to use my rescue medication because I will take my preventive medication without fail"), but the more typical reason for less-than-optimal asthma control is low goals and expectations. Patients may have low expectations for control, for example, assuming that recurrent asthma episodes are inevitable or that vigorous exercise is not possible when one has asthma. Others may be bothered by the side effects or inconvenience of treatment, but have not made a goal to address their concerns. Clinicians should make it clear by their questioning and feedback that balancing quality of life, optimal asthma management, and a healthy lifestyle is an appropriate overarching goal and the team is expecting to work with the patient to achieve this goal.

Example probes:

If you did not have asthma, how much physical activity would you like to do?

Do you think of yourself as a healthy person or more of a sickly person? If sickly, is this related to your asthma?

Is there a part of your asthma treatment regimen that feels very burdensome?

What is your goal for asthma control?

What would you like to do that asthma is interfering with?

SCHEDULING

Scheduling problems that interfere with asthma management may represent specific problems with asthma control scheduling or a more general scheduling issue. For patients who are unemployed or not going to school and/or live alone, schedules may not have much role in their lives and therefore, the scheduling of preventive routines will be more difficult to establish. Even for those with regular routines adding a new element, such as asthma medication to the routine may require some effort over time. Reminders or cues such as putting the medication next to the toothbrush can be helpful (see Chapter 48, Education Strategies). Conflicts with the patient's schedule may interfere with taking medications regularly. The clinician can get a sense of this by asking which dose is the hardest for the patient to take consistently. Conflicts with scheduling may reflect a difficulty in the situation at that time. For example, a child may take medication more reliably at lunchtime with the structured supervision of a school nurse, or an hourly worker may take medications better at home when he does not have to request a break to do so. Discussion about conflicts and the possibility of schedule flexibility will once again show the patient that the clinician is interested in making asthma control work for the patient's lifestyle. Especially for people who have difficulties with daily scheduling, difficulties with long-term regimens should be expected and explored. Follow-up appointment and failure to recognize when refills will be needed are two longer-term scheduling issues that will impact long-term management, but for which reminder processes can be put into place to avoid.

Example probes:

How do you know when you need to refill your albuterol inhaler?

Is there a dose of daily medicine that you find hard to remember to take? If so, why?

How do you keep track of your follow-up appointment?

COGNITIVE SKILLS

A chronic condition such as asthma requires the long-term application of self-regulation skills to obtain optimal control.[1,4,6] This is in contrast to the treatment of an acute condition where a diagnosis is made and a treatment prescribed, the patient adheres to the treatment for a brief period, and the condition is resolved. With a chronic condition the patient ideally engages in a cycle of symptom monitoring, problem identification, problem remediation (treatment), and reflection/reevaluation. Using their knowledge of asthma symptoms, triggers, and control strategies, patients are encouraged to recognize a change in symptoms early, decide what trigger avoidance and/or medication is necessary, and then assess if that intervention is working effectively. Without this active self-management, asthma will not be as well controlled. For example, asthma episodes will be more severe, side effects may be more bothersome, and triggers will be harder to identify. Self-management also implies the ability to observe the asthma care process and troubleshoot potential obstacles to assure long-term adherence. Important to this self-regulation process is the ability to communicate with the clinician in order to pass on observations, discuss hypotheses about episodes, or request modifications of therapies.

Given the variability in asthma for an individual over time, well-developed decision-making skills in self-management are needed for the best asthma management.[7] While it is not expected that all patients will achieve this level of cognitive skill, Creer has identified 12 judgment rules or strategies that are used both by gold standard physicians and patients in the management of pediatric asthma, and apply to adult asthma as well.[2] These skills represent the far end of the continuum of cognitive skills important in asthma management (Table 47-2). This list serves as a set of ideal cognitive skills to consider when assessing how well a patient manages a change in asthma control. A clinician's ultimate educational goal is to have a patient or caregiver develop competency for each of these rules. By evaluating how a patient handled a recent acute episode and how he or she communicated with the clinician about his or her assessment of asthma control, the patient's ability to meet these criteria will be evident.

Table 47-2
DECISION MAKING AND JUDGMENT RULES USED BY EXPERT ASTHMA MANAGERS

- Considers each acute asthma episode as a separate experiment
- Approaches care in a thoughtful and cautious manner
- Shows greater awareness of attacks, treatments, and potential outcomes
- Generates a number of testable treatment alternatives
- Consistently refers to personal database in making decisions
- Adjusts treatment to fit perceived severity of an asthmatic episode
- Does not misperceive severity of an asthmatic episode
- Regards events as correlated with, not causative of, asthma and asthmatic attacks
- Avoids preconceived notions in the treatment of asthma and individual attacks
- Thinks in terms of probabilities in managing asthma
- Is not overconfident
- Does not rely on memory in treating asthma

Adapted from Creer TL: Strategies for judgment and decision-making in the management of childhood asthma. Pediatr Asthma Allergy Immunol 1990;4(4):253–264.

Example probes:

Let's say you start coughing more at night, what would you do?

Have you noticed any common trigger among times you have had symptoms recently?

Tell me about the last time you had an asthma attack . . . start at the beginning and tell me what you noticed and what you did.

What kind of problems have you had to work out with your work, school, family, or friends to help you take better care of your asthma?

HANDS-ON SKILLS

Poor asthma control in an individual who already has been prescribed controller therapy should always raise questions regarding proper drug delivery. Many studies have documented errors in drug delivery for inhaled medications including the situation of confusing the bronchodilator inhaler with the corticosteroid inhaler. Both clinicians and patients make errors in use of all types of inhaled delivery devices. Since technique can deteriorate over time, ideally, one should check technique using a hands-on demonstration at each follow-up visit.

Similarly, spirometry and peak flow measures require good technique. Some electronic peak flow meters give users feedback on exhalation technique. If peak flow values are variable or seem higher or lower than expected, technique needs to be assessed. Obtaining home peak flow readings requires both skill as well as knowledge of how to interpret the results. This should be discussed in conjunction with symptom monitoring and with reference to the patient's personal best value. If peak flow measures are used, the clinician should ask about the readings and, before giving his/her interpretation of the readings, ask the patient to interpret the peak flow results.

Example probes:

Please show me how you take your inhaler medication.

Which inhaler do you use to prevent asthma problems? Have you found peak flow readings to be helpful at home? How?

CHILD COOPERATION

Inducing another person to take care of asthma adds a layer of complexity to asthma management. A parent may appear to have adequate knowledge and skills and have beliefs compatible with good management, but if the parent cannot ensure that the child engages in asthma management behaviors, poor outcomes will result. Lack of child cooperation may occur in multiple realms depending on the child's developmental level. Young children may refuse to take medication or medication administration may require such a struggle that the parent is exhausted by the effort and does not maintain the regimen over time. Older children and teens may not overtly protest medication use, but may be given responsibilities to take medication that they do not fulfill. Although it may be possible to oversee the environment of young children to prevent or at least reduce exposures to some triggers, adolescents may have multiple competing interests and not be attentive to avoidance of triggers to the extent necessary. Older children and teens may also at times be motivated to not report or to hide symptoms if, again, competing interests motivate them to appear symptom free. Observation of parent-child interaction within the medical encounter will often provide hints that child cooperation is a determinant of poor asthma management. If a parent is having difficulty getting the child to comply in this setting, it is very likely that cooperation in the home is worse. If the parent gets the child to comply only with a great deal of cajoling, one might expect that the parent will not be able to keep up that level of inducement in order to support a long term regimen.

A corollary to child cooperation is the child's ever-changing developmental level with regard to self-management. While it is appropriate that young children merely cooperate with treatments, by school age children with asthma should be taking a more active role in symptom monitoring and guided decision making. Through the adolescent years, teens should be taking increasing responsibility for self-management until they are independent self-managers as they are ready to leave home. As part of the needs assessment, clinicians should ascertain the level of self-management that the child has achieved as well as the parents' strategies for encouraging an increasingly active role in their children. This type of assessment can be done as the clinician observes who in the family responds to questions about symptoms and treatments, as well as with more direct questioning.

Example probes:

How well does your child cooperate with taking medications?

How long does it take to give your child the asthma medication?

Does your child let you use the facemask spacer?

Is your child getting into the habit of taking the medication regularly without protest?

Do you always have to remind him or her?

Has your child showed effort to notice and avoid some triggers?

How have you tried to encourage taking more responsibility for symptom reporting or medication taking?

Does your child wash his or her hands without reminders?

Can your child tell you when he or she is having asthma symptoms?

Do you allow your child to carry his or her own inhaler?

FINANCES

Poor adherence with asthma therapy or appointment keeping may be because of problems with finances directly or indirectly related to medical care. Some may be uninsured while others are underinsured or have restrictive insurance with respect to drug formulary and/or access to certain providers. Medication costs, even copays alone, may lead some individuals to try to get by with less medication or fail to fill some prescriptions. Sometimes a family will want information on whether a generic product can be substituted for a brand name or whether an over-the-counter product will work instead. The patient may reduce the dose to save medication and stretch the need for refills. A patient may forego use of a valved holding chamber because of lack of insurance coverage. The indirect costs of asthma nationally are impressive and are likely to influence decisions about therapy and perhaps result in accepting less-than-optimal asthma control. Indirect costs include not only medication copays, but missed work and child care costs. An individual may have transportation problems getting to visits or may have concern about environmental risks with the use of public transportation.

Example probes:

Do you have concerns about medication costs?

How do you get to clinic visits?

ASSESSMENT STRATEGIES

Interviews

In a typical clinical practice, an interview with the patient or family is the primary way in which an educational needs assessment is made. In the early postdiagnostic period, perhaps after some basic or standard reading materials or verbal instructions are given, the clinician may spend some time asking about the patient's understanding of symptoms, triggers, and interventions. Questions requiring the verbalization of information such as, "Tell me the names of your asthma medications and how they work to control your symptoms," produce a better assessment than questions that merely require assent, such as, "Do you understand that you need to take your anti-inflammatory medications daily?" While requiring the patient to "teach you back" will be initially more time consuming and more anxiety arousing for the patient, this type of questioning will better reveal educational deficiencies and reinforce for the patient that the clinician believes that this information is important.

After the early postdiagnostic period, educational needs assessment may be triggered in the course of the clinical encounter by revelations of less than optimal control. The preceding section on Determinants gives suggestions for assessing various factors that may influence asthma self-management and result in poor control.

Using Assessment Measures

There is growing support for the use of written surveys and brief questionnaires to measure patient-reported asthma control and quality of life in clinical practice. Such measures ensure that core variables that define asthma control are reviewed.

While there are a number of measures of asthma knowledge that have been published, as well as some measures of other determinants such as self-efficacy, these are not a substitute for an interactive needs assessment between the clinicians and patient and family.

Indirect Assessment

While educational needs may be assessed formally through interview or written instruments, maintaining an awareness of educational deficits should be ongoing in all aspects of the medical visit. Informal assessment is particularly useful in assessing the application of knowledge. A patient may be able to answer a direct question about a treatment or a symptom; however, in talking to the same patient about an episode and the response to an episode, the patient may have not put that knowledge into effect. When deficits in applied knowledge are identified, it is typically helpful to explore further the source of the confusion. All team members should be responsible for indirect assessment of educational needs, and it is helpful to have some way to communicate these findings to other team members so that all are aware of educational needs.

Being a Role Model during Needs Assessment

It may be of value to think about how the clinician actually is modeling the same processes that one does in asthma self-management while assessing educational needs. Reviewing asthma control and care during symptom episodes and learning from one's experiences are key steps to becoming an expert asthma manager. Needs assessment follows the same model of self-regulation through monitoring, intervention, and reevaluation.

In addition, successful clinicians need to have good communication skills including active listening.[8] Patients also require good skills to communicate with others who assist them in asthma care in the home, workplace, school, and health care settings. Through the process of needs assessment, the clinician helps the patient and family refine these communication skills and models what information is important to cover, including how one thinks and feels about carrying out self-management.

The health care provider team needs to set up a plan to act on what is learned through needs assessment. This might occur by doing a preclinic huddle before the next visit to decide what to follow up on and/or by debriefing at a point in the visit to decide what else is needed and to plan follow-up visits or phone encounters. Document needs assessment findings and the intervention plan in the patient's chart.

Throughout the encounter, one should provide reinforcement for positive behavior and attitudes. Feedback can be given for active monitoring, medication adherence, and good decision making. Acknowledge improvement in asthma control as a consequence of self-management rather than just luck or fate. A simple positive message recognizing good self-management can be a powerful reinforcement.

SUMMARY

There are many factors that can influence asthma control and self-management by patients and families. In addition, there are different ways to approach the assessment of individuals to best evaluate obstacles that need to be eliminated and positive behaviors that need to be reinforced. One would like to help each patient and family become the best self-manager possible and collaborate actively and effectively with the health care team. These "expert" self-managers recognize the chronic nature of asthma, its intrinsic variability and need for flexibility, active monitoring, and decision making with input from asthma specialists in the health care team.

REFERENCES

1. Bartholomew LK, Parcel GS, Kok G, Gottlieb NH: Step 1: Needs assessment. In Planning Health Promotion Programs: An Intervention Mapping Approach, 2nd ed. San Francisco, Jossey-Bass, 2006, pp 129, 207–233, 555.
2. Creer TL: Strategies for judgment and decision-making in the management of childhood asthma. Pediatr Asthma Allergy Immunol 1990;4(4):253–264.
3. Shegog R, Bartholomew LK, Czyzewski DI, et al: Development of an expert system knowledge base: a novel approach to promote guideline congruent asthma care. J Asthma 2004;41(4):385–402.
4. Clark NM, Valerio MA: The role of behavioral theories in educational interventions for paediatric asthma. Paediatr Respir Rev 2003;4(4):325–333.
5. Cabana MD, Slish KK, Lewis TC, et al: Parent management of asthma triggers within a child's environment. J Allergy Clin Immunol 2004;114(2):352–357.
6. Clark NM, Partridge MR: Strengthening asthma education to enhance disease control. Chest 2002;121(5):1661–1669.
7. Wade SL, Holden G, Lynn H, et al: Cognitive-behavioral predictors of asthma morbidity in inner-city children. J Dev Behav Pediatr 2000;21:340–346.
8. Clark NM, Gong M, Schork MA, et al: A scale for assessing health care providers' teaching and communication behavior regarding asthma. Health Educ Behav 1997;24(2):245–256.

Educational and Communication Strategies and Resources

Christine Waldman Wagner

- Asthma education is an ongoing process that must be integrated into asthma management at every visit.

- Learning styles, cognitive levels, and readiness to change behavior are fluid and must be reassessed frequently during the course of education.

- Telling is not teaching. The asthma educator must possess knowledge of educational principles as well as asthma care.

- Asthma education can reduce the morbidity and mortality of asthma.

- Asthma educators with national certification are being recognized as the ideal individuals to provide competent, valid asthma education to patients and families affected by asthma.

It doesn't matter how brilliant the diagnosis, how cutting edge the treatment, or how innovative the therapy, if the patient will not agree to and implement the plan of action, the disease remains untreated and potentially fatal. Studies on the effects of patient education on asthma outcomes have been sporadic and often inconclusive, frequently because of poor study design and/or inadequate follow-up. However studies do exist to support the benefits of patient education. Fireman and colleagues reported that an educational program performed by a nurse-educator resulted in reduced hospitalizations and emergency room visits, improved school attendance, and fewer asthma attacks.[1] Guevara and associates found that asthma education was associated with improved lung function, reduced school absenteeism, fewer days of restricted activity, and, in some cases, a reduced number of disturbed nights.[2] This chapter will discuss educational/learning theories, how individuals learn, and how the asthma educator can maximize the effects of patient and family education.

COMPLIANCE VERSUS ADHERENCE

While the terms compliance and adherence are frequently used interchangeably in the medical field, there are vast differences between the two terms. Compliance is defined as the act or process of conforming or adapting one's actions to a desire, demand, proposal, or coercion of another. Adherence is defined as the act of holding fast or sticking to a concept or plan.[3] Clearly, the patient is not involved in the evaluation or planning of their health care when compliance is the goal. The clinician makes all decisions and recommendations and the patient is expected to follow those directions. Adherence

implies that the patient is an active member of the educational health care team, helping to make the diagnosis and develop and implement the treatment plan. Additionally, the patient should also be involved in evaluating the treatment plan and assisting the health care providers to make appropriate adjustments to maintain asthma control.

Nonadherence can take many forms, from failure to fill a prescription to improper dosing, incorrect use of devices (inhalers, peak flow meters) or asthma action plans, and early termination of therapy.[4] Other forms of nonadherence include improper use of medications due to misunderstandings about the purpose of each medication. It is not unusual for patients or parents to report the asthma medication "doesn't work" when they are using the controller inhaler only for relief of acute asthma symptoms. Without education, the other three components of asthma care—measures of assessment and monitoring, control of factors contributing to asthma severity, and pharmacologic therapy established by the National Asthma Education and Prevention Program (NAEPP)[5] — cannot be implemented.

THEORETICAL FRAMEWORKS FOR EDUCATION

Theoretical frameworks abound and a discussion regarding the benefits and barriers of a multitude of theories would be a chapter in itself. The Health Belief Model and the Transtheoretical Model/Stages of Change are the ones this author finds most helpful when developing educational interventions and will be the basis for recommendations in this chapter.

Simply stated, the Health Belief Model states that individuals are most likely to change health-related behavior if they believe that:

- They are susceptible or vulnerable to the disease (do they have asthma or a risk of developing asthma?)
- The disease could have serious, negative impact on their lives (could they miss school, work, be hospitalized or even die from their asthma?)
- Following positive health care recommendations would reduce the risks associated with the disease (do they have confidence in the efficacy of medical intervention?)
- The benefits of following the health care recommendations outweigh the cost (physical, emotional, and financial).[6]

Each belief is supported by the previous belief. It is the job of the educator to determine, through working with the patient and family, if they are incorporating each concept into their health care plan. Often failures in therapy will be related to the lack of acceptance of one or more of the above statements.

The patient who does not believe they have asthma will not perform the skills necessary to achieve asthma control because they do not agree with the diagnosis. Frequently, the first step of the educator is to identify false beliefs ("it's just allergies, not asthma"), convince the patient that it is a false belief (by identifying reduced pulmonary function tests when the patient feels well, problems with exertion, and so forth) and then lead the patient to acceptance of the correct diagnosis. Only when false beliefs are discarded can new information be accepted, internalized, and used in the development of an appropriate plan of action.

The transtheoretical model/stages of change theory was developed by James Prochaska[7] as a synthesis of 18 major theories of psychotherapy and behavioral change, hence the term *transtheoretical*. He identified six stages of change used by individuals to facilitate smoking cessation:

- *Precontemplation*—the patient has no intention of taking any action within the next 6 months
- *Contemplation*—intends to take action within the next 6 months
- *Preparation*—intends to take action within the next 30 days and has taken some behavioral steps in this direction
- *Action*—has changed overt behavior for less than 6 months
- *Maintenance*—has changed overt behavior for more than 6 months
- *Termination*—overt behavior will never return and there is complete confidence that the patient can cope without fear of relapse.[7]

This theory was quickly found to be applicable to other disease states and can easily be applied to asthma. For example, in the *Precontemplation* stage, asthma patients are not ready to change their asthma management; they are likely to miss follow-up appointments and continue with uncontrolled asthma until their next acute exacerbation. Patients in the *Contemplation* stage might ask others about asthma, read articles, or search online. They are starting to think there might be a better way to manage their asthma but are not ready to act in the near future. Similarly, individuals in the *Preparation* stage are gathering information and anticipating taking action. They might be the ones we see in the clinic, still gathering information but not yet ready to act upon it. This is why it is a grievous error for a clinician to say, "I gave them my recommendations and they didn't act on them so I'm not going to bring it up again." Some people can remain in the contemplation stage for years before moving into the preparation stage. In the *Action* stage, the patient and/or family incorporate the information and education they have obtained into their asthma management plan. They begin taking the medications, monitoring symptoms, and instituting avoidance measures. They are also monitoring the results of their actions so it is critical that the educator meet with them often to determine what is working and what is not. For patients to reach *Maintenance* stage, the plan must be successful, easy to follow and produce benefit. Regular follow-up visits should focus on reinforcing education, offering encouragement and praise for a job well done (even if the outcomes are not optimal) and discussing new therapies that might be appropriate for the patient. The *Termination* stage is difficult if not impossible to determine in asthma care due to the variability of the disease and ever-changing treatments available.

Knowing the patient's status in these two theories can help the educator to implement a plan of action when designing educational interventions. While that task might seem formidable, asking a few questions can often begin the evaluation process. First, the educator must determine what disease the patient thinks he or she has, whether the patient believes there are risks associated with that disease, and whether the patient thinks he or she is susceptible to those risks. Identifying patient/family goals for therapy is an important step. Simply asking, "What do you want to accomplish with this visit today?" can help the patient and clinician begin to work on developing reasonable asthma management goals. Asking what therapies, medications, and actions they have tried in the past (both successful and unsuccessful) should help to direct interventions. A final question is, "When do you want to start?" This might seem to be a foolish question but patients may not be ready to begin immediately and if the educator knows this, it will reduce the frustration and enhance communication.

To begin the educational process, false information must be discarded and replaced with valid information. If this sounds time consuming, it can be. Education does not occur in one visit. It is not possible to change patient behavior and complete an educational process in one or two visits. New data, new medications, and new issues with patients make ongoing education critical. Patients can "obtain" false data at any time, which must be dealt with by the asthma educator. Lay media may be a source of false or distorted information, especially about potential side effects of medications and patients must be asked about new information gained since the last visit.

Additionally, simply supplying information is NOT providing education. Until patients incorporate the information into their health care practices, they are not educated. It is often difficult for a patient to understand why certain recommendations are being made. It is the role of the educator to explain why those recommendations are important to the patient's health and help the patient to not only recognize the need but also to determine how it can be done.

LEARNING MOTIVATION

Understanding what motivates a patient to seek care and information is an important step in effective asthma education. Information seeking is motivated by a current need or interest. Adults are unlikely to learn information that they do not feel is relevant to their current situation. Adult learning is self-directed and goal oriented and most often aimed at solving an actual or perceived problem.

Children learn differently from adults. Most of what children learn is determined by outside sources and not based on a current need. Pediatric education in the formal setting is learning to be used at some point in the future and, therefore, not related to personal goals or issues. Informal pediatric education is often goal oriented and self-motivated. A child who wants to learn a skill related to playing (e.g., sports, video games) or other self-motivated interests will learn quickly and with much less outside teaching. Telling children or adolescents that if they control their asthma they will be able to attend school might not be a motivation to take their medications. Explaining that they will be able to do the things they enjoy (fully participating in sports, playing outside with their friends, and so forth) might be a better motivator.

Individuals who deal with children are familiar with Erikson's psychosocial stages of development that focus on emotional identity stages. Piaget developed a developmental framework for cognitive abilities. Following this framework, the educator can identify educational approaches best suited for the specific child. When providing education to a parent and child it is essential to teach to the level of the child. Parents are perfectly capable of understanding information at a lower cognitive level; children (and adults) cannot assimilate information provided at a higher cognitive level.

Piaget's stages are compared to Erikson's in Table 48-1. The stages are:

- *Sensorimotor* (birth to 18 months)—during this stage of intellectual development learning takes place through sensations. Children progress from reflex activity to simple repetitive behaviors and then to imitative behavior. A sense of cause and effect is developed as they learn to problem solve through trial and error. During this stage children develop object permanence, the concept that an object exists even when it is no longer visible. This is a prerequisite for future mental activity.
- *Preoperational* (2 to 7 years)—during this period of intellectual development the predominant characteristic is egocentricity in that the child is completely incapable of placing himself in the place of another. Objects and events are not understood in general terms, only in terms that relate specifically to the child. They cannot see things from any perspective but theirs and they cannot see another's point of view. During this stage thinking is concrete, with an inability to reason beyond what is observed. They are not capable of making deductions and generalizations. Associations between ideas are best learned through imaginative play, questioning, and interacting.
- *Concrete operational* (7 to 11 years)—during this period thought becomes more logical and more coherent. The ability to sort, classify, order, and organize information is developing during this time. They can deal with several different aspects of a situation simultaneously. In this stage the ability to deal in abstraction is still not present but they can recognize points of view other than their own.
- *Formal operational* (12 to 15 years)—this stage is characterized by flexibility and adaptability. They can think in abstract terms and make logical conclusions from observations. Hypotheses can be made and tested.

Learning is accomplished more easily if the learner can relate new information and concepts to already established knowledge and routines. Using these concepts can make teaching much easier.[8]

LEARNING STYLES

There are three ways individuals learn: visually, auditorily, and kinesthetically.

- The *visual* learner must see the information to understand
- The *auditory* learner must hear (or read) the information to understand
- The *kinesthetic* learner must experience the information to understand

This is probably the basis for the old adage "See one, do one, teach one." Most individuals have one learning route that is their main way of learning and that route is augmented by the others.[9] A simple question to ask at the beginning of an educational session is, "What format makes it easiest for you to learn?" This can help the educator deliver the information in a format that is most acceptable to the patient. Unfortunately in a busy clinic setting it is difficult to fully evaluate learning styles and quickly adapt the information into the best format. The easier way is to deliver each lesson in such a way that each learning style is used. For example, when teaching inhaler techniques, first tell the patient the proper way to use an inhaler; second, show the patient the proper technique (without speaking) and provide written instructions to take home; then have the patient demonstrate the technique back to you. In this way, all three styles are covered and the patient has received the information in a variety of ways. Additionally, by having the patient return demonstration, it gives the educator the opportunity to correct faulty techniques immediately before they can become imbedded in the patient's practice. It is important that this teaching occurs at every visit because patients will develop bad techniques over time that can be discovered and corrected quickly during a visit.

Children of different ages learn through different methods and mediums. Preschool children like bold bright colors, pictures they can relate to, and play-acting. Reading a story about a child having an asthma attack and then role playing with the child about what to do if he or she were having trouble breathing can help teach a small child when to seek help from an adult. School-age children like games and do well with group learning. Children of this age learn well in a small group setting in which they recognize that the others in the group have the same issues and problems that they have. Preadolescents prefer skill learning, interactive, hands-on learning. Video games are a favorite way of learning and having fun for these

	Table 48-1		
	ERIKSON'S AND PIAGET'S DEVELOPMENTAL THEORIES		
Age	Erikson's Psychosocial Stages	Age	Piaget's Cognitive Stages
Birth to 1 yr	Trust vs mistrust	Birth to 18 mo	Sensorimotor
1 to 3 yr	Autonomy vs shame and doubt	18 mo to 2 yr	Preoperational thought, preconceptual phase
3 to 6 yr	Initiative vs guilt	4 to 7 yr	Preoperational thought, intuitive phase
6 to 12 yr	Industry vs inferiority	7 to 12 yr	Concrete operations (inductive reasoning and beginning logic)
13 to 19 yr	Identity and repudiation vs identity confusion	13 to 19 yr	Formal operations (deductive and abstract reasoning)

children. Adolescents may not respond to formal educational programs. They interact well with peers and respond to people they respect. Using peers who have successfully learned to manage their asthma can facilitate learning. Helping adolescents identify individuals they look up to who have learned to successfully manage their asthma can be very beneficial.

When teaching, remember that attention spans vary according to age: 2 to 3 minutes for a preschooler, 5 to 10 for school-aged children, and 15 to 20 for adolescents and adults. For this reason, short interventions are best. Another option is to vary the educators. Brief sessions with several educators over a visit can enhance learning even more. However, it is critical that each educator is delivering the same message.

It is important to remind parents that their child needs the parent to be involved as a guide and supervisor. Frequently, parents are tired of being "in charge" by the time a child reaches early adolescence. It is not unusual for a parent to state that the child is "old enough" to manage the asthma by himself. Developmentally, an adolescent is often unable to consistently remember everything he or she needs to manage asthma. Parents must constantly remind, supervise, and ensure medications are being refilled in a timely fashion. I have found it helpful to ask parents if during their child's sporting events they still call out instructions and encouragement from the sidelines. I have yet to find a parent who responds negatively. Explaining to the parents that giving instructions and encouragement in asthma management is the same thing often helps them to understand their role.

THE ROLE OF THE EDUCATOR

In the past, health care professionals did not receive much education on how to be an educator. Fortunately, this is changing in many institutions. Telling is not teaching and information is not education. To educate someone, the teacher must not only give information but also help the patient see how it is important to incorporate it into their life.

Assessing barriers to changing health behavior is also part of the role of the educator. Maslow established a hierarchy of needs stating that, until more basic needs were met, individuals could not work on higher needs (Fig. 48-1).[10] If a patient or parent is worrying about how they are going to pay for the medication, they will not be able to concentrate on how, when, or why to administer that medication. Discovering barriers to care may take multiple visits before the patient is comfortable revealing them to the provider. Knowing about insurance issues and copays may seem like an issue for only the front office but it also affects patient care. Helping patients by providing samples and identifying and helping them access finan-

cial assistance programs or other resources can help patients obtain the tools needed to better manage their disease.

Without effective communication, education cannot occur. Communication is not just talking, it's asking the right questions, listening to the responses, and verifying what you have heard by paraphrasing the statement back to the patient. Reading your notes back to the patient is an excellent way to show you were listening and to verify that you have captured the patient's feelings and thoughts. If your setting uses electronic medical records, try to make eye contact with your patient during conversations. Talking to someone who is staring at a computer screen is not conducive to communication.

Make sure you are being understood by the patient. For patients whose primary language is not yours, using an interpreter might be necessary. Try to avoid using a child as the interpreter. Adult patients often do not want their children hearing about their concerns and symptoms. When the child is the patient, the child may not always be thorough or honest about what the clinician is saying. Try to have a staff member act as an interpreter whenever possible. Being understood by the patient includes avoiding unfamiliar terms. Even a patient with training in the health care field should be treated as a novice. Never assume a patient "knows" something because it is not a new diagnosis.

ESTABLISHED KNOWLEDGE

To retain a new skill or new information, it is helpful if the learner can relate the new information to information already established.[10] Identifying a health care action the patient already practices can expedite the incorporation of a new preventive behavior. A good example is the use of fluoride to reduce the number of cavities. Encouraging the use of fluoride to prevent tooth decay was probably one of the most successful health education programs in the United States. Programs were presented in schools, in the written media, and through advertising on television. Everyone was inundated with the simple message: fluoride prevents tooth decay. It was a mass media campaign on the benefits of preventive health care.

The concept of decay prevention can easily be transferred to asthma care. Explaining that controller asthma medications are like fluoride is an easy concept to grasp. Everyone understands that using fluoride toothpaste on a regular basis prevents cavities. Patients do not feel the fluoride working when it is used; they know the fluoride works because when they visit the dentist they are cavity free. When using controller asthma medication daily, patients don't feel the medication working. They know it is working when they visit their asthma care provider and have improved by obtaining normal or near normal lung function; sleeping through the night; exerting without wheezing, tight chest, or shortness of breath; or by not needing reliever asthma medications.

Reliever asthma medications can be compared to repairing a cavity. The repair or filling helps the current situation (the cavity) but it does not treat the cause of the problem. If a patient uses only the reliever medication, it takes care of the immediate problem but endangers the long-term health of the patient.

Terminology is important when talking about asthma medications. The NAEPP guidelines use the terms "long-term control" and "quick relief" to differentiate the actions of the medications used to treat asthma. Somewhere along the way asthma specialists fell into the practice of using the term "rescue" interchangeably with "relief." Often patients fail to

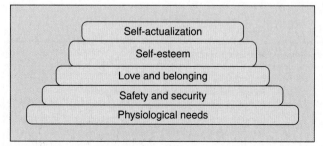

Figure 48-1 Maslow's Hierarchy of Needs.

- Self-actualization
- Self-esteem
- Love and belonging
- Safety and security
- Physiological needs

use reliever medications early in the exacerbation of asthma. When asked why they delayed using the reliever often the response was "I didn't think I was that bad." It seems apparent by these patient responses that they were waiting to need to be rescued rather than taking the medication to relieve symptoms. Reliever is a much better description of when we want patients to use these medications and should be the preferred term when teaching about medications.

When explaining why it is important to exhale fully and then take slow deep breaths when inhaling asthma medications, several points can be used. Emptying the lungs before inhaling asthma medication allows one to get more medication deeper into the lungs. Ask a child what the child would do if he or she had a half glass of water and wanted a full glass of Coke. Every child will tell you that he or she would pour the water out of the glass; no one wants watered-down Coke. Explaining that emptying their lungs first will allow them to get a full dose of medicine instead of a watered-down dose of medicine makes the lesson visual and easier to grasp.

When teaching about allergen avoidance it is sometimes hard for patients to understand about dust mites and mold spores. Convincing patients who are allergic to dust mites to get dust-proof encasings can be an ongoing process for the asthma educator. Dust mites are perceived as something only people with dirty houses have. Explain that dust mites are microscopic (you can't see them), they eat the skin we flake off (not the skin we are still using), pull their water from the air (mites like high-humidity areas), are photophobic (they like to burrow down into dark areas like pillows, mattresses, carpet pads, and upholstered furniture), and are present everywhere these conditions exist. This information can help patients understand why dust mites are present in their environment regardless of how vigorously they might clean.

Next, explain that only extremes in hot or cold temperature will kill dust mites. Since it's not possible to wash the mattress in hot water or to freeze it, it is essential to put a barrier between the patient and the allergen. The next step is to relate having dust mites in the pillow and mattress to having another allergen in there. I have found telling a dust mite–allergic patient sleeping on an uncovered pillow and mattress is like being allergic to ragweed and going out, picking some ragweed, and then stuffing it into their pillow and mattress. This is a very visual way to explain dust mite avoidance and it frequently works.

It is also important to mention that the encasings do not have to be removed every week to be washed. Recommendations range from laundering every few months to only annually. Showing the patient a sample of the encasing materials can also encourage purchase. Many patients remember the cold, noisy plastic encasings of their childhood and won't even consider buying them. Once they see and feel the fabrics used today for encasings they are much more inclined to purchase them. Many companies that sell these encasings are happy to send free booklets, tear-off sheets, and samples for you to have in your office. They can be located by Internet search using the term "allergy products."

ASSOCIATING NEW ACTIVITIES WITH EXISTING PRACTICES

Adding new activities to a daily routine can be cumbersome and difficult for anyone. A patient dealing with asthma often feels it is not possible to add anything more to their daily routine. Teaching patients to tie new activities to already practiced activities can make additional health care behaviors easier to incorporate into a daily schedule. Teaching patients to take controller medications immediately before brushing their teeth links the two activities. Some patients even need to make a physical link between the two. If a patient cannot remember to take controller medicine before brushing his or her teeth, instruct the patient to take a piece of ribbon or yarn and actually tie the inhaler to the toothbrush. After about 2 weeks the two activities will become one in the mind of the patient.

TEACHABLE MOMENTS

While much emphasis has been placed upon finding the "teachable moment," every patient encounter should be considered a time to teach. Identifying teaching tools is an important part of the educator role. Having brief, easy-to-read asthma information to give patients is a good way to initiate discussions of different aspects of asthma care. If possible, don't recreate the wheel. There is a vast amount of material available that can easily be adapted to your practice (Table 48-2). Simple nonbranded booklets like "One Minute

Table 48-2
ASTHMA EDUCATIONAL RESOURCES

Organization	Description	Contact Information
Association of Asthma Educators	Multidisciplinary organization of asthma educators	www.asthmaeducators.org
National Asthma Educator Certification Board	Certifying board of asthma educators in the United States	www.naecb.org
Allergy and Asthma Network/Mothers of Asthmatics	Newsletter/support group for patients	www.aanma.org
American Academy of Allergy, Asthma and Immunology	Professional organization of allergists, immunologists and allied health members	www.aaaai.org
American Association of Respiratory Therapists	Professional organization for respiratory therapists	www.aarc.org
American College of Allergy, Asthma and Immunology	Professional organization of allergists, immunologists and allied health members	www.acaai.org
American Thoracic Society	Professional organization for pulmonologists and allied health members	www.thoracic.org
American Lung Association	Lay organization for patients with pulmonary diseases	www.lungusa.org
Asthma and Allergy Foundation of America	Lay organization for patients with allergies and asthma	www.aafa.org
Local and state asthma coalitions	Coalitions of individuals and organizations working to improve the status of asthma care	Local listings

Patient DOB			
Date of encounter			
Patient learning preferences			
Pathophysiology			
Goals of therapy			
Early warning signs			
Asthma triggers			
Avoidance measures			
Medications/purpose			
Controller medications			
Reliever medications			
Dosage/time			
Potential side effects			
Rules of Two ©			
Inhaler technique			
Spacer			
Inhalation therapy			
Peak flow monitoring			
Written materials			
Videos			

Figure 48-2   Educational Flow Sheet. (Adapted from Wagner C: Asthma Care and Patient Education: The Nurse's Role. Houston, University of Texas Medical Center, Copyright 1985; revised 1993. May be reproduced for educational purposes.)

Asthma" (Pedipress.com) can be given to a patient or parent during a nebulizer treatment with only one or two pages identified as something the patient should read. Ask them to make notes of any questions that arise so that they can be discussed afterwards.

CONTRACTS

While contracts are most often discussed in relation to older children and adolescents, they can work well with adults too. With children, a written contract is much more effective: write down what is expected of the child, the parent, and the educator; what the positive outcome for the patient will be; and the consequences of breaking the contract. The contract should be for a specific, short (4 weeks or less typically) period of time and the method of evaluating the outcome should be specifically stated in the contract. Each party should sign the contract and a copy be given to everyone involved with the original going into the chart. All involved parties should be present when the outcome is discussed. With adults, a verbal agreement is usually adequate.

There are as many educational techniques as there are educators and students. Styles will change for each educator based on new data and experiences. As education is an ongoing process for our patients, it should also be for us as educators. Sharing our experiences will broaden our knowledge and provide us with new tools for helping our patients to manage their health successfully.

DOCUMENTATION

Current Procedural Terminology (CPT) codes exist for educational and training services. These codes are applicable to asthma education. The codes are used to report services "prescribed by a physician and provided by a qualified, non-physician healthcare professional using a standardized curriculum to an individual or a group of patients for the treatment of established illness(s)/disease(s) or to delay comorbidity(s)."[11] The code further states that the qualifications of the individual providing the education "must be consistent with guidelines or standards established or recognized by a physician society, non-physician healthcare professional society/association, or other appropriate source."[11] There is only one certifying board for asthma educators: the National Asthma Educator Certification Board (NAECB). It is essential that certified asthma educators (AE-C) work with their professional organizations to encourage third-party payers to approve reimbursement for asthma education.

CPT Codes for health education are as follows:
98960: one patient for 30 minutes
98961: two to four patients for 30 minutes
98962: five to eight patients for 30 minutes

These codes also specify that the education must be provided using a standardized curriculum.[11] As with all other health care, proper documentation will be critical. The curriculum should be well documented and the education provided. Each AE-C is responsible for developing and documenting the content of their asthma program. Figure 48-2 shows an example of an asthma education flow sheet that can be used to document asthma education provided by an AE-C within the office setting.[12]

REFERENCES

1. Fireman P, Friday GA, Gira C, et al: Teaching self-management skills to asthmatic children and their parents in an ambulatory care setting. Pediatics 1981;68(2):341–348.
2. Guevara JP, Wolf FM, Grum CM, Clark NM: Effects of educational interventions for self management of asthma in children and adolescents: systematic review and meta-analysis. BMJ 2003;326(7204):1308–1309.
3. Webster's Dictionary. New York, Harper-Collins Publishers, 2003.
4. Fish L, Lum Lung C: Adherence to asthma therapy. Ann Allergy Asthma Immunol 2001;86:24.
5. National Asthma Education and Prevention Program (NAEPP): Expert Panel Report 3 (EPR3): Guidelines for the Diagnosis and Management of Asthma (Pub. No. 08-4051). Washington, DC, U.S. Department of Health and Human Services, Public Health Services, National Institutes of Health, National Heart, Lung, and Blood Institute, 2007.
6. Rosenstock I: Historical Origins of the Health Belief Model. The Health Belief Model and Personal Health Behavior. Thorofare, NJ, Charles B. Slack, 1974.
7. Prochaska JO: Systems of Psychotherapy: A Transtheoretical Analysis. Homewood, IL, Dorsey Press, 1979.
8. Wadsworth BJ: Piaget's Theory of Cognitive and Affective Development, 4th ed. New York, Longman, 1989.
9. Siegel D: Keys to compliance through patient education. Houston Nursing, October, 1992.
10. Babcock DE, Miller MA: Client Education Theory and Practice. St. Louis, Mosby-Year Book, Inc., 1994.
11. American Medical Association: CPT Changes 2006—An Insider's View. Chicago, IL, AMA Press, 2006.
12. Wagner CW: Asthma Care and Patient Education: The Nurse's Role. Houston, University of Texas Medical Center, 1993.

Education and Support for Larger Groups

Sandra R. Wilson and Sarah B. Knowles

CLINICAL PEARLS

- Small group asthma education that is behaviorally based and uses evidence-based behavior change strategies can be equally, if not more, effective in improving patient self-management and outcomes than comparable patient education delivered individually.

- Close integration between asthma education (group or individual) and the patient's medical care has significant benefits, including the opportunity to ensure that the regimen is medically appropriate and accommodates the patient's goals and preferences.

- Newer models of health care, such as shared appointments, provide a means of delivering small group asthma education closely coordinated with the patient's medical care.

- While group programs may reduce per-patient instructional time, they pose significant challenges in staffing, scheduling, and recruiting and retaining patients. Physician referral and support are very important in recruiting patients.

- Limiting the number of sessions of a group education program may encourage attendance but limits the time available to practice new skills and address individual needs of participants, suggesting a potential benefit of individual telephone/in-person follow-up.

Patient education is recognized as a critical component in the medical management of asthma and other chronic diseases.[1-3] The value of asthma patient and/or parent education as a means of improving a variety of health outcomes has been well established.[4,5] Education is one of the four key components of care in national guidelines for the diagnosis, treatment, and management of asthma.[6,7] Educational interventions have been shown to enhance clinician-patient communication, improve patient self-management (including adherence to the treatment regimen), and improve disease outcomes.

Meta-analyses of multiple randomized control trials of asthma and other chronic disease self-management education programs have identified the key characteristics of more successful educational programs, and have shown that such programs are most effective, in terms of a full range of behavioral, clinical, and health resource utilization outcomes, when they (1) are based on clear behavioral goals, and (2) employ behavior change strategies that have a solid theoretical foundation in the behavioral sciences—strategies that address patient knowledge, attitudes/motivation, and any barriers to effective self-management. Effective educational programs go beyond the presentation of facts and concepts (supplying the necessary information); they motivate patients to engage in effective self-management and achieve/maintain control of their condition, and give them specific skills they need, such as the ability to monitor and evaluate their own condition and the ability to recognize and overcome the internal and external barriers they face to making the necessary changes in order to control their disease.

There is a further growing recognition that patient adherence to medical treatment is influenced by whether the *treatment regimen* itself is tailored to the goals and preferences of the individual patient. Such a patient-centered approach is recommended in asthma clinical guidelines[6,7] and as a general model for the health care system.[8] However, it is rarely implemented in practice. Most asthma and other chronic disease patient education programs take the treatment regimen as a given, and focus on other strategies, as noted above, to improve patient adherence. However, their success may be inherently limited if the patient did not participate actively in the treatment choice and if their own goals and preferences are not being well met. Until recently, asthma education and self-management programs have not focused on this issue, and hence meta-analyses of the available scientific evidence are mute on whether it plays (or could play) an important role in improving treatment outcomes. If this strategy is important, this fact may have significant implications for the educational process, and also increase the need to integrate patient self-management education with the patient's medical care.

SMALL GROUP VERSUS INDIVIDUAL EDUCATION PROGRAMS

One of the most obvious differences among educational programs, and a difference with significant practical implications, is whether the program is delivered to patients individually or in small groups. The benefits of asthma self-management education noted earlier have been observed both when the education was delivered to small *groups* of patients and when it was delivered individually.[9-11]

In one of the first formal, head-to-head comparisons of educational formats targeting persons with asthma, Wilson and colleagues[11] delivered the same self-management education curriculum to adults with asthma in three formats: individually, in small groups, or via a self-study workbook. These were compared with usual medical care in terms of psychological, behavioral, and clinical outcomes in a randomized control trial. All three formats delivered exactly the same information and all three used very similar strategies intended to improve self-management behavior, but adapted to the differing formats. Both the individual and small group formats were associated with significantly greater improvement in inhaler use technique, self-management behaviors, and knowledge compared with usual care; the self-study manual was not. Only for the small group program was there evidence of a significant reduction in health care utilization for asthma. On balance, the group program appears to have been at least as, and possibly more, effective than the individual program, presumably because it was better able to take advantage of the group processes that can support behavior change, and was more cost effective.

The conduct of such comparative trials is difficult and infrequent. More often, it is left to meta-analysis to try to discern whether educational format plays a role in the relative success of different programs. Given the number of differences among interventions and study designs, it remains nearly impossible, as it was a decade ago,[10] to draw firm conclusions regarding the specific features that make an individual or a small group format more effective or the desired outcomes for which one or the other format might be most advantageous. It also remains difficult, if one takes into account all of the various logistic requirements of these two approaches, to conclude that the group approach is always more efficient.

This chapter is not concerned primarily with the comparative question of the relative effectiveness of group versus individual education. Its focus is on the potential benefits and the specific limitations of small group education programs, the variations among such programs (e.g., number of sessions, degree of integration with participants' medical care), and the practical requirements and implementation issues with respect to group programs. Finally, it considers the potential integration of small group asthma and other chronic disease self-management education into newer models of health services delivery, chronic disease-care management, and shared medical appointments.

POTENTIAL UNIQUE BENEFITS OF SMALL GROUP EDUCATION

Education of patients in small groups has been posited to be more cost-effective than an individually delivered program and to have other distinct features that may better support behavior change. Thinking only of a didactic presentation (i.e., a health professional talking to several patients at a time rather than repeating the same messages to an equal number of patients individually), it would seem self-evident that the group approach would be more efficient. Moreover, providing the *comprehensive* asthma education that patients require to manage any complex health problem necessarily requires more time than is available in the typical clinical encounter. In theory, the longer the time requirement per patient, the greater might be the efficiency in education of groups rather than individuals. Small group classes for newly diagnosed type 2 diabetic patients, for example, are well accepted as an efficient educational approach.

Beyond the simple numbers issue, a hypothesized benefit of small group education is the opportunity it offers for participants to provide mutual support, empathy, and reinforcement to each other and to share experiences, concerns, and coping strategies.[12–14] Meeting others who struggle with the same problems also presents the opportunity for social comparison—a chance to evaluate the severity of one's own condition relative to that of others, consider how well controlled their condition is relative to one's own, and to see how and how well others approach both the fact that they have asthma and the specific problems it presents. Group education sessions offer the opportunity to engage such motivators and to employ specific skill-building strategies, such as role playing, which are somewhat more difficult to incorporate into one-on-one sessions between an individual patient and a health professional.

MODELS OF GROUP EDUCATION PROGRAMS

Asthma Education/Self-Management Classes

Small group asthma education classes, taught by a nurse, clinical pharmacist, respiratory therapist, or other educator, are offered in many community settings (e.g., voluntary health associations, Head Start programs, schools) and in clinical settings, most often by clinics and larger health care systems. Increasingly, the courses are taught by asthma educators who have been certified for this role (http://www.naecb.org/). They may consist of a single session or a multisession series (generally two to four sessions) that are generally structured on the premise that patients will attend all of the sessions. Some such classes use professionally developed and scientifically evaluated curricular/materials, typically tailored in some way to the local situation, or they may be locally developed and may or may not have had any evaluation.

The curriculum of such classes typically includes some or all of the following: didactic presentations about asthma and its treatment (i.e., pharmacotherapy, environmental control, treatment of contributory conditions such as allergic rhinitis and gastroesophageal reflux disease [GERD]); discussion of asthma control, how it is evaluated, and how well-controlled is the participants' asthma; instruction on the use of devices for administration of inhalant medications; development of individual asthma management and action plans; instruction on self-monitoring of asthma symptoms and/or lung function; problem-solving with regard to asthma management problems and relevant health behaviors (environmental exposures, smoking, medication adherence, patient-physician communication, and so forth); and development of plans/behavioral contracts for specific behavior changes aimed at improving asthma control and quality of life.

A composite content outline of topics from the Breathe Easier and Peak Flow group education programs is shown in Table 49-1.[15,16] Although it is preferable that the program content remain consistent, the specific topics can be ordered in different ways.

Participants may be newly diagnosed patients, patients who have been identified on institutional asthma registries as having some characteristic suggesting their asthma is poorly controlled (e.g., overuse of reliever relative to controller medications, emergency room or hospital visits), patients recruited from within a health care system through newsletters and signs, or individuals recruited from the community by advertising or physician referral.

Table 49-1
TOPICS COVERED IN COMPREHENSIVE ASTHMA EDUCATION PROGRAMS

Understanding Asthma
Facts about asthma
Pathophysiology
Symptoms
Early warning signs
How and Why to Monitor your Asthma
Evaluating how well controlled your asthma is
Proper use of peak flow meter (if applicable)
Understanding Medications
Preventive and symptomatic relief medications (classes of medications)
Proper used of prescription inhaled medical devices
Medications as part of the asthma management plan
Solutions to problems with medications
Analyzing attitudes about medications
Asthma Management and Action Plan (AAP)
Prevention and Environmental Control
Stress and asthma management
Prevention of symptoms through avoidance
Common types of problematic triggers
Exercise and asthma
Using prescribed asthma control medications
Being prepared for symptom management

From National Heart, Lung, and Blood Institute: Breathe Easier: An Adult Asthma Education Program (Publication No. 55-724). Bethesda, MD, U.S. Department of Health and Human Services; National Institutes of Health; National Heart, Lung, and Blood Institute, 1997; and Buist AS, Vollmer WH, Wilson SR, et al: A randomized clinical trial of Peak Flow versus symptom monitoring in older adults with asthma. Am J Respir Crit Care Med 2006;174:1077–1087.

Asthma Support Groups

Asthma support groups typically meet on a regular basis without necessarily any expectation that a given individual will attend every session. Sessions may include any of the elements found in an asthma self-management education class, but typically emphasize mutual support coupled with education/discussion of topics of potential interest. They tend not to have a formal "curriculum," as is typical of an asthma class, and are not primarily aimed at behavior change.

Shared Medical Appointments Involving Group Self-Management Education

Shared Medical Appointments (SMAs), and the similar Drop-in Group Medical Appointments (DIGMAs),[17-19] represent a newer model of health care delivery. They are included here because of their significant focus on patient education in a small group context. Among their distinguishing features and potential advantages are that they closely integrate education with patients' medical care, and have the ability to address both issues common to most patients with a given medical problem, as well as to address individuals' unique situations. SMAs, generally of 90-minute duration, are usually offered by larger health care systems that have sufficient numbers of patients with similar conditions. They have become increasingly popular over the past 10 years.

Shared medical appointments are currently being used effectively as part of chronic disease management, including in asthma.[20,21] For example, within the Palo Alto Medical Foundation (PAMF), a large multispecialty health care system in the San Francisco Bay Area, SMAs are offered for patients with congestive heart failure, dermatology problems, diabetes, pre-diabetes, and behavioral health diagnoses. For the subset of the latter patient population, SMAs are also offered to patients receiving treatment for psychiatric diagnoses who have any of a wide range of other chronic diseases, including asthma, and to pre- and post-bariatric surgery and vasectomy patients. Asthma patients have also been included in SMAs in other settings (e.g., Cleveland Clinic in Cleveland, OH, and the Kaiser Cooperative Health Care Clinic in Denver, CO, among others).

The PAMF SMAs are typical in emphasizing the educational element, combining face-to-face health care in a group setting with activities that enable patients to learn from each other and gain a greater understanding of their own medical conditions. During SMAs, patients benefit from listening to each other's questions while experiencing the support of a group environment. SMAs are staffed by health care providers including physicians, nurses, and medical assistants. In addition, a behaviorist, a licensed clinical social worker, or a marriage and family therapist is often present to facilitate the meeting and address any emotional concerns related to the patients' health and well-being. Patients of participating physicians can attend SMAs for the purpose of having medical questions answered, changing or renewing prescriptions, ordering tests or procedures, receiving test results, and discussing medications and treatment options. Patients' vital statistics and other information are gathered at these appointments by a medical assistant, as they would at any medical visit. Private examinations and new patient evaluations may also occur during an SMA. Use of trained asthma educators and of demonstrated effective educational materials and strategies in the context of such SMAs would appear to offer the potential for bridging the gap that may otherwise exist between group asthma education programs and personal health care by offering both in a small group setting.

BASIC REQUIREMENTS OF EFFECTIVE GROUP PROGRAMS

As already noted, effective small group and individually administered asthma education programs have the following characteristics:

- Are *behaviorally based*, meaning that the *instruction is designed to accomplish specific, measurable goals* with regard to self-management practices that are known to affect important clinical outcomes;
- Use *evidence-based behavior change strategies* and tools (i.e., asthma management and action plans);
- *Address practical needs:* those of which individuals are already aware and others about which the program can increase their awareness (e.g., the extent to which their asthma is not well controlled);
- *Actively involve patients in learning and doing*, using age-appropriate tools and activities, rather than them being passive recipients of a lecture/talk.

- ○ Success in this regard is dependent on having a group of feasible size, typically no more than 8 to 12 participants and fewer in the case of children.
- ○ The literature contains many ideas for creative activities for children, as well as specific considerations in planning programs for older adults.[5,16]

- *Integrate the program* with the patient's medical care to make it easier to ensure that the treatment regimen is appropriate and takes into account the patient's own goals and preferences.

Whenever possible, it is advisable to use existing programs with documented effectiveness that meet these criteria. Existing programs can be updated and modified as needed for a new setting, keeping in mind that altering the curriculum may alter its effectiveness. The US Centers for Disease Control and Prevention (CDC) has carefully selected and maintains a list of potentially effective asthma education interventions. Information can be found at http://www.cdc.gov/asthma/interventions.htm.

CHALLENGES AND SOLUTIONS

Small group asthma education programs offer unique advantages, but also very real challenges, notably in recruitment, scheduling/location, and staffing, that differ from, and in many respects are more challenging than, those of individually administered programs. These challenges may not be as obvious as the apparent advantages of group programs in instructional efficiency and group support. Furthermore, these challenges translate into real costs, primarily in personnel time, that must be recognized and addressed if a group asthma education program is to achieve its potential benefits and continue to be offered.

Recruitment and Retention

To consider offering a group program at all, there obviously must be a sufficient number of people who fit the description of the targeted population within the service area/population of the program sponsor. In urban areas of high asthma prevalence, a clinic or voluntary health association may easily serve a sufficiently large population that it makes sense to offer basic asthma education classes for newly diagnosed individuals and those with established disease who lack such education. In a smaller service area/population, one where asthma prevalence is not especially high, or when the target population is more specific (e.g., older adults), an individually delivered program or one that couples periodic offerings of a single, initial small group session with subsequent follow-up on an individual basis may be more feasible.

Even with a sufficiently large number of potential participants, one of the most frequent complaints of those who have offered group programs is, "We had a really good program, but we gave up because not enough people attended; it just wasn't worth it!" The challenge of recruiting patients for both single- and multisession small group asthma education programs should not be underestimated. Without significant attention to the identification and recruitment of participants, disappointing results are virtually assured. Despite the validity of the needs that motivated the program in the first

place, if attendance is poor, no one will be able to justify its continuation. This also may have a chilling effect on other, subsequent asthma education efforts as well.

There are many causes of poor attendance. Patients may not see the value in such a program and may not give attendance at such classes a priority in their lives, even if they are experiencing frequent symptoms or have had a serious, even life-threatening, asthma crisis. Transportation, child care, and other barriers may exist. For programs that include working adults or parents, and those designed for both the parent and asthmatic child to attend, scheduling conflicts with employment, children's extracurricular activities, or finding child care for nonasthmatic siblings are attendance barriers that need to be addressed.[22] By their nature, asthma classes must be held at specific, prearranged times and locations. The educator's or institution's preferred schedule may not match patient scheduling preferences, and considerable flexibility is required on the part of those offering the program in order to maximize accessibility and attendance.

Many long-standing small group programs have recruited patients by systematic promotion and announcements in health care system or voluntary health association newsletters, presentations to community groups, parent-teacher associations, and so forth, and through posters and other types of advertisements. Additionally, those based in a health care system can use a variety of methods to identify prospective participants including physician referral and screening of electronic records to identify patients who have had frequent emergency department or urgent care visits or who overuse asthma rescue medications. In our experience, physician referral of patients has been one of the most successful strategies for actually getting patients to participate in formal asthma education programs. However, it is not always easy to get this to occur, given the conflicting demands of patient care. Referral of patients from community physicians to programs offered by health associations, hospitals, and other agencies can be developed but requires effort and the establishment of professional respect, good communication, and collaboration between the educational program and physicians, as well as an alignment of incentives (e.g., physician confidence that referral will not lead to a loss of their patients).

When asthma classes are offered to its own patients by a health care system, considerable planning and preparation are still needed in order for referral and subsequent enrollment and attendance to actually occur. A common strategy is for a physician "champion" within the institution,[18,23] possibly working with an asthma quality improvement team, to foster understanding and endorsement of the program by other physicians. A consensus development process may be necessary to establish referral as a part of the standard of care; for example, a standard might be established whereby all newly diagnosed patients or those who show evidence of poor control or other problems are referred. The referral and registration process itself needs to be straightforward for both physician and patient, which can be accomplished by assigning staff to handle the process, which is facilitated by the availability of electronic medical record, scheduling, and communication systems. And, in keeping with the principle that what gets measured gets done,[24] it is important to establish a mechanism to monitor referral and patient participation at the aggregate and/or individual provider level.

A case study, reported by the CDC as part of its search for effective asthma education interventions, illustrates the value of implementing education in the context of an overall asthma quality improvement strategy, and particularly illustrates the importance of establishing an expectation and process for obtaining physician referral to such a program. In this case, a modified version of the Wee Wheezers program[25] was implemented at the Darnell Army Community Hospital (DACH) in Ft. Hood, Texas, as part of an overall quality improvement effort that included addressing other gaps in care. It involved an automatic process of referral for children with asthma. Any Ft. Hood physician who diagnosed a child with asthma or who treated a child who had not previously attended an asthma education program was required to refer the child to the DACH Asthma Information and Resources Group. This allowed all families with asthmatic children the opportunity to participate in the multisession Wee Wheezers program. Although the referral was mandatory, parental participation was voluntary. Parental participation has been very strong, and the effort, both on the health care system and patient education fronts, was associated with a substantial decrease in hospitalizations and costs of care for pediatric asthma. A small portion of the saved costs was used to fund continuation of the program and nurse educator.

Multisession group education programs, such as Wee Wheezers, offer the opportunity to have patients work on asthma management goals between classes (e.g., self-monitoring or diary-keeping, environmental control, enrolling in smoking cessation programs or taking other preparatory steps toward cessation, or trials of routine use of asthma controller medications if adherence has been poor). Progress can then be reported and assessed in subsequent sessions and the educator can provide reinforcement, assist in interpretation (e.g., of self-monitoring results), and contribute to problem solving or reevaluation of goals when difficulties are encountered.

Retention of patients through all sessions of a multisession program, however, is typically incomplete and poses significant challenges. Some proportion of people who register for a class do not show up at all, even when reminder phone calls are made by the educator the previous day and a commitment is obtained. Such "no-shows" can be a particular frustration in trying to reach some of the most at-risk populations, and require creative persistent approaches and the ability not to take such behavior as a personal rejection. Poor attendance over the course of a group program may reflect many problems that are potentially avoidable or correctable, and involving members of the target population in the development of the program, as well as debriefing those who did and did not attend sessions, can be extremely helpful. In our experience, the greatest success in retaining patients in a multisession program has involved adults older than 65, most of whom were retired. Even the final fourth session, for example, was attended by 89% of those who enrolled.[16]

In some cases, however, it may be more feasible to plan a single, longer session than to hold multiple sessions. While the evidence suggests that multiple sessions often achieve significant behavior change, it may be possible to offer a single group session that addresses a set of core behavioral goals and prepares participants for subsequent additional focus on individually relevant goals and activities, either in face-to-face or phone contacts on an individual basis. This requires a particularly clear and realistic selection of behavioral goals for the initial session as well as clarity about which goals will require subsequent follow-up activities. This format appears more feasible for programs offered within a health care setting, where an asthma educator or care manager can be employed to conduct the class and carry out the follow-up activities, potentially with the assistance of health information technology (see "Further Considerations").

Location and Scheduling

Location and scheduling are important for the program's success. The program should be offered on a day and at a time suitable for the target population, potentially varying the day and time in successive offerings. One should avoid offering programs, especially in the evening, at locations difficult to access by available means of transportation or to which participants must travel through unsafe areas. For seniors, consider offering the program during the daytime, rather than in the evening. Finally, to accommodate group participants' work, school, and other commitments, consider offering on-site child care.

Staffing

Group asthma education programs are best taught by a certified asthma educator (http://www.naecb.org/). In addition to experience with clinical care for asthma and with educational methods, the individual should enjoy and be skilled in working with small groups and effectively using the various behavior change methods of the curriculum. If the program is to include instruction of children directly, the educator must be effective and experienced in teaching and holding the attention of children in groups.

Financing

Even in situations in which volunteer educators are involved, adequate financial resources and infrastructure must be provided for promotion, recruitment, administration, oversight, and evaluation of the program. Some costs may be reimbursable under various insurance plans or covered by managed care contracts. To offset the costs of implementation, requiring a small payment/copayment by participants may actually contribute to participation in that patients may devalue free programs.

TAILORING THE CURRICULUM

In choosing or developing the curriculum, it is very important to know the target population from which the group participants are drawn. This includes their level of education and the general circumstances of their lives, including such things as financial resources, housing and living conditions, social support, and other social or cultural factors that may directly or indirectly affect asthma control and asthma self-management. Much has been written on this extremely important topic, not only with regard to asthma but health care and health education in general (http://www.nhlbi.nih.gov/about/naepp;

http://www.cdc.gov/asthma/interventions.htm) and hence will not be addressed here in detail.

Educating asthma sufferers from disadvantaged populations requires additional forethought in planning the curriculum. Whether the condition is poverty, low education level, language barriers, or lack of access to health care, developing group asthma education programs given these conditions requires the consideration of a multilevel approach. Public agencies, community organizations, and professional associations can be valuable resources in reaching low-income, multicultural communities with a high prevalence of asthma.[22,26] By collaborating with these important role players, those who offer small group programs can identify solutions to several potential barriers. These include training bilingual group facilitators, providing either multilingual learning materials at an appropriate reading level or more pictorial learning materials, an easily accessible group meeting place, free parking or transportation vouchers for participants to attend, and culturally appropriate curricula. In some cultures, for example, traditional treatments for asthma may need to be recognized, and even the format modified if families want all members to participate rather than just the patient or the parent.

Although there is evidence that school-based asthma education programs can be beneficial for children with asthma, it is unrealistic to expect that such programs can successfully address factors beyond the child's control (e.g. parental smoking, environmental mold). For that reason, and because parents of young children are ultimately responsible for administering asthma medications, education of parents is critical as well.

The CDC's asthma program is a useful resource for finding cultural- and age-appropriate educational resources. These resources can serve as a general starting point, although a review of the published literature is best for additional information about tailoring interventions to a specific target audience. Programs developed for children can be found at http://www.cdc.gov/asthma/interventions/children.htm, and include community-based and school-based programs. Additional school-based program information can be found at http://www.cdc.gov/asthma/interventions/children.htm#schools. Programs targeting parents of children with asthma can be found at both http://www.cdc.gov/asthma/interventions/mothers.htm and at http://www.cdc.gov/asthma/interventions/parents.htm.

FURTHER CONSIDERATIONS

Health Information Technology

The use of electronic medical records and other health information technology is increasingly widespread, and now has the capability of allowing patients access to their personal health records and secure Web-based communication with their health care providers. As a result, electronic systems are being developed that can assist patients with routine self-monitoring and interpretation of the results, allow this information to be shared with their physician, and provide individually appropriate reminders of tests and visits as well as disease, treatment, and risk-related information necessary to make and sustain changes that will improve their disease control. Coupling such innovations with changes in service delivery, such as small group education or shared medical appointments with individual follow-up, may lead to more efficient and effective patient education and better overall management of asthma and other chronic health problems.

Coordination with the Patient's Medical Care

However useful asthma education may be, whether in groups or individually, it is not a substitute for proper medical care. If the educational program is not formally associated with the participant's usual asthma medical management, every effort should be made to ensure that participants are receiving appropriate medical management for their asthma.

Most asthma classes and small group education programs offered in a community setting are not integrated with the patient's medical care, and hence are limited in what they can do to address the medical needs of patients. Such needs may relate to not being on an adequate treatment regimen, having unrecognized, and therefore unaddressed, environmental exposures or allergies, or having coexisting medical problems that are not being addressed, such as chronic obstructive lung disease, allergic rhinitis or GERD, or depression.

In such situations, educators can advise and encourage a participant to seek appropriate medical care or they may serve an ombudsman role and assist the patient in accessing adequate care. Additionally, they may provide assistance in resolving medication or other cost issues for individual participants. Even these care-facilitating activities presuppose a class format that elicits and addresses individual patient concerns and questions such that the educator becomes familiar enough with participants to understand their needs. Of course, it also presupposes sufficient expertise on the part of the educator to be able to discern such needs and potential problems.

Small group educational programs that are offered by a health care system to its own patients are more readily coordinated with the patient's ongoing care. However, coordination is not automatic and typically requires attention at the clinic, department or system level, and/or consideration of work flow issues. It also involves the same sorts of professional education and consensus-building processes described above, with regard to encouraging physicians to refer patients for asthma education, in order to achieve effective and efficient integration.

A true team approach to care—one that includes the patient educator—is very difficult to accomplish in a non–health care setting. However, such programs may fulfill a critical need when health care system sponsorship of asthma education for the target population is not possible.

CONCLUSION

Group asthma education is an effective and potentially efficient educational approach. In a clinical setting, such group programs enable patients to receive more education regarding self-managing their asthma than they otherwise would in a typical one-on-one medical appointment. The groups can, and should, be structured to allow for addressing individual asthma self-management needs and goals. However, as described above, group asthma education poses significant challenges including recruitment, staffing, and other issues such as location and scheduling.

For many participants, group asthma education may need to be supplemented by individual sessions, either with an asthma care manager or a health educator.[10] When coordinated with appropriate medical care, including newer models of care, such as shared medical appointments or care management, the effectiveness and financial viability of group asthma self-management education may be further enhanced. The efficiency of these newer models, and of group education in those settings, may be further improved as it plays a larger role in patient-centered care. Group asthma education has the potential to enhance patients' self-efficacy, reduce perceived barriers to self-management, and hone their decision-making abilities (Box 49-1).

BOX 49-1 Small Group Asthma Education

- Small group asthma education is an effective and potentially efficient approach.
- The challenges involved in designing and implementing an effective small group education program should not be underestimated, including recruitment and retention, location and scheduling, staffing, and financial support.
- Basic requirements for effective education programs include:
  - Behaviorally based and designed to meet measurable goals;
  - Use of evidence-based behavior change strategies and self-management tools such as self-monitoring aids and written asthma management and action plans;
  - Preferably, integration with the patient's medical care;
  - Actively involve patients in setting goals and practicing self-management skills; and
  - Use of culturally and age-appropriate activities.

REFERENCES

1. Friedman RH, Kazis LE, Jette A, et al: A telecommunications system for monitoring and counseling patients with hypertension. Impact on medication adherence and blood pressure control. Am J Hypertens 1996;9:285–292.
2. Piette JD, Weinberger M, McPhee SJ, et al: Do automated calls with nurse follow-up improve self-care and glycemic control among vulnerable patients with diabetes? Am J Med 2000;108:20–27.
3. Osterberg L, Blaschke T: Adherence to medication. N Engl J Med 2005;353:487–497.
4. Gibson PG, Powell H, Coughlan J, et al: Self-management education and regular practitioner review for adults with asthma. Cochrane Database Syst Rev 2003;(1):CD001117.
5. McGhan SL, Cicutto LC, Befus AD: Advances in development and evaluation of asthma education programs. Curr Opin Pulm Med 2005;11:61–68.
6. Global Initiative for Asthma (GINA): Pocket Guide for Asthma Management and Prevention, 2006. Available at http://www.ginasthma.org/Guidelineitem.asp??l1=2&l2=1&intId=37, accessed November 28, 2007.
7. National Asthma Education and Prevention Program. Expert Panel Report 3: Guidelines for the diagnosis and management of asthma (NIH Publication No 08–4051). Bethesda, MD, U.S. Department of Health and Human Services; National Institutes of Health; National Heart, Lung and Blood Institute, 1997.
8. Institute of Medicine. Crossing the Quality Chasm: A New Health System for the Twenty-first Century. Washington, DC, National Academy Press, 2001.
9. Bailey WC, Richards JM Jr., Manzella BA, et al: Promoting self-management in adults with asthma: an overview of the UAB program. Health Educ Q 1987;14:345–355.
10. Wilson SR: Individual versus group education: is one better? Patient Educ Couns 1997;32:S67–S75.
11. Wilson SR, German DF, Lulla S, et al: A controlled trial of two forms of self-management education for adults with asthma. Am J Med 1993;94:564–576.
12. Lepore SJ, Helgeson VS, Eton DT, Schulz R: Improving quality of life in men with prostate cancer: a randomized controlled trial of group education interventions. Health Psychol 2003;22:443–452.
13. Zabalegui A, Sanchez S, Sanchez P, Juando C: Nursing and cancer support groups. J Adv Nurs 2005;51:369–381.

14. Spiegel D, Bloom JR, Kraemer HC, Gottheil E: Effect of psychosocial treatment on survival of patients with metastatic breast cancer. Lancet 1989;2:888–891.
15. National Heart, Lung, and Blood Institute: Breathe Easier: An Adult Asthma Education Program. (Publication No. 55–724). Bethesda, MD, U.S. Department of Health and Human Services; National Institutes of Health; National Heart, Lung, and Blood Institute, 1997.
16. Buist AS, Vollmer WH, Wilson SR, et al: A randomized clinical trial of peak flow versus symptom monitoring in older adults with asthma. Am J Respir Crit Care Med 2006;174:1077–1087.
17. Bronson DL, Maxwell RA: Shared medical appointments: increasing patient access without increasing physician hours. Cleve Clin J Med 2004;71;369–377.
18. Noffsinger EB: Will drop-in group medical appointments (DIGMAs) work in practice? Permanente J 1999;3:58–67.
19. Scott JC, Robertson BJ: Kaiser Colorado's Cooperative Health Care Clinic: a group approach to patient care. Manag Care Q 1996;4:41–45.
20. Trento M, Passera P, Bajardi M, et al: Lifestyle intervention by group care prevents deterioration of type II diabetes: a 4-year randomized controlled clinical trial. Diabetologia 2002;45:1231–1239.
21. Wagner EH, Grothaus LC, Sandhu N, et al: Chronic care clinics for diabetes in primary care: a system-wide randomized trial. Diabetes Care 2001;24:695–700.
22. Wilson SR, Scamagas P, Grado J, et al: The Fresno Asthma Project: a model intervention to control asthma in multiethnic, low-income, inner-city communities. Health Educ Behav 1998;25:79–98.
23. Noffsinger EB: Establishing successful primary care and subspecialty drop-in group medical appointments (DIGMAs) in your group practice. Group Pract J 1999;48:202,20–28.
24. James BC: Quality Management for Health Care Delivery. Chicago, The Hospital Research and Educational Trust, 1989.
25. Wilson SR, Latini D, Starr NJ, et al: Education of parents of infants and very young children with asthma: a developmental evaluation of the Wee Wheezers program. J Asthma 1996;33:239–254.
26. Zayas LE, McLean D: Asthma patient education opportunities in predominantly minority urban communities. Health Educ Res 2007;22:757–769.

Special Populations with Asthma

Maureen George

CLINICAL PEARLS

- Recognizing biases and implementing simple culturally sensitive behaviors are the first steps that an educator takes in developing cultural competency.

- In special populations where low literacy and limited English language proficiency are operative, oral instruction by a native speaker, followed by hands-on practice, is always preferable.

- The best way to evaluate whether knowledge was transmitted and interpreted correctly is to have the patient apply the information in a problem-based situation.

- The ability to evaluate the readability of educational materials is a skill that every educator must develop.

- The success of educational interventions in special populations may be measured by unique metrics, such as increased use of free clinics for well visits.

In the United States, asthma prevalence, morbidity, and mortality continue to rise in racial/ethnic minority groups as compared to whites despite effective treatments. In the Latino community, Puerto Ricans are disproportionately burdened by asthma with a 13.2% prevalence rate compared with a 5.3% asthma rate for Dominicans and Mexicans. Differences in prevalence rates among Latino groups cannot be explained by household size or location, use of home remedies, educational attainment, or country in which education was completed. In addition, the age-adjusted death rate for Puerto Ricans is nearly three times that of Cuban Americans and four times that of Mexican Americans. Overall, death rates for Latinos were 14% higher than for whites. Of all racial/ethnic groups however, blacks have the highest prevalence rates for asthma with hospitalization rates and age-adjusted death rates three times that of whites. In fact, one quarter of all asthma deaths occur in blacks although they represent less than 13% of the U.S. population. Of particular concern, black females experience the highest asthma mortality.[1]

Poverty is associated with the greatest health inequalities.[2] Poor minorities are less likely to receive continuity of care,[2] asthma education, or specialist care and are less often prescribed inhaled corticosteroids (ICSs) even among those with health insurance.[3] Together, inadequate medical management and low socioeconomic status contribute to excessive disease burden and the observed disparities in health outcomes.

In summary, the greatest asthma burden occurs in U.S. racial/ethnic populations with the fewest medical and financial advantages. As such, it is important that the clinician recognizes and responds to the increased risk for inadequate asthma outcomes common to low-income minority communities.

ASSESSMENT

The ability to deliver effective self-management educational programs may be impeded in low-income minority groups by a variety of factors including poverty and inadequate health insurance, literacy and low educational attainment, limited English language proficiency and immigration status, and distrust of the medical establishment, as well as alternative beliefs and attitudes. The failure to identify and address these barriers may result in low participation and ineffective and culturally insensitive interventions.

Poverty and Lack of Health Insurance

Thirty-seven million (12.7%) Americans lived in poverty in 2004, up from 12.5% in 2003. The percentage of the population without health insurance coverage and the proportion of uninsured children remained unchanged at 15.7% and 11.2% respectively. As seen in Table 50-1, blacks and Latino populations have lower median incomes and greater uninsurance rates compared with whites.[2,4] Importantly, even when insured, low-income minority patients may experience poorer asthma outcomes.[3] Focus groups with low-income blacks who receive government-subsidized health care have highlighted the impediments to effective asthma self-management.[5] These barriers include difficulty in obtaining prescription medications due to restricted formularies, prior authorization procedures, mandatory wait periods for refills, lapses in insurance eligibility, and limited income to cover copays. When patients experienced these obstacles, ICS doses were omitted to conserve medications and short-acting beta$_2$-agonists were substituted.[5] Underuse of controller ICSs and overreliance on rescue medicines have been implicated as two of the causative factors for increasing asthma disparities.[6]

Table 50-1
INCOME, UNINSURANCE, AND POVERTY RATES BY RACIAL/ETHNIC GROUPS

	Blacks	Latinos	Non-Latino Whites
Median income ($)	30,134	34,241	48,977
Uninsured (%)	19.7	32.7	11.3
Poverty rate (%)	24.7	21.9	8.6

Data from DaNavas-Walt C, Proctor BD, Lee CH: US Census Bureau, Current population report, P60-229, Income, poverty, and health insurance coverage in the United States, 2004. Washington DC, U.S. Government Printing Office, 2005.

Limited expendable income and inadequate insurance coverage therefore can present a considerable barrier to obtaining prescription medication necessary for disease control in this group.

Literacy and Low Educational Attainment

In 2003, the National Center for Educational Statistics surveyed American adults to compare current literacy to 1992 literacy rates.[7] The National Assessment of Adult Literacy (NAAL) survey was a nationally representative assessment of literacy among more than 20,000 adults older than 16 residing in households and prisons. In this survey, literacy was defined as "using printed and written information to function in society, to achieve one's goals, and to develop one's knowledge and potential." Three types of literacy tasks were evaluated by the NAAL:

- *Prose skills*—ability to search, comprehend and apply material extracted from continuous texts, e.g., reading a patient instruction sheet to identify food and exercise restrictions prior to a pulmonary function test
- *Document tasks*—ability to find, interpret and use information from discontinuous texts, e.g., ability to decipher data from an asthma action plan
- *Quantitative literacy*—the ability to perform numeric calculations, e.g., the ability to calculate 80% of one's personal best peak flow reading.

NAAL survey scores were characterized as *below basic, basic, intermediate*, and *proficient*. Fourteen percent of all participating adults had *below basic* scores in prose, 12% in document, and 26% in quantitative literacy. Further, 29% of adults were characterized as having *basic* literacy levels in prose, 22% in document, and 33% in quantitative literacy. Taken together, the NAAL survey suggests that approximately 45% of US adults perform at a *basic* or *below basic* literacy level and nearly 60% demonstrate *basic* or *below basic* quantitative abilities.

Striking disparities can be found in the NAAL results for those with lower educational attainment and racial/ethnic minority status compared to more highly educated whites. For example, in the *below basic* category, nearly 55% of respondents had less than a high school education. The percentage of Asians/Pacific Islanders and whites at the *proficient* level for all three scales was significantly higher than Latinos or blacks although Latinos were more likely to be *proficient* than blacks.

How might limited literacy affect the patient with asthma? In a cross-sectional survey, 112 adults with asthma were given a brief health literacy assessment tool and asked to read and interpret standard instructions for an inhaled corticosteroid and rescue albuterol inhaler[8] (Fig. 50-1). Forty-three percent of the sample had scores indicative of low literacy and 18% made errors in reading or interpreting standard directions appearing on the prescription asthma medication labels. Low literacy groups had greater difficulty reading and interpreting the labels compared with the higher literacy groups and those individuals with a high school education or less were more likely to have low literacy and more likely to make errors in reading and interpreting prescription labels compared to those with more than a high school education. Since low literacy is a problem for a significant number of individuals, careful attention needs to be directed toward assessment of an individu-

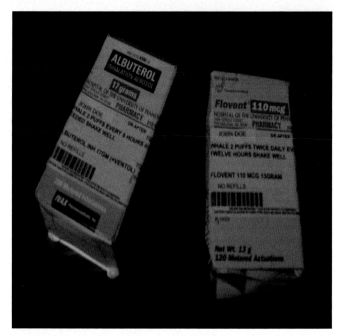

Figure 50-1 Standard labels for ICS and rescue therapies. Patients' ability to interpret prescription instructions accurately is integral to any asthma self-management plan.

al's ability to read and to follow medication directions during clinical encounters. Health care providers must consider the possible contributions of low literacy to inadequate disease management particularly in underserved minority populations where lower educational attainment is more common.

English as a Second Language (ESL) and Immigration Status

The national asthma guidelines state that asthma education and care are best conducted in a patient's primary language.[6] In the United States, 92% of the population age 5 and older are characterized as having no difficulty speaking English[9] leaving 22 million people with limited or no proficiency in English. Linguistic barriers pose significant challenges to patients who will require health care and to providers who work in a system short on time, resources, and the diversity to meet the needs of the non–English-speaking community.

Of all the uninsured in the United States, an estimated 10 million individuals (25%) are illegal aliens; Mexico is the primary source country. Drawn by high standards of living and stable political and legal systems, aliens enter the United States looking for a better life. Unfortunately, aliens who are unable to secure medical insurance place increased stress on an overburdened medical system.[10,11] Having no legal immigration status, no medical insurance, and limited English-language proficiency poses a considerable challenge to the implementation of an optimal asthma self-management plan.

Mistrust

Racial/ethnic minorities' mistrust of the medical establishment is rooted in historical and personal experiences with racism and segregation (legal or de facto) in this country.[2] Examples of racism masquerading as medical science are easily found. For example, Charles Darwin used Linnaeus's classification taxonomies to "prove" that blacks were more susceptible to disease, fostering his theory that blacks were an intermediary evolutionary step between monkeys and man, doomed for extinction.[12,13] In 1839, Samuel Morton, a prominent Philadelphia physician, published *Crania Americana*, a popular scientific treatise on craniometry, or brain-size measurements.[2] Based on head circumference measurements, Dr. Morton offered "evidence" of whites' superiority over Native Americans and blacks.[13] The 20th century also saw the rise of eugenics, in which the improvement of the human race was linked to the extermination of "inferior" races. Eugenics led policymakers to stem the tide of immigration to the United States after World War I and led to the extermination of racial and ethnic groups in Nazi Germany.[13]

The U.S. government has also been complicit. During the Civil War, the government commissioned Sanford Hunt, a Union army surgeon, to compare the brain weights of 24 deceased white soldiers to 381 black soldiers. Dr. Hunt concluded that the heavier weight of whites' brains demonstrated an endowed intellect.[13] Further, it was not until after World War II that the U.S. Armed Forces ceased procuring and separating blood products by race. Finally, government funding of the Tuskegee project (a nontherapeutic observation of the natural history of syphilis in black men) allowed the trial to continue even after the discovery of an antibiotic cure.[13] As a result of both historical and personal experiences, mistrust of the medical establishment is common[5,14] and serves as an additional barrier to improving health outcomes.

Complementary and Alternative Medicine (CAM) and Alternative Beliefs

Perhaps due to mistrust, limited expendable incomes, or culturally bound traditions, racial/ethnic minorities are more likely to refuse conventional treatment, particularly invasive interventions, than whites.[2] In asthma, lower adherence to conventional ICS therapy has been associated with black race, Spanish-language speakers, and low income.[15] Although individual preferences for care do not fully explain treatment refusal or the observed health disparities, the choice of less conventional therapy is likely one contributing factor to poor clinical outcomes.[2]

In the United States, complementary and alternative medicine (CAM) is becoming increasingly popular.[16] CAM, a group of practices and products not presently considered part of conventional medicine, may offer patients an alternative approach to managing symptoms or disease states.[16] The National Center for Complementary and Alternative Medicine (NCCAM) categorizes CAM into five domains (Table 50-2).[17] Using these domains, researchers characterized the prevalence and preferred CAM modalities of more than 31,000 U.S. adults in 2002. Black adults were more likely to use mind-body interventions including prayer, but less likely to use biologically based treatments including megavitamins, alternative medical systems, energy therapies or body-based remedies than whites or Latinos.[16] CAM use was also less common in higher income groups than in the poor or near-poor groups when megavitamins and prayer for health were excluded from the analysis.[16]

Asthma is one of the most common diseases for which CAM is used[16] and CAM is primarily used as a supplement to, rather than replacement for, conventional care.[18] Unfortunately, providers rarely inquire about a patient's alternative health beliefs during the clinical encounter,[17] perhaps due to insufficient time, assumptions about nonuse, or unfamiliarity with CAM. Providers may have particularly limited knowledge

---

Table 50-2
CAM DOMAINS AS DEFINED BY NCCAM

1. Alternative Medical Systems
Alternative medical systems are built upon complete systems of theory and practice. Often, these systems have evolved apart from and earlier than the conventional medical approach used in the United States. Examples of alternative medical systems that have developed in Western cultures include homeopathic medicine and naturopathic medicine. Examples of systems that have developed in non-Western cultures include traditional Chinese medicine and Ayurveda.

2. Mind-Body Interventions
Mind-body medicine uses a variety of techniques designed to enhance the mind's capacity to affect bodily function and symptoms. Some techniques that were considered CAM in the past have become mainstream (for example, patient support groups and cognitive-behavioral therapy). Other mind-body techniques are still considered CAM, including meditation, prayer, mental healing, and therapies that use creative outlets such as art, music, or dance.

3. Biologically Based Therapies
Biologically based therapies in CAM use substances found in nature, such as herbs, foods, and vitamins. Some examples include dietary supplements, herbal products, and the use of other so-called natural but as yet scientifically unproven therapies (for example, using shark cartilage to treat cancer).

4. Manipulative and Body-Based Methods
Manipulative and body-based methods in CAM are based on manipulation and/or movement of one or more parts of the body. Some examples include chiropractic or osteopathic manipulation and massage.

5. Energy Therapies
Energy therapies involve the use of energy fields. They are of two types:
- Biofield therapies are intended to affect energy fields that purportedly surround and penetrate the human body. The existence of such fields has not yet been scientifically proven. Some forms of energy therapy manipulate biofields by applying pressure and/or manipulating the body by placing the hands in, or through, these fields. Examples include qi gong, Reiki, and therapeutic touch.
- Bioelectromagnetic-based therapies involve the unconventional use of electromagnetic fields, such as pulsed fields, magnetic fields, or alternating current or direct-current fields.

From National Center for Complementary and Alternative Medicine. What Is Complementary and Alternative Medicine (CAM)? Available at: http://nccam.nih.gov/health/whatiscam.

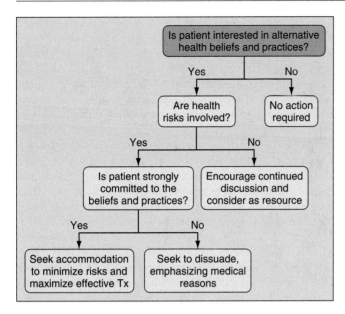

Figure 50-2 Decision tree for evaluating a patient's willingness to negotiate use of CAM. Tx, treatment.

of culture-bound healing traditions, such as those found in the Catholic-rooted African religions (e.g., Candomblé from Brazil or Santeria from the Caribbean), Latino healing traditions (Curanderismo from Mexico), or endemic practices, such as Kampo from Japan. Yet these religious and endemic traditions, complete with their own preferred providers and therapies, are practiced in the United States, often under the radar of, but in concert with, mainstream medicine.[19]

In the absence of open communication, the failure to identify alternative beliefs may lead providers to assign treatments to which the patient is unwilling or unable to adhere. Perhaps the most drastic and irreconcilable uses of CAM can be found in life-threatening diseases in which miraculous healing through faith-based programs or alternative treatment centers has led patients to uniformly reject conventional care. In asthma, for which patient acceptance of orthodox treatment is already suboptimal, the failure to identify, discuss, and reconcile preferred treatment options may also be of great consequence. Alternatively, patients and providers who engage in these discussions may establish a therapeutic alliance that supports a jointly developed integrated treatment plan. A decision-making algorithm is offered to assist providers in accommodating, negotiating, and reconciling patients' CAM use (Fig. 50-2).[19]

AGE-, GENDER-, AND DISABILITY-SPECIFIC CHALLENGES

Certain asthma subpopulations create unique challenges to the effective implementation of an asthma management plan. These groups include the young, the elderly, women, and people with disabilities.

Age

Asthma currently affects more than 6 million children and is a common cause of school absenteeism and physical limitation in childhood.[20] Young children may be ineffectively managed due to inadequate communication or suboptimal delivery of topical medication due to lower inhalation flow rates, device-related dexterity and coordination issues, or inability/unwillingness to fully participate in the treatment.[21]

An additional 2 million people older than 65 have asthma. The elderly are more likely to die from asthma[20] perhaps due to comorbidities or as a result of greater severity and lower lung function associated with long-standing disease. The elderly may experience greater difficulty achieving optimal disease control because of comorbidities, memory lapses, or, as in young children, inadequate drug deposition from lower inspiratory flow rates, dexterity, and coordination difficulties.

Gender

In children 0 to 17 years of age, males are more likely to have an asthma diagnosis, but among adults, females are 7% more likely than males to ever have been diagnosed with asthma.[20] In addition, females experience more asthma morbidity as measured by hospitalization rates and have an asthma death rate about 40% higher than males.[20] The increased morbidity and mortality in women may be explained, in part, by lower prescription fill rates for controller medications in women compared with men.[22]

Physical Disabilities

Insufficient fine motor skills, hand-mouth coordination, strength, or visual or mental acuity may all serve as impediments to adequate asthma self-management particularly as it relates to drug delivery devices. For example, tremors may make it difficult to prepare devices for inhalation and poor vision may prevent an individual from accurately assessing whether a full dose has been delivered or if a device is empty. Such disabilities require that providers perform a detailed assessment of an individual's ability to correctly prepare a dose, accurately administer the dose, and properly care for the device before dispensing a device for home use. In summary, the design of a tailored educational plan for the asthma patient must begin with an assessment of individual and environmental factors that may impede the transmission or retention of knowledge or the ability of an individual to implement the management strategy. For example, a self-management plan will be constrained by the cost of its implementation in low-income groups where limited expendable income and inadequate health insurance present formidable barriers to obtaining medications and making environmental modifications, such as obtaining mite-proof covers. In addition, an individual's ability to comprehend, interpret, and implement a set of highly varied and complex skills, such as symptom assessment, peak flow monitoring, multiple inhaler techniques, daily and rescue medication routines, and environmental trigger reduction will be considerably more difficult in the setting of low literacy and limited English language proficiency. Patients who are illegal aliens or who are distrustful of the medical establishment may experience more inconsistency in primary care and greater skepticism regarding medical advice, creating a significant obstacle to adequate disease management. Further, alternative beliefs and attitudes may serve as an impediment to acceptance of the medical plan. Finally, special populations, such as the young and the elderly, women, and those with disabilities may face specific challenges. Strategies to address these barriers are offered in the sections that follow.

EDUCATION

When given a choice, patients prefer to receive care and education in the community in which they reside and from individuals of the same race and ethnicity.[2] For this reason, community-based programs using peers as health educators are particularly popular. Greater acceptability, attendance, and credence may be given to an educational health initiative coordinated through community-based organizations (CBOs), such as churches, mosques, barbershops, or retail stores, compared to efforts organized by "outsiders." Challenges to effective CBO-based initiatives however, must be considered, such as the fact that few peer educators are licensed health care professionals and many are volunteers. For example, members of black churches are frequently lay educators interested in health but without the requisite training or time to effectively deliver a complex health initiative, such as asthma self-management training, without intensive training, support, and access to resources themselves. This may be particularly evident when the health initiative is part of a research study and includes tasks unfamiliar to peer educators, such as obtaining informed consent, collecting data, or performing data entry.

If it is not possible to have providers who are racially or ethnically concordant with the patient population they care for, then providers should receive cultural sensitivity training, the first step in the lifelong learning process of developing cultural competency. Structured training is important because negative stereotypes towards racial/ethnic minorities exist even among health care providers.[2] National standards on Culturally and Linguistically Appropriate Services (CLAS) have been developed by the Institute of Minority Health for voluntary adoption by health care organizations (Table 50-3).[24] Individual providers are also encouraged to voluntarily comply with these standards to create care environments that are "more culturally and linguistically accessible."[24] The principles and activities of CLAS are meant to be integrated at every point of contact within a practice and in concert with the community. Detailed recommendations for the delivery of culturally and linguistically accessible asthma education are described in the following section.

TECHNIQUES

Asthma Education in Low-Income, Underinsured, or Uninsured Populations

The poor and near poor populations face substantial obstacles to obtaining medical and prescription coverage. In the context of a patient's inability to access primary care or prescription therapy, the value of asthma education is greatly diminished. Therefore, an educational program targeted to those living in poverty might require substantial amounts of time allocated to the identification of affordable health care (e.g., free clinics) and assistance in insurance applications. Further, the provision of asthma edu-

cation in populations with limited expendable incomes or inadequate insurance will require that the educator have greater resources available for training purposes. Typically, less expensive spacers and peak flow meters will cost between $10 and $20 and one-way valved holding chambers, preferred for inhalation therapy, will range from $25 to $60. If these devices are not a part of a patient's prescription or durable medical equipment plan, then these may be prohibitively costly, hindering the acquisition of devices necessary for symptom management and optimal medication delivery. In this situation, the patient would be well served by an educational program that provides complimentary devices as a benefit of participation. Alternatively, if the educator's resources are limited, a written action plan based on daytime and nighttime symptoms (rescue doses required/week and nocturnal awakenings/month) may be an adequate substitute for peak flow monitoring.[25]

Asthma Education in Populations with Low Literacy or Low Educational Attainment

Asthma educators are resourceful individuals, looking to stretch precious dollars whenever and wherever possible. A common error, however, is made when the educator relies on donated educational materials that are written at too high a reading level for the group with whom they are working. Educators may recognize that informational pamphlets supplied by the pharmaceutical industry are frequently written at a high school reading level but may erroneously assume that patient education materials from nonprofit organizations are of a low reading level. The ability to assess the reading level of materials, therefore, is a key skill for the asthma educators.

Different reading formulas are available to the educator. Two approaches to calculate readability are presented in Tables 50-4 and 50-5. If the material is available as a Word document, the reading level can be automatically calculated after spelling and grammar have been checked. Conversely, if the material is a print piece, then the simplified measure of gobbledygook (SMOG) formula can be used.[26]

Importantly, in low literacy groups, perhaps the best education will not be conveyed with printed materials but rather orally. This can be done by either using a live instructor or a videotape and should be followed with hands-on practice, a question-and-answer period, and assessment of comprehension. To enhance comprehension and retention, information is best presented in small "chunks," with the most important information presented initially and repeated frequently.[27] Multiple short teaching sessions are more likely to result in greater comprehension of materials and are therefore preferable to the one-day "get-it-all" program. Comprehension is best evaluated not by testing knowledge, but by testing the individual's ability to apply the information in a real-life situation. Application therefore, is best assessed using problem-based approaches. For example, if you want to assess the patient's ability to implement an asthma action plan, ask the patient to imagine they are experiencing asthma symptoms. Ask them, what should they do first and why? What will they do if the initial steps they take fail to relieve their symptoms? Although time consuming, this approach of tailored individual education and assessment provides much more convincing evidence that knowledge was transmitted and interpreted correctly and can be implemented.

Table 50-3
NATIONAL STANDARDS ON CULTURALLY AND LINGUISTICALLY APPROPRIATE SERVICES (CLAS)[24]

Standards 1-3: Culturally Competent Care
Standard 1.
Health care organizations should ensure that patients/consumers receive from all staff members effective, understandable, and respectful care that is provided in a manner compatible with their cultural health beliefs and practices and preferred language.

Standard 2.
Health care organizations should implement strategies to recruit, retain, and promote at all levels of the organization a diverse staff and leadership that are representative of the demographic characteristics of the service area.

Standard 3.
Health care organizations should ensure that staff at all levels and across all disciplines receive ongoing education and training in culturally and linguistically appropriate service delivery.

Standards 4-7: Language Access Services
Standard 4.
Health care organizations must offer and provide language assistance services, including bilingual staff and interpreter services, at no cost to each patient/consumer with limited English proficiency at all points of contact, in a timely manner during all hours of operation.

Standard 5.
Health care organizations must provide to patients/consumers in their preferred language both verbal offers and written notices informing them of their right to receive language assistance services.

Standard 6.
Health care organizations must assure the competence of language assistance provided to limited English proficient patients/consumers by interpreters and bilingual staff. Family and friends should not be used to provide interpretation services (except on request by the patient/consumer).

Standard 7.
Health care organizations must make available easily understood patient-related materials and post signage in the languages of the commonly encountered groups and/or groups represented in the service area.

Standards 8-14: Organizational Supports for Cultural Competence
Standard 8.
Health care organizations should develop, implement, and promote a written strategic plan that outlines clear goals, policies, operational plans, and management accountability/oversight mechanisms to provide culturally and linguistically appropriate services.

Standard 9.
Health care organizations should conduct initial and ongoing organizational self-assessments of CLAS-related activities and are encouraged to integrate cultural and linguistic competence-related measures into their internal audits, performance improvement programs, patient satisfaction assessments, and outcomes-based evaluations.

Standard 10.
Health care organizations should ensure that data on the individual patient's/consumer's race, ethnicity, and spoken and written language are collected in health records, integrated into the organization's management information systems, and periodically updated.

Standard 11.
Health care organizations should maintain a current demographic, cultural, and epidemiological profile of the community as well as a needs assessment to accurately plan for and implement services that respond to the cultural and linguistic characteristics of the service area.

Standard 12.
Health care organizations should develop participatory, collaborative partnerships with communities and utilize a variety of formal and informal mechanisms to facilitate community and patient/consumer involvement in designing and implementing CLAS-related activities.

Standard 13.
Health care organizations should ensure that conflict and grievance resolution processes are culturally and linguistically sensitive and capable of identifying, preventing, and resolving cross-cultural conflicts or complaints by patients/consumers.

Standard 14.
Health care organizations are encouraged to regularly make available to the public information about their progress and successful innovations in implementing the CLAS standards and to provide public notice in their communities about the availability of this information.

From National Standards on Culturally and Linguistically Appropriate Services (CLAS), available at http://www.omhrc.gov/.

Education in ESL and Alien Populations

Since health-related topics are complex, same-language instruction is preferable. Speakers however must have command of more than just conversational skills. For this reason, using a family member or community volunteer as a translator is not recommended unless a native-speaking trained medical person is unavailable.[24] Non-English versions of educational materials should be available although care must be taken to ensure that they are not written at too high a reading level for the population and that the translation was done adequately. Translation usually requires that one native-speaking individual does the initial translation from English, which is then given to a second native speaker who back-translates the material into English. Then both documents are compared and discrepancies addressed. Frequently, several rounds of translations and back-translations are necessary before translated materials accurately represent the original material.

Table 50-4
CALCULATING THE READING LEVEL OF A MICROSOFT WORD DOCUMENT USING THE FLESCH-KINCAID GRADE LEVEL (UP TO GRADE 12)

Setting Up Your Computer to Calculate Reading Level
1. From the Toolbar, select Tools.
2. From the Tool drop-down menu, select Options.
3. From the Options function, select the Spelling and Grammar tab.
4. Under the options for grammar, select (check) "Show readability statistics".
5. Click OK.

Calculating Reading Level
1. From the Toolbar, select Tools.
2. From the Tool drop-down menu, select Spelling and Grammar.
3. After completing the Spelling and Grammar check, the Readability Statistics will appear in a pop-up window.
4. The Flesch-Kincaid Grade Level will be displayed in the last row.

The primary challenge in providing asthma education to an illegal alien population is finding the audience. Because of their illegal status, aliens tend to make less use of routine primary care and more use of acute care services. The Emergency Department therefore might be a more appropriate setting for an educational intervention in this group. Alternatively, CBOs may be effective in locating an alien population but their program participation will be poor unless anonymity and safety can be assured. In addition, alien populations will often have the same need for educational programs that address

Table 50-5
CALCULATING THE READING LEVEL OF PRINT PIECES USING THE SMOG FORMULA (UP TO THE GRADUATE LEVEL—GRADE 18)

1. Mark off 10 consecutive sentences at the beginning, middle and end of the document
2. Count the total number of words that are three syllables or more
3. Use the conversion chart to determine reading level

SMOG Conversion Table I (For Longer Materials)		SMOG Conversion Table II (Use on Material with < 30 Sentences)	
Word Count	Grade Level	# of Sentences	Conversion No.
0–2	4	29	1.03
3–6	5	28	1.07
7–12	6	27	1.1
13–20	7	26	1.15
21–30	8	25	1.2
31–42	9	24	1.25
43–56	10	23	1.3
57–72	11	22	1.36
73–90	12	21	1.43
91–110	13	20	1.5
111–132	14	19	1.58
133–156	15	18	1.67
157–182	16	17	1.76
183–210	17	16	1.87
211–240	18	15	2.0
		14	2.14
		13	2.3
		12	2.5
		11	2.7
		10	3.0

low literacy, limited expendable incomes, and limited English language proficiency as described previously. In addition, mistrust of the medical establishment, as described in the next section, may be operative and must be addressed if effective health education is to be delivered.

Education in Distrustful Populations

One of the most effective methods of delivering care and education to groups that perceive medicine as racist is to match the race and/or ethnicity of the provider with that of the patient.[2] When race or ethnicity concordance is not possible, then providers should receive training to increase their cultural sensitivity. The evolution from cultural sensitivity to competency is not always linear. Generally, cultural sensitivity begins with the educator recognizing that they are not immune from racial/ethnic stereotyping but desire to mitigate the influence of these biases in their practice. To accomplish this, the provider invites their patients to explain their views of health in a safe environment that encourages disclosure. Whenever possible, nonconventional approaches to health promotion and disease management should be integrated into the medical plan. A model for accommodation is depicted in Figure 50-2.[19]

As the educator works to develop cultural competency, relatively easy-to-adopt behaviors promote culturally sensitive interactions with patients. These include the recognition of and respect for traditions in which the individual is not the decision maker for his or her own health. In Asian populations, for example, the family or council of elders frequently makes decisions regarding an individual's health care. In Latino populations the decision maker may be the male head of the household. Conversely, in black communities, the influential decision makers may be the mother and grandmothers. In fact, individual decision making is a decidedly white American value.

Other behaviors that can demonstrate cultural sensitivity include the manner in which the health care professional addresses the patient, as well as body language and gestures.[23] For example, patients should always be addressed initially by their surname with the use of the first name reserved for those individuals who invite its use. When a patient invites the use of his or her first name, the educator may in turn, choose to be addressed by his or her first name. First-name familiarity may be a helpful strategy to bridge the patient-provider gap particularly when the patient and educator are not racially or ethnically concordant. Further, although blacks and Latinos may enjoy close social spaces and physical contact with their provider, this would be a culturally incorrect approach for Asian populations. As a great deal of diversity exists within racial/ethnic groups, no "cookbook" approach can be recommended. Rather, patients should be asked about their preferences.

Asthma Education in the Context of Alternative Beliefs and Practices

As shown in Figure 50-2,[19] patient-provider partnerships are less fractious when there is agreement over the medical plan. However, this should not be misconstrued to suggest that complete agreement is possible or desirable. Rather, partnership necessitates that compromises be made. Fortunately in the area of CAM, most patients prefer to use a combination of alternative and conventional approaches.[18] Identifying unsafe practices and dissuading patients from their use, perhaps by substituting a safe CAM, suggests how this type of partnership might be executed. Take for example the patient who wants to use biologically based asthma treatments to complement the use of ICSs. An educator willing to partner with the patient will spend less time exhaustively lecturing the patient on the lack of scientific evidence in support of herbs (a brief statement should suffice) and more time helping the patient select a safe product. For the patient with asthma this may mean encouraging peppermint tea and discouraging echinacea, a member of the ragweed family.

Individuals who reject the medical plan completely in favor of CAM present the educator with particular challenges. Their decision to reject conventional care may be based on inaccurate beliefs about prescription medicine or faulty beliefs regarding the efficacy of CAM. Although knowledge in and of itself is necessary, it is often insufficient to effect a change in health behaviors. Therefore, individuals who are resistant to conventional medications should be followed over time so that if the door opens for a trial of prescription medicine, trust has already been established.

Age-, Gender-, or Disability-Specific Asthma Education

The In-check Dial is a tool that assesses the adequacy of inspiratory flow rate by simulating the resistance of eight different inhalational devices. As such, the In-check Dial is invaluable when working with young and elderly patients. In addition to adequacy of inspiratory flow rate, fine motor skills, hand strength, and hand-mouth coordination should also be assessed to determine if the individual has the physical ability to prepare and deliver a dose of medication. For example, if the patient has intentional tremors, removing a capsule from a foil package and loading it in a chamber may be more difficult than using a device that has self-contained drug. Similarly, dry-powder inhalers may be easier to activate than traditional metered-dose inhalers if hand strength and flexibility are diminished, as in arthritis. Providers may want to consider an assistance device that will help administer the medication, such as is used with patients that have arthritis to actuate a metered-dose inhaler or the use of an alternate delivery device (e.g., breath-actuated inhaler).

Patients with poor visual acuity may experience other difficulties in using inhalational devices. For example, many dry powder devices require that the medication chamber be visually inspected after inspiration to determine if any powder remains. If powder is visible in the chamber, it is recommended that a second inhalation be performed. Those with poor eyesight may have difficulty in making this determination. In addition, although dry powder devices have the advantage of dose counters, many patients with poor eyesight complain that the counters are too small to be easily read. Using a magnifying glass may seem a logical approach to correct this problem; however, magnification causes additional distortion in some devices, such as the Diskus. Moreover, several devices use red ink to warn of low doses, which is more difficult to read against a white background than is black ink.

Finally, evidence suggests that women experience a greater asthma burden than men,[20] perhaps because of lower adherence rates to controller therapies[22] or poorer inhaler technique.[23] Whatever the cause, it is imperative that both ability and willingness to perform self-management be assessed before a tailored educational plan is initiated.

In summary, a variety of key educational strategies have been suggested for use in special populations. Assessing their success, an integral component of any educational program, is discussed in the final section of this chapter.

OUTCOMES

The goal of asthma education is to improve the patient's quality of life (QOL) and increase the acceptance of the medical plan. Short of administering QOL questionnaires (designed to measure group and not individual changes) and objectively monitoring the use of peak flow meters and inhalational therapies, how could we measure success in special populations? The metrics of success in these populations may look quite unconventional. For example, successful outcomes might be demonstrated by an increase in the number of individuals obtaining and maintaining insurance, by more frequent and routine attendance at free health clinics or educational programs, or by more risk-taking disclosure during the clinical or educational encounter.

To successfully intervene in special populations, the educator must "think outside the box" of traditional education where one describes anatomy ("These are the lungs. Their function is to bring oxygen in and move carbon dioxide out."), disease ("Asthma is a chronic disease characterized by airway inflammation, bronchoconstriction, and hyperreactivity.") and management ("Inhaled corticosteroids are the cornerstone of treatment."). Rather, the educator working with special populations concentrates their efforts on identifying resources for their clients and relies on oral instruction and hands-on training. When written materials are used they have been fully evaluated for their readability and cultural appropriateness. Finally, the successful educator will solicit patients' alternative beliefs and integrate safe CAM into the patient's comprehensive management plan. Together, these approaches are likely to enhance trust, the foundation of all future health behaviors.

REFERENCES

1. American Lung Association: Lung Disease Data in Culturally Diverse Communities, 2005. Available at www.lungusa.org.
2. Smedley BD, Stith AY, Nelson AR (eds): Unequal Treatment: Confronting Racial and Ethnic Disparities in Health Care. Washington, DC: National Academies Press, 2002.
3. Krishnan JA, Diette GB, Skinner EA, et al: Race and sex differences in consistency of care with national asthma guidelines in managed care organizations. Arch Int Med 2001;161:1660–1668.
4. DaNavas-Walt C, Proctor BD, Lee CH: U.S. Census Bureau, Current population report, P60-229, Income, poverty, and health

insurance coverage in the United States, 2004. Washington, DC, U.S. Government Printing Office, 2005.

5. George M, Freedman TG, Norfleet AL, et al: Qualitative research-enhanced understanding of patients' beliefs: results of focus groups with low-income, urban, African American adults with asthma. J Allergy Clin Immunol 2003;111(5):967–973.

6. National Asthma Education and Prevention Program Expert Panel Report II: Guidelines for the Diagnosis and Management of Asthma (Publication No. 97-4051). Bethesda, Md, Public Health Service, National Institutes of Health, Heart Lung Blood Institute, 1997.

7. National Assessment of Adult Literacy. Available at http://nces.ed.gov/naal.

8. George M, Albert C, Fein DG, Apter, AJ: Low literacy and inhaler prescription reading and interpretation errors in adults with asthma. Am J Respir Crit Care Med 2005;2:A587.

9. United States Bureau of the Census 2000. Available at http://www.ccnsus.gov/main/www/cen2000.html.

10. Edwards JR: Two Sides of the Same Coin. The connection between legal and illegal immigration. Available at www.cis.org/.

11. Cosman MP: Illegal aliens and American medicine. J Am Phys Surg 2005;10:6–10.

12. Kreiger N: Shades of difference: theoretical underpinnings of the medical controversy on black/white differences in the United States. Int J Health Serv 1987;17:259–278.

13. Manning KR: Race, science and identity. In Early G (ed): Lure and Loathing. New York, Penguin Books, 1994, pp 317–336.

14. Brandon DT, Isaac LA, LaVeist TA: The legacy of Tuskegee and trust in medical care: is Tuskegee responsible for race differences in mistrust of medical care?. JAMA 2005;97(7):951–956.

15. Apter AJ, Reisine ST, Affleck G, et al: Adherence with twice-daily dosing of inhaled steroids. Socioeconomic and health-belief differences. Am J Respir Crit Care Med 1998;157(6 Pt 1):1810–1817.

16. Barnes PM, Powell-Griner E, McFann K, Nahin RL: Complementary and alternative medicine use among adults: United States, 2002. Advance data from vital and health statistics, No. 343. Hyattsville, MD, National Center for Health Statistics, 2004.

17. National Center for Complementary and Alternative Medicine. What Is Complementary and Alternative Medicine (CAM)? Available at:http://nccam.nih.gov/health/whatiscam.

18. Eisenberg DM, Davis RB, Ettner SL, et al: Trends in alternative medicine use in the U.S. 1990–1997: results of a follow-up national survey. JAMA 1998;280(18):1569–1575.

19. Hufford DJ: Folk medicine and health culture in contemporary society. Prim Care 1997;24(4):723–741.

20. Lethbridge-Cejku M, Rose D, Vickerie J: Summary health statistics for US adults: National Health Interview Survey 2004. National Center for Health Statistics. Vital Health Stat 2004;10(238):200. Available at http://www.cdc.gov/.

21. Dolovich MB, Ahrens RC, Hess DR, et al: Device selection and outcomes of aerosol therapy. Chest 2005;127(1):335–371.

22. Boulet L: Perception of the role and potential side effects of inhaled corticosteroids among asthmatic patients. Chest 1998;113:587–592.

23. Goodman DE, Israel E, Rosenberg M, et al: The influence of age, diagnosis and gender on proper use of metered-dose inhaler. Am J Respir Crit Care Med 1994;150:1183–1187.

24. National Standards on Culturally and Linguistically Appropriate Services (CLAS). Available at http://www.omhrc.gov/.

25. National Asthma Education and Prevention Program: Expert Panel Report: Guidelines for the Diagnosis and Management of Asthma-Update on Selected Topics 2002 (EPR-Update 2002) (Publication No. 02-5075). Bethesda, Md, National Institutes of Health, 2002.

26. McLaughlin G: SMOG grading: a new readability formula. J Read 1969;12(8):639–646.

27. George M: Culturally competent asthma education. Houston, Texas, Association of Asthma Educators, 2002.

Improving Adherence

Elizabeth L. McQuaid, Karen J. Tien, and Andrea J. Apter

CHAPTER

51

CLINICAL PEARLS

- Low adherence to medications is common. Providers have an important role in facilitating communication that will identify barriers and result in improved adherence.

- Low adherence to environmental recommendations is also common. Nonjudgmental discussions between provider and patients may help to reduce these exposures.

- Simplify asthma management regimens to facilitate adherence. Self-management recommendations must be negotiated between patient and physician and individualized to each patient.

- Preventing decline in adherence over time is a critical task; adherence must be addressed and negotiated with patients and their families at every visit.

Despite the array of pharmacological options and environmental control strategies available to treat asthma, adherence to asthma regimens remains a critical clinical problem. In this chapter, we present a brief overview on adherence, examine the methods available to assess adherence, review interventions aimed at improving asthma management and adherence, and provide recommendations regarding how practitioners can collaborate with patients to improve adherence to asthma regimens in the clinical setting.

THE DEFINITION OF ADHERENCE

In contrast to the term *compliance*, *adherence* suggests a therapeutic alliance or contract between the patient, family, and physician in treatment planning and a more active role for the patient and family in treatment-related decisions. Concerns regarding generally accepted definitions of adherence and how the term has been used, however, have been noted. For example, although adherence is thought of as the extent to which a patient's behavior coincides with medical advice, adherence often is not measured in relation to a prescribed regimen, but rather is evaluated against a standard or ideal regimen. Current definitions of adherence may imply that the physician recommendation is the gold standard to which the patient must adhere, regardless of how much adherence actually may be needed for clinical benefit. Additionally, in current models the onus to adhere is placed on the patient, even though provider factors (e.g., communication style, cultural competence) should be acknowledged as having a joint role in the process.

In general, we recommend that adherence be (1) recognized as a complex behavior with many considerations involved; (2) viewed on a continuum, with an understanding that perfection not only is unrealistic, especially for lifelong conditions, but may not be necessary for every patient and illness; (3) appreciated as an active, constantly evolving process that can be negotiated and renegotiated reasonably by the patient and family, in consultation with the medical provider; and (4) understood as a process for which patients, families, and providers share responsibility. This approach may be more likely to promote a true patient-family-provider alliance in adherence decisions, greater patient and family investment in adherence agreements and, in turn, greater rates of adherence overall.

NONADHERENCE TO ASTHMA REGIMENS

Poor adherence to medications has been implicated in disease decline and death across numerous medical conditions. In asthma, poor treatment adherence has been related to increased symptoms, decreased pulmonary function, and worse control.[1] Nonadherence to asthma regimens may result in increased emergency department visits and is implicated in increased asthma mortality.[2]

A wealth of research consistently has demonstrated poor adherence to controller medications for asthma in both children and adults. These findings are more pronounced when objective measures, as opposed to self- or parent reports of adherence, are used. Advances in technology have provided multiple methods for the objective assessment of patient adherence to inhaled asthma medications. Research using electronic monitoring devices for preventive medications suggests that children and adults generally take 50% to 65% of prescribed doses,[3,4] much less than recommended by their health care providers.

Although there has been much less research on adherence to environmental control recommendations, adherence in this area also appears to be low. As an example, adherence to recommendations to quit smoking or limit environmental tobacco smoke exposure is poor. In a large multi-center study, Kattan and colleagues[5] found that many urban parents of children with asthma were smokers, with as many as 48% of children regularly exposed to environmental tobacco smoke. Lemiere and Boulet[6] identified similar rates of smoking among adults with asthma as among those without asthma, suggesting that having asthma does not prompt most people to stop smoking. Approximately two thirds of families of children with asthma have household pets.[7] Joseph and associates[8] found that allergen-control bedding encasing adherence for children with asthma was 50%.

DISEASE AND REGIMEN BARRIERS TO ADHERENCE

Many features of asthma, including its chronicity, variable symptom presentation, and in some cases, regimen complexity, present barriers to adherence. Medical conditions with intermittent symptoms and variable symptom severity, such as asthma, may lead to treatment nonadherence, because medications are less likely to be taken during periods with fewer symptoms. Adherence may be lower with more complex regimens, such as those that involve greater frequency of medication administration.

INDIVIDUAL/FAMILY BARRIERS TO ADHERENCE

Nonadherence to asthma treatment has been associated with several demographic factors including limited financial means, less educational achievement, Spanish as a primary language, and minority status.[4,9,10] Individuals with lower financial status may have limited access to care and more difficulty affording treatment copays. Individuals with less education and less English proficiency may have trouble comprehending asthma treatment plans, and this lack of comprehension may be unrecognized by the health care provider. If such vulnerable individuals are the caretakers of an asthmatic child, communicating medical instructions to alternate care providers, such as day care centers and schools, may be difficult.

Among youth, age (and stage of development) is an important demographic factor that is relevant to adherence. It is well-established that nonadherence often becomes more pronounced in adolescence compared to earlier childhood, in spite of the more sophisticated cognitive abilities of adolescents and greater expectations that parents tend to have for them.[10] McQuaid and co-workers[10] found that older children were less adherent to preventive medications for asthma than younger children, in spite of having more knowledge about asthma and responsibility for asthma management. Possible explanations for the pattern of poor adherence in adolescence include less motivation to take medications in the face of competing developmental tasks; less attention on bodily cues that would indicate the need for treatment given greater focus on developmental changes (e.g., puberty) and tasks (e.g., dating); increased likelihood of forgetting medications with less parental supervision of older children; and a sense of immortality, which could lead to risk taking.

Certain individual health beliefs also seem to play a role in adherence. For example, greater perceived severity of child illness by mothers has been related to greater adherence in pediatric asthma.[11] Additionally, greater perceived benefit of treatment by pediatric patients and parents has been associated with greater adherence to asthma regimens.[11] Similarly, Apter and colleagues[9] found that medication adherence by adults with asthma was associated with better "attitude," which was defined as belief in treatment benefits with less fear of side effects. Other studies have shown that a lack of perceived benefits and greater perceived costs of treatment serve as detriments to adherence.[12]

Poor adherence may also be linked to both a lack of information regarding medical treatment and a lack of skills to perform a particular regimen. Along with behavioral skills, behavioral consequences can influence adherence. Negative consequences of adherence (e.g., having an asthma attack after taking controller medication as prescribed) as well as a lack of positive consequences for adherence (e.g., no immediate perceivable benefit to taking controller medication) may decrease the likelihood of future adherence.

The available literature consistently documents some associations between mental health difficulties and problems in adherence. Pediatric nonadherence has been related to psychological difficulties among children,[13] parents,[14] and families.[15] Depressive symptoms and stress are related to poor adherence.[16] Stress may contribute to nonadherence, perhaps through perceived lack of time and competing concerns. Through focus groups with low-income, African American adults with asthma, George and colleagues[12] found that one challenge to taking preventive medications is remembering, especially in the context of competing distractions (e.g., numerous social demands) in large households.

CULTURAL BARRIERS TO ADHERENCE

It is increasingly understood that cultural norms and values may influence patient and family acceptance of medical treatment. Studies have shown that various cultural groups have concerns about standard medical treatment for asthma. Apter and collaborators[9] found that African-American adults with asthma have greater fear about the use of inhaled corticosteroids than white adults with asthma. George and associates[12] found that some African Americans reportedly fear perceived side effects of inhaled corticosteroids such as weight gain, organ damage, infertility, cancer, somatic complaints (e.g., headaches), hyperactivity, tolerance, and addiction. Other research has shown that Dominican mothers' preferred first response to asthma symptoms is the use of alternative medications, such as herbal remedies,[17] as opposed to conventionally prescribed medications. With the increasing diversity of the U.S. population, more research on cultural barriers experienced by different ethnic groups is needed.

HEALTH CARE SYSTEMS BARRIERS TO ADHERENCE

Access to health care is thought to be related to adherence. Managed care, with its emphasis on cost containment and profitability, encourages shortened medical appointments and less personal care, neither of which is likely to be promote adherence. Furthermore, there are numerous, additional health care access barriers for patients and families who lack financial means, transportation, English proficiency, knowledge of the American health care system, and/or equal treatment by others based on discrimination. It is well established that racial and ethnic minorities receive poorer health care than nonracial and nonethnic minorities.[18] Poor access to (quality) care likely may explain some of the relation between minority status and nonadherence. Additionally, many insurance approval policies for medications are restrictive, confusing, and time-consuming for patients with managed Medicaid health plans. Without insurance coverage, the high cost of medications may be prohibitive, and even with insurance coverage, expensive copays for medication may hinder adherence.

Research has shown that certain provider factors, specifically those relating to lack of continuity of care,[19] poor communication, and lack of cultural competence[12] are related to poor adherence. Aspects of provider communication that may hinder adherence include unclear recommendations, lack of repeat instructions, failure to discuss treatment risks and benefits, lack of friendliness and empathy, and criticism.[12] Some researchers have suggested that lack of cultural awareness and consideration of the patient's circumstance may impede adherence.[12] An Institute of Medicine report[18] provides a summary of research indicating less preferential treatment of ethnic and racial minorities and individuals with lower socioeconomic status by health care providers, which suggests that patient/provider interactions may play a critical, yet understudied role in nonadherence.

ASSESSMENT

Before intervening to address adherence difficulties, it is important to assess the nature and extent of the problem. In the following section we provide a summary of the most commonly used methods to assess adherence to asthma regimens, including clinical interviewing, self-report instruments, and objective methods such as drug assays or electronic monitoring of medication consumption.

Clinical Interviewing

Informal clinical assessments of adherence to prescribed treatment regimens are commonly made within the context of medical encounters. Clinical assessment is a key component of patient-provider communication, yet the validity of clinical judgment to obtain precise information regarding asthma management is questionable. First, clinical interviewing is rarely performed in a systematic manner and questions are often issued in a close-ended fashion (e.g., "Are you taking your medicine?"), rather than using an open-ended technique that promotes further exploration (e.g., "Most people find it challenging to take medications every day; I am wondering what has been difficult for you?"). Health care providers are not necessarily accurate in assessing patient adherence to treatment recommendations. Research indicates that physicians tend to be more accurate when identifying highly adherent patients, compared to identifying those who are nonadherent to treatment plans.[20] The quantity and accuracy of information gleaned during clinical assessment may be confounded by the quality of the patient-physician relationship. Specifically, patients may be more likely to acknowledge difficulties with adherence when they perceive the provider to be generally supportive and nonjudgmental. Clinical interviews that are specifically tailored to identify patient health beliefs regarding medications and promote open-ended discussion of adherence barriers may lay the groundwork for promoting adherence.

Self-Report Instruments

Patient self-report of specific asthma management behaviors are commonly used in clinical trials and interventions, and are appealing because of their low cost and ease of use. Numerous self-report measures are available to assess variables related to asthma management such as asthma knowledge, self-efficacy to manage asthma symptoms, and quality of life related to asthma. Self-report measures such as these

may be helpful when assessing patient beliefs, attitudes, and experiences regarding medications and asthma management in general. For specific behaviors such as medication use, however, self-reports such as asthma diaries have been shown to overestimate adherence to treatment regimens by as much as 30%. Patients' reports of *nonadherence* may be more useful than reports of *adherence*, as it is less likely to find patients motivated to misrepresent themselves as nonadherent than adherent. Self-reports of medication use may be helpful if they are employed in the service of attempting to identify adherence barriers (e.g., pinpointing times of the day or week that medications are typically missed), yet clinicians must be aware that such reports may be influenced by social desirability (i.e., the desire to show the health care provider that they are actively cooperating with treatment goals).

Objective Assessment Tools

Objective methods of assessing asthma management behavior have generally been limited to (1) assessments of medication levels, and (2) electronic monitoring of medication use or peak flow meter use. Drug levels can be assessed directly or measured through metabolic indicators by use of laboratory assays of bodily fluids, including serum, urine or saliva. These assays are only available to determine the usage of some less commonly used asthma medications, such as theophylline and oral corticosteroids. This approach has the advantage of providing direct confirmation of medication use. Results, however, may be confounded by diet, metabolism, and use of other medications. Additionally, this approach fails to capture patterns of day-to day adherence, and yields no information regarding what barriers may have impeded consistent adherence.

Electronic monitoring devices have been increasingly used to assess patterns of medication use and adherence to medication regimens. Electronic devices that measure inhaler use have been employed widely in clinical trials and research settings.[3,4,10] Devices that measure tablet consumption by recording opening and closing of medication bottles have also been used to assess adherence to oral asthma medications. Last, peak flow monitors that provide an electronic record of use have been implemented to assess adherence to recommendations for peak flow monitoring.[21]

Many of these devices are prohibitively expensive for regular use in a clinical setting. Additionally, devices vary in terms of the precision of the behavior that is measured. For example, whereas some devices may measure only the opening of a pill bottle, or the actuation of an inhaler, other devices measure whether or not a dose of an inhaled medication actually was inhaled. As with direct metabolic indices of medication use, electronic monitoring methods, when used alone, do not provide any information regarding the context in which medication use (or failure to take medication) is taking place. Additionally, using only electronic monitoring methods constrains the definition of adherence to a very specific behavior such as taking a certain medication or using a peak flow meter. This may be useful if that particular behavior is a target of intervention. If an assessment of adherence to an overall management plan is desired, additional areas must be assessed, including avoiding or attempting to control asthma triggers, responding appropriately to symptoms, and maintaining an ongoing relationship with a health care provider.

TECHNIQUES FOR IMPROVING ADHERENCE: OVERVIEW OF EXISTING INTERVENTIONS

A number of different approaches to improving adherence have been proposed and studied, including educational and behavioral approaches (Table 51-1), physician-based and organizational strategies, multicomponent approaches, and individualized methods. The following section reviews the empirical data supporting each of these options and ultimately encourages clinicians to strongly consider multi-faceted and individualized interventions on both a theoretical and empirical basis.

Educational Approaches

One of the most common interventions for difficulties in medication adherence is to provide asthma education, either in the office setting or through referral to a formal asthma education program. These programs typically provide information regarding the physiology of asthma, medications and their use, and strategies for environmental control. The effects of asthma education on adherence have been mixed, as most programs do not specifically target adherence. A Cochrane database review of patient education programs for adults with asthma that provided information only (without self-management strategies) indicated virtually no improvements in health outcomes.[22] Overall, basic educational programs have not translated into substantially better health outcomes, including adherence, even when knowledge has improved.[23] To sum, educational programs are considered necessary and an essential component of an intervention to improve adherence, but not sufficient (i.e., they are passive and do not require a commitment on the part of the patient or provider).

Behavioral Approaches

A behavioral strategy is any strategy that targets or manipulates factor(s) thought to be contributing to a behavioral problem (e.g., nonadherence) in an effort to reduce that problem.

Table 51-1
BEHAVIORAL INTERVENTIONS TO IMPROVE ADHERENCE THAT CAN BE USED SINGLY OR AS PART OF A MULTICOMPONENT INTERVENTION

Patient or Patient/Family Centered
Self-monitoring
Behavioral contracting and incentives
Social support
Problem-solving
Provider-Centered
Appropriate asthma education
Organizational strategies
Cultural competence training
Patient/Family- and Provider-Centered
Skills training
Reminders
Supervision
Feedback
Identification and removal of barriers
Communication training

Broadly, factors that contribute to a problem may be classified as antecedent factors (i.e., factors that precede and lead to a problem) or consequent factors (i.e., factors that follow a problem but serve to reinforce or maintain it). In the case of nonadherence, antecedent factors could be a lack of skills necessary for adherence, forgetfulness, and disbelief in a medication's effectiveness. Examples of consequent factors that could reinforce nonadherence include a lack of perceived benefit following adherent behaviors, symptoms after adhering to a medical regimen, and an absence of positive attention for adherence. Different behavioral approaches are described below.

SKILLS TRAINING

Teaching the necessary skills to adhere to a particular regimen is one approach that can be used to complement basic asthma education. Skills training typically involves instruction, modeling, behavioral rehearsal (i.e., practice), feedback, "teach-back," and shaping (i.e., reinforcing successive approximations of a skill until it is learned). In a clinical setting, modeling and feedback regarding specific skills, such as use of peak flow meters and medication delivery devices, may be a useful adjunct to providing asthma education.

SELF-MONITORING

Another important behavioral strategy is self-monitoring of symptoms and/or adherence. Baum and Creer[24] compared the effect of self-monitoring of asthma symptoms (via peak flow) versus self-monitoring plus education and reinforcement of adherence in youth with asthma and found that both treatments led to similar improvements in adherence. Other research suggests that self-monitoring alone is not likely to increase adherence to complex regimens and incentives may be needed.[25] One issue is whether the patient will adhere to the self-monitoring itself. Indeed, adherence to peak flow monitoring when measured electronically is poor.[21] Although self-monitoring may not consistently result in better adherence, it often is useful for identifying nonadherence patterns (e.g., times of day when adherence is poor).

In terms of symptom monitoring, peak flow monitoring may be helpful for certain patients. It may help parents understand their child's asthma control, particularly if the child is young but can perform the maneuver appropriately. It also may be useful for promoting communication with the health care provider when medication regimens are changed for an adult or a child. Reviewing results of peak-flow monitoring can help a patient and their physician understand the patient's asthma state more fully when symptoms do not match lung exam or spirometry.

REMINDERS

Reminders to follow medical recommendations have been shown to increase adherence. Specific types of reminders that have demonstrated effectiveness include oral reminders, such as clinic telephone calls; written reminders, such as postcards and Post-its; and visual reminders, such as putting medicine in a conspicuous place and posting one's medication schedule on a clock. New technological approaches such as message-based pagers with reminders to take medicine, instructions regarding which medicines to take, and information on proper technique also have shown preliminary effectiveness in improving adherence.[26] Although reminders have been shown to be helpful, most of their support stems from their use with acute illness regimens (e.g., cues for a limited course of antibiotics),[27] as opposed to chronic illness regimens. Pairing medications with daily routines also may increase medication adherence.

SUPERVISION

Different types of supervision may be instrumental for adherence. For pediatric patients, parental supervision may entail an increased degree of monitoring and tracking adherence and checking medication supplies and devices. In one randomized clinical trial, Adams and co-workers[28] found that a parent-youth teamwork intervention involving parental supervision of child medication use resulted in significantly greater adherence to inhaled corticosteroids than asthma education or standard care. For pediatric patients with asthma, appropriate levels of parental monitoring based on the child's adherence pattern may benefit overall adherence. Physician supervision also may benefit patients with asthma. For example, Eney and Goldstein[29] found that patients with asthma who had physician monitoring of theophylline levels were significantly more likely to achieve therapeutic levels than those in the control group. More research examining the influence of physician and/or family supervision of adult adherence to asthma regimens is needed.

FEEDBACK

Providing feedback on actual adherence appears to be a promising approach. Nides and colleagues[30] demonstrated that patients with asthma who received feedback on their medication use (based on electronic monitoring) adhered significantly better to their medications than control patients. More recently, Onyirimba and associates[31] found that direct clinician-to-patient feedback on inhaled corticosteroid and beta-agonist use according to electronic monitors improved adherence in high-risk adults with asthma. Given patients' tendency to overestimate their own medication adherence, using electronic monitoring or obtaining pharmacy records to assess refill rates can provide useful clinical information. In some areas of the country, health plans are increasingly providing information to health care providers about the utilization and medication refill patterns of their "high risk" patients. In a clinical setting, health care providers who are able to use objective information on medication adherence in the context of a supportive clinical encounter may be in a unique position to facilitate behavior change.

BEHAVIORAL CONTRACTING AND INCENTIVES

A behavioral contract is a written or verbal behavioral commitment. In asthma, behavioral contracts typically specify what the patient will do (e.g., take medicine), how others will help the patient achieve his or her goals, and how goal attainment will be monitored. Behavioral contracts can be made specifically for adherence goals. Behavioral contracts are more likely to be effective when rewards for adherence goals or, in other words, incentives are built in. Token reinforcement systems (i.e., incentive programs in which tokens are given for adherence, and a certain number of tokens may be exchanged for a reward) are the most validated behavioral strategy for increasing adherence to chronic regimens.[32] They may be particularly helpful when there are no perceivable and

immediate positive consequences of adherence, as often is the case with adherence to controller medications for asthma. Finney and co-workers[20] implemented a token reinforcement system with children to improve adherence to allergy/asthma clinic appointments. For three of the five participants, adherence improved throughout the intervention, but decreased once the reward system was removed. These findings suggest that reinforcement systems may improve adherence only while they are in place, and strategies for relapse prevention may be needed. Of note, token reinforcement systems need not be used exclusively with children. The well-documented problem of adherence decay over time among adults with asthma suggests that external incentives for adherence may be important for adults as well.

SOCIAL SUPPORT, PROBLEM SOLVING, AND COMMUNICATION TRAINING

Social support may foster adherence to long-term regimens. van Es and colleagues[33] conducted a randomized controlled trial with 112 teenagers with asthma to investigate the effect of an intervention consisting of extra physician and nurse education and psychological treatment to bolster positive attitudes and coping, social skills, effective communication, feelings of social support, and self-efficacy. Follow-up at 2 years demonstrated a significant improvement in teen-reported adherence.

IDENTIFICATION AND REMOVAL OF BARRIERS

Tailoring adherence interventions to patients' specific circumstances and needs, with a consideration of adherence barriers, may be a particularly useful approach. Based on prior research indicating that cost is a common barrier to adherence to allergen encasings for beds, especially among lower socioeconomic status (SES) groups, Joseph and associates[8] provided free dust mite–proof bed covers to patients of predominantly lower SES in an effort to improve adherence to their use. Participants who received the allergen-control bed covers were more likely to use them than control participants who were encouraged by their allergists to invest in the covers, but not given them for free.

OTHER BEHAVIORAL STRATEGIES

Effective consequences for adherence (e.g., social reinforcement) and nonadherence (e.g., removal of attention or a privilege) may encourage greater adherence. In cases of more serious or intractable nonadherence, consulting with or referring to a mental health professional can lead to gains in adherence. Godding and co-workers[34] investigated the impact of consultation between physicians and child psychiatrists on behavioral and health outcomes for children with asthma who were at high risk for poor outcomes. The intervention resulted in significantly better adherence and health outcomes (e.g., fewer symptoms and hospitalizations).

Physician-based and Organizational Strategies

Given asthma management difficulties may arise from problems in the patient-provider interaction, some have advocated physician-training programs to improve health care providers' skills in patient interaction.[35] Clark and colleagues[35] designed the Physician Asthma Care Education (PACE) program, an interactive seminar based on self-regulation theory, to attempt to improve pediatric asthma outcomes by improving physician knowledge of treatment guidelines and enhancing communication skills. Results of a randomized, controlled trial indicated many positive outcomes, including higher levels of prescribing inhaled anti-inflammatory medications in the intervention group, as well as patient reports of greater frequency of being asked to demonstrate use of a metered-dose inhaler.[35] Interestingly, physicians in the treatment group reported that adopting the intervention components did not result in longer patient sessions. More recently, this program has been shown to be effective in improving outcomes for patients from low-income backgrounds.[36]

Organizational strategies (e.g., how a health care setting and treatment are organized) may influence patient adherence. Part of being a "customer friendly" health care environment is a willingness to simplify medical recommendations so that adherence goals are more realistic and the "customer" is more likely to be successful. Simplifying medical regimens in a variety of different ways (e.g., introducing the simplest medication to administer first, adding additional medications one at a time, decreasing the number of medications, and using long-lasting medications) may result in better medication adherence.

Multicomponent Interventions

OVERVIEW

Because multiple factors often contribute to nonadherence, any single intervention is unlikely to result in satisfactory adherence, especially over time. Multicomponent interventions, however, may be considered more likely to lead to good adherence. One difficulty with multicomponent interventions is that it often is not clear which components are actively influencing better adherence and health outcomes, and some components may be extraneous. In actuality, most evaluations of multicomponent interventions do not include adherence as an outcome variable; rather, morbidity outcomes are measured with adherence presumed to be a contributing factor. Multicomponent interventions have had mixed results, but for the most part have demonstrated positive changes, especially those that combine different strategies or have a strong family and problem-solving component.

SELF-MANAGEMENT INTERVENTIONS

Self-management interventions focus on empowering the patient to actively take control of illness management. Typically, they involve goal setting, monitoring, information processing, decision making, action, and self-administered consequences. Nearly two dozen pediatric asthma self-management programs have been evaluated with largely positive results, though adherence is not consistently measured. These programs usually are successful at increasing asthma knowledge and perceived competence in asthma management, but are less effective at achieving adherence to treatment recommendations and controlling asthma episodes.[37] With respect to adult self-management interventions, Creer and Levstek[38] remark that several studies have reported increased medication adherence as a result. Some concerns with the literature on asthma self-management programs include difficulty recruiting and retaining patients in these programs, lack of

objective measures of adherence, lack of replication of findings, and little evaluation of long-term benefits.

Some asthma self-management programs combine education with additional components in an effort to improve overall self-management of asthma. Perez and associates[39] evaluated a self-management program consisting of six educational sessions and cognitive-behavioral strategies (e.g., relaxation, self-monitoring, communication training, decision making, practice with feedback, positive thinking, and positive reinforcement) for children with asthma. Following treatment, the treatment group had increased child and parent knowledge, better asthma self-management, and reduced morbidity compared to the control group.

Other asthma self-management programs focus specifically on asthma attack prevention, attack management, and social skills around asthma episodes. These programs typically cover how to recognize asthma symptoms, administer medications, avoid panic, respond to symptoms, lessen trigger exposure, and communicate effectively. Clark and co-workers[35] reviewed 18 child asthma self-management programs with a focus on attack prevention, attack management, and social skills. Programs varied in terms of delivery format (i.e., individual versus group), setting (e.g., outpatient clinic), and type of professional conducting the program; however, most of the programs were evaluated in randomized clinical trials. A number of positive outcomes were found including fewer school absences, reduction in emergency department and hospital usage, greater patient self-efficacy and use of self-management skills, less frequent wheezing, and better academic performance. Changes in adherence were not noted. More research on the value of these programs for adult patients with asthma is needed.

INDIVIDUALLY TAILORED PROGRAMS BASED ON PROBLEM AREAS

A newer multi-component asthma intervention described by Bartlett and colleagues[40] includes individually tailored components based on identified problems with adherence. This pilot intervention used behavioral social learning strategies (e.g., goal setting, monitoring, feedback, shaping, reinforcement, self-efficacy building, and problem solving) and targeted known barriers to medication use for 15 inner-city children with asthma. Individualized family-based asthma action plans were developed based on adherence barriers. Electronic monitors on metered-dose inhalers provided immediate feedback on medication adherence to families. Families received up to five nurse visits in the home. The percentage of children adhering to their medications as prescribed increased from 28% at baseline to 54% after one month of treatment. Although findings are preliminary, this study presents an interesting example of identifying and targeting adherence problems using feedback and behavioral strategies. Unique aspects of this study include the tailored piece of the intervention and the objective measurement of adherence.

Conclusions

Numerous asthma interventions aimed at improving adherence and/or other outcomes for patients with asthma (e.g., morbidity) have been developed and evaluated. Although many single-component interventions have resulted in better adherence, multicomponent interventions generally are considered more likely to influence optimal adherence outcomes. The true benefits of multicomponent asthma interventions, however, are not well understood due to a number of limitations in the literature. Studies using objective measurements of adherence to various medical recommendations, including retaining nonadherent patients, evaluating treatment integrity and changes in variables directly targeted by treatment (e.g., problem solving), and examining the long-term effects of treatment are all needed. Additionally, research should focus on interventions that are feasible for adaptation in a busy clinical practice with limited resources.

PROMOTING ADHERENCE IN A CLINICAL PRACTICE SETTING: THE PREVENTION MODEL

Rapoff[41] proposes a prevention model that has significant applicability for transforming the assessment and management of nonadherence in a clinical setting. Using a public health framework, he delineates a three-tiered approach to identifying and preventing nonadherence. *Primary prevention* involves strategies to prevent nonadherence from occurring before it begins. *Secondary prevention* refers to clinical strategies that can be used to detect the problem early, before clinically significant health difficulties have occurred. *Tertiary prevention* involves techniques that can be used to prevent further declines in health functioning and well-being for those who are currently experiencing the problem.[41] We discuss the applicability of this model in facilitating adherence to asthma regimens in clinical practice, and offer concrete suggestions regarding what practitioners can do to improve adherence to asthma regimens.

Primary Prevention

Primary prevention strategies can be used for individuals who recently have been diagnosed with asthma, with parents of children with asthma that has been newly identified, or with patients who are new to a practice. Strategies with this group involve modifying provider factors or clinical approaches to facilitate collaboration in the patient-physician relationship. Given that the literature indicates that adherence to medication regimens and strategies for environmental control is generally low, a first step is to *assume that it will be difficult for most, if not all, patients to adhere to their asthma regimens*. Beginning with this assumption transforms the frame of every visit to include questions regarding adherence, including an assessment of adherence barriers and potential strategies to address them.

Due to the benefits of educational programs, all patients should receive asthma education, which should optimally include information regarding the disease, treatment approach, and benefits of consistent adherence. Within a clinical setting, reinforcing specific educational messages (e.g., the concept of symptom prevention), is necessary. Given that techniques of medication administration may decline over time, modeling and observation of technique should be used for teaching concrete skills such as peak expiratory flow rate meter use, as well as use and cleaning of medication delivery systems.

Given research indicating that treatment complexity is related to poor adherence, health care providers should consider simplifying the regimen as much as possible by considering coordinating timing of medication dosages and administering combination medications, when appropriate. Once a treatment approach has been proposed, a critical step is assuming that the patient and family will have concerns about medications and eliciting these concerns directly. Research shows that various cultural groups have concerns about the use of inhaled corticosteroids[12] and may prefer to use alternative medications for acute asthma treatment.[17] Assessing concerns about controller medications and the use of complementary alternative medications (CAM) in a culturally sensitive manner will be important in facilitating medication adherence.

Health care providers should have an ongoing dialogue with patients and families about treatment adherence at every visit. For patients who are just beginning treatment, it will be important to anticipate with them that it will be difficult to be perfectly adherent with a medication regimen, and/or challenging to follow all strategies for environmental control. This can set the stage for addressing barriers to following treatment recommendations that will arise. At follow-up visits, discussing barriers to adherence in an open-ended manner (e.g., "How did you do taking your medicine this past month? When were you most likely to miss doses?") can help health care providers offer suggestions and tailor the regimen to the patient's lifestyle.

Secondary Prevention

Secondary prevention for adherence problems can be conceptualized as identifying and assisting patients who are having some difficulties that have not yet resulted in significant disease expression, such as very poorly controlled symptoms or impaired quality of life.[41] Patient-provider discussions can be supplemented by additional discussion with other members of the medical team such as allied health care professionals. Specialists and primary care practitioners may want to collaborate in this endeavor. Adherence barriers can be identified and self-monitoring discussed. Discussions with patients should be open-ended and nonjudgmental. For more intensive follow-up, allied health care providers, such as nursing staff, respiratory therapists, or certified asthma educators (AE-Cs) also can implement these strategies.

Approaches to maintaining adherence can be negotiated initially between patient and provider, and should be reassessed at each visit. It is not necessary to accomplish all of the educational objectives in one visit. Educational components should be repeated and embellished and supplemented over a series of visits.

Tertiary Prevention

There are some patients who, either consistently or at certain times, find it extremely difficult to adhere to treatment regimens. For these patients, tertiary prevention efforts[41] or strategies aimed at remediating significant nonadherence and preventing further decline are needed. We propose implementation of a "safety net" approach, with substantially increased coordination among health care providers, family, and for children, school personnel such as teachers and nurses. If asthma control is poor and adherence is poor or if practitioners are concerned about depression, stress, or other factors beyond their expertise, the help of a social worker or other experts in behavioral health can be considered.

THE "SAFETY NET"

For patients with significant nonadherence that is affecting their disease course, they may need to be seen more frequently. We recommend significantly increased coordination among health care providers and other relevant professionals to intensify the monitoring and oversight of care. For patients who are seen by multiple providers in a group practice (such as a large community-based practice, or a training setting with medical residents), making sure that the primary physician is contacted every time the patient is seen can enhance coordination of care. Communication between specialists and primary care providers should be intensified (e.g., through regular phone contact). For children with asthma, the physicians coordinating care should be in regular contact with not only the parents, but also those who may observe asthma symptoms and administer medications in other settings, such as day care providers or school nurses. Concerted efforts to improve the "safety net" around patients with asthma with significant nonadherence can help to identify declines in health status more readily and address them more promptly.

Additionally, there are some cases in which referral to a mental health professional who has particular expertise in medical issues can be a useful adjunctive approach. When available, such professionals can work to identify individual, family, and systems barriers to adherence, and implement a collaborative plan with the primary care provider or asthma specialist to address these issues. Such referrals can be particularly useful when psychiatric issues such as depression or anxiety are impeding adherence to the treatment plan.

SUMMARY

Adherence in all chronic diseases is difficult to achieve and maintain. In each patient there are myriad individual influences on this complex behavior. We need to better understand the continuum of adherence and what minimal medication and environmental interventions are necessary and acceptable to the patient to maintain lung function and quality of life. This patient plan must be formulated through negotiation with and agreement of the patients and must be individualized and tailored to each patient's unique social and economic context. A lasting patient-provider alliance must be built so that the plan can be constantly modified and renegotiated as the patient's social, health, and asthma status change.

REFERENCES

1. Bender B, Milgrom H, Rand C: Nonadherence in asthmatic patients: is there a solution to the problem? Ann Allergy Asthma Immunol 1997;79:177–186.
2. National Institutes of Health: Asthma management in minority children: Practical insights for clinicians, researchers and public health planners (DHHS Publication No. 95-3675). Washington, DC, U.S. Government Printing Office, 1995.
3. Bender B, Wamboldt FS, O'Connor SL, et al: Measurement of children's asthma medication adherence by self report, mother report, canister weight, and Doser CT. Ann Allergy Asthma Immunol 2000;85:416.
4. Apter A, Reisine S, Affleck G, et al: Adherence with twice-daily dosing of inhaled steroids. Socioeconomic and health-belief differences. Am J Respir Crit Care Med 1998;157(6 Pt 1):1810–1817.
5. Kattan M, Mitchell H, Eggleston P, et al: Characteristics of inner-city children with asthma: The national cooperative inner-city asthma study. Pediatr Pulmonol 1997;24:253–262.
6. Lemiere C, Boulet LP: Cigarette smoking and asthma: a dangerous mix. Can Respir J 2005;12:79–80.
7. Wamboldt FS, Ho J, Milgrom H, et al: Prevalence and correlates of household exposures to tobacco smoke and pets in children with asthma. J Pediatr 2002;141:109–115.
8. Joseph KE, Adams CD, Cottrell L, et al: Providing dust mite-proof covers improves adherence to dust mite control measures in children with mite allergy and asthma. Ann Allergy Asthma Immunol 2003;90:550–553.
9. Apter AJ, Boston RC, George M, et al: Modifiable barriers to adherence to inhaled steroids among adults with asthma: It's not just black and white. J Allergy Clin Immunol 2003;111:1219–1226.
10. McQuaid E, Kopel SJ, Klein RB, et al: Medication adherence in pediatric asthma: reasoning, responsibility, and behavior. J Pediatr Psychol 2003;28:323–333.
11. Radius SM, Marshall HB, Rosenstock IM, et al: Factors influencing mothers' compliance with a medication regimen for asthmatic children. J Asthma Res 1978;15:133–149.

12. George M, Freedman TG, Norfleet AL, et al: Qualitative research-enhanced understanding of patients' beliefs: Results of focus groups with low-income, urban, African American adults with asthma. J Allergy Clin Immunol 2003;11:967–973.
13. La Greca AM, Bearman KJ: Adherence to pediatric treatment regimens. In Michael C. Roberts (ed): Handbook of Pediatric Psychology. 3rd ed. New York, Guilford Press, 2003, pp 119–140.
14. Bartlett SJ, Krishnan JA, Riekert KA, et al: Maternal depressive symptoms and adherence to therapy in inner-city children with asthma. Pediatrics 2004;113(2):229–237.
15. Bender B, Milgrom H, Rand C: Psychological factors associated with medication nonadherence in asthmatic children. J Asthma 1998;35:347–353.
16. Cluley S, Cochrane GM: Psychological disorder in asthma is associated with poor control and poor adherence to inhaled steroids. Respir Med 2001;95:37–39.
17. Bearison DJ, Minian N, Granowetter L: Medical management of asthma and folk medicine in a Hispanic community. J Pediatr Psychol 2002;27:385–392.
18. Institute of Medicine: Unequal treatment: confronting racial and ethnic disparities in health care. Washington, DC, The National Academies, 2002.
19. Lieu TA, Finkelstein JA, Lozano P, et al: Cultural competence policies and other predictors of asthma care quality for Medicaid-insured children. Pediatrics 2004;114:102–110.
20. Finney JW, Lemanek KL, Brophy CJ, et al: Pediatric appointment keeping: improving adherence in a primary care allergy clinic. J Pediatr Psychol 1990;15:571–579.
21. Burkhart P, Dunbar-Jacob J, Rohay J: Accuracy of children's self-reported adherence to treatment. J Nurs Scholar 2001;33:27–32.
22. Gibson PG, Powell H, Coughlan J, et al: Limited (information only) patient education programs for adults with asthma. Cochrane Database Syst Rev 2002;(2):CD00105.
23. Bernard-Bonnin A, Stachenko S, Bonin D: Self-management teaching programs and morbidity of pediatric asthma: a meta analysis. J Allergy Clin Immunol 1995;95:34–41.

24. Baum D, Creer TL: Medication compliance in children with asthma. J Asthma 1986;23:49–59.
25. Wysocki T, Green L, Huxtable K: Blood glucose monitoring by diabetic adolescents: compliance and metabolic control. Health Psychol 1989;8:267–284.
26. Erikson SR, Ascione FJ, Kirking DM, et al: Use of a paging system to improve medication self-management in patients with asthma. J Am Pharmaceut Assoc 1998;38:767–769.
27. Lima J, Nazarian L, Charney E, et al: Compliance with short-term antimicrobial therapy: some techniques that help. Pediatrics 1976;57:383–386.
28. Adams CD, Joseph KE, MacLaren JE, et al: Parent-youth teamwork in pediatric asthma management. Poster presented at the 60th annual meeting of the American Academy of Allergy, Asthma, and Immunology (AAAAI), March 2004, San Francisco, California.
29. Eney RD, Goldstein EO: Compliance of chronic asthmatics with oral administration of theophylline as measured by serum and salivary levels. Pediatrics 1976;57:513–518.
30. Nides MA, Tashkin DP, Simmons MS, et al: Improving inhaler adherence in a clinical trial through the use of the nebulizer chronolog. Chest 1993;104:501–507.
31. Onyirimba F, Apter A, Reisine S, et al: Direct clinician-to-patient feedback discussion of inhaled steroid use: its effect on adherence. Ann Allergy Asthma Immunol 2003;90:411–415.
32. Rapoff MA: Adherence to Pediatric Medical Regimens. New York, Kluwer Academic/Plenum Publishers, 1999.
33. van Es SM, Nagelkerke AF, Colland VT, et al: An intervention programme using the ASE-model aimed at enhancing adherence in adolescents with asthma. Patient Educ Counsel 2001;44:193–203.
34. Godding V, Kruth M, Jamart J: Joint consultation for high-risk asthmatic children and their families, with pediatrician and child psychiatrist as co-therapists: model and evaluation. Family Process 1997;36:265–280.
35. Clark NM, Gong M, Schork MA, et al: Impact of education on patient outcomes. Pediatrics 1998;101:831–836.
36. Brown R, Bratton SL, Cabana MD, et al: Physician asthma education program improves outcomes for children of low-income families. Chest 2004;126:369–374.
37. Klingelhofer EL, Gershwin ME: Asthma self-management programs: premises, not promises. J Asthma 1988;25:89–101.
38. Creer TL, Levstek D: Adherence to asthma regimens. In Gochman DS (ed): Handbook of Health Behavior Research II: Provider Determinants. New York, Plenum Press, 1997, pp 131–148.
39. Pérez MG, Feldman L, Caballero F: Effects of a self-management educational program for the control of childhood asthma. Patient Educ Counsel 1999;36:47–55.
40. Bartlett SJ, Lukk P, Butz A, et al: Enhancing medication adherence among inner-city children with asthma: results from pilot studies. J Asthma 2002;39:47–54.
41. Rapoff MA: Facilitating adherence to medical regimens for pediatric rheumatic diseases: primary, secondary, and tertiary prevention. In Drotar D (ed): Promoting Adherence to Medical Treatment in Chronic Childhood Illness. Mahwah, N.J., Erlbaum, 2000, pp 329–346.

Development, Implementation, and Evaluation of an Asthma Management Plan	CHAPTER 52

Laurel R. Talabere

CLINICAL PEARLS

- Build an active, ongoing partnership, grounded in a caring relationship.
- Recognize that the final decision for appropriate self-management belongs to the person with asthma.
- Give careful attention to cultural and developmental considerations when formulating the asthma action plan.
- Adapt the asthma action plan to fit the person's lifestyle and work or school schedule.
- Emphasize the importance of having a readily accessible current asthma action plan at work or school as well as at home.
- Be proactive in the early identification of barriers that may compromise adherence.

This chapter describes the development, implementation and evaluation of an asthma management plan. The overriding goal of asthma management is to engage persons with asthma in the process of taking the informed actions necessary to control their asthma. This approach combines the regular use of preventive measures, including medications and environmental control, with accurate monitoring of signs and symptoms and the appropriate implementation of rescue actions. To meet the Healthy People 2010 goals,[1] increased emphasis has been placed on the need for written asthma management plans from health care providers that include information on early symptoms identification, peak flow monitoring, use of inhalers, medication regimens that reduce the need for rescue medications, follow-up care, and environmental measures.

This increased attention to the importance of asthma management plans underscores the need for asthma education that is provided by health care professionals who have met a quality standard. According to the National Asthma Educator Certification Board (NAECB),[2] "Asthma certification is an evaluative process that demonstrates that rigorous education and experience requirements have been met."

Many episodes of asthma are thought to be preventable. However, lack of adherence to an asthma management plan is all too common. The Asthma in America National Population Study found that only 20% of persons with asthma reported using anti-inflammatory drugs.[3] In a study by LaRocco,[4] almost 43% of persons with a chronic illness, including asthma, did not follow their treatment plan. The person who has asthma may have inadequate or incorrect information about managing their asthma, misunderstand or deny their asthma, have

unrealistic expectations for treatment, fail to implement fully or accurately the measures necessary to prevent an asthma episode, delay their response when an episode occurs, lack family support or economic resources, or find the treatment regimen too complex or "at odds" with their lifestyle.

The health care provider may under- or misdiagnose the asthma or its severity, lack adequate knowledge about asthma education, or allot insufficient time and attention to the asthma management plan. A study by Doerschug and colleagues[5] found that physicians accurately estimated asthma severity in only 43% of patients. This error often leads to inappropriate or inadequate treatment. Clark and Gong[6] described the "asthma knowledge gap" as the disparity between the knowledge of the health care provider and the resulting behaviors of the person with asthma. Thus, the need for improved asthma management to reduce both morbidity and mortality and to provide optimum outcomes is clearly evident.[7]

The critical components of effective asthma management include early and accurate diagnosis, individualized treatment matched to the level of severity, consistent follow-up care, and education tailored to the particular needs of the person with asthma and their family with due consideration for developmental level, culture, and comorbidity. Furthermore, it is essential that asthma management is built on accepted guidelines that offer rational strategies that encompass the best evidence-based practices available.

CHANGING BEHAVIOR

As a chronic illness, the trajectory of asthma is characterized by symptom-free periods interspersed with asthma episodes. A central goal of asthma management is to extend the symptom-free periods and minimize both the frequency and severity of the asthma episodes. Achievement of this goal requires clear objectives, stated in behavioral terms, which are mutually agreed on by the person with asthma and the health care provider. The management plan, including asthma education, must be carefully designed and individualized with provision for long-term follow-up care and ongoing evaluation of behavioral outcomes. Both the plan for care and the educational component must be revised and updated on a regular basis.

Effective asthma management requires changes in behavior that must be integrated into the person's lifestyle and sustained over time. The Stages of Change Model,[8] shown in Table 52-1, provides an excellent framework for understanding and fostering the incremental process of behavioral and lifestyle modification that is key to learning how to manage a chronic illness.

Table 52-1
STAGES OF CHANGE MODEL

Stage of Change	Behavioral Characteristics of a Person with Asthma	Techniques to Foster Change in a Person with Asthma
Precontemplation	Does not think about change or may be resigned to having asthma "Ignorance is bliss"—denies asthma Does not believe having asthma or needing control applies to self Believes consequences of having asthma are not serious	Validate lack of readiness Encourage evaluation of current behavior Encourage awareness and self-reflection, not action Explain and personalize risks
Contemplation	Ambivalent about changing current asthma behaviors Weighs benefits and costs of current asthma behaviors versus proposed asthma management changes	Emphasize: decision belongs to the person with asthma Encourage evaluation of pros and cons of behavior change in asthma management Identify expectations for new outcomes
Preparation	Experiments with small changes in asthma management plan Interested in "testing the waters"	Identify barriers and assist in problem solving Help identify social supports Verify underlying skills for behavior change Encourage small initial steps
Action	Takes definitive actions to change behaviors in asthma management Consistently practices new asthma management behaviors	Restructure social support if needed Bolster self-efficacy for dealing with barriers Identify and combat feelings of loss Reiterate long-term benefits
Maintenance	Maintains new asthma management behaviors over time Gives evidences of ongoing commitment	Plan for follow-up support Reinforce internal rewards Discuss coping with relapse
Relapse	Resumes "old" behaviors Usually feels demoralized May perceive change process as abnormal	Identify trigger for relapse Reassess motivation and barriers Plan stronger coping strategies

Adapted from Prochaska and DiClemente's Stages of Change Model, UCLA Center for Human Nutrition. Available at http://www.cellinteractive.com/ucla/physcian_ed/stages_change.html.

FOSTERING A PARTNERSHIP IN ASTHMA MANAGEMENT

The person with asthma must be an informed participant in his own plan of care, which means mutual determination of goals and decisions about asthma management. It is imperative that the action plan be perceived as realistic, effective and "doable" by both the person with asthma and the health care provider. Furthermore, a person's adherence—willingness to follow health care instructions on a voluntary basis—is likely to be enhanced if it is grounded in a relationship with the clinician that is characterized by caring and trustworthiness. It has been said that "patients may be better served if they first know how much we care rather than caring how much we know."[9] Therefore, an active partnership between the health care provider and the person with asthma is fundamental to effective asthma management.

According to the Expert Panel Report 3 (EPR3) Guidelines,[10] building and maintaining an active partnership with the person with asthma remains the cornerstone of asthma management. Clark and associates[11] emphasized that the joint development of and agreement to short- and long-term goals encourages active participation, enhances the provider-client relationship, and improves the actual management of asthma. This partnership should be established at the time of diagnosis and continued throughout the therapeutic relationship so that key educational messages can be integrated into every step of care, expanded or updated as needed, and reinforced at every opportunity. These key educational messages, listed in Box 52-1, provide a basis for sound management decisions for the

---

BOX 52-1 Seven Key Educational Messages Central to an Asthma Action Plan

- The disease process including risk factors
- Monitoring of signs and symptoms
- Triggers and trigger control measures including environmental control
- Controller and rescue medications
- Skills: correct technique for peak flow monitoring and medication delivery devices
- When and how to implement the rescue plan
- Ongoing, follow-up care

---

person with asthma. It is essential that they include information that is both developmentally and culturally appropriate.

DEVELOPMENT OF AN ASTHMA MANAGEMENT PLAN

An action plan is an individualized set of "instructions both for daily actions to keep asthma controlled and for actions to adjust treatment when symptoms or exacerbations occur."[10] Action plans are also called self-management guidelines and management plans. The most recent EPR3 Guidelines[10] recommended the inclusion of a written action plan as part of the overall approach to asthma management, primarily because it enhances communication between the clinician and the person with asthma. Furthermore, a written plan is particularly indicated for persons with moderate or severe persistent asthma or a history of severe exacerbations.

According to Lorig,[12] the three most important components of a model for self-management of a chronic illness include:

- How to handle illness consequences from both a physiologic and lifestyle perspective,
- How to solve problems and make informed decisions, and
- How to maintain an effective partnership between the practitioner and the person with asthma.

The facilitation of self-efficacy for the person with asthma, that is, the individual's belief that they are able to take appropriate actions and control their disease, plays a central role in moving the person with asthma toward desired behaviors and outcomes through consistent application of knowledge and skills.

The asthma action plan should be congruent with the overall goals of therapy.[10] These principles include:

- Minimal or no chronic symptoms during the day or night
- Minimal or no asthma episodes
- Peak expiratory flow rate (PEFR) = 80% of personal best, if used
- Minimal use of inhaled or oral short-acting beta$_2$-agonist (<1 per day)
- No or minimal adverse effects from medications

Although some studies are inconclusive about the benefits of written action plans, the Cochrane Collaboration,[13] a review of 25 studies that compared asthma self-management education interventions for adults with and without written asthma action plans, showed that those interventions with written action plans were the most beneficial in terms of fewer asthma-related hospitalizations and emergency room visits and improved lung function. Further evidence supporting written action plans was found in a study by Abramson and associates,[14] which demonstrated that written action plans in adults with severe persistent asthma resulted in a 70% reduction in mortality risk.

Written action plans serve two purposes. First, a daily self-management plan is intended for day-to-day monitoring and the implementation of control procedures including pharmacologic and environmental measures. Second, an action plan for asthma episodes focuses on rescue measures and includes specific approaches for managing worsening signs and symptoms as well as explicit criteria and steps for obtaining urgent/emergent care. Most action plans combine the protocols for control and rescue into a single document. By outlining these precise procedures for managing asthma, an action plan can alleviate anxiety for the person with asthma or the caregiver of a child with asthma as well as increase the likelihood that well-defined steps will be followed.

Content and Format

Both the content and the format of the asthma action plan are important considerations. The content is the requisite information generated by the regimen. It must be accurate, current, and individualized for the particular care needs and circumstances of the person with asthma including cultural considerations. An effective plan addresses these content areas:

- Specific suggestions for preventive measures including environmental control and avoidance, reduction, or modulation of other risk factors, such as exercise and influenza
- Explicit, step-by-step procedures for appropriate use of controller and rescue medications and delivery devices
- Assessment of signs and symptoms including early recognition of changes as well as appropriate use and correct interpretation of peak flow monitoring
- A specific course of action to be taken in an emergency, including criteria for seeking urgent care and contact information

It is important to adapt the content to meet a particular cultural perspective. For example, in the Hispanic community, it is a prevailing health belief that illnesses are "hot" or "cold" and should be treated with the opposite modality. Thus, asthma is a "cold" illness requiring a "hot" treatment. This belief can be incorporated into the action plan by affirming the common practice of giving oral medications with a hot drink such as tea. This culturally sensitive modification strengthens the partnership between the clinician and the person with asthma and fosters increased adherence to the asthma management plan.

The format of the written action plan is designed to communicate information in a manner that corresponds to the educational and developmental characteristics of the person with asthma as well as any specific language needs. Font style and size, text organization and density, illustrations, and color are important considerations. Easy-to-read fonts such as Arial and Tahoma (sans serif fonts) or Courier New and Times New Roman (serif fonts) in size 11 or 12 are preferred. The text should be arranged with attention to appropriate spacing and allow for sufficient blank space. Illustrations must be carefully selected to reinforce the text message. They should be clear, black and white or color line drawings. Colored text and illustrations add interest and emphasis, but the colors should provide good contrast.

Peak flow zones and colors are often used as the organizing framework for asthma action plans. For example, many asthma action plans for children combine the stoplight colors of green, yellow, and red to reinforce the messages of "go," "caution," and "stop" in relation to actions that need to be taken under differing circumstances. The action plan shown in Figure 52-1 is actually a magnet that can be placed on the refrigerator door or inside a school locker. There are many online sources for templates for Asthma Action Plans that are appropriate for both children and adults, as listed in Table 52-2. Although they vary in format, educational level, and use of color, all of these templates include the essential elements.

Reading Level and Language Considerations

It is standard practice for health education materials to be written at the sixth grade reading level.[15] However, if the person's reading level is at the lower elementary grade level or English is a second language, further modifications are needed. A number of scoring formulas are available to calculate the reading level, as summarized in Table 52-3.[16] The Flesch-Kincaid Grade Level Index is the formula used by Microsoft Word to automatically calculate the grade level of selected text.

ASTHMA ACTION PLAN

Plan for: _____

(Child's Full Name)

Doctor's Name: _____

Doctor's Phone: _____

My PERSONAL BEST
peak flow reading is _____

Date: _____

Medical Record #: _____

☎ Emergency 911 or: _____

Asthma Type:
- ☐ Exercise Induced ☐ Moderate Persistent
- ☐ Mild Intermittent ☐ Severe Persistent
- ☐ Mild Persistent

GREEN = GO

☐ Breathing is good
☐ No cough or wheeze
☐ Can work or play

OR

Peak Flow Number
above _____
{Greater than 80% of BEST}

Use these medicines every day!

Medicine   How much to take   When to take it
_____
_____
_____
_____
_____

15 minutes before sports or play: _____

YELLOW=CAUTION

☐ Cough
☐ Mild Wheeze   Call Doctor
☐ Tight Chest   ☐ Yes
☐ Wake up at night   ☐ No
☐ Mucus or sputum
☐ Short of breath
☐ First sign of a cold

OR

Peak Flow Number
_____ to _____

Take these medicines to relieve these symptoms.

Medicine   How much to take   When to take it

• **Start taking Albuterol Aerosols 4 times a day OR Take 2
puffs of Albuterol with a Spacer 4 times a day**

• **Call your doctor**

Special Instructions: _____

RED = STOP

☐ Albuterol **not** helping or lasting 4 hours, call doctor
☐ Medicine is **not** helping, call doctor
☐ Heart rate or pulse is very fast
☐ Nose open wide when breathing
☐ Hard to walk
☐ Ribs or neck muscles show when breathing in
☐ It is hard to talk
☐ Lips or fingernails turn gray or blue

OR

Peak Flow Number
below_____

Get help from a Doctor now!

Medicine   How much to take   When to take it

• **Take Albuterol Aerosol *right now***

• **Go to the doctor or ER!!**

STOP! MEDICAL ALERT. This could be a life-threatening emergency. Get Help. Your symptoms are serious. Call your doctor. You may need to go to the nearest emergency room or call 911.

Figure 52-1   An asthma action plan in colors that correspond with a stoplight format (2006). *(Used with permission from Nationwide Children's Hospital, Columbus, Ohio.)*

For persons who are not proficient in English, the action plan should be in their first language. Health care should be provided "in a manner compatible with [the] cultural health beliefs and preferred language" of the client. Furthermore, "easily understood patient-related materials" must be made available in the languages of the major population groups in the service area of the health care agency.[17] Table 52-4 lists Web sites for online asthma action plans in languages other than English. Obviously, health care providers must obtain the asthma action plan in their own language and review it for appropriate content before giving it in another language to a person with asthma.

Developmental Considerations

An action plan must also take into consideration developmental milestones and any physical limitations of the person with asthma. For example, the delivery device for inhaled bronchodilators and corticosteroids must be tailored to the individual's particular capabilities and needs. Aerosolized medications have become the mainstay of pharmacologic management for adults, and more recently for children, because they can be delivered rapidly and effectively, they act quickly, and the lower dosages compared with oral delivery often result in fewer side effects. However, the disadvantages

Table 52-2
ONLINE SOURCES FOR TEMPLATES FOR ASTHMA ACTION PLANS

Source	Web Site	Title of Document(s)
AIM: Asthma Initiative of Michigan	http://www.getasthmahelp.org/actionplan_components.asp	Asthma Action/Control Plans for Child, Student, Child Care Setting
American Academy of Allergy, Asthma, and Immunology	http://www.aaaai.org/members/allied_health/tool_kit/handouts/my_action_plan.pdf	My Asthma Action Plan
	http://www.aaaai.org/patients/topicofthemonth/0901/managementplan_pt1.html	Asthma Action Plan, Part 1
	http://www.aaaai.org/patients/topicofthemonth/0901/managementplan_pt2.html	Asthma Action Plan, Part 2
Amer. Academy of Family Physicians	http://familydoctor.org/696.xml	Asthma Action Plan
American Lung Association	http://www.lungusa.org	
Cleveland Clinic	http://www.webmd.com/content/article/46/1660_51181	Your Asthma Action Plan (Adults & Teens)
Columbus Children's Hospital		See Fig. 52-1.
National Heart, Lung, and Blood Institute	http://www.nhlbi.nih.gov/health/public/lung/asthma/asthma_actplan.htm	Asthma Action Plan
National Jewish Medical and Research Center	http://www.nationaljewish.org/diseaseinfo/diseases/asthma/living/tools/action/index.aspx	Asthma Self-Management Asthma Action Plans for Fall, School, Summer Fun, Under Age 5
New York State Health Department	http://www.health.state.ny.us/diseases/asthma/pdf/4850.pdf	Asthma Action Plan

Table 52-3
FORMULAS FOR DETERMINING THE READING LEVEL OF AN ASTHMA ACTION PLAN

Formula	Calculation	Comments
Flesch Reading Ease Score	Formula: $206.835 - (1.015 \times ASL) - (84.6 \times ASW)$ where: ASL = average sentence length (# of words divided by # of sentences) and ASW = average # of syllables per word (# of syllables divided by # of words)	Rates text on a 100-point scale. The higher the score, the easier to understand the text. Aim for score of 60 to 70.
Flesch-Kincaid Grade Level Score	Formula: $(.39 \times ASL) + (11.8 \times ASW) - 15.59$ where: ASL = average sentence length (# of words divided by # of sentences) and ASW = average # of syllables per word (# of syllables divided by # of words)	Rates text on U.S. school grade level. Score of 8.0 means an 8th grader can understand it. Aim for score of 7.0 to 8.0.
Fog Index	Select sample of 100 words. Divide 100 by # of sentences to get average sentence length. Divide 100 by # of "big" words* to get percentage of "big" words. Add average sentence length and % of "big" words. Multiply this sum by 0.4 to get grade level.	Rates text by U.S. grade level. No specific score is recommended by the source.
SMOG Readability Formula	Formula: Count 30 sentences: 10 at beginning, 10 in middle, 10 at end. Count "big" words, even if a word is duplicated. Total word count is converted to grade level. Word count of 3 to 6 = 5th grade, 7 to 12 = 6th grade, 13 to 20 = 7th grade.	For text with > 30 sentences. Rates text by US grade level. Aim for 6th grade or less. Person reading at or above grade level understands 90 to 100% of material.

*"Big" words are defined as 3 or more syllables; acronyms and proper names are not included.

Table 52-4
ONLINE RESOURCES FOR ASTHMA ACTION PLANS IN LANGUAGES OTHER THAN ENGLISH

Source of Document	Web Site	Title of Document	Available Languages
Asthma Focus Program	http://www.programstogo.com/zones/multilanguage/asthmafocus/1001-MultilanguageAsthma_inc.html	Asthma Action Plan Using an Asthma Action Plan	Arabic, Armenian, Bosnian, Cambodian, Chinese, Farsi, French, Haitian Creole, Hmong, Japanese, Korean, Lithuanian, Polish, Portuguese, Russian, Somali, Spanish, Tagalog, Vietnamese
Lung Assn., Canada	http://www.on.lung.ca/asthmaaction/action_plan.html	Asthma Action Plan Asthma Action Diary	French, Hindi, Punjabi
National Jewish Medical & Research	http://www.nationaljewish.org/diseaseinfo/diseases/asthma/living/tools/action/index.aspx	Spanish Asthma Action Plan	Spanish
Regional Asthma Management & Prevention	http://www.rampasthma.org/AAP%20page.htm	Asthma Action Plans (adult, child > 5 yr, child 0 to 5 yr)	Chinese, Spanish, Vietnamese

must be considered. Any delivery device is technique dependent, which means effective use requires attention to correct and sequential steps as well as cooperation and coordination. In children, these requisite conditions can make effective delivery of inhaled medications particularly challenging.

There are many specific considerations for the preschooler or child with asthma who attends a daycare center or school. For example, when selecting delivery devices, the following questions must be answered:

- What is the knowledge and skill level of the person assisting the child?
- Do family resources allow for a medication and device to be kept at school and another "set" to be kept at home, or do these items need to be carried back and forth?
- What is the policy about the child's access to the medication and delivery device in the daycare/school setting?

Whether or not children are permitted to carry and self-administer asthma rescue medications is determined by state statute as shown in Figure 52-2. Building active participation by the child into the action plan is an effective way to foster self-management. Table 52-5[18] summarizes developmentally appropriate asthma management activities for selected age groups. For example, a preschooler can learn to seek adult help when breathing problems occur, a young school-aged child can

Table 52-5
A DEVELOPMENTAL APPROACH TO ASTHMA MANAGEMENT

Age Group	Asthma Management Activities
3- to 4-year-olds can...	Hold a spacer/holding chamber while an adult activates the inhaler Wash a spacer/holding chamber and/or nebulizer parts Learn the names of allergens Tell an adult when wheezing or other breathing problems occur
5- to 6-year-olds can...	Blow a party favor horn Blow into a peak flow meter and write down the numbers Help set up a nebulizer treatment or connect an inhaler to a spacer/holding chamber Learn names of medications
7- to 11-year-olds can...	Use inhalers correctly without assistance Know when to use which medications Think through criteria for using rescue medications Track the use of their peak flow meter and medications

Adapted from Growing up with Asthma. Allergy & Asthma Network Mothers of Asthmatics. MA Report 2004:19(7):1–2, www.aanma.org.

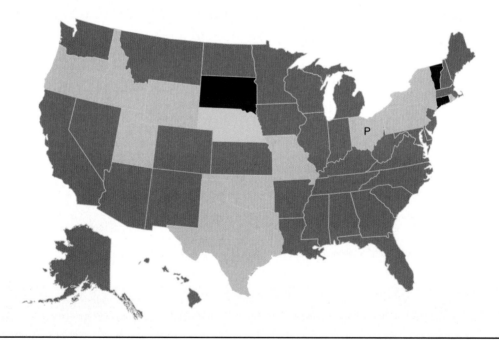

Color Key:

■ States that protect student rights to possess and self-administer prescribed life-saving asthma and anaphylaxis medications.

▢ States that protect student rights to possess and self-administer prescribed lifesaving asthma medications.

⊡P States that protect student rights to possess and self-administer prescribed lifesaving asthma medications and have pending legislation also allowing anaphylaxis medications.

▢ States that have pending legislation.

■ States that do not have statues protecting student rights to possess and self-administer prescribed lifesaving asthma and/or anaphylaxis medications.

Figure 52-2   United States map showing state statutes protecting student rights to carry and use prescribed asthma and anaphylaxis medications. *(From Allergy & Asthma Network: Mothers of Asthmatics. Retrieved November 8, 2007, http://www.aanma.org/pdf/ch_ColorMap.pdf)*

connect a spacer/holding chamber to an inhaler canister, and an older school-aged child can learn when and how to self-administer a rescue inhaler. Adolescents are capable of taking increased responsibility for all dimensions of their action plan. However, concerns about peer group acceptance may lead to denial of their asthma and interfere with adherence to their action plan. They need ongoing reinforcement of previous teaching with special emphasis on trigger management, avoiding smoking at all costs, and appropriate use of both controller and rescue medications. In the older adult, diminished fine motor skills secondary to arthritis, for example, may interfere with effective actuation of a metered-dose inhaler (MDI), making a dry powder inhaler (DPI) a better choice.

Medication Schedules and Delivery Devices

Lifestyle must be taken into account when designing an asthma action plan. Whether the individual with asthma is a student in school or a working adult, medication times need to be adjusted to fit the school or work day as much as possible without compromising pharmacological effectiveness. The medication timetable must take into account the individual's schedule in relation to meals, leaving and returning home, bedtime and other regular occurrences. For example, the adult who works evenings or nights will likely take medications on a different schedule than one who is employed during daytime hours. Working swing shifts or irregular hours may require further flexibility.

It is generally accepted that spacers or holding chambers should be a part of the delivery system for MDI medications for all persons, regardless of age. A wide variety is available. The most important criteria for selection include fit with the MDI canister or mouthpiece, ease of use and cleaning, cost, and durability. A one-way valve near the spacer/holding chamber's exit prevents medication backflow on expiration. For children too young to create a tight seal around the mouthpiece with their lips, a facemask with a flexible seal to prevent air leaks is necessary. Crying in a child is characterized by irregular, shallow inspirations and prolonged expirations which result in less aerosolized medication reaching the lungs. Therefore, to insure increased efficacy, calming and distraction activities during medication administration need to be incorporated into the asthma action plan for a young child.

Environmental Control

While much attention is given to clinical and pharmacologic management, environmental assessment and intervention deserve equal billing in the development of an asthma action plan. There are two important dimensions: (1) an environmental history to determine triggers with possible referral for allergy testing, and (2) information provided to the person with asthma and their family that describes measures for eliminating or reducing exposure.[19]

The environmental history must be thorough with careful attention to all of the places in which the person with asthma spends time on a regular basis. For children these settings may include home, daycare, school, childcare locations, camp, and various outdoor venues. For some children, shared custody arrangements or living part of the time with extended family must be considered. For adults, the home, workplace, the car or other vehicles (if long commutes are a usual occurrence), and other frequented sites must be discussed as possible sources of environmental triggers. It is important to remember that there may be seasonal variations with exposure to both indoor and outdoor allergens. Also, viral illnesses are a frequent trigger for asthma, especially in children.

Once the triggers have been identified, a comprehensive asthma management plan must provide targeted information about how to best manage the triggers. The recommended measures are much more likely to be carried out if they are perceived as realistic and "doable" by the person with asthma and their family. Instructions for managing ubiquitous allergens such as dust mites and mold spores are usually long and tedious. Advice for other allergens such as animal dander and cockroaches may be more specific but no less daunting. Suggestions for dealing with environmental tobacco smoke and indoor and outdoor air pollution may seem beyond the control of the individual. Therefore, it is crucial that the health care provider carefully select those measures deemed most effective. *Environmental Management of Pediatric Asthma: Guidelines for Health Care Providers: Part 3: Environmental Intervention Guidelines*[19] is an excellent resource for prioritizing interventions and can easily be adapted for adults.

Peak Flow Monitoring

Peak flow meters are portable devices for measuring peak expiratory flow rate (PEFR) or how much air a person with asthma can move out of their lungs in one quick, forced expiration. Because asthma is an obstructive lung disease, exhaling air becomes increasingly difficult as an asthma episode progresses. Thus, a decreasing peak flow indicates more air trapping and diminished air exchange. Usually, peak flow values will drop before symptoms of wheezing and coughing occur, making a peak flow meter a valuable adjunct to asthma management. To give a useful picture over time, peak flow values should be recorded twice daily, morning and evening, and whenever signs and symptoms of an asthma episode develop. Used correctly and regularly, peak flow meters can (1) provide early detection of worsening changes in lung function; (2) indicate one's response to rescue medication during an acute asthma episode; (3) monitor the overall response to treatment; (4) provide a pattern of data that can help determine whether one's asthma is under "good control" or adjustments are needed in the management plan; and (5) evaluate the severity of asthma.[20]

Peak flow meters are packaged with a chart that gives baseline values based on height, gender and age. However, an individual's personal best must be established by using the same peak flow meter twice a day for two weeks. Conducting these tests after the person has been awake for a few hours will result in the highest peak flow readings. During this testing time the person's asthma must be under good control. The highest number achieved is one's personal best, although unusually high or low values should be ignored. This value becomes the reference point for interpreting changes in the peak flow numbers as indicated in Figure 52-3.[21] To increase reliability, the same peak flow meter should be used over time. In addition, the peak flow meter needs to be cleaned periodically according to manufacturer instructions to maintain accuracy. It is also important to remember that the personal

If your child's best peak flow* is normally one of the following	A reading in this column indicates GREEN ZONE	A reading in this column indicates YELLOW ZONE	
100	80–100	50–80	
200	160–200	100–160	
300	240–300	150–240	
400	320–400	200–320	
500	400–500	250–400	
600	480–600	300–480	

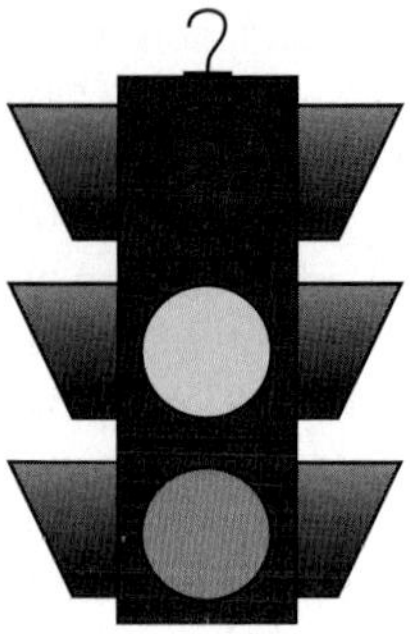

Figure 52-3 Peak flow meter zones.

best value will change as the severity of the asthma changes. If the peak flow meter is being used with a child, the personal best value will change as the child grows.

A variety of templates are available. Peak flow zones are designated green, yellow, and red to correlate with a stoplight, a familiar reference point for children. A person is in the *green or "go" zone* if the peak flow value is 80% or more of personal best. These numbers suggest "good control." There are no signs or symptoms, and only the medications for prevention, if prescribed, need to be taken. If a person on daily medication remains in this zone for a period of time, the health care provider may consider a gradual reduction in medication. Numbers that are 50% to 80% of personal best fall in the *yellow or "caution" zone*. Symptoms of respiratory distress are present, requiring immediate administration of a rescue inhaler. These values suggest a lack of "good control" and may signal the need for an increase in controller medications. The *red or "stop" zone* with numbers below 50% of personal best means a medical alert. In addition to immediately taking a rescue inhaler, a clinician or emergency care facility must be contacted without delay.

An additional use of peak flow meters is to measure peak flow variability. Because most people with asthma have more symptoms at night, it is particularly important to compare evening peak flow values. Peak flow numbers that vary less than 15% within a 24-hour period indicate that one's asthma is under "good control."

IMPLEMENTATION OF AN ASTHMA MANAGEMENT PLAN

When the asthma action plan has been laid out and agreed on by the practitioner and the person with asthma, it is ready to be launched. Successful implementation requires a proactive approach built on open, ongoing communication between the person with asthma and the health care provider.

Once an asthma action plan has been developed, it is intended to be readily accessible and usable in a variety of venues. Every person with asthma should have an asthma action plan for use, not only at home, but also in all other locations frequented by that person including school and work settings.

The NAEPP Resolution on Asthma Management at School (2005)[22] recommended four essential policies that focus on student safety and balance a student's active involvement in asthma self-management while participating in school activities. These policies, which should be adopted by all schools, provide strong support for the implementation of

an asthma action plan in the school setting. They must be consistent with both the needs of the students with asthma and the safety of others. The policies include:

- A smoke-free environment for all school activities
- A written medication policy providing safe, prompt, and reliable access to medications during all school-related activities. Students should carry and self-administer rescue medications whenever possible.
- A school-wide emergency plan for handling asthma episodes
- Professional development for all school personnel on school medication policies, emergency procedures, and process for communicating health concerns about students

Five additional policies deemed highly desirable include:

- Access to health services under school nurse supervision throughout the day and appropriately delegated
- Services including:
  ○ Identification, assessment and monitoring students with asthma
  ○ A current, written asthma action plan for each student
  ○ Availability of resources for emergency care including a rescue inhaler and a spacer/holding chamber
  ○ Procedures for reporting and documenting medication administration
- Provision of asthma awareness and education for school staff and other students
- Provision of appropriate physical education options for students with asthma
- Development of a supportive and healthy environment that fosters respect for each student with asthma including:
  ○ Indoor air quality management
  ○ Use of appropriate pest control techniques
  ○ Minimal exposure to diesel exhaust from school buses

These policies are most likely to be successful if they are put forth at the beginning of each school year, if all staff are made aware of them, and if they are reinforced throughout the year.

Perhaps the most important component of these policies for children in educational settings is to have an asthma action plan readily accessible on site. The action plan should be signed by the parent (or other legal caregiver) as well as the child's health care practitioner, kept on file, and updated at least annually but more often if warranted by a change in either the child's level of severity or the asthma management plan. The school nurse or other health personnel as well as the classroom teacher and the coach or physical education instructor need to be familiar with the plan. All too often the school nurse is not informed of the child's diagnosis of asthma, the treatment modalities, or the steps to take should an asthma episode occur.

For many adolescents and young adults with asthma, going away to college brings a new level of responsibility in managing their asthma. Advance preparation can help the student anticipate how to handle new surroundings, demands, and activities and adjust the asthma action plan accordingly. "The Freshman 15: Top tips for allergy and asthma control"[22] lists 15 specific steps a young adult with asthma should take before leaving for college to ensure a smooth and safe transition.

Working adults should have a copy of their asthma action plan in their immediate workplace setting. Also, they should inform coworkers of their asthma and let them know there are specific written steps to follow, should an acute episode occur. In addition, a current copy of the asthma action plan should be on file in the office of the occupational health nurse. Adults with asthma, whether they have occupational asthma associated with specific workplace triggers or asthma that preceded their entry into their present work setting, need to avoid exposure to second-hand smoke as well as other environmental substances that may trigger an acute episode. If that is not possible and continued exposure leads to increased severity, they should be advised either to explore relocating within their job facility or to consider a job change.

An effective asthma management plan is greatly enhanced by a daily journal that can reveal patterns of "good" and "bad" days, symptom experiences, the relationship between symptoms and triggers, frequency of medications, and peak flow readings. Tips for making regular entries include writing in it at the same time every day and keeping it in the same place, preferably a visible location like a refrigerator door or kitchen bulletin board. The asthma journal should be brought to each visit with a health care provider. Such a record provides valuable longitudinal information between follow-up visits and can lead to evidence-based decisions about whether to adjust the asthma management plan. Many easy-to-use templates are available, such as the one shown in Figure 52-4.[23]

EVALUATION OF AN ASTHMA MANAGEMENT PLAN

Quality asthma management requires regular, consistent follow-up care by accessible, available, and responsive health care providers. These encounters must include confirmation at each visit that the individual understands and is able to implement the plan of action, including the correct use of medications and medication delivery devices. The importance of this ongoing assessment has been underscored by many studies providing evidence that less than half of all prescribed asthma medications are ever used.[24] Furthermore, the use of inhaled corticosteroids, particularly in children, may be less than effective due to suboptimal dosing which in turn can lead to decreased adherence and cessation of treatment.[25] A person may understandably question the reason for maintaining a treatment regimen if he or she perceives that it doesn't seem to make a difference because no signs of a problem exist! Obviously, the absence of symptoms is the hallmark of success, but a person with asthma who is symptom free

may perceive that the controller medications "don't make any difference" and decide to discontinue them or take them less frequently.

Consistent adherence to the management plan is imperative. It has been suggested that nonadherence is the most common reason for suboptimal asthma control. Thus, it is essential to anticipate possible barriers that may interfere with implementation and explore ways to offset them. Perhaps the most common barrier relates to the medication regimen. The central principle of asthma management, that is the prevention of episodes primarily through the regular use of corticosteroids and environmental control, is an abstract concept. It requires the person with asthma to regularly implement actions in the absence of signs and symptoms or other concrete evidence that such choices are worth the time, effort and money that may be involved. Thus, taking medication on a regular basis when the person with asthma "feels fine" may not command a high priority, particularly if cost is a concern, the medicine is used up and has not been refilled, or the medication schedule is perceived as a "hassle." Side effects may also be a concern. For example, some parents may confuse corticosteroids with anabolic steroids, or they may worry that corticosteroids will affect their child's growth. Some adolescent girls may be concerned about gaining weight. Least-demand dosing, that is, using the longest-acting medications possible to achieve efficacy combined with the least complicated delivery devices, can help remove some of the barriers to adherence.

Other barriers may include lack of easy access to the health care setting or provider; lack of provider continuity; lack of interest on the part of the clinician or the person with asthma; language and cultural barriers; inadequate comprehension of the treatment modalities and the severity of the asthma; actual or perceived adverse effects of treatment; treatment expenses; inadequate self-efficacy; an eroding partnership; and psychological alterations in the person with asthma and the family.[26]

It is important to note the underlying concept: that asthma can be controlled through appropriate adjustment of the asthma action plan, based on periodic evaluation of outcomes. Once the management plan has been implemented, it is essential that the health care provider and the person with asthma mutually review it every 1 to 6 months to determine its degree of effectiveness and any indications for revision. This review should include a candid discussion of specific behavioral outcomes. Control that is sustained for at least 3 months warrants consideration of a gradual reduction in treatment. On the other hand, if there is evidence of poorly controlled asthma, both the use of medications and the application of environmental controls must be explored in depth. Inadequate control signals the need to evaluate several areas for possible change or improvement: delivery device technique; adherence to the prescribed regimen; environmental control; and the need for more aggressive pharmacological management.

A change in delivery devices requires special attention. For example, the differences in technique between the use of an MDI and a DPI are critical. Most MDIs require two actuations for each dose, waiting at least 1 minute between puffs. Each actuation is coordinated with a slow, deep breath with a spacer/holding chamber. The aerosolization provides

TWO WEEK ASTHMA RECORD FOR _____ FROM_____ TO_____

Figure 52-4 Asthma track: Asthma chart. *(Adapted from Loyola Asthma Program, Loyola University Medical Center, Maywood, Illinois by G. Fisher and E. Gyllenhaal (2000). Retrieved March 6, 2007, from http://asthmatrack.org/tips_ forms.html.)*

Directions: Enter check marks for symptom categories and times for treatments or other symptoms. Use comment section and back to elaborate.

	Date:														
Wheezing or short of breath	None														
	Some of the day														
	Most of the day														
Cough	None														
	A little														
	Some of the day														
	Most of the day														
Other symptoms	Vomiting														
	Cold symptoms														
	Other														
Peak flow meter reading	Morning														
	Afternoon														
	Bedtime														
Night (night before date at top)	No problem														
	Awoke once														
	Awake most of the night														
Daily activity	Normal														
	Problems after activity														
	Problems with daily routine														
	Missed work or school														
	Extra doctor/ER visit														
Inhaler treatment	Reliever puffs														
Nebulizer treatment	Reliever via nebulizer														
Other treatment															

Comments:

"evidence" that the device has produced the medication. On the other hand, most DPIs require one quick, deep inhalation twice a day. Because DPI medication is not visible on the "shelf," is not delivered in a visible "puff," and is a minute amount of a tasteless substance, the individual does not have the same "evidence" that the medication is actually there. Without proper understanding of these differences, an individual might take a second inhalation of a DPI "just to be sure." Improper inhalation technique with either device might result in most of the medication being deposited in the oropharyngeal cavity rather than in the lungs. Thus, transitioning from one delivery device to another requires careful instruction and monitoring to be sure desired outcomes are not compromised.

Another point to be clarified if delivery devices are changed is that DPI medications, which usually combine a long-acting beta$_2$-agonist and a corticosteroid, are used only for prevention and never for rescue. On the other hand, the medications contained in an MDI may be used for either rescue or prevention. Thus, it is imperative that the action of a specific

medication is clearly understood so that it is taken for the correct reason.

Tools are available to assist in the evaluation process. For example, *A Tool for School Nurse Assessment* (Fig. 52-5) provides a template that can be used by school nurses, primary care providers, asthma educators, and asthma specialists to determine the effectiveness of an asthma action plan for a given student. It includes criteria that indicate whether or not a student's asthma is under "good" control as well as a checklist of assessment questions related to medications, monitoring, and trigger awareness and avoidance.

SUMMARY

Asthma is a chronic respiratory disease that levies a significant disease burden on children and adults alike. Although there is no cure, an asthma management plan that is developed collaboratively by the person with asthma and the health care provider, implemented consistently, and evaluated and updated as the person's condition or environment changes

IS THE ASTHMA ACTION PLAN WORKING?
A tool for school nurse assessment

Assessment for: _____ Completed by:_____ Date:_____
(Student)   (Nurse or parent)

This tool assists the school nurse in assessing if students are achieving good control of their asthma. Its use
is particularly indicated for students receiving intensive case management services at school.

With good asthma management, students should:
- Be free from asthma symptoms or have only minor
  symptoms:
  ○ no coughing or wheezing
  ○ no difficulty breathing or chest-tightness
  ○ no wakening at night due to asthma symptoms.
- Be able to go to school every day, unhampered
  by asthma.

- Be able to participate fully in regular school and daycare activities,
  including play, sports, and exercise.
- Have no bothersome side effects from medications.
- Have no emergency room or hospital visits.
- Have no missed class time for asthma-related interventions or
  missed class time is minimized.

Signs that a student's asthma is not under good control:
Indicate by checking the appropriate box whether any of the signs or symptoms listed below have been observed or reported by
parents or children within the past 6 months. If any boxes are marked, this suggests difficulty with following the treatment plan
or need for a change in treatment or intervention (e.g., different or additional medications, better identification or avoidance of
triggers).

☐ Asthma symptoms more than twice a week that require
  quick-relief medicine (short-acting beta-agonists, e.g. albuterol):
☐ Symptoms get worse even with quick relief meds
☐ Waking up at night because of coughing or wheezing
☐ Frequent or irregular heartbeat, headache, upset stomach,
  irritability, feeling shaky or dizzy

☐ Missing school or classroom time because of asthma symptoms
☐ Having to stop and rest at PE, recess, or during activities at
  home because of symptoms
☐ Symptoms require unscheduled visit to doctor, emergency room
  or hospitalization
☐ 911 call required

If "yes" to any of the above, use the following questions to more specifically ascertain areas where intervention may be needed.

Probes	Responsible person/site	Yes	No	N/A
Medications: • Are appropriate forms completed and on file for permitting medication administration at school?	By school staff	☐	☐	☐
	Self-carry	☐	☐	☐
• Has a daily **long-term-control** medication(s) (controller*) been prescribed?		☐	☐	☐
• Is **controller** medication available to use as ordered?	Home	☐	☐	☐
	School	☐	☐	☐
• Is the student taking the **controller** medication(s) as ordered?	Home	☐	☐	☐
	School	☐	☐	☐
• Has a **quick-relief** (short-acting B$_2$-agonist) medication been prescribed?		☐	☐	☐
• Is **quick-relief** medication easily accessible?	Home	☐	☐	
	Personal inhaler(s) at school health office	☐	☐	
	Self-carry	☐	☐	
• Is the student using **quick-relief** medication(s) as ordered... ○ Before exercise?	Home	☐	☐	☐
	School	☐	☐	☐
○ Immediately when symptoms occur?	Home	☐	☐	☐
	School	☐	☐	☐
Medication administration: • Does the student use correct technique when taking medication?		☐	☐	☐
• Does the person administering the medication use correct technique?		☐	☐	☐

Figure 52-5 A tool for school nurse assessment. *(From National Heart, Lung, Blood Institute: National Asthma Education and Prevention Program and the National Association of School Nurses. Retrieved March 6, 2007, from http://www.nhlbi.nih.gov/health/prof/lung/asthma/asth_act_plan_frm.pdf)*

(Continued)

	Responsible person/site	Yes	No	N/A
Monitoring • Can the student identify his/her **early** warning signs and symptoms that indicate onset of an asthma episode and need for **quick-relief** medicine?		☐	☐	☐
• Can the student identify his/her asthma signs and symptoms that indicate the need for help or medical attention?		☐	☐	☐
• Can the student correctly use a peak flow meter or asthma diary for tracking symptoms?		☐	☐	☐
• Are the students' asthma signs and symptoms monitored using a peak flow, verbal report or diary? ○ Daily?	Home	☐	☐	☐
	School	☐	☐	☐
○ For response to **quick-relief** medication?	Home	☐	☐	☐
	School	☐	☐	☐
○ During physical activity?	Home	☐	☐	☐
	School	☐	☐	☐
Trigger awareness: • Have triggers been identified?		☐	☐	
• Can student name his/her asthma triggers?		☐	☐	☐
• Can parent/caregivers list their child's asthma triggers?		☐	☐	
• Are teachers, including physical educators, aware of this student's asthma triggers?		☐	☐	
Trigger avoidance: • Are triggers removed or adequately avoided or managed?	Home	☐	☐	☐
	School	☐	☐	☐

Figure 52-5, cont'd

will likely lead to asthma control. To be effective, an asthma management plan must be tailored to the individual's needs with due consideration for developmental and reading levels, cultural and linguistic factors, anticipated barriers, and the stages of behavioral change. Many available resources are identified in this chapter, including asthma action plan templates in several languages and formulas for scoring the reading level of selected materials.

Effective asthma management is built on a trusting and respectful partnership. The person with asthma must perceive the plan as realistic, "doable," and adaptable to one's lifestyle. The health care provider must formulate the plan according to "best practices" from both a clinical and educational perspective. Ultimately, a successful asthma plan depends on individualized development, consistent implementation, and regular evaluation.

REFERENCES

1. Healthy People 2010: Washington, DC, Office of Disease Prevention and Health Promotion, U.S. Department of Health and Human Services. Available at http://www.healthypeople.gov/.
2. National Asthma Educator Certification Board: 2005. Available at http://www.naecb.org.
3. Adams RJ, Fuhlbrigge A, Guilbert T: Inadequate use of asthma medication in the United States: results of the Asthma in America National Population Survey. J Allergy Clin Immunol 2002;110:58–64.
4. LaRocco LA: Outcomes management for patients with asthma. Outcomes Manag Nurs Pract 1999:3:175–180.
5. Doerschug KC, Peterson MW, Dayton CS, Kline JN: Asthma guidelines: an assessment of physician understanding and practice. Am J Respir Crit Care Med 1999:159(6):1735–1741.
6. Clark NM, Gong M: Management of chronic disease by practitioners and patients: Are we teaching the wrong things? BMJ 2000:320:572–575.
7. Gibson PG, Boulet L: Role of asthma education. In Fitzgerald JM, Ernst P, Boulet L, O'Byrne PM (eds): Evidence-based Asthma Management. London, B.C. Decker, Inc., 2001, pp 275–290.
8. Prochaska and DiClemente's Stages of Change Model, UCLA Center for Human Nutrition. (n.d.) Available at http://www.cellinteractive.com/ucla/physician_ed/stages_change.html.
9. Marvin NG: Patient education. J Kans Med Soc 1980:81:115–117.
10. National Asthma Education and Prevention Program: Expert Panel Report 3 (EPR3): Guidelines for the diagnosis and management of asthma. Washington, DC, U.S. Department of Health and Human Services, Public Health Service, National Institutes of Health, National Heart, Lung, and Blood Institute, 2007, Pub. No. 08-4051, p 115.
11. Clark NM, Nothwehr F, Gong M, et al: Physician-patient partnership in managing chronic illness. Chest 1995:70(11):957–959.
12. Lorig K: Patient Education—A Practical Approach. 3rd ed. Thousand Oaks, Calif, Sage Publications, Inc., 2001.
13. Gibson PG, Coughlan J, Wilson AJ, et al: Self-management education and regular practitioner review for adults with asthma. Cochrane Database Syst Rev 2002;(2):CD001117.
14. Abramson MJ, Bailey MJ, Couper FJ, et al: Are asthma medications and management related to deaths from asthma? Am J Respir Crit Care Med 2001:163(1):12–18.
15. The SMOG Readability Formula: 2006. Available at http://uuhsc.utah.edu/pated/authors/readability.html.
16. Fog Index: 2006. Available at http://process.umn.edu/groups/ppd/documents/information/writing_tips.cfm.
17. National Standards for Culturally and Linguistically Appropriate Services in Health Care: Washington, DC, US Department of Health and Human Services, Office of Minority Health, 2001.
18. Growing Up with Asthma. Allergy & Asthma Network Mothers of Asthmatics. MA Report 2004:19(7):1–2. www.aanma.org.

19. Roberts JR, McCurdy LE: Environmental management of pediatric asthma: guidelines for health care providers. Washington, DC, The National Environmental Education & Training Foundation, 2005. Available at http://www.neetf.org/Health/asthma_resources.htm.
20. American Academy of Allergy Asthma & Immunology: Tips to Remember: What Is a Peak Flow Meter? 2003. Available at http://www.aaaai.org/patients/publicedmat/tips/whatispeakflowmeter.stm.
21. State statutes protecting student rights to carry and use prescribed asthma and anaphylaxis medications: Allergy & Asthma Network: Mothers of Asthmatics. Available at http://www.aanma.org/pdf/ch_ColorMap.pdf.
22. National Asthma Education and Prevention Program (NAEPP): Resolution on Asthma Management at School. Washington, DC, U.S. Department of Health and Human Services, Public Health Service, National Institutes of Health, National Heart, Lung, and Blood Institute, 2005.
23. American Academy of Allergy Asthma & Immunology: The Freshman 15: Top tips for allergy and asthma control. 2004. Available at http://www.aaaai.org/patients/topicofthemonth/0704.
24. Asthma Track: Asthma Chart. 2005. Available at http://asthmatrack.org/tips_forms.html.
25. Milgrom H, Bender BG: Factors affecting compliance and safety. Symposium: Improving outcomes in asthma: Concepts in clinical application. Program and abstracts of the 1999 Annual meeting of the American College of Allergy, Asthma, and Immunology, November 12–17, 1999, Chicago, Illinois.
26. Camargo CA Jr, Patel P: Reducing the risk of asthma exacerbations. J Respir Care Pract 2005:18(4):26, 29–30.
27. Musto PK: General principles of management: Education. Nurs Clin North Am 2003;38:621–633.

Asthma Self-Management

Susan L. Janson

CLINICAL PEARLS

- Collaboratively develop goals for self-management of asthma.
- Provide skills in self-assessment of asthma control.
- Teach and reinforce a correct inhaler technique for all medications and devices.
- Teach self-monitoring and interpretation of symptoms and/or peak flow trends.
- Write a self-management plan that includes daily steps to control asthma and actions to take when asthma worsens.

There is abundant evidence that educating people with asthma to be actively involved in their own care is effective in improving health outcomes. Self-management education for both children and adults includes specific training in the skills of self-assessment, use of medications, and actions to prevent or control exacerbations, in addition to information about asthma. Information alone improves knowledge but is not sufficient to produce the behaviors necessary to improve asthma outcomes. Expert care through regular planned visits with a consistent clinician is necessary but also not sufficient to control asthma. Patient-centered care means that patients and their families are actively involved in controlling asthma by minimizing exposure to factors that make asthma harder to control and taking prompt actions when asthma worsens by adjusting medications. The benefits of providing self-management education and support to patients and their families include reduced hospitalizations, emergency department and urgent care visits, asthma-related health care costs, and improved quality of life and health status. Other proven outcomes of value to patients are reduced symptoms and nighttime awakenings, fewer days of restricted activity, and improved perception of asthma control. These outcomes lead to better quality of life.

The overall goal of self-management education is to improve the patient's ability to live a full life with asthma. It is critical for clinicians to understand the important role patients play in the management of their own asthma on a day-to-day basis and during exacerbations and to provide ongoing self-management support to patients and their families. The key elements of self-management support are: (1) helping patients to acquire the skills and confidence to participate in their own care; (2) providing self-assessment tools and teaching patients to interpret their own data; (3) evaluating problems and praising accomplishments; and (4) referring patients to community resources. When the clinician and patient are working together collaboratively to make joint treatment decisions, asthma can be controlled more effectively, with better adherence and improved outcomes.

The methods for providing education can be structured or unstructured, brief or comprehensive, in one session or many sessions, or delivered individually or in groups through any mode (verbal, written, video, audio, or computer). Regardless of the format, self-management education must include teaching age-appropriate behaviors and skills that will allow patients and their caregivers to recognize worsening asthma and take actions to control the disease. Given the opportunity, both children and adults can learn these skills and use them appropriately. Depending on the age of the patient, some will require direct assistance with self-management. For young children and elderly patients, caregivers must be trained to assist or take over care when necessary. With the exception of children under the age of 4 years, most patients can learn to manage their asthma appropriately. However, a trained patient (or caregiver) is not sufficient to control asthma alone. Clinicians must also be trained to recognize the changing levels of asthma severity and control and to adjust treatment accordingly. This type of surveillance is achieved through regular planned visits aimed at specific goals to keep asthma under control.

ASSESSMENT

Self-monitoring requires recognition of signs and symptoms, interpretation of the meaning of these symptoms, the actions to take control of them, and the skills to evaluate the response and resolution. In order to provide the education necessary for a patient to follow their self-management plan, their specific health concerns and learning needs must be assessed. In assessing the patient's learning needs the provider must consider what information the patient needs, the specific health and illness attitudes and beliefs the patient may have, what skills are necessary to perform health care behaviors, and any barriers there may be to achieving the desired behavior. The provider should determine what the patient already may know about asthma and assess the accuracy of the patient's knowledge. If the patient is misinformed the provider should incorporate specific detail where knowledge is incomplete. In the same way self-assessment skills must be honed.

Providers may use health assessment instruments to gather and organize data. The "Patient Self-Assessment Form" from the NAEPP Practical Guide for the Diagnosis and Management of Asthma (list www.nhlbi.gov/health/prof/lung/asthma/practgde/practgde.pdf) can be used to gather information on the history of present illness and allows the patient to identify any current concerns or questions they may have about asthma. The "Patient Self-Assessment Form for Environmental and Other Factors" that can make asthma worse (also from the NAEPP Practical Guide) allows the patient and clinician to identify any environmental factors and potential comorbidities that may make asthma more difficult to control.

Self-management education targets the asthmatic patient and/or the caregiver when the patient is a young child. Therefore, it is important to understand the learning preferences of the target audience. A study on the learning preferences of caregivers of asthmatic children showed that a kinesthetic learning method was preferred, suggesting that role-playing or problem-solving scenarios may be the most effective teaching strategy for this group. However, individual learning assessments may be performed using the VARK Questionnaire. The questionnaire is available for adults and children and can be obtained in 15 different languages (http://www.vark-learn.com/english/index.asp). This approach may be useful as tailored educational programs have been shown to be more effective in achieving positive health outcomes.

It is important to recognize that self-management may not be actualized by the patient due to unmet basic needs. The provider must use the assessment period to identify barriers and to design an individualized self-management plan with negotiated goals that the patient agrees with and can meet reasonably. The ability to learn may be affected by physical discomfort, denial, anxiety, dependency needs, and cognitive/developmental factors. The most significant barrier to learning self-management is lack of self-confidence. Patients should be encouraged to identify their own short-term goal(s) while long-term goals should be developed mutually by the patient and clinician and should involve collaboration with family members when appropriate.

EDUCATION

When patients and their families are capable of self-management, they have information about the chronic nature of asthma and the central role of airway inflammation. They understand how prescribed daily medications work to control asthma and the actions and timing of rescue medications. They have the skills necessary to inhale medications correctly so they receive maximum benefit. Inhaled medications are marketed with many different types of devices and each one requires different skills and practice to achieve proficiency. As the ability to perceive symptoms varies widely, objective measures of lung function, such as peak flow, may be helpful for some patients to monitor and evaluate the status of their asthma. When asthma worsens, patients and their caregivers need to know what actions to take, including manipulation of doses of medications and when to seek urgent medical care without delay.

The following outline addresses the information and skills that each patient should possess to engage in asthma self-management (items 1 to 3). The written components of the self-management plan are established collaboratively between the patient and the clinician (item 4).

Asthma Self-Management for the Adult

1. KNOWLEDGE AND INFORMATION
- *Asthma and Inflammation.* Describe the chronic nature of asthma and the role of inflammation. Emphasize that the inflammation is in the airways (bronchial tubes), which is why correct inhalation of medications is so important. A picture of the human head and torso, showing the lungs with bronchial airways connected to the upper airways is essential (Fig. 53-1). Models of airways showing what inflammation looks like can be used to illustrate where the problem is and the site of medication action.
- *Signs and Symptoms of Worsening Asthma.* The sensation of chest tightness, wheezing, and difficulty breathing during days or nights are important signs that asthma is getting worse. Patients need to know that these symptoms are not "normal" for people with asthma and their appearance means that asthma is not under control. Emphasize key times of symptom worsening; being awakened from sleep or symptoms during the early morning means that asthma is flaring.
- *Asthma Triggers.* Describe the aggravating role of relevant factors that make asthma harder to control, such as exposure to allergens, irritants (tobacco smoke, household cleaners, fumes and aerosols), uncontrolled allergic rhinitis, or gastric reflux. These factors must be controlled to achieve asthma control. The patient's role is to use the prescribed treatments for these conditions appropriately. For patients with allergic rhinitis, particularly those who complain of post-nasal drip, consider antihistamines, nasal steroid sprays, and nasal lavage.

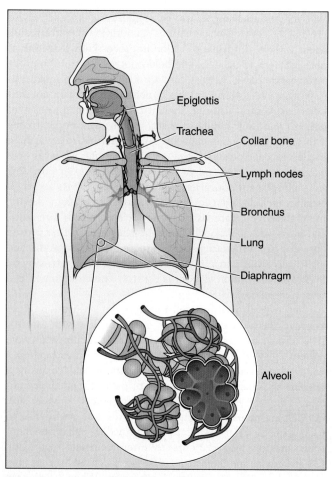

Figure 53-1   Model of the human airways.

2. PATIENT COLLABORATION—THE ROLE OF ATTITUDES, BELIEFS, AND VALUES

- *Long-Term Goals.* Discussing and establishing long-term treatment goals for asthma control may improve adherence. Emphasize that medication may be adjusted over time based on the individual's level of control. The ultimate goal is to control asthma with the lowest dose of inhaled medications with few to no side effects. This means symptom-free days and nights, optimal lung function, participation in desired activities, minimal need for rescue medication, and satisfaction with quality of life and asthma care.

- *Decision Making.* Allow the patient to participate in decisions about therapy as much as they are able. Identify any attitudes or beliefs about asthma that may become barriers to implementing self-management behavior. For example, patients who believe it is unhealthy to take regular daily medication will need discussion and time to reframe need to control asthma through preventive steps. By helping them to see that they are healthier when controlling airway inflammation with daily medication, the clinician can engage the patient by focusing on short-term valued goals. A common belief of both asthmatic adults and parents of children with asthma is that taking the medication every day will cause tolerance so that it doesn't work when needed. Such misconceptions will need to be carefully discussed in nonjudgmental terms to arrive at a mutually acceptable agreement. When patients experience difficulty participating in self-management decisions, screen the patient for depression, one of the most common barriers to self-management of chronic diseases.

- *Medication Taking.* Describe the role of each medication and the component of asthma it addresses. Explain why taking controller medication is the healthiest approach to managing asthma. The patient should be able to explain why increased or continuous use of quick-relief medication is a sign that their asthma is not well-controlled. Fears about long-term effects of medications should be openly discussed. Some patients will respond well to facts but others will need to develop an approach based in mutual trust.

3. SKILLS AND PERFORMANCE

- *Correct Inhalation Technique.* Patients need to be shown how to entrain the puff of medication directly into the airway with a deep breath. Demonstration, repetition, and practice are required and must be repeated often. Break the maneuver down into simple steps. Table 53-1 reviews correct technique and identifies key mistakes for the use of metered-dose and dry powder inhalers. Figure 53-2 shows appropriate inhalation techniques for metered-dose and dry powder inhalers.

- *Self-Adjusting Medication Dose.* Inhaled short-acting beta$_2$-agonists should be described to patients as "rescue" medication. Describe the action, onset (10 minutes) peak effect (20 minutes) and duration (3 to 4 hours) of the usual dose (two puffs). Using either peak flow and/or symptoms, teach the patient how to increase the dose safely to manage an acute episode of symptoms. As a general guide, two puffs of the short-acting beta$_2$-agonist can be repeated if needed every 20 minutes within an hour

---

Table 53-1
INHALERS: CORRECT TECHNIQUE AND KEY MISTAKES

Metered-dose inhaler: Remove the cap. Attach the inhaler to the holding chamber if using one. Shake the inhaler. Breathe out. Close the lips over mouthpiece tightly, activate the inhaler (press down) while slowly breathing in, and hold the breath for several seconds.

Key Mistakes: Failure to breathe out first, breathing in before actuation of the inhaler, breathing in too fast, failure to hold the breath, and activating the inhaler more than one time per breath.

Dry powder inhalers: Load the dose according to the type of device prescribed, keeping the device level and horizontal, seal the lips tightly around the mouth piece, breathe in rapidly and forcefully, hold the breath for several seconds.

Key mistakes: Failure to load the dose correctly, shaking the inhaler, breathing in too slowly without enough effort, and swallowing the dose.

Inhaler instructions in various languages can be found on the Community Action to Fight Asthma Web site: www.calasthma.org.

---

for an acute episode at home or work or school, but if symptoms are not improved, the patient should seek medical care without further delay. Other individualized steps include increasing the dose or potency of the inhaled corticosteroid medication, or starting prednisone by following an agreed-on written plan.

- *Peak Flow Monitoring.* If peak flow monitoring is used, patients must be able to accurately and reliably perform measurements. They must be able to compare their daily peak-flow readings to their established personal best and make care decisions based on a corresponding written or verbal action plan. For some patients, following trends in morning peak flow values over a period of time may be useful, especially when they are assessing their response to new treatments or to environmental triggers.

4. THE WRITTEN PLAN FOR SELF-MANAGEMENT OF ASTHMA

- *Recommended Doses and Frequencies of Daily Medications.* All information about dosing and frequency must be clearly written on the self-management plan. Include information about refilling medication(s) in this section. It is important to note that the provider's instructions for medication dosing are often affixed as a printed label to the medication packaging and not on the inhaler itself; therefore it is important to rewrite the instructions as part of the written self-management plan. Using colored stickers to identify the rescue versus daily control medications is helpful to many patients who become confused by the myriad of inhalers.

- *Managing Exacerbations.* When asthma worsens, patients need to take actions based on specific signs, symptoms, sensations, or peak flow measurements that indicate loss of asthma control. Signs and symptoms are individual but generally include the sensation of chest tightness, increasing difficulty breathing, wheezing, and falling peak flow. Clear and simple action steps should be written down that will guide the patient in the actions to take when asthma worsens. Initiation of each step is based on recognition of worsening asthma as well as knowledge of what treatments to use, and how to evaluate response to these treatments. Patients and their families need to be able to identify key warning

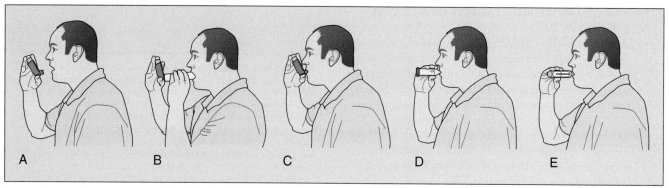

Figure 53-2 Inhaler techniques. **A,** MDI with open-mouth technique. **B,** MDI with spacer. **C,** Close-mouth technique. **D,** Dry Powder Turbuhaler. **E,** Dry Powder Diskus Inhaler.

signs, such as difficulty talking or walking, grey or bluish lips and nail beds, and finding it harder and harder to breathe, that indicate the need to seek urgent medical care without delay. Self-management of acute episodes depends on practicing these skills and building the confidence to carry them out effectively. These skills should be rehearsed at every opportunity. Exacerbations should be reviewed at the next follow-up visit to evaluate the patient's self-management knowledge, the actions taken by the patient during the exacerbation, and to provide support, reinforcement, and praise for appropriate self-management. Write down for the patient emergency telephone numbers for the clinician, emergency department, prompt transportation, and for family or friend who can provide aid and support.

- *Environmental Trigger Management.* All identified allergens, airway irritants, and asthma triggers can be listed on the daily self-management plan with control interventions that the patient and clinician have agreed upon. Before allergen environmental control strategies can be implemented, it may be necessary to identify sensitivities through limited allergy testing in order to convince the patient that the allergen is related to their (or their child's) degree of asthma control.

Asthma Self-Management for the Child

Asthma self-management in children is complex; its success hinges on several key variables, which include the age of the child, the child's caretakers' abilities, and the time spent at home, school, and outside activities. With school and extracurricular activities, educating a single caretaker is often not enough. In addition to the parents/family members, teachers, coaches, and childcare workers need to know how to respond when asthma is uncontrolled or suddenly worsens. The self-management plan, including actions to manage acute asthma, should be shared with these other adults.

The most important consideration in writing the asthma self-management plan for children is simplicity. Children should be told that difficulty breathing and/or wheezing is not normal and that when this happens they must tell an adult. The management plan must be shared and understood by the child (when age appropriate), the parents, other family, school administrators, and any other secondary caregivers.

Peak flow monitoring with a simple action plan based on a "traffic light" analogy (Fig. 53-3) can be useful for school-age children. Children 4 years and older can be taught to use a peak flow meter appropriately.

The NAEPP Practical Guide includes a simple "School Self-Management Plan" that identifies the child, current medications, environmental triggers, an emergency plan, and signs to get help. The clinician should complete this form with the primary caregiver and instruct her/him to provide a copy to all secondary caregivers and school personnel.

Special Considerations

INFANTS AND TODDLERS

Since peak flow monitoring and standard inhaler techniques may not be feasible in this population, alternative management techniques should be used. Infants will need nebulized medication but for toddlers, a holding chamber equipped with a mask should be considered for use with metered-dose inhalers as an alternative to the nebulizer; inhaler technique should be reviewed frequently. An action plan based on a "traffic light" analogy may also be used for this population, however the zones and action cut-points should be dictated by signs (coughing, labored breathing, wheezing), and breathing rate (Fig. 53-4). The attention span for toddlers is about 2 to 3 minutes so choose a simple task, such as opening the inhaler or breathing in on command, to teach skills. Preschool children are attracted to bright colors and pictures. They like to explore tools and "play-act" with dolls. When confronted with a new situation, they will defer to parents until comfortable. These attributes can be used to tailor asthma self-management education to young children. Self-management may be as simple as, "Tell someone when you can't breathe."

SCHOOL-AGED CHILDREN

School-aged children have an attention span of 10 to 15 minutes and have the verbal skills to report asthma symptoms. They may have difficulty with verbal descriptions so consider asking the child to draw a picture of what it feels like to have asthma; this may provide useful insight into the child's experience. School-aged children respond well to pictures, cartoons, videos, books with large print, and computers. They especially like games and learning in groups so asthma self-management is best taught in structured group situations.

ENGLISH

My Asthma Plan

Patient Name: _____

Medical Record #: _____

Physician's Name: _____   DOB: _____

Physician's Phone #: _____   Completed by: _____   Date: _____

Controller Medicines	How Much to Take	How Often	Other Instructions
		_____ times per day **EVERYDAY!**	
		_____ times per day **EVERYDAY!**	
		_____ times per day **EVERYDAY!**	
		_____ times per day **EVERYDAY!**	
Quick-Relief Medicines	**How Much to Take**	**How Often**	**Other Instructions**
		Take ONLY as needed	NOTE: If this medicine is needed frequently, call physician to consider increasing controller medications.

Special instructions when I feel ● *good,* ○ *not good,* and ● *awful.*

GREEN ZONE

I feel *good.*

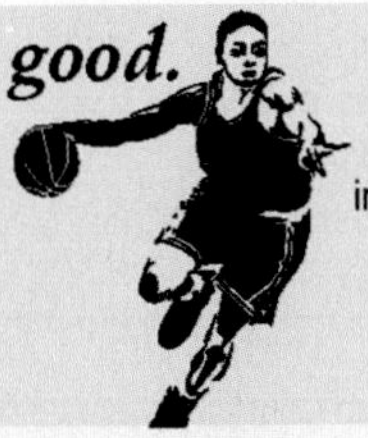

(My **peak flow** is in the GREEN zone.)

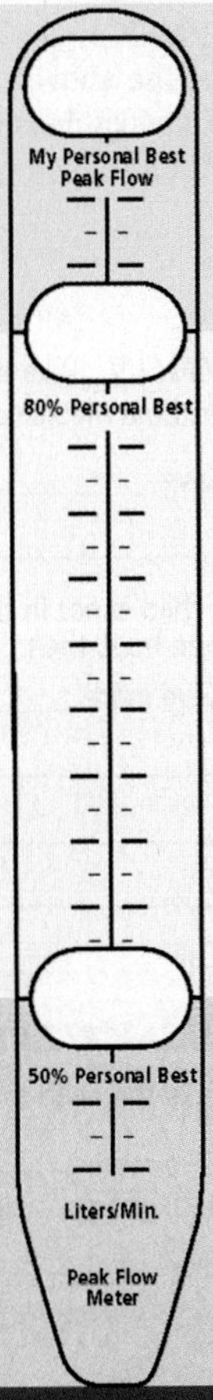

My Personal Best Peak Flow

80% Personal Best

PREVENT asthma symptoms everyday:

☐ Take my controller medicines (above) everyday.

☐ Before exercise, take _____ puffs of _____

☐ Avoid things that make my asthma worse like:

YELLOW ZONE

I do *not* feel *good.*

(My **peak flow** is in the YELLOW zone.)

My symptoms may include one or more of the following: 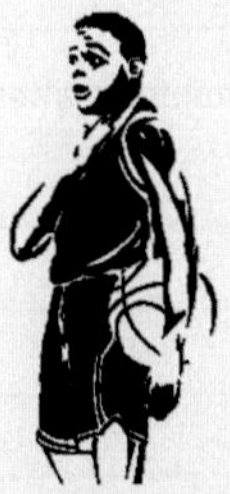
- Wheeze
- Tight chest
- Cough
- Shortness of breath
- Waking up at night with asthma symptoms
- Decreased ability to do usual activities
- _____
- _____

CAUTION. I should continue taking my everyday controller asthma medicines AND:

☐ Take _____

If I still do not feel good, or my peak flow is not back in the *Green Zone* within one hour, then I should:

☐ Increase _____
_____

☐ Add _____
_____

☐ Call _____

RED ZONE

I feel *awful.*

(My **peak flow** is in the RED zone.)

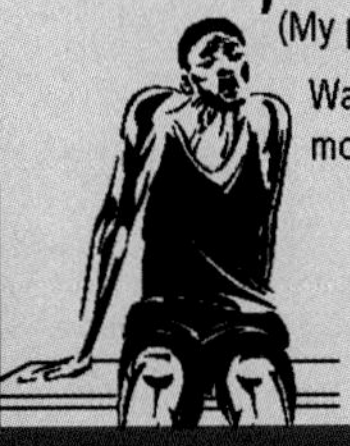

50% Personal Best

Liters/Min.

Peak Flow Meter

Warning signs may include one or more of the following:
- Its getting harder and harder to breathe
- Unable to sleep or do usual activities because of trouble breathing

MEDICAL ALERT! Get help!

☐ Take _____
until I get help immediately.

☐ Take _____
_____

☐ Call _____

Danger! Get help immediately!   Call 911 if trouble walking or talking due to shortness of breath or lips or fingernails are gray or blue.

ORIGINAL (Patient)   /   CANARY (School / Child Care / Work / Other Support Systems)   /   PINK (Chart)   ©2001, Public Health Institute (RAMP)

Figure 53-3   Regional Asthma Management and Prevention Initiative (RAMP). Asthma action plan for adults and children over 5 years of age. (Available at: *http://www.rampasthma.org/actionplanpdf.pdf*).

ENGLISH

Child Asthma Plan
0-5 year olds

Patient Name: _____

Medical Record #: _____

Healthcare Provider's Name: _____   DOB: _____

Healthcare Provider's Phone #: _____   Completed by: _____   Date: _____

Controller Medicines (Use Everyday to Stay Healthy)	How Much to Take	How Often	Other Instructions (such as spacers/masks, nebulizers)
		_____ times per day EVERYDAY!	
		_____ times per day EVERYDAY!	
		_____ times per day EVERYDAY!	
		_____ times per day EVERYDAY!	

Quick-Relief Medicines	How Much to Take	How Often	Other Instructions
		Give ONLY as needed	NOTE: If this medicine is needed often (_____ times per week), call physician.

GREEN ZONE

Child is **well** and has no asthma symptoms, even during active play.

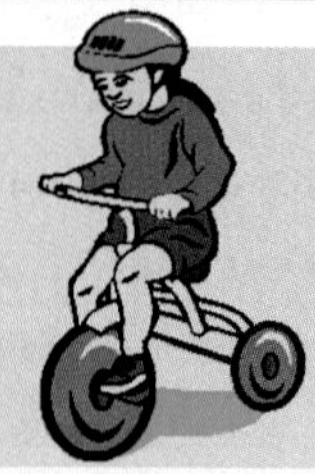

PREVENT asthma symptoms everyday:
- **Give the above controller medicines everyday.**
- Avoid things that make the child's asthma worse:
☑ Avoid tobacco smoke; ask people to smoke outside.
☐ _____
☐ _____

YELLOW ZONE

Child is **not well** and has asthma symptoms that may include:
- Coughing
- Wheezing
- Runny nose or other cold symptoms
- Breathing harder or faster
- Awakening due to coughing or difficulty breathing
- Playing less than usual
- _____
- _____

Other symptoms that could indicate that your child is having trouble breathing may include: difficulty feeding (grunting sounds, poor sucking), changes in sleep patterns, cranky and tired, decreased appetite.

CAUTION. Take action by continuing to give regular **everyday** asthma medicines AND:

☐ Give _____
_____
(include dose and frequency)

If the child is not in the **Green Zone** and still has symptoms after one hour, then:

☐ Give more _____
_____
(include dose and frequency)

☐ _____
_____
(include dose and frequency)

☐ Call _____

RED ZONE

Child **feels awful!** Warning signs may include:
- Child's wheeze, cough or difficulty breathing continues or worsens, even after giving yellow zone medicines.
- Child's breathing is so hard that he/she is having trouble walking / talking / eating / playing.
- Child is drowsy or less alert than normal.

Danger! Get help immediately!

MEDICAL ALERT! Get help!

☐ Take the child to the hospital or call 911 immediately!

☐ Give more _____ until you get help. *(include dose and frequency)*

☐ Give _____ *(include dose and frequency)*

Call 911 if:
- **The child's skin is sucked in around neck and ribs; or**
- **Lips and / or fingernails are grey or blue; or**
- **Child doesn't respond to you.**

ORIGINAL (Patient) / CANARY (Child Care / School / Other Support Systems) / PINK (Chart)

Figure 53-4   Regional Asthma Management and Prevention Initiative (RAMP). Asthma action plan for children ages 0–5 years. *(Available at: http://www.rampasthma.org/actionplanpdf.pdf).*

TEENAGERS

Managing a chronic illness, such as asthma, can further intensify the difficulties of the teenage years. Special focus on the dangers of smoking with asthma is needed, as adolescents will likely be exposed to tobacco smoke and may even experiment with smoking. However, adolescents may not respond to formal didactic education. They seek independence in decision-making and yet lack the knowledge and maturity to self-manage asthma entirely alone. They may respond well to peer education or peer idols who have asthma. Control of medications and asthma self-management should be gradually transferred to the adolescent during this stage. Parents should remain involved and support the teenager's efforts at self-management. Simple, discreet medication regimens are likely to be better tolerated. Dry powder inhalers and/or once-daily regimens may suit teenagers better. They are active problem solvers, computer savvy, and knowledgeable about the Internet. Web-based self-management programs with problem-solving scenarios and teen bulletin boards for posting anonymous questions may ultimately prove to be the most useful approach for this age. It is important to provide some adult oversight and regular, planned evaluation visits with an interested clinician, especially if symptoms are persistent.

OLDER ADULTS

Older adults tend to be particularly interested in detail and in understanding the rationale for health-related recommendations. They may require adaptation of learning materials and self-management plans when visual or auditory impairments interfere with learning. Providers should consider group education as older adults tend to be more willing to attend and participate due to available time, interest, and need for socialization. Older adults are quite capable of self-management as long as cognitive problems are not present and should be respectfully included in all treatment decisions. It is important to remember that medication-taking skills can wane over time in all people but reinforcement of skills is especially important in elderly patients.

PREGNANT WOMEN

Pregnant women with asthma will need special attention to asthma self-management to keep asthma under control and avoid exacerbations. Asthma may improve, get worse, or stay the same during pregnancy and women need to be trained in self-assessment techniques in order to adjust treatment promptly. They should be told that to have a healthy baby it is critical to keep asthma under control with appropriate medications. Fears about the effects of medications should be discussed openly with emphasis placed on preventing severe bronchospasm and episodes of hypoxemia. All pregnant patients need a self-management plan and prompt access to medical care if asthma worsens. After the baby is born, the postpartum period represents another period of vulnerability for women with asthma. Hormone fluctuations and changes in continuity of care between obstetricians and primary care clinicians can occur at this time when the woman will continue to need close monitoring.

CULTURAL NEEDS

When patients and providers are of different backgrounds or cultures it is important that communication be clear,

---

Table 53-2
QUESTIONS FOR UNDERSTANDING CULTURAL ATTITUDES AND BELIEFS ABOUT ASTHMA

- What do you call your problem? What name does it have?
- What do you think caused this problem?
- Why do you think it started?
- What does your asthma do to you? How does it work?
- How bad is it? Will it have a short or long course?
- What fears do you have about your asthma?
- What are the major problems that your asthma causes?
- Is there anything you do to treat your asthma?
- What kind of treatment do you think you should use?
- What are the most important results you hope to receive from the treatment?

Adapted from Kleinman's Tools to Elicit Health Beliefs in Clinical Encounters, in Kleinman A: Patients and Healers in the context of culture. Berkeley, University of California Press, 1981.

---

effective, and respectful when designing and implementing a self-management plan. Providers should use formal address unless the patient says otherwise. Language abilities should be assessed in order to determine language barriers or literacy needs. Identifying the patient's specific beliefs and attitudes about their asthma is essential and must be incorporated into the self-management plan. Table 53-2 suggests questions to ask, adapted from *Kleinman's Tool to Elicit Health Beliefs in Clinical Encounters*, when assessing individual patient's cultural beliefs and attitudes. Patients from some cultures will not want to agree that they have asthma or any chronic disease due to stigma. If reasonable, providers should try to elicit the descriptors that the patient uses in talking about their asthma. If language ability poses a significant barrier to successful communication between the patient and the provider, interpreter services should be sought. The Federal Interagency Working Group on Limited English Proficiency has developed a Web site called "Let Everyone Participate" that lists several translator and interpreter organizations that specialize in medical translation (http://www.lep.gov/medtrans.html). When using an interpreter to teach self-management, be careful to speak directly to the patient, not the interpreter. Thoese with hearing deficits who use American Sign Language will need to be positioned so that they can see both the ASL interpreter and the clinician who is speaking. Deaf patients can use visual cues, sensations, and peak flow to monitor their asthma and will need active demonstrations of inhalers.

LITERACY NEEDS

A report generated by the U.S. Department of Education found that about 13.4 million U.S. adults are not able to perform even simple health literacy tasks proficiently. Inadequate health literacy indicates limited ability to read and comprehend prescription bottles, appointment slips, and other important health-related materials. The Harvard School of Public Health offers a plain language glossary for improving communication about asthma (http://www.hsph.harvard.edu/healthliteracy/asthma/asthma3.pdf). Providers should note that people who are illiterate may learn differently; they may not necessarily understand diagrams or figures. The clinician should check that a patient comprehends and can express their self-management plan in their own words. Even patients with limited literacy may want educational materials, booklets, and written plans to take home, where family or friends can read to them. The Community Action to Fight Asthma Web site (www.calasthma.org) provides several low-literacy instructions and fact sheets about asthma in multiple languages.

SOCIOECONOMIC STATUS

Patients of lower socioeconomic status are less likely to seek treatment when ill and access health care later than those of higher socioeconomic status. Patient education in self-management can help by focusing on health risks that can be modified with healthier lifestyles and practices. Community-based approaches using local pharmacists, community health workers, and neighborhood leaders may be the most effective approaches to implementing asthma self-management programs. Clinicians can identify community resources and engage pharmacists to help teach self-management skills. It is important to ask the patient which pharmacy they use to fill prescriptions and communicate with that pharmacy at regular intervals. This team approach helps to support patient self-management.

USE OF ALTERNATIVE OR COMPLEMENTARY CARE

Alternative or complementary therapy may interfere with recommended or prescribed therapies but patients may not tell their clinicians about these treatments. Clinicians should ask patients what other approaches they are using to promote or control health, but should avoid implying judgment. The mechanisms and effects of therapy in question should be assessed. Many complementary therapies are not harmful and should not be discouraged if the patient finds them helpful. When the patient has a therapeutic relationship with an alternative or complementary health provider, ask the patient for permission to contact that person to coordinate asthma care.

Adherence is Key to Successful Self-Management

Information on how and why the medication(s) work can improve adherence to prescribed treatment. However, cost-effectiveness, simplicity of regimen, clear cues for actions, and medication-taking skills can also influence adherence. Persistent symptoms, missed appointments, and infrequent refills can indicate nonadherence to prescribed medications. Take time to decide whether nonadherence is an issue in achieving successful self-management. Table 53-3 addresses different types of nonadherence and suggests specific interventions for each type.

TECHNIQUES

Teaching and Learning Activities

Several strategies may be used to teach self-management skills and knowledge. Some are more effective than others at teaching specific components of self-management. A successful self-management educational plan will likely use two or more teaching strategies.

Table 53-3
DEFINING AND TREATING NONADHERENCE

Intermittent Nonadherence: Forgetting to take medication or missing doses at times while taking medication correctly at other times.
Reasons: Busy work/life schedule, inconvenient dosing schedule, forgetfulness, fatigue, and depression.
Interventions: Cues, reminders, minimal daily dosing, integrating medication taking with daily activity pattern, treating depression.

Unwitting Nonadherence: Taking the wrong dose, taking the medication incorrectly or at the wrong dose intervals.
Reasons: Language barriers, communication problems, misunderstanding, lack of a written plan, inadequate demonstration and practice of skills.
Interventions: Careful instruction, demonstration of skills, written instructions, pictures.

Purposeful Nonadherence: Not filling the prescription or purposefully not taking the medication even after filling the prescription.
Reasons: Beliefs, attitudes, concerns, cost, and access.
Interventions: Open communication and discussion of issues and concerns, contracting, planned evaluation of progress and benefit.

---

1. *Lecture (talking)*. Use of succinct messages is highly effective for teaching information and knowledge but not effective for teaching behaviors, skills, and actions, nor for eliciting attitudes, health beliefs, and values about health care.

2. *Group discussion*. Active participation by group members with the educator is useful in the application of knowledge, shaping attitudes or dispelling myths. It requires at least two participants plus the educator.

3. *Demonstration*. Active demonstration is most effective for teaching psychomotor skills. Providers should allow time for observation of the skill, practice, and reinforcement of techniques.

4. *Role Play*. Demonstration can be followed by potential scenarios; the two are often used in combination to practice applying knowledge, attitudes, and skills in life-like situations under supervision. Role-playing is especially useful for teaching patients to implement action plans for self-management of exacerbations or exposure to triggers.

5. *Age-Appropriate Video/Pictures/Graphics/Models*. Learning enhancements that provide visual, auditory, and tactile cues to reinforce all three types of learning should be used as adjuncts and are not substitutes for a live teacher. Learning skills still require return demonstration not provided by media.

6. *Computer-Assisted Instruction*. Software or Web-based programs can be used to simulate potential situations, practice lessons, teach facts, and as tutorials to individualize lessons, problem-solve, test knowledge and attitudes, and provide feedback. Simulations and games can help patients learn information and practice decision-making skills. Some Web-based programs also allow trending of symptoms and peak flow over time in graphic displays.

7. *Printed Materials*. These are the most commonly used tools for patient education and are important as they can be language specific. They are important in emphasizing essential information. However, while printed materials can reinforce learning they do not ensure learning.

Table 53-4
ADVANTAGES AND DISADVANTAGES OF TEACHING AND LEARNING FORMATS

Individual Teaching	Group Teaching
Advantages	*Advantages*
• Allows tailoring of the intervention to the specific needs of the patient and capitalizes on "teachable moments" when the patient is more open to learning, e.g., after recovery from a life-threatening asthma exacerbation.	• Economical in targeted populations within health centers/agencies.
	• Patients learn from one another and derive support/inspiration.
• Allows ongoing assessment and reinforcement of technical skills.	• Family members can be present to hear the information and adapt it to their family and cultural functioning.
Disadvantages	*Disadvantages*
• May be more costly than group formats if the educator is not the primary provider of care.	• Group size affects the educator's ability to meet individual learning needs. Small group (2 to 5 patients) is best for teaching and learning skills.
• Lack of peer group support.	• Group dynamics may not be conducive to learning. Competition among group members may impede discussion.
• Family members and partners often not present.	• Group teaching works best if members meet the target criteria for the group before enrollment. Diversity in age, language skills, or literacy may impede learning in groups.

Table 53-5
DETERMINING THE EFFECTIVENESS OF A SELF-MANAGEMENT INTERVENTION

1. Format
   • How was the patient taught? Was it compatible with the patient's learning style and needs?
2. Content
   • Was the necessary information received and did it result in behavior change?
3. Teaching-learning activities
   • Did the patient participate, ask questions, and practice skills?
   • Was the learning problem-centered and immediately applied by the learner?
   • Was the method of teaching/learning appropriate?
4. Media
   • Were the media resources appropriate and understandable to the patient and family?
5. Patient and family satisfaction
   • Which activities did they find most and least useful?
   • Were their concerns addressed?
   • Do they believe what they learned is useful?
6. Time, cost, and resources used
   • Were the resources adequate?
   • Were there unmet needs due to lack of resources?
   • Did deficits in resources for patient education create barriers for patient learning?

Table 53-6
EVALUATING THE OUTCOMES OF A SELF-MANAGEMENT INTERVENTION

1. Patient's participation during the intervention
   • Does the patient ask questions, seem alert and interested?
   • Does the patient actively participate in discussion and goal-setting?
2. Patient's performance immediately following the learning experience
   • Were performance objectives met and to what extent?
   • What modifications are needed for reinforcement of learning or improvement in performance?
3. Patient's performance at home
   • Does the patient perform the learned behaviors at home?
   • Were difficulties encountered (misunderstandings, inability to perform skills, problems remembering)?
4. Patient's overall self-care and health management
   • Did the management and education approaches resolve and/or control asthma?
   • Did objective markers (e.g., peak flow, lung function, hospital utilization) reflect successful self-care?
   • What are the long-term results of patient's individual self-management plan? Is adherence or skill performance maintained?

8. *Games and Simulations.* Games of strategy give patients the opportunity to use problem-solving strategies in a parallel, entertaining, competitive situation. This technique may work well with adolescents. Simulations provide the opportunity to apply new skills in lifelike situations where coaching and encouragement are available from the educator.

Individual and group formats have advantages and disadvantages as listed in Table 53-4. These features should be weighed when selecting an appropriate format.

Evaluation of Self-Management Educational Interventions

Routinely assessing the effectiveness of a prescribed self-management plan is paramount to its success. Rating the patient's participation, immediate performance, performance at home, and overall self-care are required. Identifying difficulties and praising successes are part of the process of arriving at a successful self-management plan. Tables 53-5 and 53-6 are assessment tools to gauge the effectiveness of the intervention and to evaluate its outcomes, respectively.

OUTCOMES

When asthma self-management education is successful, patients and their families will be able to:

• Maintain communication with regular provider of health care.
• Attend planned clinic visits for review of asthma status.
• Take asthma medications appropriately, perform self-assessments, and respond to symptoms at home, work, or school with appropriate actions.
• Participate fully in age-appropriate, valued activities.
• Keep asthma under control and recognize when asthma is going out of control.
• Implement the action steps of the self-management plan when asthma worsens without delay.
• Achieve satisfactory quality of life and satisfaction with asthma care.

The outcomes of asthma self-management training for individuals and groups are decreased asthma-related hospitalizations, emergency department visits, urgent care visits, and fewer missed work/school days due to symptoms. Adult individuals will achieve a sense of control and self-confidence for living with and managing the variations of asthma over time. Children will demonstrate increasing ability to manage their own asthma medications. Group sessions often produce awareness of others who have similar experiences with asthma and can offer helpful suggestions. Networks of people are often created in group education, providing support to each other in managing asthma. Peer support groups are especially useful for teenagers and older individuals because they decrease the isolation of living with a chronic disease.

SUGGESTED READING

Academy of Allergy, Asthma, and Immunology: Pediatric Asthma: Promoting Best Practice. Guide for managing asthma in children. Milwaukee, WI, Academy of Allergy, Asthma, and Immunology, 1999.

Community Action to Fight Asthma: A site for people working to address asthma in California. Available at: http://www.calasthma.org/resources/, accessed January 8, 2008.

Farber HJ, Boyette M: Control Your Child's Asthma: A Breakthrough Program for the Treatment and Management of Childhood Asthma. New York, Harold Holt and Company, 2001.

Fleming, N: VARK—A Guide to Learning Styles. 2006. 31 May 2006. Available at http://www.vark-learn.com/english/index.asp.

Kleinman A: Patients and Healers in the Context of Culture. Berkeley, University of California Press, 1980.

Rodriguez J, Valderrama Y, Surkan P, et al. Asthma Glossary: Key Words in Plain English. Health Literacy Studies: Innovative Materials. Harvard School of Public Health. May 31, 2006. Available at http://www.hsph.harvard.edu/healthliteracy/asthma/asthma3.pdf.

Rudd R: Adult education and public health partner to address health literacy needs. Adult Learning 2007;15:7–9.

Translator and Interpreter Organizations—Medical. 31 October 2001. Let Everyone Participate. 1 Jun 2006. Available at http://www.lep.gov/medtrans.html.

U.S. Department of Health and Human Services: National Asthma Education and Prevention Program. Asthma Management in Minority Children: Practical Insights for Clinicians, Researchers, and Public Health Planners. Bethesda, MD, National Institutes of Health, 1995.

U.S. Department of Health and Human Services: National Asthma Education and Prevention Program. Nurses: Partners in Asthma Care. Bethesda, MD, National Institutes of Health, 1995.

U.S. Department of Health and Human Services: National Asthma Education and Prevention Program. Practical Guide for the Diagnosis and Management of Asthma (Publication Number 97–4053). Bethesda, MD, National Institutes of Health; National Heart, Lung, and Blood Institute, 1997.

BIBLIOGRAPHY

Bodenheimer T, Wagner EH, Grumbach K: Improving primary care for patients with chronic illness. JAMA 2002;288(14):1775–1779.

Clark NM: Management of chronic disease by patients. Annu Rev Public Health 2003;24:289–313.

Gibson PG, Howell H, Coughlan J, et al: Limited (information only) patient education programs for adults with asthma. Cochrane Database Syst Rev 2002;(2):CD001005.

Gibson PG, Howell H, Coughlan J, et al: Self-management education and regular practitioner review for adults with asthma. Cochrane Database Syst Rev 2003;(1):CD001117.

Greene J, Yedidia MJ: Provider behaviors contributing to patient self-management of chronic illness among underserved populations. J Health Care Poor Underserved 2005;16(4):808–824.

Janson S, Becker G: Reasons for delay in seeking treatment for acute asthma: the patient's perspective. J Asthma 1998;35(5):427–435.

Janson SL, Fahy JV, Covington JK, et al: Effects of individual self-management education on clinical, biological, and adherence outcomes in asthma. Am J Med 2003;115(8):620–626.

Murphy VE, Gibson PG, Talbot PI, et al: Asthma self-management skills and the use of asthma education during pregnancy. Eur Respir J 2005;26(3):435–441.

Perneger TV, Sudre P, Munter P, et al: Effect of patient education on self-management skills and health status in patients with asthma: a randomized trial. Am J Med 2002;113(1):7–14.

Powell H, Gibson PG: Options for self-management education for adults with asthma. Cochrane Database Syst Rev 2003;(1):CD004107.

Toelle BG, Ram FS: Written individualised management plans for asthma in children and adults. Cochrane Database Syst Rev 2004;(2):CD002171.

Evaluating Individual and Program Outcomes

Lynn B. Gerald and Joan M. Mangan

- The evaluation of individual or program outcomes determines the value or worth of an intervention provided to persons with asthma and their families.

- An evaluation may examine the process of delivering an intervention and/or the impact an intervention has on a person with asthma and their families.

- The ability to detect changes brought about by a program will depend on (1) the operational definition of a physiologic marker, behavior, or event to be evaluated; (2) the precision of the measure used; (3) effect size; and (4) the sample size.

- The goals of asthma therapy provide a basis for what is evaluated when assessing individual patient and program outcomes.

- The strategies used to gather data for an evaluation are guided by the resources available to conduct the evaluation and the nature of the evaluation's goals.

Advances in medical technology as well as the drive to ensure access to quality health care for all citizens have led, in part, to the escalating costs of health care. In turn, these costs have highlighted the need for evidence-based medicine, generated calls for greater accountability for the dollars spent on patient care and health promotion programs, and have raised concerns for documenting the worth of program expenditures in relation to their costs. Accordingly, the evaluation of individual and program outcomes has become paramount.

Entire textbooks have been dedicated to the topic of evaluation; the challenge is to present key issues related to the evaluation of individual and program outcomes in one chapter. In an attempt to meet this challenge the first portion of this chapter highlights approaches for evaluating outcomes and detecting changes brought about by an intervention. The second half of the chapter presents a synopsized discussion of clinical measures of asthma, asthma events, and behavioral measures that might be incorporated into the evaluation of patient or program outcomes, as well as a discussion of data collection.

EVALUATION

A Definition of Evaluation

At its core, the term *evaluation* speaks to the value or quality of a program for people with asthma, or the care and services provided to individual patients. In order to establish value or judge the level of quality, a systematic assessment of an asthma program or patient outcomes is compared to a set of explicit or implicit standards.[1]

Explicit standards may be found in clinical practice guidelines or case management protocols, while the explicit standards for a program or research study are usually developed by program/study leaders and set forth in the program's/study's objectives. Examples of explicit standards include: the change expected in spirometry measures before and after a patient inhales a short-acting bronchodilator; an average 2-point change in overall score on a questionnaire measuring depressive symptoms; the reduction in days per week a person experiences asthma symptoms; or the number of missed doses per month of daily inhaled corticosteroids.

Implicit standards are generally understood and can be harder to define because they may vary by people or groups based on personal interests, or overlap based upon shared aims. Examples of implicit standards include: the expectations a patient brings to a clinical encounter; a health care team's aspiration to help their patients attain a better quality of life; or a health organization's goal to motivate patients to engage in healthy behavior changes.

Why Evaluate?

The underlying reasons why an evaluation is conducted can vary. Generally, an evaluation of an individual patient may be conducted in order to:

- Monitor the clinical progress of individual patients.
- Identify factors impacting the clinical progress of patients.
- Determine the effectiveness of an intervention.

An evaluation of an entire program may focus on the same issues, as well as:

- Explore ways to increase efficiency in the delivery of a program.
- Determine the effectiveness of attempts to improve an existing program.
- Satisfy accountability requirements of a sponsor or stakeholder.
- Examine the allocation of resources.
- Justify the expansion, reduction or abandonment of a program or services.
- Determine approaches to decrease the costs associated with the provision of services.[2,3]

As this list illustrates, the evaluation of program outcomes is often a political activity. Unless programs have a demonstrable effect, it is difficult to garner the support needed to maintain them. Knowledge of a program's effect may still be insufficient to justify its continuation. Decisions related to a program are often made based on the program's *benefits* in relation to its *costs*. However, estimating costs can be extremely difficult and often requires input from individuals with a financial background since the process requires assumptions to be made about the dollar value of program-related activities and the benefits of the program[3].

Because the information obtained from an evaluation of patient and program outcomes helps to guide and justify future decisions, the following criteria should be met prior to initiating formal evaluation activities. First, the goals, objectives, and informational needs of an evaluation must be well defined. Next, program leaders must ascertain that these goals and objectives are reasonable, that the needed data can be obtained, and how the data will be obtained. Finally, the intended users of the evaluation results should agree on how the findings will be used.

Nevertheless, it is important to recognize that evaluation is a dynamic process and involves frequent modification of the original plan. Often, this is because evaluation occurs in a continually changing political and administrative climate with frequent changes in resources, priorities and political interests. Furthermore, there may be unanticipated problems in implementing the intervention or evaluation design, creating the need to alter the original plan. Another unique feature of evaluation plans is that they must consider the financial and resource constraints of the organization implementing the program and evaluation as well as the interests of all stakeholders (which may include a combination of any of the following groups: patients, patient families, health care providers, health care institutions, program sponsors, insurance providers, policy makers); thus, the data collected must yield useful results for all persons with a vested interest in the program (stakeholders).

Approaches to Evaluation

An evaluation may focus on the process of delivering an educational program, patient care, or services and/or the immediate and long-term outcome that these programs, services, or approaches to care may have on people with asthma. A discussion of these modes of evaluation follows. Interventions provided to asthma patients in an inpatient or outpatient setting, as well as efforts designed to enhance asthma self-management or improve asthma outcomes in the community, workplace, or a school environment will be referred to collectively as "programs." The individuals eligible to receive care or services through these programs are referred to as the "recipients."

PROCESS EVALUATION

The primary objective of a *process evaluation* is to document the extent to which a program is implemented as planned. This entails collecting data to describe (1) how much of the program has been implemented, (2) who the program was provided to and whether the program reached the intended recipients, (3) when program activities were conducted, and (4) who conducted program activities.

To address these issues both qualitative and quantitative data may be gathered. When collecting qualitative data, the process of collecting, analyzing, synthesizing, and evaluating information may take place more or less simultaneously. *Qualitative data* may be collected through the observation of program activities as they occur, the staff as they carry out their responsibilities, and/or recipients' responses to the program. Discussions with program staff and recipients

related to program processes and any problems they may have encountered are also extremely useful. This information allows program leaders to make adjustments, solve problems, and avoid future problems that could jeopardize program success. In contrast, *quantitative data* focuses on information that can be expressed in numerical terms, counted or compared on a scale. Quantitative data that may be collected as part of a process evaluation includes audits of preliminary data, program records, and budgets.

Before initiating data collection for a process evaluation it is helpful to work with program leaders to create a description of the program itself. The description should outline all program components including: an explanation of the target population; strategies for implementing the program; day-to-day activities and the circumstances surrounding these activities; intended behaviors of program staff and recipients; the educational products and technologies needed to deliver the program; and explicit standards by which success will be measured. This description illustrates the complexity of the program and provides a reference for persons conducting the evaluation as they assess the delivery of the program.[2,4]

An appraisal of each program component facilitates a better understanding of which components contribute to program success and which are not performing as expected. Accordingly, the second objective of a process evaluation is to identify ways in which the program design and operational plan may be improved. Suggestions for improvements may be provided by staff involved in delivering the program, program recipients, community collaborators, or by comparing the quantitative and qualitative data collected with standards outlined through policy and procedure manuals or guidelines available from professional associations or accrediting agencies.[2]

Table 54-1 provides a description of program components for a school-based program designed to teach daily

---

Table 54-1
EXAMPLE PROCESS EVALUATION FOR A PROGRAM

1. Within classrooms, children logged onto a program Web site each day.
2. The children then blew into a peak flow meter.
3. The children noted the peak flow result by "zones." A green zone indicated 81% to 100% of the expected reading, a yellow zone indicated 50% to 80% of the expected reading, and a red zone indicated less than 50% of the expected reading.
4. Teachers visually verified the peak flow reading result.
5. The children then recorded their peak flow reading into the computer program by the color of the zone.
6. Children then used the computer to point and click on any asthma symptoms they were currently experiencing.
7. The computer provided feedback to each child, with directions to "go play it is a good day" or "slow down and talk to an adult about your asthma."
8. Teachers documented verification of the child's peak flow rate in the system. If a child was absent, the teacher recorded the absence in the computer program with a reason for the absence upon the child's return to school.
- If a child reported a yellow or red zone peak flow reading, school staff assisted the child in following their asthma action plan; this too was documented on a separate form.

Data from Mangan JM, Gerald LB: Asthma agents: monitoring asthma in school. J Sch Health 2006;76:300–302.

self-management skills to children with asthma. The description reveals that the program is moderately complex. After participating in an interactive educational session with project staff and a computer program in which children were taught to use a peak flow meter and metered-dose inhaler, there were eight general activities to be carried out each day and one additional activity in the event a child's peak flow reading was low. Program leaders decided to set the following goal for implementation: 95% or more of the children enrolled in the program will have a record of their daily peak flow rate and symptoms or a teacher report of an absence.

A process evaluation of this program might look at the students' peak flow meter skills, ability to interpret peak flow meter results, capacity to maneuver through the system, and understanding of icons used to represent asthma symptoms. Feedback might also be solicited from teachers regarding the level of interruption the program caused to classroom activities; technical difficulties encountered logging into the program's website, and whether the program appeared to maintain the children's interest. Also an evaluator would want to request a school calendar with school holidays, teacher work days, and field trips in order to identify those days low log-in rates would be expected.

OUTCOME EVALUATIONS

While process evaluations generally review the delivery of a program, the objectives of an *outcome evaluation* are to assess the immediate and continuing changes a program may have (intended and unintended), and to gauge the extent to which the program causes a desired change. Examples of immediate changes include changes in a person's asthma knowledge and self-management skills. Conversely, continuing changes may be physical or social-behavioral in nature, or may refer to events. For example, a physical change might be an improvement in daily peak flow rate among patients following an asthma self-management program; while a social-behavioral change would be a person's level of adherence to a daily controller medication. A decrease in emergency room visits or asthma exacerbations are examples of a change in an event.

Outcome evaluations may use an experimental or quasi-experimental design. The purpose of an *experimental design* is to test a cause-and-effect relationship between a treatment or some other type of intervention and an outcome. The key feature of an experimental design is the random assignment of program recipients to a treatment group or a control group. A comparison of these two groups helps to control potential biases and ensure that only one factor (such as a medication or patient education program) is what causes the groups to differ. If the number of individuals in the treatment and control groups is large enough, then differences such as gender and age should be relatively small and due to chance.[5]

The purpose of a *quasi-experimental design* is the same as an experimental design; the major difference is that random assignment is not possible. To emulate an experimental design, pre- and post-treatment observations are made of a program's recipients. Another approach is to compare program recipients to a second group of individuals who do not receive the treatment, but are not quite the same as the program's recipients. The credibility of this approach may be contingent on the inclusion and exclusion criteria used to select persons in the comparison group.[5]

Qualitative approaches to data collection include the use of focus groups, one-on-one interviews, and key informant interviews. Quantitative approaches may include medical record abstractions, measures of airflow obstruction and inflammation in the lungs (e.g., forced expiratory volume in 1 second [FEV_1] or exhaled nitric oxide levels), electronic monitoring systems to determine medication adherence, patient diaries, and interviewer or self-administered questionnaires. The pros and cons of these approaches to data collection are discussed later in this chapter.

Regardless of the design chosen, the ability to detect changes brought about by a program will depend on four main factors. First, each physiological marker, behavior, or event (commonly referred to as *variables*) must be operationally defined. In essence, the definition provides a precise description of how these variables will be measured or observed. These measures or observations may then be compared in a meaningful way to the standards that will denote the success or failure of a program.

An *operational definition* may vary based on the program being evaluated and the type of data that is available. Table 54-2 provides two different operational definitions of an asthma exacerbation. The first definition was used to evaluate a school-based program designed to increase children's adherence to controller medications, while the second definition was used in a National Institutes of Health–sponsored research study to determine whether treating gastroesophageal reflux disease would reduce the frequency of asthma exacerbations among people with inadequately controlled asthma.

The second critical factor for detecting a change is the precision of the measurement used. For example, if the variable of interest is a measure of lung function, the spirometer that is used must be maintained and regularly calibrated. Likewise, if the variable is social-behavioral, such as quality of life (QOL), the questionnaire used to assess recipient's QOL should be evaluated and found to be valid, reliable and sensitive prior to being used as part of an evaluation.

Lastly, the *effect size* and the *sample size* are important. These two factors influence the possibility of finding a change when one truly exists. The effect size is the amount or level of change that would be clinically meaningful. This effect size is then used to determine the number of individuals that must be observed in order to statistically determine whether an effect of such magnitude is achieved by the intervention.

Table 54-2
EXAMPLES OF AN OPERATIONAL DEFINITION
Operational Definitions of an Asthma Exacerbation
Definition 1: The primary outcome to be evaluated will be the number of asthma exacerbations among the schoolchildren participating in this program. For the purposes of this evaluation, an asthma exacerbation is defined as any one of the following: a teacher-verified red or yellow peak flow meter reading, school absence due to respiratory illness or an increased use of rescue medication while at school.
Definition 2: An asthma exacerbation will be defined by one or more of the following: decrease of ≥ 30% AM peak expiratory flow (from personal best) for 2 consecutive days, addition of oral prednisone to treat asthma symptoms, unscheduled visit with a health care provider for asthma symptoms.

To conduct analyses to measure change, the *unit(s) of analysis* must be clarified. The unit of analysis is often defined by the goals of the evaluation itself. For instance, if the evaluation aims to evaluate the effect of a treatment regimen, the units of analysis are individual patients. This is a simple example. In reality, the choice of a unit of analysis may be more difficult, particularly if an evaluation requires different levels of analysis. For example, if an evaluation seeks to determine how patients feel about a particular medication regimen and the patient education program that was provided within a hospital district prior to the medication being prescribed, the source of the education would be one level of the analysis. In order to evaluate the educational program itself, the decision that must be made is whether the units of analysis are the hospitals and clinics within the district or the individual health educators who delivered the educational program. Likewise, individual patients or educational sites might be chosen as the unit of analysis so as to assess patients' perceptions of the medication regimen.[4]

It is important to recognize that when the components of a program are complex, the delivery of the program is an equally important aspect of an evaluation. For this reason process evaluations are often conducted to support the findings obtained through an outcome evaluation.[2] For example, in the program described in Table 54-1, the goal was to collect data each day for 95% or more of the children enrolled in a moderately complex program. However, if the program yielded reports for only 65% to 70% of the children each day, the question is, why? Did the computer program fail to record the information entered? Were some teachers opposed to having their classroom activities interrupted by this program? Were some teachers unable to operate the computer? Did the children simply not like the program and therefore were not motivated to logon to the program each day? A process evaluation could identify a myriad of possible reasons for this outcome and eliminate the need to speculate as to the reasons for missing data.

Optimally a program and the evaluation plan are designed simultaneously. This allows time to select an evaluation design, select the method for data collection, choose or develop data collection instruments as needed, and organize for the work to be done. A plan should also be developed for analyzing the data collected. This planning allows program leaders to clarify how information will be used and which data are needed, and helps to avoid gathering too much data as well as the expense of collecting information that will not be used.

In some cases, evaluations that are planned once a project is underway often find it is extremely difficult to obtain needed data or find it impossible to gather unbiased information. As a result, the findings of these evaluations are less credible.

WHAT IS EVALUATED

For a long time, health care professionals have recognized that asthma does not have a single phenotype but is expressed in a variety of ways. Studies have demonstrated differences in asthma based on environmental and genetic factors, triggers that induce symptoms, and patients' responses to medications. Despite these differences, the goals of asthma therapy are the same: to prevent chronic and troubling asthma symptoms and asthma exacerbations; maintain near-normal parameters of pulmonary function and normal levels of physi-

cal activity; provide optimal medication therapy with minimal adverse effects; and deliver care that meets patients' and families' expectations.[6]

These goals provide the basis for what is evaluated when assessing individual patient outcomes and some of the changes a program might bring about. The following pages briefly discuss traditional measures as well as the behavioral outcomes programs often aim to achieve and measure. These discussions are by no means exhaustive and not all outcomes or mediating factors that can impact patient and program outcomes can be addressed in one chapter. In light of this, we have attempted to provide a more comprehensive list of outcomes and mediating factors in Table 54-3 along with issues to consider when evaluating these outcomes and approaches to data collection. This table groups patient and program outcomes into three major categories: clinical measures, measures of asthma events, and behavioral and psychosocial measures. Accordingly, we have separated this section into these three categories.

Clinical Measures of Patients and Asthma

Other chapters in this text discuss in detail the clinical measures of patients' asthma; therefore we will briefly mention those most commonly incorporated into the evaluation of clinical, community, and work- or school-based programs.

ASTHMA SYMPTOMS
Because every patient with asthma should be taught to recognize asthma symptoms and symptom patterns that indicate asthma is not in control, asthma symptoms are the most frequent outcome measure in the evaluation of individual patients and program impact.[6] In addition to the assessment of a person's symptom history, programs may gather data related to: symptom patterns; the onset, duration and frequency of symptoms; symptom triggers; diurnal variations; and symptom response to pharmacotherapy. These data may be collected via patient or caregiver interviews, questionnaires, asthma diaries, and/or medical record reviews.

PULMONARY FUNCTION
Objective measures of pulmonary function are commonly included in the evaluation of patient or program outcomes as a measure of asthma control. As described in Chapter 8, spirometry measurements, in particular, a person's FEV_1, are compared to reference or predicted values based upon the individual's age, height, and gender and used to determine the degree of airflow obstruction. Spirometry can be done in children as young as 4 years of age although many cannot adequately conduct the maneuvers until after age 7.

PEAK EXPIRATORY FLOW (PEF)
Peak expiratory flow is a simple measure of airflow obstruction that can be done by the patient themselves. Monitoring peak expiratory flow (PEF) can increase patient awareness of disease control, help patients detect significant changes in symptoms and make self-management decisions, assist in evaluating the decisions made, and enhance patient-provider communications. For these reasons, PEF monitoring is frequently included in outcome evaluations, and is often examined in conjunction with symptom monitoring.

Table 54-3
INDIVIDUAL AND PROGRAM OUTCOME MEASURES

		Measure	Considerations/ Potential Mediators*	Measurement Approaches
Clinical Measures of Patients and Asthma	**Physical Variables**	**Signs and Symptoms of Asthma** ■ Cough ■ Wheezing ■ Shortness of breath ■ Chest tightness ■ Sputum production	**History of Symptoms** **Pattern of Symptoms** ■ Perennial, seasonal, or both ■ Continual, episodic, or both **Symptom Onset, Duration, Frequency** ■ Number of days or nights per week or month **Diurnal Variations in Symptoms** ■ Nocturnal ■ Upon awakening ■ Early morning ■ Daytime **Pharmacotherapy and Symptoms** ■ Symptoms not improved 15 minutes after short-acting beta$_2$-agonist **Symptom Triggers/Antecedents** **Poor Perception of Symptoms***	■ Asthma diary 　° Pen and paper 　° Internet/Web-based ■ Self-report: questionnaires and interviews ■ Caregiver Report questionnaires and interviews ■ Medical record review
		Pulmonary Function	**Spirometry** ■ FEV$_1$ ■ FVC ■ FEV$_1$\FVC **Age of Patient***	■ Spirometry 　° Initial assessment 　° After treatment is initiated and patient is stable 　° Every 1 to 2 years
		Peak Expiratory Flow	**Frequency of Monitoring** ■ One measure a day ■ Multiple measures to capture diurnal variations **Duration of Monitoring** ■ Prolonged monitoring is not recommended **Age of Patient***	■ Peak flow meter ■ Asthma diaries
		Inflammation	**Inflammatory Markers** ■ Exhaled nitrous oxide ■ Sputum eosinophils	■ Exhaled breath condensate ■ Sputum samples
Measures of Asthma Events Indicative of Asthma "Out of Control"	**Events**	**Asthma Exacerbations**	**History of Exacerbations** ■ Exacerbation frequency ■ Patterns to exacerbation ■ Antecedents Note: Exacerbation may be defined based on program or treatment being evaluated and the type of data available	■ Self-report: questionnaires and interviews ■ Asthma diaries ■ Medical record review
		Healthcare Utilization	**Types of Utilization** ■ Urgent physician office/ outpatient clinic visits ■ Emergency room Visits ■ Overnight hospitalizations **Level of Clinical Intervention** ■ Intubation ■ Admission to an intensive care unit **Delays in Seeking Care*** ■ Knowledge, attitudes, beliefs ■ Coping styles ■ Insurance/access	■ Self-report: questionnaires and interviews ■ Asthma diaries ■ Medical record review
		Asthma Mortality		■ Death certificates
Behavioral and Psychosocial Measures	**Behavioral Variables**	**Knowledge**	**Factual Knowledge** ■ Asthma pathophysiology ■ Signs and symptoms of asthma out of control ■ Medication ■ Asthma triggers **"How To" Knowledge** ■ Recognize and respond to asthma symptoms ■ Use an asthma action plan ■ Use medications appropriately ■ Control exposure to triggers **Functional Literacy/Health Literacy*** **Patient-Provider Communication***	■ Questionnaires and interviews ■ Responses to hypothetical scenarios ■ Skill demonstration

(Continued)

Table 54-3
INDIVIDUAL AND PROGRAM OUTCOME MEASURES

Measure	Considerations/ Potential Mediators*	Measurement Approaches
Self-Efficacy	**Self-Efficacy Specific to Asthma Self-Management** ■ Recognize and monitor symptoms ■ Control triggers to symptoms ■ Monitor physical indicators ■ Use medications ■ Follow an asthma action plan ■ Manage acute episodes and emergencies ■ Maintain nutrition and diet ■ Maintain adequate exercise/activity ■ Quit smoking	■ Self-administered questionnaires

Treatment Adherence
■ Quick relief medication
■ Daily control medication
	History of Adherence/Nonadherence
	■ Patterns in Adherence Levels
	■ Ratio of controller medication dispensed to quick relief medication dispensed
	Barriers to Adherence*
	■ Medication side effects
	■ Insurance coverage
	■ Copayment costs
	■ Access to a healthcare home
	■ Patient-provider communication
	■ Attitudes and beliefs related to medications
	■ Misperceptions related to asthma symptoms
	■ Home remedies
	■ Over the counter remedies
		■ Self-report: questionnaires and interviews
		■ Prescription records
		  ° Controller medication
		  ° Quick relief medication
		■ Electronic medication monitoring devices
		■ One-on-one interviews
		■ Focus groups

Control Asthma Triggers	■ Secondhand smoke ■ Cockroaches and other pests ■ Dust mites and house dust ■ Molds ■ Pets and other animals ■ Strong odors and fumes ■ Chemicals ■ Allergens **Socioeconomic Status***	■ Self-report questionnaires and interviews ■ Environmental assessments
Lifestyle Changes	**Exercise** ■ Level of activity ■ Types of physical activity ■ Appropriate use of asthma medication prior to physical activity **Smoking** ■ Smoking Cessation	■ Self-report questionnaires and interviews ■ Physiologic monitoring ■ Endurance ■ Diaries ■ Measures of nicotine and nicotine metabolites
Healthcare	**Appointment Keeping** ■ Missed appointments **Healthcare Home** ■ Regular Provider ■ Provider specialized in asthma care **Socioeconomic Status***	■ Self-report questionnaires and interviews ■ Clinic records ■ Insurance records
Quality of Life	**General Health Related Quality of Life** **Asthma Quality of Life** **Individual Perspective** ■ Patient ■ Caregiver ■ Family **Possible Mediators*** ■ Stress ■ Depression ■ Limitations on physical functioning ■ Effect on growth, development, behavior, school or work performance, and lifestyle ■ Impact on family routines, activities, or dynamics ■ Family Support	■ Self-report questionnaires and interviews
Economic Impact	■ Number of days missed at work/school	■ Self-report questionnaires and interviews ■ Records of absenteeism

Side labels: Behavioral and Psychosocial Measures—cont'd | Behavioral Variables | Impact of Asthma on Patient or Family

* Denotes some potential mediators—factors that may influence an outcome

PEF monitoring is inexpensive and can be done anywhere by persons with asthma. Currently, the guidelines recommend that peak flow monitoring be done in the morning. Children as young as 5 can be taught to measure their PEF using peak flow meters (PFM). These devices are produced by a number of companies and models are available for children and adults. It should be noted that when PEF is incorporated into an evaluation of programs for children with asthma, a child's personal best PEF should be assessed at least once every six months while they are growing, thereby ensuring accurate interpretation of a PEF result. To check the accuracy of the PFM, periodic comparisons of the readings from the PFM and spirometry may be useful.

Measures of Asthma Events

ASTHMA EXACERBATIONS

Exacerbations are generally thought of as the worsening of asthma symptoms. As described earlier in this chapter the definition of an exacerbation must be operationalized for evaluation purposes. That is, the features of an *asthma exacerbation* must be specified in detail with respect to what one wants to capture, together with one or more measurable criteria. Many different definitions of exacerbations have been used to evaluate individual and program outcomes. The choice of definition and measurement should be related to the intervention and the capacity for measurement. An evaluation may also inquire about the frequency of exacerbations, exacerbation antecedents, and patterns. These data may be collected using medical records, asthma diaries, questionnaires, and patient interviews.

HEALTH CARE UTILIZATION

Evaluations of asthma exacerbations are often conducted in conjunction with an assessment of patients' *health care utilization*. In order to quantify health care utilization as accurately as possible, specific information about scheduled and urgent visits to physicians, scheduled and urgent visits to outpatient clinics, emergency room visits, and hospitalizations are collected separately. This information may be collected using medical records, asthma diaries, questionnaires, and patient interviews.

Behavioral and Psychosocial Measures

Efforts put forth to assist patients and their families in attaining optimal outcomes has led to the study and identification of a broad array of behavioral and psychosocial factors that influence outcomes. A number of these factors have been addressed elsewhere in this text; therefore we will limit our discussion to the three most commonly integrated into evaluation activities.

KNOWLEDGE

Knowledge is not sufficient to change behavior, yet it is recognized as a necessary antecedent for behavior change. More specifically, knowledge is essential to several processes required for effective asthma self-management. Therefore, the evaluation of patient and caregiver knowledge is one of the most common indicators used to evaluate programs that provide patient education.

In addition to measuring changes in a person's understanding of their condition and treatment, knowledge questions may be used to help explain an individual's attitudes and behavior. This may be accomplished by examining an individual's grasp of knowledge about asthma and "how-to" knowledge. Knowledge about a disease or a component of a regimen helps patients understand their condition or the reasons why a treatment may be prescribed, yet this form of knowledge is not as critical to behavior change as the how-to knowledge needed to act on medical recommendations and solve problems.

In the course of evaluating knowledge, special consideration must be given to reducing guessing, overstatements of knowledge, and the perceived threat for those respondents who do not want to appear foolish or ill informed when responding to knowledge questions.[7] The perceived threat knowledge questions may pose can be reduced using preparatory phrases such as, "Do you happen to know?" or "Can you recall, offhand?" The addition of "I don't know" as an answer choice also helps to reduce the threat, helps to control overstatements of knowledge, and reduces the incidence of guessing. The inclusion of these statements or response items sends the message that a lack of knowledge is acceptable. Asking a detailed follow-up question to the original question may control overstatements of knowledge.[7] When additional questions are not appropriate, the use of a "sleeper" response is helpful. Sleeper responses are plausible false answers, that when chosen, signal probable overstatements of knowledge by a respondent. Finally, the reliability of respondents' scores on tests and scales increases with the number of items, so more reliable assessments of knowledge may be obtained if multiple questions are used. As a rule, knowledge questions are best asked face-to-face or on the phone.

A search of the literature reveals numerous questionnaires designed to measure patient and caregiver's asthma knowledge. However, the best measures of knowledge for a program evaluation would most likely be developed to reflect the program's content.

SELF-EFFICACY

Self-efficacy was defined by Albert Bandura[8] as an individual's confidence in his or her ability to regulate his or her motivation, thought processes, and environment in order to attain "designated types of performances." Self-efficacy influences a number of aspects of behavior, including the selection of specific behaviors a person is willing to attempt, the amount of effort a person will expend to master a behavior, and the thought processes a person experiences when enacting or anticipating the behavior.

Self-efficacy is often measured in conjunction with knowledge because, as some researchers point out, a baseline level of knowledge may be necessary to enable some actions to occur but after this threshold has been met additional information does not automatically bring about added behavioral change. Also, the predictive quality of self-efficacy as well as its positive correlation with self-management and adjustment to chronic illness makes it a potentially useful measure of patients' transition to active self-management following educational interventions. Self-efficacy may also be measured independently if a program's goal is to raise a person's perceived self-efficacy. Self-efficacy is a particularly desirable outcome since a number of research studies have indicated people with a higher level of perceived self-efficacy attempt more, accomplish more, and persist longer at a specific task compared to individuals with lower perceived self-efficacy. Conversely, individuals with low self-efficacy tend to avoid difficult tasks and will often give up sooner if the activities are challenging.

As asthma self-management includes diverse behaviors, a person's self-efficacy to carry out each of these behaviors is measured individually. This is done for two main reasons. First, self-efficacy is specific to a given behavior and challenge a patient faces. Second, medical prognoses and therapeutic interventions can alter beliefs of personal efficacy, which have the potential to impact health outcomes. For instance, if a patient suffers a severe asthma exacerbation, he or she may retain the self-efficacy to adhere to a daily medication regimen, but lack the self-efficacy to engage in an exercise program for fear exercise would trigger another severe exacerbation.

Questions used to evaluate self-efficacy should be written at the reading level of the target population, and technical jargon and double-barreled questions need to be avoided. General questions should be asked first, followed by specific questions. The strength of peoples' self-efficacy beliefs can be evaluated in one of three ways. First, separate questions can be used to assess the strength of the belief. Second, a series of independent questions can be asked, each question reflecting the general belief. The total number of items a respondent agrees with theoretically reflects the strength of their belief. Third, strength dimensions can be built into the questions themselves.[9] For example, asthma patients might be asked, "How much do you dislike inhaled corticosteroids (none, a little, somewhat or very much)?" Because of its ability to predict patient outcomes, some instruments to measure self-efficacy have been developed specifically for asthma patients and caregivers.

Quality of Life

Most interventions aim to minimize symptoms, reduce exacerbations and limitations imposed by asthma, and improve quality of life. QOL is recognized to be both multidimensional and subjective. Because it is multidimensional, a measure of QOL may examine functional ability and physical, emotional, and social well-being. Its subjective nature requires that it is measured from the perspective of the patient. Because QOL is dependent on the patient's perspective, it can be strongly influenced by family, social, and behavioral factors. A person's adherence to their treatment plan is one example of a behavioral factor that may influence QOL. For example, patients who frequently skip daily doses of corticosteroids and use their rescue medication may experience a lower QOL due to their nonadherence. At the same time, QOL measures are only weakly associated with traditional measures of physiologic impairment such as spirometry. For this reason, QOL is often measured in conjunction with clinical measures. Over the last two decades, a number of generic and asthma-specific QOL measures have been created. The choice of which type of measure should be used in an evaluation will depend in part on the questions to be answered as part of the evaluation. Often, outcome evaluations will incorporate both a generic and asthma-specific measure. The advantage to generic measures of QOL is that they have often been tested in a variety of clinical settings, thereby enabling a comparison to be made of patients with different conditions as well as revealing important but unexpected effects of a program or treatment. Asthma-specific measures of QOL are more likely to detect small changes specific to asthma. Further information regarding patient-oriented QOL measures that have been used in the study and management of patients with pulmonary disease (including adult and pediatric asthma) are available through the American Thoracic Society Web site (www.atsqol.org).

GATHERING EVALUATION DATA

As the previous sections have illustrated, an evaluation requires planners to make a number of decisions, including the selection of a data collection method. This decision is, in large measure, guided by the resources available to conduct the evaluation and the nature of the evaluation's objective. The objective will often prescribe the selected data collection strategy. For example, if program leaders sought to evaluate the impact of a case management program on hospitalizations over a six-month period, program recipients may be contacted at the end and asked whether or not they had been hospitalized. Conversely, an evaluation of more mundane events such as daily use of a corticosteroid may be influenced by recipients' poor recall or desire to be socially acceptable. To circumvent these problems a variety of approaches exist (discussed in Chapter 50). These may be used separately or in combination with each other to facilitate measures of reliability and comprehensive data collection for analysis.

Details related to the performance and interpretation of measures of lung function have been addressed in Chapter 8; therefore, the following sections describe the most common approaches to gathering data, as well as some of the benefits and barriers to these methods (Table 54-4).

Questionnaires and Surveys

A broad range of questionnaires and surveys have been created specifically to evaluate outcomes for persons with asthma and their family members. Often, these existing questionnaires, surveys, or scales (hereafter referred to as *measures*) will meet the evaluation needs of many programs. However, in the event existing measures do not completely meet program evaluation needs, it may become necessary to create a new measure. This usually involves considerable effort and skill, not to mention a commitment of resources.

Unfortunately, space constraints prohibit a detailed discussion of existing measures or guidelines for constructing a new measure for the evaluation of patient and program outcomes. Instead, the following sections describe desirable characteristics of measures used as part of an evaluation and potential problems associated with self-reported data collected through a questionnaire or survey.

DESIRABLE CHARACTERISTICS OF MEASURES

Regardless of whether a new measure has been created or an existing measure is used, there are a number of characteristics, or *psychometric properties*, that are looked for in the measures

Table 54-4
ADVANTAGES AND DISADVANTAGES TO DIFFERENT MODES OF DATA COLLECTION

Mode Of Data Collection	Advantages	Disadvantages
Diaries	■ Reduce a person's need to rely on memory ■ Minimize the incidence of recall bias ■ Provide more accurate information related to low saliency and routine events ■ Increase the amount of data collected without the associate cost or time commitment ■ May help overcome problems associated with collecting sensitive information ■ Data collected through this method may be used to supplement information obtained through an interview, or to guide an interview	■ Patients or caregivers may be reluctant to adhere to the requirements of diary entry ■ May lead to insufficient cooperation or participant attrition ■ Potential for sample selection bias ■ May lead to errors caused by respondents changing their behavior as a result of keeping the diary or becoming less conscientious than when they started the diary, leading to incomplete information and underreporting of data ■ Require respondents to possess a certain level of literacy ■ Data processing can be labor intensive, especially when unstructured diaries are used or a pen-and-paper method is employed with structured diaries ■ Difficulty to implement with populations that are somewhat mobile
Self-administered surveys	■ Economical ■ Respondent may control the pace and time ■ Reduce respondent apprehension of being evaluated/judged by an interviewer ■ May be conducted during an encounter with respondent or via mail, e-mail, the Internet	■ Recall bias ■ Functional illiteracy and cultural norms may prohibit use ■ Questions may not be explained ■ Slow ■ Without an interviewer's encouragement, increased risk of skipping questions ■ Respondent may solicit other's opinions when answering questions on mail or computer-based surveys
Interviewer-administered surveys	■ Increased response rate to individual questions, compared to self-administered survey ■ Respondent feedback may be obtained ■ Questions may be clarified for respondent	■ Recall bias ■ Personnel costs associated with administration of survey ■ Respondent may feel pressure to answer questions in a socially acceptable manner ■ Respondent may experience apprehension over being evaluated/judged by an interviewer ■ Interviewer may lead respondent to "correct" or "expected" answer
One-on-one interviews	■ Remove barriers due to respondent's literacy level ■ Flexible structure ■ In-depth/rich data ■ Information collected may be supplemented by impressions of the interviewee	■ Time consuming ■ Expensive ■ Data quality depends on quality of interaction between interviewer and interviewee, and quality of the interviewer ■ Risk of bias introduced by the interviewer ■ Requires extra steps before data can be entered ■ Coding data
Medical record abstraction	■ Clinical documentation of events ■ Source of objective, clinical indicators ■ Records that incorporate structured checklists provide data that is gathered consistently	■ Information contains little/no contextual information ■ Some information may not be consistently incorporated into the medical record
Medication Event Monitoring System (MEMS)	■ Collects date and time data on an ongoing basis ■ Storing, retrieving and reporting information in a format convenient for use	■ Expensive ■ Researchers must assume that patients have actually taken all missing medication ■ Limited in providing accurate adherence information ■ May cause underreporting of adherence in patients who remove more than one dose at a time ■ Loss of data due to device damage, device failure, and data loss

used as they influence the credibility of an evaluation report. Particularly important are the validity, reliability, and responsiveness of a measure. Briefly, *validity* is the extent to which a questionnaire, survey or scale measures what it is intended to measure. The validity of a measure may be assessed in a number of ways; the method used depends on the purpose of the questionnaire, survey or scale and the topic to be measured. *Face validity* is the extent to which a questionnaire

or survey *appears* to measure what it is supposed to measure.[10] Face validity is also referred to as *clinical credibility*, since this form of validity is inferred from the comments of experts or patients who review the measure for both clarity and completeness[11]. *Content validity* refers to the extent to which the included questions are representative of the concepts they are intended to reflect, or more specifically, how well items reflect the theoretical subject they are supposed to

represent.[12] *Construct validity* and *criterion validity* assume
that there are well-developed theories or hypotheses regarding the relationships of one variable to the other variables
being measured.[12] More specifically, *construct validity* exam-
ines whether, and how many of, the relationships predicted
by theories or hypotheses are supported when the data are
analyzed.[13] *Criterion validity* refers to the comparison of a
measure against a gold standard or some type of indicator. To
establish the criterion validity of a measure, the results of the
measure might be compared to a diagnostic test, such as FEV_1
or compared to a future event (i.e., future emergency room
visits) to determine if the measure can predict a future event.
In establishing the criterion validity of a measure the *sensitivity* and *specificity* of the measure are assessed. Traditionally,
sensitivity assesses the number of people who truly have the
disease and are correctly classified as having the disease by the
measure (questionnaire), while specificity measures the number of people who do not have the disease and are classified
as negative by a measure (questionnaire). *Reliability* refers
to the extent to which a measure produces the same results
repeatedly in a given situation.[3] Consequently, the reliability or consistency of a questionnaire is considered the most
essential issue in a questionnaire, survey or scale development
by some since the focus is on error in measurement. The use
of a measure in which the validity and reliability are considered poor or have not been established calls into question any
reported results.

Responsiveness is another key component of a measure.
Responsiveness refers to whether a measure can distinguish
small, but clinically important, changes over time. Small but
significant changes in traditional clinical tests such as FEV_1 are
readily understood. However the minimal clinically important difference in a health status measure, such as those that
examine quality of life or depression, is not always understood and must be delineated by the individuals who created
and evaluated the measure.

POTENTIAL PROBLEMS WITH SELF-REPORTED DATA

Patients and their caregivers are frequently asked to report on
their experiences, practices, knowledge, attitudes and beliefs
as part of the evaluation of a program. When responding to
a question, a person will interpret the question posed, search
his or her memory for the appropriate information, evaluate
the information retrieved, and determine the relevance to
the question asked. When appropriate, this information may
be combined with other information in order to provide an
answer. Finally, the person will assess the sensitivity or threat
a question poses, by considering whether there is a "right"
or "wrong" answer, whether a particular response would be
viewed as *socially acceptable* or desirable, as well as the probable accuracy of the formulated answer. Only after a person
has completed these mental processes will he or she decide
what answer to provide.

These processes and potential biases must be taken into
consideration during the design and evaluation of questions
included in the interviews, surveys, and diaries used to obtain
self-reported data related to asthma symptoms, self-management behaviors, or self-care decisions a patient or caregiver is
asked to provide. To minimize the potential of a person sac-
rificing the accuracy of a reply in lieu of a socially acceptable
response, questions that may be viewed as having a right or

wrong answer, as well as questions that may explore sensitive
topics or be viewed as threatening, must be carefully worded.
Often the use of open-ended questions rather than closed
questions, familiar words to describe a situation or event,
embedding a question in a list of less threatening topics, or
asking a sensitive question last may help obtain more accurate
data.

Additionally, different types of questions may place different demands on a person at the different stages involved in
formulated an answer.[12] Retrieving information from memory
regarding an event or behavior is often the most important
step and also the one most prone to a *recall bias*. People's ability to recall information is limited. Consequently, the more
current and specific the question, the greater the likelihood
of obtaining an accurate answer.

When patients or caregivers are asked to recall information related to factors such as symptom frequency, symptom
duration, or medication use, the time frame should be as
recent as possible. The primary factor to consider when
determining a time frame is that forgetting is related to the
amount of time elapsed and the saliency of the event. The more
important the event, the easier it is to remember. Events that
occur rarely in a person's life or historical events are more
likely to be remembered indefinitely. Memory of highly
salient events such as a protracted illness or hospitalization
is adequate for periods of a year or more. Conversely, incidents that may be considered to have an intermediate level
of saliency, such as an emergency visit or unscheduled visit
to a doctor, may be accurately remembered for a time frame
of 1 to 3 months. Periods of 2 weeks to a month appear to
be appropriate to ask a person to recall an experience with
a lower level of saliency, such as an asthma exacerbation for
a person with persistent asthma; while routine events such
as taking medication, monitoring symptoms, or avoiding specific asthma triggers may be difficult to remember for more
than a few days.[7]

Asthma Diaries

A data collection approach that reduces a person's need to
rely on memory, minimizes the incidence of recall bias, and
provides more accurate information related to low saliency
and routine events is the use of *asthma diaries*. Patients or
caregivers are asked to use diaries to collect information
about events, behaviors, thoughts or other aspects of life in a
structured manner; thereby providing researchers an opportunity to collect a more complete picture of what occurs on
an everyday level.

Diaries may employ an open format, allowing people to
record activities and events in their own words, or they may
be highly structured, containing a form or "log" that allows
a person to record the incidence of events, such as symptoms and medication use in categories. Others researchers have used diaries in what is called the "diary-interview"
approach, in which a person is asked to answer questions
after submitting their diary, so that the internal consistency
of the diary accounts may be checked, and omissions or gaps
in information may be filled in.

The primary advantage to using diaries is the volume and
type of data that may be collected. Diaries also enable data
collection surrounding a process or a sequence of activities,

such as the activities involved in asthma self-management. Other advantages to the use of diaries include (1) less opportunity for memory lapses; (2) greater reliability in data collected; and (3) the ability to increase the amount of data collected without the associated cost or time commitment; (4) similar to other self-completion methods, can help to overcome problems associated with collecting sensitive information by personal interview; and (5) may be used to supplement information obtained through an interview or to guide an interview.[7]

Diaries can also help a patient or caregiver form a link between what has been explained to them about controlling their asthma and their personal experiences with symptoms or exacerbations. If a patient with a history of uncontrolled asthma is asked to keep a diary documenting medication use and asthma symptoms and is able to view a pattern of decreased symptoms related to medication adherence, the experience may be more persuasive than a patient-counseling session alone.

As with any other form of data collection, the literature cites a number of potential disadvantages to the use of diaries. These disadvantages include (1) reluctance of patients or caregivers to adhere to the requirements of diary entry; (2) insufficient cooperation or participant attrition; (3) sample selection bias (e.g., a person who is willing to fill out a diary is likely to be different from other individuals); (4) errors due to people changing their behavior as a result of keeping the diary or becoming less conscientious than when they started the diary, leading to incomplete information and underreporting or recall bias; (5) requires people to possess a certain level of literacy; and (6) processing is labor intensive, especially when unstructured diaries are used.[7]

Researchers have also suggested the more narrow the focus of the diary, the more likely a person will record relevant events. It is important to note however that this does not mean a diary should focus on just one type of behavior or event. When a diary keeper is asked to report on only one behavior or event, the tendency is for the diary keeper to focus on the behavior, thereby increasing the likelihood of a change in behavior.[7] Finally, diaries should be kept short; 5 to 20 pages is recommended, with each page denoting either a week, a day of the week or a 24-hour period or less. The time period over which a diary is kept needs to be long enough to capture the behavior or events of interest without jeopardizing successful completion by imposing an overly burdensome task. A number of studies report using 7- to 14-day recording periods with success.

Medical Record Abstractions

Medical records are viewed as an objective source of data. However, medical records are intended for patient care and information is not systematically recorded. Consequently the review of these records may find them incomplete and can be time-consuming, and thus an expensive form of data collection. The advent of electronic medical records has led to the creation of templates in which reports on diagnostic studies or interventional treatments are more standardized. These templates facilitate an evaluation of the quality of care, services provided, and patient outcomes. Yet, contextual information may still be lacking.

Electronic Monitoring Systems

Advances in computer technology have led to the development of electronic tools to measure adherence. Two systems often employed in asthma research are *Medication Events Monitoring Systems (MEMS)* in which computer chips are embedded in medication bottle cap and the *Metered Dose Inhaler Logs (MDILog) or Electronic-Doser*, small devices containing a computer chip and attached to metered dose inhalers (Note: the MDILog may also be used with inhalers that use spacers). These devices have the capacity to record the date and time of day each time the medication bottle is opened or an inhaler is actuated, counting each event as a dose.

The primary factor that limits the use of both electronic systems is the costs of the devices. Another drawback to the use of both the MEMS Caps and Digi-dosers is that the researcher must assume that patients have actually taken all missing pills or inhaled all actuated medicine. The literature has reported incidents in which the MEMS devices may underreport adherence among patients who remove more than one dose at a time to avoid meddlesome pill bottle caps, conceal medication use from others, or transfer pills from bottles to pill organizer boxes to facilitate personal adherence. Studies have also described incidents where overreporting has occurred due to "dumping" of medication or actuating the device without inhaling medication as well as difficulties due to device damage, device failure, and data loss.

The Effect of Endogenous Events on Data Collection

Many asthma programs operate in environments in which ordinary or "natural" events may influence the outcomes of interest. For example, seasonal changes, such as a spring season with an above-average pollen count may mask the effect of a program that aims to decrease seasonal asthma exacerbations. Likewise, a mild winter may enhance outcomes of the same program. These effects are referred to as *endogenous changes*.

Endogenous changes may be overt, resulting from an interfering event such as a hurricane that hampers the delivery of medicines, thereby interfering with a program aimed at improving medication adherence. Endogenous changes may be much more subtle, such as maturational trends that produce changes in individuals that mimic or mask the effects of the program. For example, results of a program designed to teach adolescents to self-manage exercise-induced asthma may be masked by a general decline in playing sports that occurs when teens enter the work force. The confounding effect these changes may have on an evaluation requires program leaders to be especially attentive when designing an evaluation and when summing up evaluation findings.

SUMMARY

For many individuals working in the health arena, the focus is on the provision of services. Staff members may believe so strongly in the worth of the services provided, they might not recognize the need to evaluate a program or services provided. However, limited resources, calls for accountability, and the need to demonstrate program value have increased the visibility of evaluations.

Optimally evaluations are planned at the same time a program is designed. However this may not always be feasible. Regardless of when an evaluation is planned, program leaders must first identify the goals of the evaluation and how the information gained through an evaluation will be used. Next a myriad of decisions must be made related to whether a program's delivery processes and outcomes will be evaluated, the design used, when and what data will be collected, and how this data will be gathered. All the while, program leaders need to remain aware of potential pitfalls that may undermine the credibility of the results obtained.

REFERENCES

1. Weiss CH: Evaluation: Methods for Studying Programs and Policies, 2nd ed. Upper Saddle River, NJ, Prentice Hall, 1998.
2. Windsor R, Baranowski T, Clark N, Cutter G: Evaluation of Health Promotion, Health Education, and Disease Prevention Programs. 2nd ed. Mountain View, CA, Mayfield Publishing Company, 1994.
3. Rossi PH, Freeman HE: Evaluation: A Systematic Approach 5. Newbury Park, CA, Sage Publications Inc, 1993.
4. Wholey JS, Hatry HP, Newcomer KE (eds): Handbook of Practical Program Evaluation. San Francisco, Jossey-Bass Publishers, 1994.
5. Bickman L, Rog DJ (eds): Handbook of Applied Social Research Methods. Thousand Oaks, CA, Sage Publications, 1998.
6. The National Asthma Education and Prevention Program (NAEPP): Practical Guide for the Diagnosis and Management of Asthma, Based on the Expert Panel Report 2: Guidelines for the Diagnosis and Management of Asthma (NIH Publication No. 97–4053).
National Heart, Lung, and Blood Institute, 1997, www.nhlbi.gov/health/prof/lung/asthma/practgde/practgde.pdf.
7. Sudman S, Bradburn NM: Asking Questions: A Practical Guide to Questionnaire Design. San Francisco, Jossey-Bass Publishers, 1982.
8. Bandura A: Self-Efficacy: The Exercise of Control. New York, W.H. Freeman, 1997.
9. Bandura A: Guide for Constructing Self-Efficacy Scales. Stanford, CA, Stanford University, Department of Psychology, 2001.
10. Anastasi A: Psychological Testing, 5th ed. New York, McMillan, 1982.
11. McDowell I, Newell C: Measuring Health: A Guide to Rating Scales and Questionnaires. New York, Oxford University Press, 1996.
12. Aday LA: Designing and Conducting Health Surveys: A Comprehensive Guide. San Francisco, Jossey-Bass Publishers, 1989.
13. Carmines EG, Zeller RA: Reliability and Validity Assessment. Beverly Hills, CA, Sage, 1979.

Index

Note: Page numbers are followed by *b* for boxes, *f* for figures, and *t* for tables.